COMPREHENSIVE CARDIAC CARE

P9-BZF-619

COMPREHENSIVE CARDIAC CARE

EDITED BY

Kathleen Gainor Andreoli, D.S.N., F.A.A.N.

Vice President of Educational Services, Interprofessional Education and
International Programs
The University of Texas Health Science Center at Houston
Houston, Texas

Douglas P. Zipes, M.D.

Professor of Medicine, Indiana University School of Medicine
Senior Research Associate,
Krannert Institute of Cardiology
Indianapolis, Indiana

Andrew G. Wallace, M.D.

Vice Chancellor for Health Affairs, Chief Executive Officer, Hospital
Duke University Medical Center
Durham, North Carolina

Marguerite R. Kinney, R.N., D.N.Sc., F.A.A.N.

Professor of Nursing
School of Nursing
The University of Alabama at Birmingham
Birmingham, Alabama

Virginia Kliner Fowkes, F.N.P., M.H.S.

Director, Primary Care Associate Program and
Stanford Area Health Education Center, Division of Family Medicine
Stanford University School of Medicine
Stanford, California

SIXTH EDITION

with 1063 illustrations

The C. V. Mosby Company

ST. LOUIS • WASHINGTON, D.C. • TORONTO 1987

MOSBY

A TRADITION OF PUBLISHING EXCELLENCE

Senior editor: Barbara Ellen Norwitz
Developmental editor: Sally Adkisson
Project editor: Carlotta Seely
Production editor: Radhika Rao Gupta
Design: Rey Umali

SIXTH EDITION

Previous editions copyrighted 1968, 1971, 1975, 1979, 1983

Printed in the United States of America

The C.V. Mosby Company
11830 Westline Industrial Drive, St. Louis, Missouri 63146

Library of Congress Cataloging-in-Publication Data

Comprehensive cardiac care.

   Includes bibliographies and index.
   1. Cardiovascular disease nursing.   2. Coronary
care units.   I. Andreoli, Kathleen G.   [DNLM:
1. Coronary Care Units.   2. Heart Diseases—nursing.
WY 152.5 C737]
RC674.C65   1987   616.1'2   87-1533
ISBN 0-8016-0250-5

GW/VH/VH   9 8 7 6 5 4 3 2 1   03/B/313

Kathleen Gainor Andreoli, D.S.N., F.A.A.N.

Vice President of Educational Services, Interprofessional Education and International Programs, The University of Texas Health Science Center at Houston, Houston, Texas

James A. Blumenthal, Ph.D.

Associate Professor, Division of Medical Psychology; Assistant Professor, Department of Medicine, Duke University Medical Center, Durham, North Carolina

Martha E. Branyon, R.N., Ed.D.

Associate Professor, School of Nursing, University of Alabama at Birmingham, Birmingham, Alabama

Elizabeth Darling, R.N., M.S.N.

Clinical Research Assistant, Electrophysiology Laboratory, Indiana University School of Medicine, Indianapolis, Indiana

Edwin G. Duffin, Jr., Ph.D.

Bakken Fellow and Manager of Special Devices, Medtronic, Inc., Minneapolis, Minnesota

Sue Faust, R.N., M.S.N.

Electrophysiology Nurse, Indiana University School of Medicine, Indianapolis, Indiana

Virginia Kliner Fowkes, F.N.P., M.H.S.

Director, Primary Care Associate Program and Stanford Area Health Education Center, Division of Family Medicine, Stanford University School of Medicine, Stanford, California

Ruth A. Giebel, B.S.N.

Division of Cardiology, Department of Internal Medicine, The University of Texas Health Science Center at Houston, Houston, Texas

Susan J. Hasselman, R.N.

Cardiac Intensive Care Unit, Duke University Medical Center, Durham, North Carolina

James J. Heger, M.D.

Associate Professor of Medicine, Indiana University School of Medicine; Research Associate, Krannert Institute of Cardiology, Indianapolis, Indiana

Paula Hindle, R.N., M.S.N.

Department of Nursing Services, New England Medical Center, Boston, Massachusetts

Marguerite R. Kinney, R.N., D.N.Sc., F.A.A.N.

Professor of Nursing, School of Nursing, The University of Alabama at Birmingham, Birmingham, Alabama

F. Paul Koisch, B.A., B.S.

Administrative Director, DUPAC, Duke University Medical Center, Durham, North Carolina

Lori B. Maloy, R.N.

Head Nurse, Coronary Care Unit, University Hospital, Indiana University School of Medicine, Indianapolis, Indiana

Elaine G. Martin, R.N.

Head Nurse, Duke University Medical Center, Durham, North Carolina

Helene S. Mau, R.N.

DUPAC Activity Center, Duke University Medical Center, Durham, North Carolina

John C. McMahon, Ph.D.

Professor of Physiology Dental Branch, and Coordinator of Sports Medicine, The University of Texas Health Science Center at Houston, Houston, Texas

Miriam C. Morey, M.A.

Clinical Coordinator, Gerofit, Geriatric Research, Education and Clinical Center, Veterans Administration Center, Durham, North Carolina

Leigh Anne Musser, M.P.H.

Research Associate, Office of Educational Services, Interprofessional Education and International Programs, The University of Texas Health Science Center at Houston, Houston, Texas

Gerald V. Naccarelli, M.D., F.A.C.C.

Associate Professor of Medicine and Director, Clinical Electrophysiology, Department of Internal Medicine, Division of Cardiology, Medical School, The University of Texas Health Science Center at Houston, Houston, Texas

Akira Nishikawa, M.D.

Director of Coronary Care Unit, Department of Internal Medicine, Division of Cardiology, Medical School, The University of Texas Health Science Center at Houston, Houston, Texas

Debra L. Peeples, R.N., M.S.N.

Educational Projects Manager, Regional Medical Education Center, Veterans Administration Medical Center, Birmingham, Alabama

Eric N. Prystowsky, M.D.

Professor of Medicine and Director, Clinical Electrophysiology, Duke University Medical Center, Durham, North Carolina

Cynthia M. Schuch, R.N., M.S.N., C.C.R.N.

Cardiac Intensive Care Unit, University of Alabama at Birmingham, Birmingham, Alabama

Nancy L. Stephenson, R.N., B.S.N.

Manager of Physician Relations, Medtronic, Inc., Minneapolis, Minnesota

Elizabeth Wagner, R.N.

DUPAC Activity Center, Duke University Medical Center, Durham, North Carolina

Andrew G. Wallace, M.D.

Vice Chancellor for Health Affairs, Chief Executive Officer, Hospital, Duke University Medical Center, Durham, North Carolina

Jennifer J. Williams, P.A.

DUPAC Activity Center, Duke University Medical Center, Durham, North Carolina

R. Sanders Williams, M.D.

Associate Professor, Departments of Medicine and Physiology, Division of Cardiology, Duke University Medical Center, Durham, North Carolina

Douglas P. Zipes, M.D.

Professor of Medicine, Indiana University School of Medicine; Senior Research Associate, Krannert Institute of Cardiology, Indianapolis, Indiana

The sixth edition of *Comprehensive Cardiac Care* reflects continued advancement and expansion of knowledge related to the care and rehabilitation of persons with coronary artery disease and the prevention of this disease in the population as a whole. Since diseases of the heart remain the leading cause of death in the United States, new diagnostic and treatment modalities continue to be introduced and adopted, with technology becoming increasingly sophisticated. At the same time preventive strategies are receiving increasing attention as part of the health professional's responsibility in controlling the disease. The risk factor data base for coronary artery disease continues to grow, providing more substantiated clinical data on which to base decision-making related to preventive strategies for avoiding the premature onset of coronary atherosclerosis. Finally, methods of care and rehabilitation continue to evolve to ensure both the quality of care and the best quality of life for patients who have had a cardiac incident.

The contributors to the sixth edition of *Comprehensive Cardiac Care* have grown in number from nineteen to twenty-five, continuing to represent the multiplicity of disciplines that contribute to the health and welfare of patients with coronary artery disease and individuals seeking to reduce their risk. Further, a new name has been added to the editor list. We welcome Dr. Marguerite Kinney to the post. Dr. Kinney's reputation in nursing is well known, and her presence on our editorial board has been important in the production of this new edition.

The sequencing of chapters follows the general pattern of former editions, a pattern that we believe facilitates incremental learning. Each chapter, however, is also capable of providing an independent learning experience. Although there is some overlapping of content, we believe this serves to reinforce the importance of the material. The book moves quickly from the basic facts of anatomy, physiology, and pathology of the heart and coronary artery disease to the clinical application of current knowledge and its application to prevention, diagnosis, and treatment, including medical and surgical management, psychologic considerations, nursing care, and rehabilitation. Two chapters, one on surgical management and angioplasty and the other on coronary artery disease in the elderly, have been added to make the book a truly comprehensive text. As in the past, this text will remain responsive to trends, issues, and changes in the field of coronary artery disease.

As with any truly multidisciplinary effort, organizing and generating the sixth edition of *Comprehensive Cardiac Care* was challenging. We extend our sincere thanks to those who made this production a first rate experience—contributing authors, typists, illustrators, and editorial assistants. We also thank you, our readers, for supporting this endeavor and encouraging us to continue it. It has been a stimulating and satisfying experience. Moreover, we believe the end product has been and will continue to be a valuable resource for health professionals who practice comprehensive cardiac care.

Kathleen Gainor Andreoli
Douglas P. Zipes
Andrew G. Wallace
Marguerite R. Kinney
Virginia Kliner Fowkes

CONTENTS

9   Sudden Cardiac Death, 279

Eric N. Prystowsky
Elizabeth Darling

10   Cardiovascular Drugs, 297

James J. Heger
Sue Faust

11   Artificial Cardiac Pacemakers, 328

Edwin G. Duffin, Jr.
Nancy L. Stephenson
Douglas P. Zipes

12   Care of the Cardiac Patient, 352

Martha E. Branyon
Cynthia M. Schuch

13   Psychologic Considerations in Coronary Artery Disease, 385

James A. Blumenthal
Helene S. Mau

14 Rehabilitation after Myocardial Infarction, 399

Elizabeth Wagner
R. Sanders Williams

15 Surgical Management and Angioplasty for Coronary Heart Disease, 411

Elaine G. Martin
Susan J. Hasselman

COMPREHENSIVE CARDIAC CARE

CHAPTER 1

Anatomy and Physiology of the Heart

Miriam C. Morey
F. Paul Koisch

This chapter briefly reviews the anatomy and physiology of the heart. It is not intended to be a detailed discussion but merely to serve as a general background.

ANATOMY

Heart muscle is composed of cells that are connected to each other end-to-end as well as side-to-side, giving any particular sample of tissue the appearance of a syncytium.

Each cell is composed of myofibrils (the contractile machinery) and mitochondriae (the energy-producing units). Under a microscope myofibrils are seen to be composed of alternating light and dark bands consisting of actin and myosin molecules (Fig. 1-1). These long proteins overlap in a highly organized manner such that they shorten following excitation, causing the cell and the myofibril to shorten and the entire syncytium to contract, thereby re-

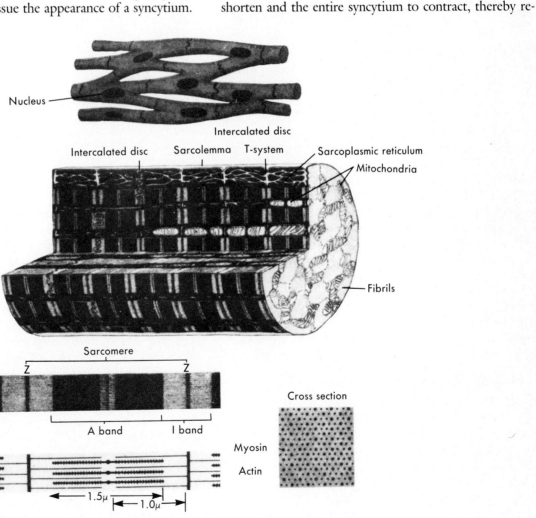

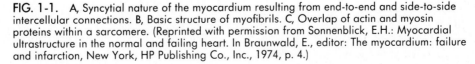

FIG. 1-1. A, Syncytial nature of the myocardium resulting from end-to-end and side-to-side intercellular connections. B, Basic structure of myofibrils. C, Overlap of actin and myosin proteins within a sarcomere. (Reprinted with permission from Sonnenblick, E.H.: Myocardial ultrastructure in the normal and failing heart. In Braunwald, E., editor: The myocardium: failure and infarction, New York, HP Publishing Co., Inc., 1974, p. 4.)

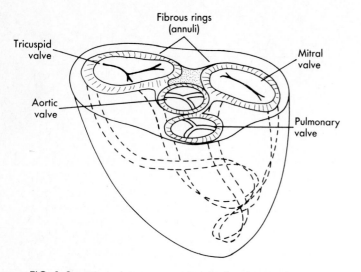

FIG. 1-2. Fibrous rings connecting the four heart valves.

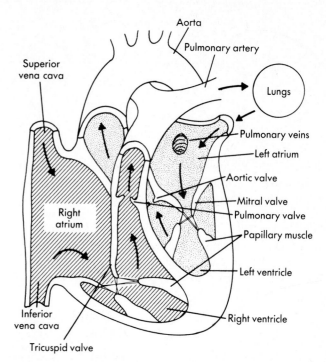

FIG. 1-3. Internal anatomy of the heart. (Modified from Guyton, A.C.: Function of the human body, ed. 3, Philadelphia, 1969, W.B. Saunders Co.)

ducing the volume of the cardiac chamber.[1] Excitation is initiated by depolarization of the cell membrane, which causes the internal release of calcium; when the calcium concentration increases to a threshold level, the actin-myosin molecules interact and shorten.[2] Because each heart cell is connected to its immediate neighbors by low-resistance couplings, the excitatory event spreads very rapidly to all cells leading to a nearly simultaneous and coordinated contractile event.

The heart has a skeleton of four fibrous rings or annuli connected into a single framework (Fig. 1-2). Each annulus is the supporting structure for one of the four valves of the heart and the connecting site of the muscular network that comprises the four chambers. This fibrous skeleton is nonconductive, and the atrial syncytium is separate from the ventricular syncytium. The specialized conduction system responsible for initiating electrical depolarization and conducting the impulse through the fibrous skeleton from atrium to ventricle and throughout the endocardial shell of the ventricles will be discussed later in the chapter.

BLOOD FLOW

The heart, a muscular pump, divided anatomically into right and left sides propels blood into the arterial (delivery) system and receives blood from the venous (return) system (Fig. 1-3). Each side has a receiving chamber, the atrium, and a pumping chamber, the ventricle. The right atrium receives desaturated venous blood from the inferior vena cava, which drains blood from the lower half of the body, from the superior vena cava, which drains blood from the upper half of the body, and from the coronary sinus, which drains blood from the heart muscle. From the right atrium the venous blood flows through the tricuspid valve into the right ventricle. Upon contraction of the ventricle,

blood is ejected through the pulmonary valve into the pulmonary artery and then into the lungs for oxygenation. Oxygenated blood returning from the lungs enters the left atrium through four pulmonary veins. It passes from the left atrium through the mitral valve to the left ventricle. Upon contraction the left ventricle ejects oxygenated blood through the aortic valve into the aorta, which then distributes this blood to the peripheral tissues.

The leaflets of the tricuspid and mitral valves are attached by chordae tendinae to the papillary muscles that lie in the floor of the ventricles. Contraction of these papillary muscles prevents the leaflets from everting into their respective atria during ventricular contraction.

The pumping action of the heart includes a period of relaxation, diastole, and a period of contraction, systole. In diastole the mitral and tricuspid valves are open and blood flows freely into the atria and ventricles. The ventricles fill passively to about 70% of their ultimate end diastolic volume during this period, with the aortic and pulmonary valves closed. At the end of each diastole, the atria contract and propel a further quantity of blood into the ventricles. With atrial relaxation, a pressure gradient from ventricle to atrium develops, causing the atrioventricular valves to close.

The ventricles are the primary pumps of the heart. During the systolic portion of the cardiac cycle, the pressure in each ventricle increases, causing the aortic and pulmonary valves to open. With the valves open, 70 to 80 ml of blood is pumped out by each ventricle per contraction; this stroke volume represents about 65% of the total volume of blood in the ventricle at end-diastole. The cardiac output, the total volume of blood pumped per minute, is the product of heart rate and stroke volume and is approximately 3 to 5 liters/minute in normal adults at rest.[3] Because body size affects the adequacy of blood supply in perfusing body tissues, the cardiac index is used to express cardiac output by body surface area; it is calculated by dividing the cardiac output by the body surface area.

The major physiologic roles of the circulatory system are the delivery of oxygen and other essential substrates to the tissues of the body and the removal of carbon dioxide and other products of cellular metabolism. Many of the substances carried to and from the tissues are dissolved in plasma, and their transport depends on the volume of flow. Oxygen and carbon dioxide, however, are both transported by red blood cells bound to the hemoglobin molecules.

As the blood from the right side of the heart passes through the pulmonary capillaries, red blood cells exchange carbon dioxide for oxygen within pulmonary alveoli in preparation for returning to the systemic circulation. As blood from the left side of the heart passes through the systemic capillary bed, red cells surrender their oxygen to metabolizing tissues and accumulate carbon dioxide. The transport of these gases to and from tissues is affected not only by the volume of blood flow but also by the metabolic rate of specific tissues at any given time. The local rate of metabolism is probably the most important determinant in the distribution of cardiac output. During exercise, for example, blood flow increases in areas involved in the activity—such as specific muscle groups and the skin—and decreases in areas of little metabolic activity—such as the kidneys, stomach, and intestines. Blood flow to the brain remains nearly the same at rest or during exercise.

SYSTEMIC CIRCULATION

The systemic circulation is comprised of the arteries, arterioles, capillaries, and veins. Blood flows through the system because of a continuing gradient of pressure along these conduits. Pressure is highest at the arterial level, and it progressively decreases until the blood reaches the right atrium.[4] When blood is pumped from the left ventricle into the aorta, a high arterial pressure is created, and the aorta becomes distended (Fig. 1-4). As a consequence of the cyclic pumping action of the heart, arterial pressure normally fluctuates between approximately 120 mm Hg (systolic pressure) and 80 mm Hg (diastolic pressure).

The arteries begin branching at the arch of the aorta and continue branching until they become small arterioles. These arterioles have muscular walls that can dilate or con-

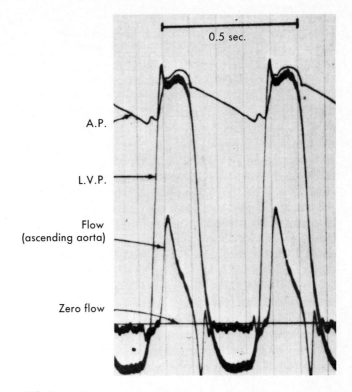

FIG. 1-4. Cardiac cycle. *LVP,* left ventricular pressure, *AP,* aortic pressure, flow. Ascending aortic flow velocity curve. (From Spencer, M.: Circ. Res. 10:275, 1962.)

strict, controlling blood flow into the capillary bed. Vasodilatation or vasoconstriction is usually dictated by the needs of the tissues for oxygen or other nutrients. Vascular resistance is highest at the arteriolar level in the systemic circuit causing a drop in pressure to less than 30 mm Hg as the blood enters the capillaries.[5]

Once the blood is inside the capillary bed, its rate of flow is at its slowest. This allows sufficient time for the blood and the interstitial space to exchange fluid, gases, and nutrients. Capillary walls are very thin, and most exchanges occur by diffusion. Since the total surface area of the capillary walls is extensive, adequate exchange of nutrients is ensured. When oxygen demand is low, much of the capillary surface is not needed and individual capillaries within a network are closed. Conversely, these capillaries open during a period of metabolic need. This is a dynamic process with capillaries opening and closing continuously.

Blood flows from the capillaries into venules, which converge to form larger veins. At this level of the systemic circuit, pressure is very low (about 5 to 10 mm Hg). Venous walls are thin and compliant yet muscular and contractile, which allows them to accommodate to large variations in blood flow and volume while still facilitating the return of blood to the right atrium.

PULMONARY CIRCULATION

Like systemic circulation, pulmonary circulation is a continuous circuit. Blood is pumped by the right ventricle into the pulmonary arteries, which branch into pulmonary arterioles and capillaries, where oxygen is extracted from pulmonary air spaces and carbon dioxide is released from the blood. The pulmonary capillaries converge into pulmonary veins and return oxygenated blood to the left atrium.

Gas exchange between the pulmonary capillaries and the alveolar spaces takes place through a thin pulmonary-alveolar membrane. When the body is at rest, blood usually traverses the pulmonary capillaries in about 1 second. When oxygen demand increases, the increased rate of blood flow through the pulmonary capillaries can shorten the diffusion time to less than half a second. Since the equilibrium time for gas exchange across the alveolar-capillary membrane is less than 0.3 seconds, enough time is available for capillary blood to come into near-equilibrium with alveolar air. Pulmonary circulation can also adjust to an increased oxygen demand, such as during exercise, by opening capillaries that are normally closed at rest.

An important feature of pulmonary circulation and of the distribution of flow is the ability of pulmonary vessels to regulate blood flow through the lungs. Since gas exchange is the major reason blood flows through the lungs, pulmonary blood vessels must ensure that blood flows only through adequately ventilated areas. When certain alveoli become blocked or damaged, the local pulmonary vessels normally constrict and force the blood through a properly aerated area of the lungs.

Pulmonary blood vessels are thin-walled and offer a low resistance to flow; these two characteristics allow blood to flow through the lungs with only a modest pressure gradient. Because the pulmonary and systemic circulations occur in series, the volume of blood flowing through the lungs per unit of time is the same as the volume flowing through the systemic circulation. The lungs must therefore be prepared to accept as much as a fivefold increase in blood flow during strenous exercise without putting additional strain on the right ventricle. At rest, pulmonary artery mean pressure is about 20 mm Hg, and only a small increase in required to augment flow to the levels observed during exercise.

CORONARY CIRCULATION

The function of the coronary artery system is to maintain an adequate blood supply to the heart muscle (myocardium). Two major coronary arteries, the left and right, arise from the aorta immediately behind their respective cusps of the aortic valve.[6] Shortly after its origin, the left coronary artery divides into two branches (Fig. 1-5), the anterior descending branch and the circumflex. The anterior descending branch passes down the groove between the two ventricles on the anterior surface of the heart. From it arise diagonal branches, which supply the left ventricular wall, and septal perforating branches, which supply the anterior portion of the interventricular septum and the anterior papillary muscle of the left ventricle. The anterior

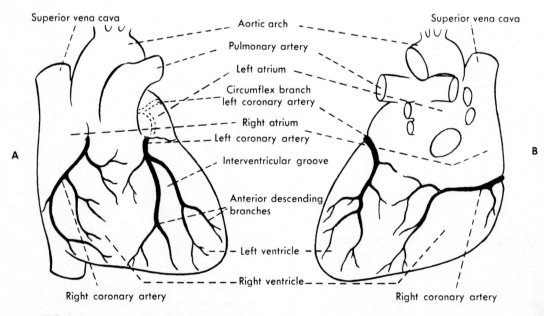

FIG. 1-5.   A, Coronary arteries supplying the anterior aspect of the heart. B, Coronary arteries supplying the posterior aspect of the heart.

descending artery usually supplies the entire apical portion of the interventricular septum before turning at the apex to terminate in channels that anastomose with the posterior descending coronary artery. The circumflex branch of the left coronary artery passes posteriorly and to the left in the groove between the left atrium and left ventricle. It gives off several small and one or two large marginal branches that supply the lateral aspects of the left ventricle.

The right coronary artery passes around the right atrioventricular (AV) groove, giving off branches to the right ventricle, and then turns at the crux of the heart to descend into the posterior interventricular groove. The posterior descending artery supplies the posterior aspect of the septum and the posterior left ventricular papillary muscle before terminating in channels that anastomose with the anterior descending branch of the left coronary artery. The right coronary artery gives off important branches that supply the sinoatrial (SA) node in 50% to 60% of human hearts (the other 40% to 50% from left circumflex, CX) and the AV node in 90% of human hearts (the other 10% from branch of CX). If the right coronary artery turns at the crux and supplies the posterior aspect of the left ventricle and interventricular septum, the coronary circulation is said to be *dominant right*. About 80% to 90% of the population have a dominant right coronary circulation. When the posterior aspect of the ventricle is supplied by the left circumflex artery, the coronary circulation is then referred to as *dominant left* circulation.[7]

Coronary blood flow at rest averages about 220 ml/minute, which represents about 5% of the total cardiac output. It is controlled primarily by the local rate of metabolism and therefore responds proportionally to the oxygen demand of the myocardium. With normal activity, about 70% of the arterial oxygen content is extracted by the myocardium, which leaves only a small oxygen reserve available in the blood if the oxygen demand increases. Thus the local rate of metabolism dominates in regulating coronary vascular resistance, and an increase of coronary blood flow is the principal mechanism to provide an increase in oxygen when myocardial work is augmented. With strenuous activity coronary blood flow can increase up to five times to ensure adequate oxygen supply to the myocardium.

Impairment of the coronary circulation by atherosclerosis constitutes the most frequent cause of heart disease. The atherosclerotic process causes a decrease in the diameter of the coronary vessels, which compromises normal blood flow. Blood flow is reduced, at least during exertion, when the lumen of a coronary artery is reduced by 50% or more.

EXCITATION OF THE HEART

The normal cardiac impulse arises in specialized pacemaker cells of the sinoatrial or sinus node, located about 1 mm beneath the right atrial epicardium at its junction with the superior vena cava (Fig. 1-6). Spontaneous diastolic depolarization in these cells causes a wave of excitation (depolarization) to spread over the atrial myocardium, to the left atrium via Bachmann's bundle and to the region of the AV node via the anterior, middle, and posterior internodal

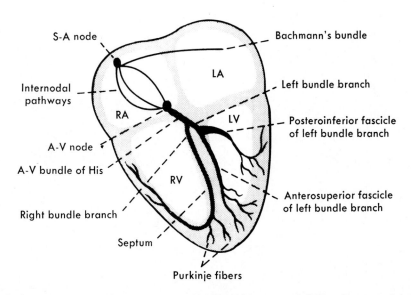

FIG. 1-6. Transmission of the cardiac impulse from the sinoatrial (SA) node over atrial myocardium, Bachmann's bundle, and internodal pathways, then through the AV node and bundle of His and down the left and right bundle branches, emerging into the Purkinje fibers, which distribute the impulse to all parts of the ventricle.

tracts connecting the sinus and AV nodes. When the impulse reaches the atria, it depolarizes electrically, producing the P wave on the electrocardiogram (ECG) (see Chapter 6). Contraction of the atria produces the A wave of the atrial pressure pulse and propels blood forward into the ventricles (Fig. 1-7).

Conduction slows markedly when the impulse reaches the AV node, accounting for the P-R interval on the electrocardiogram, and allows sufficient time for blood to flow from the atria into the ventricles. After the impulse emerges from the AV node, conduction assumes a very rapid velocity through the His bundle and down the left and right bundle branches. The left bundle divides into anterosuperior, middle, and posteroinferior divisions. Left and right bundle branches supply the inner shells (endocardium) of their respective ventricles with a profusely branching terminal network called Purkinje fibers (Fig. 1-6). These fibers allow almost simultaneous deplorization of both ventricles by distributing the impulse rapidly throughout the ventricular endocardium.

All conduction prior to an impulse leaving the Purkinje fibers takes place between atrial and ventricular depolarization (P-R interval) on the ECG recording. When the impulse emerges from the Purkinje fibers, ventricular de-

polarization occurs, producing the QRS complex on the ECG and the mechanical contraction of the ventricles that propels the blood forward into the pulmonary artery and aorta. Considering the many different parts of the specialized conduction system, it is interesting that only atrial depolarization (P wave), ventricular depolarization (QRS complex), and ventricular repolarization (T wave) appear in the standard ECG recording (Fig. 1-7).[8] Sometimes atrial repolarization is recorded at the Ta wave; however, more often this wave is obscured by the QRS complex.

REGULATION OF CARDIAC FUNCTION

Among the many factors that contribute to the regulation of the heart, the autonomic nervous system plays an important role in the rate of impulse formation, the speed of conduction, and the strength of cardiac contraction.[9] It regulates the heart through both the sympathetic and the parasympathetic sets of nerves (Fig. 1-8). The sympathetic nerve fibers supply all areas of the atria and ventricles. Vagal nerve fibers primarily innervate the SA node, atrial muscle fibers, and the AV node. They supply the ventricular myocardium also, but the density of innervation there is lower than in the atrium, and the physiologic consequences of vagal innervation of the ventricles are uncertain. Recent data suggest, however, that vagal innervation may affect ventricular electrophysiology more than has been previously thought.

Within the postganglionic nerve fibers are locted neurotransmitters—acetylcholine in the vagus nerve and nor-

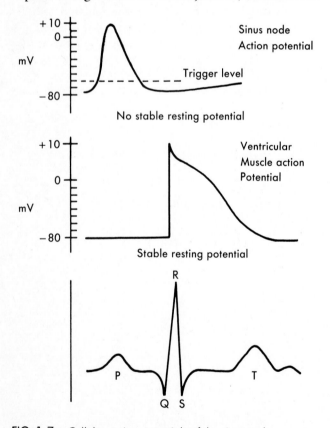

FIG. 1-7.   Cellular action potentials of the sinus node (pacemaker) and ventricular muscle and the resulting electrocardiographic tracing.

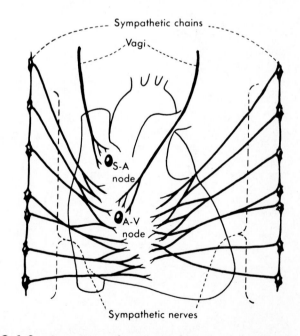

FIG. 1-8.   Connections of parasympathetic nerves (vagi) and sympathetic nerves with the heart. (Modified from Guyton, A.C.: Function of the human body, ed. 3, Philadelphia, 1969, W.B. Saunders Co.)

epinephrine in the sympathetic nerves. Electrical impulses traveling down the postganglionic nerve fibers release the neurotransmitters, which in turn mediate the influence of the autonomic nerves on the heart by binding to specific receptors on the surface membrane of myocardial cells.

Vagal nerve stimulation has the following effects on the heart: decreased firing rate of the SA node, decreased contractile force of atrial (and probably ventricular) muscle, and decreased impulse conduction speed through the AV node, which lengthens the delay period between atrial and ventricular contraction (PR interval). Vagal stimulation also speeds conduction through the atrial muscle and shortens the atrial repolarization period. Sympathetic nerve stimulation has several effects on the heart: increased heart rate, increased conduction speed through the AV node, a shortened ventricular and atrial repolarization period, and increased vigor of cardiac contraction.

Autonomic nerve activity can be modulated by the central nervous system (such as reflexes triggered by fear or pain) or by reflex changes caused by stimulation of sensors that detect changes in pressure (pressoreceptors).[10] Pressoreceptors are mechanoreceptors, chemoreceptors, and others located in the aortic arch and carotid arteries and are connected to the vasomotor center in the medulla by way of the vagus and glossopharyngeal nerves. Sudden elevation of blood pressure within the aorta or the carotid sinus (for example, by a hypertensive drug or by carotid sinus massage) stimulates the pressoreceptors in these vessels. This stimulates the cardioinhibitory center, which in turn inhibits the accelerator center. Conversely, a sudden drop in blood pressure within the aorta or carotid sinus stimulates pressoreceptors less intensely. The cardioinhibitory center is stimulated less, producing less depression of the accelerator center and consequently less reflex acceleration of the heart. This phenomenon becomes apparent during hypotension.[11]

The heart also has several intrinsic autoregulating mechanisms and can operate without nervous influence. The major intrinsic mechanism is described by Starling's law, which states that, within limits, the more the heart is filled during diastole (end-diastolic volume-EDV), the greater will be the force of contraction and the resulting stroke volume during systole. Striated muscle, such as cardiac muscle, characteristically contracts with greater force when stretched. Thus the heart automatically adapts to different incoming blood volumes by changing its force of contraction. In heart failure, however, cardiac muscle is already operating at the upper end of the Starling curve, and further dilatation will decrease the stroke volume.

Another mechanism that regulates cardiac function is based on the local rate of metabolism in peripheral tissues. Blood flow to various organs is influenced by each organ's metabolic rate, which in turn influences systemic vascular resistance, a determinant of cardiac output. Thus with anxiety, fever, and exercise, cardiac output increases because peripheral resistance drops.

Other factors that can affect either the heart rate or the contractile force of heart muscle include levels of oxygen and carbon dioxide in the blood, electrolyte disorders, and the presence of certain drugs in the body.

REFERENCES

1. Pollack, G.H., and Krueger, J.W.: Sarcomere dynamics in intact cardiac muscle, Eur. J. Cardiol. **4** (suppl.):53, 1976.
2. Fabiato, A.: Myoplasmic-free calcium concentration reached during the twitch of an intact cardiac cell and during calcium-induced release of calcium from the sarcoplasmic reticulum of a skinned cardiac cell from the adult rat or rabbit ventricle, J . Gen. Physiol. **78**:456, 1981.
3. Rushmer, R.F.: Structure and function of the cardiovascular system, ed. 2, Philadelphia, 1976, W.B. Saunders Co.
4. Katz, A.M.: Physiology of the heart, New York, 1977, Raven Press.
5. Guyton, A.C.: Textbook of medical physiology, ed. 5, Philadelphia, 1976, W.B. Saunders Co.
6. James, T.N.: Anatomy of the coronary arteries in health and disease, Circulation **32**:1020, 1965.
7. Braunwald, E., Ross, J., and Sonnenblick, E.H.: Mechanisms of contraction of the normal and failing heart, ed. 2, Boston, 1976, Little, Brown & Co.
8. Wellens, H.J.J., Lie, K.I., and Janse, M.J.: The conduction system of the heart, Leiden, 1976, Hyman, Stenfort Kroese & Zoon, N.V.
9. Braunwald, E.: Heart disease: a textbook of cardiovascular medicine, ed. 2, Philadelphia, 1984, W.B. Saunders Co.
10. Berne, R.M., and Levy, M.N.: Physiology, St. Louis, 1983, The C.V. Mosby Co.
11. Bishop, V.S., Malliani, A., and Thoren, P.: Cardiac mechanoreceptors. In Handbook of physiology, Section 2: The cardiovascular system, vol. 3, Bethesda, Md., 1983, American Physiological Society.

CHAPTER 2

Coronary Artery Disease

Jennifer J. Williams
Andrew G. Wallace

PATHOGENESIS

Despite recent declines in annual per capita mortality rates, coronary artery disease and its complications remain the leading cause of death in Europe and the Western hemisphere, responsible for 1.5 million heart attacks and 550,000 deaths in the United States each year.[1] Coronary artery disease and arteriosclerotic heart disease are essentially synonymous.

Arteriosclerosis is a chronic disease of the arteries, characterized by abnormal thickening and hardening of the vessel walls that results in loss of elasticity. There are several possible causes of the arteriosclerotic process; its manifestations differ according to the type of vessel involved and the site and extent of the disease within the vessel. It is convenient to categorize the disease into the following types[2]:

Type I: Intimal atherosclerosis. This form of arteriosclerosis affects the internal membranes (intima) of arteries and consists of irregular thickening and plaque formation. Plaques consist of lipid, proliferating smooth muscle cells, and variable amounts of collagen. Intimal atherosclerosis primarily affects the large vessels, may begin at a very young age, and to some degree is almost universally present in people over the age of 20.

Type II: Medial sclerosis. This process consists of calcification and hypertrophy of the muscular portion of the artery (media). It affects medium-sized blood vessels such as the brachial artery and the femoral artery, which become thickened, rigid, and tortuous. It is not necessarily associated with any reduction in the caliber of the involved vessel.

Type III: Arteriolar sclerosis. This type of the disease affects small blood vessels and is characterized by hypertrophy of the muscular media and thickening of the intima; it is usually seen in patients with long-standing hypertension. It often affects the small vessels in the fundus of the eye and in the kidney.

Although these three types of arteriosclerosis may exist separately, there is in fact considerable overlap. Type I, or intimal atherosclerosis, is the cause of most coronary artery disease but may be aggravated or accelerated by coexisting hypertension.

The natural history of coronary artery disease has three phases. The first phase begins with injury to the intimal endothelium, which may either heal or progress to a second phase. The second phase is the response to injury: blood platelets and other plasma constituents adhere to the site of injury, inducing proliferation of smooth muscle cells, and lipid accumulates abnormally in the arterial intima. At the earliest (and still reversible) part of this stage only a fatty streak may be produced. With more severe involvement, however, massive amounts of lipid, extensive smooth muscle proliferation, and the influx of cells, such as macrophages and collagen-producing fibroblasts, may combine to produce a full-blown atherosclerotic plaque. Although mature atherosclerotic lesions may occasionally regress, the usual course is a progressive encroachment upon the lumen of the affected artery. The third phase in the natural history of coronary artery disease is the production of clinically manifest symptoms, either angina pectoris, myocardial infarction, or, all too frequently, sudden cardiac death.[3]

Different factors may contribute to the development of clinically evident heart disease during each of these three phases. For example, homocysteine, which accumulates in patients with congenital homocystinuria, a genetic disorder characterized by the early onset of severe and diffuse atherosclerosis, has been shown to produce diffuse sites of endothelial injury. Carbon monoxide inhaled during cigarette smoking may work through similar mechanisms. On the other hand, excessive levels of low-density lipoprotein probably produce accelerated atherosclerosis by increasing the accumulation of lipid at the sites of endothelial injury. Finally, other poorly identified factors must exist to explain the tremendous variations in longevity and clinical symptoms among subjects with equivalent amounts of coronary artery disease.

A number of pathologic events, either gradual or sudden, may affect the clinical course of coronary artery disease. Ross[4] and others have emphasized the dynamic interaction between platelets and vascular endothelium, and the participation of factors released from these cells, such as platelet-derived growth factor, thromboxane A_2, and prostacyclin, as determinants of both the acute and the gradual progression of atherosclerosis. Usually a plaque enlarges slowly as fat is deposited and scar tissue develops. Sometimes blood vessels that grow into the fibrous plaque rupture, producing small hemorrhages. Such subintimal hemorrhages increase the size of the plaque and are frequently followed by scarring and fibrosis, which further enlarge the lesion. Rupture of blood vessels within the plaque also may cause a sudden major obstruction of the lumen of the vessel. The intima covering a plaque may break, causing a clot to form on the surface, which adds to the building obstruction of the vessel's lumen. The clot or plaque also may embolize and occlude the vessel distally where the lumen becomes narrow. Evidence indicates that myocardial infarction is usually produced by an acute thrombotic event complicating preexisting atherosclerosis.[5] The discovery that acute coronary thrombosis is usually present in myocardial infarction has fostered attempts to restore coronary blood flow by chemical agents that dissolve blood clots (streptokinase or tissue plasminogen activator)[6] or by mechanical disruption of the thrombus (balloon angioplasty)[7] before the myocardium supplied by the occluded vessel is irreversibly damaged.

In addition to compromising blood supply by obstruction, the atherosclerotic process may cause weakening of the arterial wall and aneurysm formation. Thus obstruction and aneurysm may coexist in the same artery.

GROSS PATHOLOGY AND PROGNOSIS

Atherosclerotic lesions usually form at branch points in the arterial tree. In the carotid and iliac arteries the disease is most prevalent at the bifurcation. Coronary arteries are particularly susceptible to atherosclerosis. Although it is unusual to have peripheral vascular disease without coronary artery involvement, coronary disease without involvement of peripheral arteries is not rare. In coronary circulation the atherosclerotic process is confined to the portions of the vessels that lie on the epicardial surface, sparing the smaller penetrating arteries. Such a pattern of distribution suggests that turbulence of flow at branch points and rhythmic torsion of untethered vessels may contribute to the genesis of the lesion.

In considering the natural history of coronary artery disease, it is important to distinguish factors that affect the underlying coronary artery disease per se, that is, the previously described accumulation of lipid, cellular material, and sometimes calcium within the vessel wall,[4] from factors that influence the occurrence of clinical complications such as sudden death, angina pectoris, or myocardial infarction. An additional discussion of pathophysiology will highlight the importance of this distinction.

Some degree of coronary artery disease is present in most individuals above the age of 30 in Western industrialized nations.[2] However, such disease is almost always clinically silent until it progresses to occlude 75% of the diameter of a major coronary vessel. Even at this degree of obstruction, blood flow to the region of the myocardium supplied by the occluded vessel is usually normal at rest, and it becomes inadequate only when the oxygen require-

ments of the heart muscle are high, for example, during strenuous exercise. Only when the vessel lumen is narrowed to less than 5% of its normal vessel diameter is the blood flow insufficient to maintain a normal oxygen supply to the myocardium in the resting state. Furthermore, even with such severe stenosis, blood from other major coronary vessels may reach the muscle supplied by the severely narrowed vessel through alternative channels, termed *collaterals,* thereby maintaining normal blood flow, even during exercise.[8]

The degree to which an individual patient's heart forms such collaterals is very unpredictable; therefore the relationship between the severity of the stenosis and the severity of symptoms is also unpredictable. Furthermore, some individuals may have serious limitations to myocardial blood flow, even developing myocardial infarction in the absence of chest pain, an occurrence that further complicates the clinical assessment of patients with coronary artery disease.

An additional anatomic feature of the coronary arteries that is clinically relevant is that they are not rigid pipes, but muscular structures capable of rapid variations in diameter under the influence of autonomic nerves that innervate them or vasoactive substances released in the vessel lumen by vascular endothelium, or by platelets.[9] The degree to which an atherosclerotic plaque present in a coronary vessel limits blood flow will be dependent not only upon the severity of the plaque itself, but upon the muscular tone of the vessel around the plaque. Thus an insignificant 25% stenosis may rapidly become a critical 99% stenosis under the influence of a vasoconstrictive stimulus. This occurrence is termed *coronary spasm* and may be suspected clinically with observation of transient ST-segment elevation on the electrocardiogram, in the absence of the release of myocardial enzymes into blood that characterizes a myocardial infarction. To further complicate matters, such limitations in coronary blood flow, and even myocardial infarction, may occasionally occur in the absence of clinically demonstrable atherosclerosis.[10]

These pathophysiologic considerations, in addition to the marked variability in the rate of progression of the underlying atherosclerosis and also in the occurrence of sudden catastrophic events such as acute coronary thrombosis of ventricular fibrillation, account for the disconcerting unpredictability of the prognosis carried by an individual patient with coronary artery disease. These considerations also explain part of the difficulty in trying to detect coronary artery disease in its early stages. However, it is possible to use anatomic and physiologic data to yield probability estimates concerning prognosis. An important variable is the number of major coronary vessels with obstructions exceeding 75% of the vascular lumen. Persons with only one involved vessel have annual mortality rates of only 1% to 3%, whereas death rates approach 10% to 15% in persons with three-vessel disease, and up to 25% to 30% in persons with a high-grade obstruction of the left main coronary artery.[11] Coronary artery disease occurs most frequently in the left anterior descending artery, less in the right coronary artery, and still less frequently (although not rarely) in the circumflex artery. Narrowing tends to be most severe in the proximal 2 to 3 cm of each artery, but distal involvement, particularly of the right coronary artery, is not uncommon. The site of vessel obstruction is clinically important, since proximal lesions are much more amenable to therapy by saphenous vein-grafting or by percutaneous transluminal coronary angioplasty with balloon-type catheters. In almost all pathologically examined cases of myocardial infarction, the vessel supplying the infarcted area demonstrates a lesion of 95% or greater. Thus significant disease of the right coronary artery is found in patients with inferior myocardial infarction and disease of the left anterior descending artery in patients with anterior infarction.[12]

A second factor with prognostic importance for the patient with coronary artery disease is the contractile function of the left ventricle, which is determined largely by the amount of muscle tissue damaged by previous myocardial infarction. Subjects with good ventricular function have a much better prognosis than those with impaired function, despite equivalent degrees of coronary obstruction.[13] The increased mortality of patients with poor ventricular function is attributable largely to a higher incidence of sudden death, presumably caused by ventricular fibrillation, rather than to recurrent infarction or to inexorably progressive congestive heart failure. Sudden death also occurs in patients with coronary disease and normal ventricular function, although with a lower incidence, and, tragically, can occur as the initial manifestation of coronary artery disease in previously asymptomatic persons. Frequent premature ventricular contractions or ventricular tachycardia in the postinfarction period also may identify persons at higher risk for sudden death.[14]

Although the number of diseased coronary vessels and left ventricular functions are powerful predictors of both symptomatic improvement and prognosis in patients with coronary artery disease, exceptions to the general trends described above occur with some frequency. Patients with severe three-vessel coronary artery disease or markedly severe left ventricular dysfunction may be asymptomatic and may survive for more than a decade. Conversely, some patients with single-vessel disease may have disabling angina pectoris or may die unexpectedly as a result of myocardial infarction or ventricular arrhythmia.

In summary, coronary atherosclerosis may be without symptoms for many years until the disease progresses to produce an obstruction that interferes with the arterial blood supply to the myocardium. If the obstruction progresses gradually over a period of years, intercoronary collateral circulation may develop, and clinical evidence of disease may be deferred or may never occur. Despite marked obstructive disease, the myocardial cells may receive adequate oxygen regardless of demands. On the other hand, when an artery is partially obstructed and sufficient collateral circulation has not yet developed, the obstruction may impair blood flow during conditions of increased demand, producing symptoms of intermittent vascular insufficiency.

INCIDENCE, PREVALENCE, MORBIDITY, AND MORTALITY

In 1985 the American Heart Association estimated that 4.67 million persons in the United States had coronary artery disease. Of the nearly 40 million Americans with some form of cardiovascular disease, coronary artery disease ranked second to hypertensive heart disease in prevalence. Of the approximately 600,000 who die annually from heart attacks, sudden death is the first clinical manifestation in 20% to 25% of the first events and is responsible for 50% to 60% of all heart attack deaths. Of those who die, 25% are under the age of 65. Furthermore, two thirds of the deaths from heart attack occur outside the hospital and within the first 2 hours of an acute attack.[1]

RISK FACTORS

Mortality for coronary heart disease increased steadily in the 1950s, reached a plateau in the 1960s, and has steadily decreased 16% to 20% since 1968.[15] At least part of this decline is attributable to an increased public awareness of cardiovascular risk factors. These have been identified by large-scale epidemiologic studies[16,17] as clinical variables that are associated statistically with the subsequent manifestation of coronary artery disease. Presumably such factors are involved in the pathogenesis of coronary atherosclerosis, and advances in basic science have helped to identify many of the mechanisms by which such factors may influence arterial plaque formation. In this context risk is viewed as the probability of developing coronary heart disease, and that probability is determined by the number of risk factors in any given individual, by the level of each factor (that is, the level of blood pressure or cholesterol) and by age is important to consider the cumulative nature of risk factors in the clinical evaluation of the patient. For example, a person who smokes and is hypertensive has approximately twice the risk as one who smokes and is normotensive. Although the disease is more common when multiple risk factors are present, it can occur in the absence of any identifiable risk factors; yet some persons may live for many years with multiple risk factors and have no manifestations of the disease. Clearly, genetic or environmental factors can act independently of established risk factors and influence the clinical outcome. Nonetheless, identification and elimination of risk factors remain the mainstay of efforts to further lower the incidence of this disease.

Risk factors are either primary or secondary. Primary factors are those that are thought to contribute to the development of coronary atherosclerosis, and secondary factors are those that are thought to enhance the risk of any specific manifestation of the disease (such as arrhythmias or myocardial infarction) in those who already have coronary atherosclerosis. Cigarette-smoking and the high intake of cholesterol clearly appear to be both primary and secondary risk factors. The likelihood of developing coronary heart disease is influenced by and can be predicted from many primary risk factors.

Age, Sex, and Race

Atherosclerosis is more prevalent in older people (see Chapter 16). It is, however, a major cause of death in men of age 35 to 45 and causes 40% of the deaths in men of ages 55 to 64. In the United States the death rate is nearly six times higher in men between 35 and 55 years of age than in white women of the same age. After menopause, however, the incidence of the disease in women rapidly approaches that in men. Prior to 1968 nonwhite males had lower death rates than white males. Since that time, however, nonwhite males have shown higher mortality up to the age of 65. Nonwhite females have higher mortality than white females.[18] A decline in deaths from coronary heart disease in recent years has been observed in whites, but not in blacks, Hispanics, and other minority groups.[19]

Blood Pressure

In the coronary heart disease study conducted in Framingham, Massachusetts, middle-aged men with arterial pressures in excess of 160/95 showed a fivefold increase in the incidence of ischemic heart disease, compared with subjects having blood pressures of 140/90 or less.[20] A man with a systolic pressure over 150 has more than twice the risk of heart attack than a man with systolic pressure under 120. Both systolic and diastolic pressure elevations correlate positively with ischemic heart disease; systolic blood pressure often increases with age, but elevated systolic blood pressure is still a risk factor in the elderly.[18]

Hyperlipidemia and Diet

The lipids in the plasma that are of general importance are cholesterol, triglycerides, and free fatty acids. Cholesterol has been studied more extensively than other lipids and, when its level is elevated, it is associated with an increased incidence of coronary heart disease.[21] Cholesterol and triglycerides are insoluble in plasma and therefore must be

transported by lipoproteins, which are soluble. These lipoproteins can be separated and measured. In the fasting state very low-density lipoproteins (VLDL) carry mostly triglyceride and lesser amounts of cholesterol. Low-density lipoproteins (LDL) are derived from the metabolism of VLDL and carry most of the cholesterol in plasma. High-density lipoproteins (HDL) are mostly protein and carry 10% to 50% of total plasma cholesterol. Numerous epidemiologic studies[22] have shown that the relationship between total serum cholesterol and risk of coronary atherosclerosis is even stronger if LDL cholesterol levels are high. A high ratio of HDL to LDL conveys protection against vascular disease. The significance of these associations is heightened by pathophysiologic studies that have shown that high levels of LDL cholesterol damage the endothelial lining of vessels and promote a proliferation of both smooth muscle cells and other components of the atherosclerotic lesion.[23] Among patients with premature atherosclerosis, the two most common patterns of hyperlipidemia are type IV (elevated level of triglycerides with a normal or only slightly elevated level of cholesterol) caused by increased VLDL, and type II (elevated levels of cholesterol with normal or only slightly elevated levels of triglycerides caused by increased LDL. Dietary and pharmacologic methods are moderately effective in lowering serum cholesterol and triglyceride.

Studies have also focused on the specific proteins that are found in circulating lipoprotein complexes. Some of these apolipoproteins are frquently elevated in persons with coronary artery disease, whereas other apolipoproteins, when present in higher amounts, are associated with a decreased risk. Some studies have suggested that measurements of plasma apolipoprotein levels may have more predictive value than measurements of total plasma cholesterol, or even of the HDL and LDL fractions, in identifying individuals with higher risks for coronary disease and its complications.[24]

The relationships between diet, plasma lipids, and coronary artery disease have been explored in many studies. Population studies have shown a relationship between the fat content of the diet and serum lipids, both in individuals and in whole countries. In 1979 a 20-nation study[25] examined the relationship between the calories from fat and high-cholesterol animal products and the risk of coronary heart disease mortality for whole countries. The United States, Finland, New Zealand, Australia, and the United Kingdom led the list of countries consuming the most calories from these products and also have the most deaths from coronary heart disease. Conversely, Japan had the least fat-related calories and the lowest mortality. Recent studies have demonstrated that lowering total serum cholesterol in humans reduces subsequent mortality from coronary artery disease.[26]

Smoking

The relationship between cigarette smoking and the development of coronary heart disease is clear. Statistical evidence supports a mean increase of about 75% in the death rate from coronary artery disease in middle-aged men who smoke one pack of cigarettes per day when compared with nonsmokers.[15] This percentage decreases with advancing age, and the relationship is more complex in women. Pipe and cigar smokers do not have an increased risk, probably because they do not inhale. The chief effects of nicotine on the cardiovascular system are cardiac stimulation and peripheral vasoconstriction. The former results in an increase in heart rate, stroke volume, cardiac output, and cardiac work. The peripheral vasoconstriction caused by nicotine is not greater in patients with vascular disease than in normal persons, but the resultant decrease in blood flow is more conspicuous in the patient with circulatory impairment and enhances the ischemia already present. Smoking causes carbon monoxide levels of possibly 5% or more to accumulate in the blood. The chief effects of carbon monoxide are the interference with oxygen binding to hemoglobin and a decrease in the threshold for ventricular fibrillation.[27]

Glucose Intolerance

Coronary heart disease is more prevalent in patients with adult onset diabetes mellitus, although the precise mechanisms is unclear. Patients with diabetes have an increased tendency toward degeneration of connective tissue, which may make them more prone to atheroma formation. Men with glucose intolerance have a 50% greater risk of developing coronary artery disease than those without it[18] whereas in women the risk is more than doubled, which equalizes the risk of CAD in men and women with diabetes.

Physical Inactivity

Many studies, but not all, have suggested that physical inactivity is associated with an increased risk of coronary heart disease. However, the strength of the relationship has generally been low in comparison with other factors such as cigarette smoking or hypertension. A study of California longshoremen[28] demonstrated a strong inverse relationship between energy expenditure at work (excessive calorie expenditure) and the incidence of fatal and nonfatal heart attacks. The reduced risk was evident in all age groups, but it was more striking in the young and was still evident after correcting for excess weight, smoking patterns, and serum cholesterol. The most significant finding of this study of over 3000 men was that habitual expenditure of about 1800 calories per day above basal level through physically demanding work reduced by nearly 50% the incidence of fatal heart attacks compared with those men who expended less than 1000 calories per day above basal level. A study of college alumni in 1978 observed a similar relationship between physical activity during leisure time and coronary risk and found a progressive decrease in risk with increased activity up to 2000 calories per week that was independent of other risk factors.[29] Regardless of whether physical activity influences the natural history of coronary artery disease independently of other known risk factors, increasing physical activity may have favorable influences on lipoprotein patterns, obesity, hypertension, and glucose tolerance.[30]

Personality Factors

For many years coronary heart disease has been thought to be more prominent among individuals subject to chronic anxiety or stress. Subsequently a personality type, called type A, more prone to coronary heart disease, was identified. The characteristics of type A behavior include aggressiveness, ambition, competitive drive, and a chronic sense of urgency (see Chapter 13). The report of a western collaborative study showed that the incidence of coronary heart disease was twice as high in type A individuals than in type B individuals (who had these traits to a lesser degree) even after correcting for other risk factors.[31] These observations are of considerable interest, but a link between the type A personality and the pathophysiology of coronary atherosclerosis has not yet been defined. Furthermore, it remains to be shown that the modification of behavioral patterns is possible or that it will be effective in altering risk.

Obesity

Although this is a controversial issue, most epidemiologic studies show a positive relationship between obesity (any weight greater than 20% over ideal weight) and morbidity and mortality from coronary heart disease among those under 50 years of age. It has primarily been considered as a risk in conjunction with its effects on other characteristics such as hypertension, but most data suggest that obesity makes an independent contribution to coronary heart disease risk, at least up to 50 years of age.[18]

Other Risk Factors

Additional signs associated with increased risk of coronary heart disease are electrocardiographic abnormalities at rest and in response to exercise and hyperuricemia. Some major risk factors may be determined by familial or genetic factors. The tendency toward development of hypertension, diabetes, and hyperlipidemia may be inherited. Also, certain habits and life-styles such as smoking, overeating, and lack of exercise may be passed down in a family. There may also be other inherited traits, currently immeasurable, that affect one's risk. It is vitally important to recognize that risk is multifactorial, that the influence of two or more factors may be synergistic, and that risk is influenced by any given factor's degree of abnormality, not just its presence or absence. The emphasis for the future is on primary prevention, which includes risk factor education, basic research support, and acceptance by the public or responsibility for their own health maintenance. (See Chapter 3 for discussion of preventive strategies.) Secondary risk factors, including myocardial infarction and arrhythmias, will be discussed in subsequent chapters.

REFERENCES

1. American Heart Association: Heart facts, 1985, American Heart Association.
2. McGill, H.C.: The geographic pathology of atherosclerosis, Lab. Invest. 18:463, 1968.
3. Wolintsky, H.: A new look at atherosclerosis, Cardiovasc. Med. 1:41, 1976.
4. Ross, R.: The pathogenesis of atherosclerosis—an update, N. Engl. J. Med. 314:488, 1986.
5. Roberts, W.C.: Coronary thrombosis and fatal myocardial ischemia, Circulation 49:1, 1974.
6. Davies, G.J., and others: Prevention of myocardial infarction by very early treatment with intra-coronary streptokinase, N. Engl. J. Med. 311:1488, 1984.
7. Papapiotro, S.E., and others: Percutaneous transluminal coronary angioplasty in acute myocardial infarction, Am. J. Cardiol. 55:48, 1985.
8. Berne, R.M., and Rubio, R.: Coronary circulation. In Berne, R.M., and others, editors: Handbook of physiology: The heart, Bethesda, Md., 1979, American Physiological Society.
9. Hillis, L.D., and Braunwald, E.: Coronary-artery spasm, N. Engl. J. Med. 299:695, 1978.
10. Rosenblatt, A., and Selzer, A.: The nature and clinical features of myocardial infarction with normal coronary angiogram, Circulation 55:578, 1977.
11. Stamler, J.: Epidemiology of coronary heart disease, Med. Clin. North Am. 1:1973.
12. Roberts, W.C.: Coronary arteries in fatal acute myocardial infarction, Circulation 45:215, 1972.
13. Harris, P.J., and others: Survival in medically treated coronary artery disease, Circulation 60:1259, 1979.
14. Bigger, J.T., and others: Prevalence and significance of arrhythmias in 24 hour ECG recordings made within one month of acute myocardial infarction. In Kulbertus, H.E., and Wellers, H.J., editors: The First Year after a Myocardial Infarction, Mount Kisco, N.Y., 1983, Futura Publishing Co., Inc.
15. Levy, R.I.: Progress toward prevention of cardiovascular disease—a 30-year retrospective, Circulation 60:1555, 1979.
16. Kaplan, N.M., and Stamler, J.: Prevention of coronary heart disease, Philadelphia, 1983, W.B. Saunders Co.
17. Kannel, W., and Gordon, T.: Evaluation of cardiovascular risk in the elderly: the Framingham Study, Bull. N.Y. Acad. Med. 54:573, 1978.
18. Levy, R.I., and Feinleib, M.: Risk factors for coronary artery disease and their management. In Braunwald, E., editor: Heart disease: a textbook of cardiac medicine, Philadelphia, 1980, W.B. Saunders Co.
19. Department of Health and Human Services: Report of the Secretary's Task Force on Black and Minority Health, vol. 1, Rep. 0-487-637(QL3), 1985.
20. Kannel, W.: Coronary risk factors: the Framingham Study, J. Occup. Med. 9:611, 1967.
21. Kannel, W.W., and others: Serum cholesterol, lipoproteins, and the risk of coronary heart disease: the Framingham Study, Ann. Intern. Med. 74:1, 1971.
22. Gordon, T., and others: High density lipoprotein as a protective factor against coronary heart disease, Am. J. Med. 62:707, 1977.
23. Goldstein, J.L., and Brown, M.S.: The low-density lipoprotein pathway and its relation to atherosclerosis, Ann. Rev. Biochem. 46:897, 1977.
24. Avogaro, P., and others: Plasma level of lipoprotein A_1 and apolipoprotein B in human atherosclerosis, Artery 4:385, 1978.
25. Stamler, J.: Research related to risk factors, Circulation 60:1575, 1979.
26. Lipid Research Clinics Program: The lipid research clinics coronary primary prevention trial results, JAMA 251:351, 1984.
27. Aronow, W.S., and Kaplan, N.M.: Smoking. In Kaplan, N.M., and Stamler, J., editor: Prevention of coronary heart disease, Philadelphia, 1983, W.B. Saunders Co.
28. Paffenbarger, R.S.: Physical activity and fatal heart attack: protection or selection. In Amsterdam, E., and others, editors: Exercise in cardiovascular health and disease, New York, 1977, Yorke Medical Books.
29. Paffenbarger, R.S., and others: Physical activity as an index of heart attack risk in college alumni, Am. J. Epidemiol. 108:161, 1978.
30. Wenger, N.K.: Exercise and the heart, Philadelphia, 1985, F.A. Davis Co.
31. Friedman, M., and others: The relationship of behavior pattern A to the state of the coronary vasculature, Am. J. Med. 44:525, 1968.

CHAPTER 3

Preventive Strategies for Coronary Artery Disease

Kathleen Gainor Andreoli
Leigh Anne Musser
Virginia Kliner Fowkes

The traditional medical approach to coronary artery disease has focused on the application of medical and/or technologic solutions in an attempt to treat the disease in patients with overt symptoms. In many cases, however, the medical approach is not optimum; it is limited by the fact that some patients need to survive a heart attack to benefit from it; it does not approach the problem at the population level; it provides no solution to the underlying disease process; it does not have long-term benefits for future generations; it often does not provide flexibility in support of individual patient belief systems; and it is often the most expensive approach.[1] Thus it is not surprising that beginning in about 1970 interest in prevention as a method of improving health status and providing cost-effective care surged dramatically[2] and that support for preventive efforts continues to grow.

Economics will probably be the major factor in establishing prevention as the principal method of dealing with coronary artery disease in the future. Health care costs have more than doubled since 1965, reaching over $365 billion in 1985. The amount spent on health care represents nearly 11% of the U.S. Gross National Product and is projected to account for 12% of the GNP by 1990.[3] The medical costs of coronary artery disease—including hospital costs, physician charges, medications, and lost productivity—have been estimated at $72.1 billion, or nearly 21% of total health care costs.[1] The fact that a single coronary bypass operation has an average price tag of $25,000[1] is a vivid illustration of the staggering costs associated with the medical treatment of coronary artery disease.

The movement toward prevention of coronary artery disease is based on the assumption that it is cheaper and more effective to prevent an illness than to attempt to treat it, and that prevention of the onset of chronic diseases, particularly cardiovascular diseases and cancer, will do much to alleviate the inflationary pressures of health care costs. Thus a change from the heavy emphasis on very expensive technologic interventions that benefit few to an increased emphasis on preventive measures that benefit large numbers of individuals both in the short-term and in the long-term is cost-effective and medically and ethically sound. A healthy balance of prevention and cure is the best strategy for effectively dealing with coronary artery disease.

There are three categories of preventive strategies: (1) primary, those implemented before overt manifestation of disease that aim to prevent or postpone new occurrences of disease, (2) secondary, those used after the onset of disease, which are efforts to detect conditions early and thus improve prognosis through early intervention, and (3) tertiary, those aimed at reducing or preventing residual defect and dysfunction and postponing death.[4] Primary prevention of coronary artery diseases will be the major focus of this chapter. Secondary and tertiary preventive strategies are described in most of the other chapters in this book.

CORONARY MORTALITY TRENDS

Between 1967 and 1982 the age-adjusted death rates for heart disease declined by 29%.[1] The decreases in mortality were not evenly distributed across all age and sex groups. While male coronary heart disease rates leveled off beginning in the 1950s, the rate for women aged 35 to 54 actually rose during this time.[5] Coronary heart disease rates have not decreased for blacks, Hispanics, Native Americans, and other minorities.[6] One indicator of the ethnic difference is that rates of coronary heart disease in black women are twice as high as in white women. The true cause of the dramatic overall decline in heart disease has not been established decisively. Many experts agree, however, that behavior and life-style changes, not medical strategies, are responsible for most of the reduction in mortality[7] and that much of the decline in heart disease mortality is related to improvements in diet with concomitant declines in serum cholesterol concentration, decreased smoking, improved hypertension control, and increased leisure-time physical exercise.[8]

RISK FACTORS FOR CORONARY ARTERY DISEASE

That individual behavior affects coronary artery disease risk as well as risk for other chronic diseases is well established. The majority of the risk factors for coronary artery disease can be prevented or modified. These include: high plasma LDL (low-density lipoproteins) cholesterol, low plasma HDL (high-density lipoproteins) cholesterol, cigarette smoking, hypertension, physical inactivity, obesity, Type

II diabetes, stress, caffeine consumption, and alcohol consumption. The major nonmodifiable risk factors are family history, male sex, and age.[1] Toxemia and the use of oral contraceptives have also been found to be risk factors for cardiovascular disease in women.[9] Modifiable coronary risk factors are discussed in detail in Chapter 2.

The following section focuses on five major behaviors that are associated with coronary artery disease risk—nutrition, smoking, exercise, stress, and caffeine/alcohol intake—and presents strategies for changing unhealthy behaviors to healthy ones. For the most part other modifiable coronary artery disease risk factors will benefit from changes in the five behaviors discussed.

Nutrition

The relationship between diet and health has been established for a number of chronic diseases. "Unhealthy" nutritional habits that prevail in the U.S. population include a high intake of saturated fats; high salt intake which contributes to elevated blood pressure; overconsumption of sugar which increases the blood triglyceride levels, requires an increased amount of insulin, and can contribute to weight increase; low levels of fiber intake; and the poor overall nutritional quality of the diet.

The association of dietary factors with coronary artery disease has been amply demonstrated and is discussed in detail in Chapter 2. Most important is the relationship between elevated serum cholesterol levels and heart disease. In more than 20 major international epidemiologic studies, a single measurement of serum cholesterol made at the time of entry into a trial has proved to be a significant predictor of the occurrence of coronary heart disease in subsequent years.[10] A recent study reported on the effect of blood cholesterol reduction on coronary heart disease mortality among 3806 asymptomatic middle-aged men with primary hypercholesterolemia followed for an average of 7.4 years. The findings indicated that lowering plasma cholesterol through diet and cholestyramine resulted in a 19% reduction in coronary heart disease risk.[11,12] Levels of serum cholesterol associated with low risk of heart disease fall below 180 mg/100 ml; the average American male has a serum cholesterol level of 220 mg/100 ml.[13]

Retrospective and prospective studies of populations across the world have demonstrated an association between intake of saturated fatty acids and dietary cholesterol and the risk of coronary heart disease.[14-17] Moreover, there is now some evidence that elevated levels of HDL cholesterol have a protective effect against heart disease,[18] although their mechanisms are not yet completely understood.[19]

Diets high in fiber have also been associated with a lower incidence of cardiovascular disease, as well as of certain cancers,[20] although the relationship is not as well defined as for lipids. Certain fibers, especially pectins and guar, are believed to assist in lowering serum cholesterol, although only slightly.[21] Morris and others[15] found an inverse relationship between fiber intake and risk of death from coronary heart disease. Kromhout and associates[22] found that men with high levels of dietary fiber intake had a mortality rate that was four times lower than that of men with low levels of fiber intake. However, other dietary factors may have been responsible for the relationship because adding these factors into the equation eliminated the relationship between fiber and all mortality except from cancer. Findings from the Ireland-Boston coronary heart disease study[17] also yielded an inverse relationship between fiber intake and coronary heart disease mortality, although the relationship was not significant after adjustment for other risk factors. Strick vegetarian diets seem to have a significant effect in lowering the likelihood of coronary lesions.[23]

The importance of effective dietary counseling to alter nutrition behavior is paramount in the prevention of coronary artery disease. The principal stages in dietary changes include conducting an inventory of foods in the household, recording daily dietary intake, making small changes in the diet by substituting healthy for unhealthy foods and modifying one food group at a time, developing family support systems, and identifying reinforcement and motivation factors (such as alleviation of physical problems, better self-image, and illness prevention.)[24]

Preventive measures that focus on nutrition typically seek to reduce total fat, saturated fat, and dietary cholesterol in the diet.[25] The Select Committee on Nutrition and Human Needs of the United States Senate[26] recommends these dietary goals to lower risk of heart disease:

Reduction of fat consumption to 30% of total calories.

Reduction of saturated fat consumption to 10% of total calories.

Balanced intake of monounsaturated and polyunsaturated fat intake to 10% of total calories.

Reduction of cholesterol intake to about 300 mg daily.

Increased complex carbohydrate consumption to 48% of total calories.

Reduction of sugar consumption to 10% of total calories.

Reduction of salt consumption to 5 g daily.

These dietary goals may be accomplished in part by lowering dietary intake of refined sugar, refined foods, desserts, and animal fats, and by increasing consumption of fruits, vegetables, whole grains, and legumes.

Diet modification also plays an important role in the secondary prevention of coronary artery disease, although studies of the degree to which the incidence of further manifestations of ischemic heart disease can be decreased through dietary modifications have not been decisive.[27]

Smoking

In 1983 the Surgeon General concluded that ". . . cigarette smoking should be considered the most important of the known modifiable risk factors for coronary heart disease in the United States."[28] Despite the known health effect, in 1983, 50 million Americans continued to smoke cigarettes regularly.[29] Between 1964 and 1983, however, over 30 million Americans quit smoking,[30] with the proportion of men who smoke dropping from 52% in 1964 to 38% in 1983 and the proportion of women smokers declining from 34% to 30%.[31] Smoking among adolescent females, however, rose dramatically, from 8% to 13% between 1968 and 1979, according to the most recent survey of adolescent smoking. It is important to note that in 1985 lung cancer was estimated to surpass breast cancer as the number one cancer-related cause of death in women.[31] Exposure to passive smoke, or inhaling smoke from the environment, also creates health risks.[32]

There has been a great deal of effort to reduce smoking in the workplace, in public, and even at home. In 1980, 34 states and the District of Columbia had statutes restricting smoking in some manner.[33] By 1984, eight states had statutes that specifically dealt with workplace smoking control.[34] The recent vote by the American Medical Association to support legislation to ban advertising of all tobacco products, prepare model state bills to prohibit cigarette sales to individuals under 21, eliminate vending machine sales, and encourage the Surgeon General to put health warnings on all tobacco products is a vivid illustration of the acknowledged health threat associated with smoking and the health professional response to it. Cigarette smoking among adults is on the verge of becoming deviant behavior. This is a healthy national trend.

Two main effects of smoking have been incriminated as factors in the development of cardiovascular disease: the effect of nicotine in constricting the blood vessels and the desaturation of hemoglobin by carbon monoxide. Other smoking-associated coronary artery disease risks include increased platelet adhesiveness[35] and a correlation between smoking and low levels of high-density lipoproteins (as discussed in the section on nutrition, high levels of HDL cholesterol appear to offer some protection against atherosclerosis).[36]

Smoking cessation is clearly associated with a decreased risk of coronary artery disease in patients with overt symptoms. Studies have found that smoking cessation is associated with a 20% to 50% decrease in the incidence of new infarction and sudden death in patients with myocardial infarction,[37,38] a reduction in the risk of nonfatal reinfarction, and an extension of the benefits into the long term. Potential adverse effects of smoking cessation, such as weight gain, depression, and irritability, can often be prevented through careful counseling. Obese and hypertensive patients, however, may require special attention from a physician, dietitian, or psychologist.[39]

The most effective preventive programs for coronary artery disease risks associated with cigarette smoking are those aimed at preventing individuals from starting, usually in childhood and early adolescence. (See the section on home and schools for information on smoking prevention in childhood.) Women, heavy smokers, individuals who smoke to relieve stress, and individuals not concerned with their health are the least likely to be successful in quitting.[40,41] Coronary artery disease patients, on the other hand, typically have high rates of smoking cessation success following an event, such as a myocardial infarction. Risk factor intervention studies indicate that up to 70% of postinfarction patients stop smoking on advice from their physician.[38] Long-term repetition of intervention measures and continued medical and family support are necessary to prevent the patient from resuming smoking.

Although smoking is a difficult behavior to change, successful programs do exist. Some of the specific methods of smoking cessation include "cold turkey," substituting other sources of nicotine such as Lobeline or nicotine chewing gum, aversion therapy, hypnosis, and acupuncture. Studies of the effectiveness of nicotine gum as a smoking cessation technique have demonstrated success rates between 35% and 70%.[42-45] Side effects from this product, such as hiccups and nausea, can be controlled by lowering the dose of nicotine in the gum and by slow and paced chewing.[45] One aversion technique, rapid-smoking, has yielded success rates from 15% to 60%.[46-48] The negative consequences of this technique have caused many physicians to discourage its use; elderly patients should not be treated with this method. Hypnosis-based smoking cessation programs have had variable success rates, ranging from 20% to 90%.[49-51] Auricular acupuncture has been an effective smoking-cessation method in some cases: a study of 300 French subjects revealed that after a 6-week period, 50% of the subjects had stopped smoking completely and 25% had reduced their cigarette use; only 25%, mostly women, did not respond to treatment.[52] Smoking cessation programs that use a variety of approaches are also often effective, with long-term success rates averaging over 40%.[53]

Exercise

Regular exercise has been associated with a reduced risk of coronary heart disease. In general, it is agreed that aerobic exercise or sustained physical activity using the large muscles of the body for a minimum of 15 to 20 minutes, three or four times a week, contributes to cardiovascular conditioning. Aerobic exercises include brisk walking, dancing, jogging, running, swimming, cross-country skiing, bicycling, tennis, and "aerobics."[20] Although some 49% of the adult population in the United

States claim to exercise every day, experts estimate that fewer than 30% of those who exercise derive any aerobic benefit.[54] The increasing popularity of jogging, with as many as 20 million who jog and 12 million who run several miles a day,[36] and the spread of "aerobics," are other healthy national trends.

The largest body of evidence on the relationship between exercise and reduced cardiovascular risk comes from a study of 17,000 Harvard alumni.[55] Regular habitual exercise was found to reduce the risk of heart disease regardless of other risk factors such as cigarette smoking or high blood pressure. Hypertension was found to be the strongest clinical predictor of coronary attack, but inadequate exercise was strongest epidemiologically. In another large study, 17,944 male British civil servants were followed over several years; results indicated that those classified as "nonvigorous exercisers" had a rate of first coronary event that was twice as high as those classified as "vigorous exercisers".[56] Paffenbarger and Hale[57] studied 6,351 San Francisco longshoremen for 22 years and found that men in jobs requiring high levels of exertion had fewer fatal heart attacks than did men in jobs that required only moderate or light activity.[57] Cooper and others[58] found physically fit men to have lower risk for coronary heart disease than those who were less fit. The fit men had lower levels of serum cholesterol, triglycerides, glucose, uric acid, lower blood pressure, and less body fat. Costas and others[59] demonstrated that physically active men have fewer, less severe, and later onset manifestations of coronary heart disease.

A notable lack of research of the relationship between exercise and coronary risk in women is apparent. One study in Finland showed a positive relationship between exercise and risk of heart disease in women similar to that in men.[60]

A variety of biologic mechanisms have been suggested to explain how physical activity may serve to prevent the manifestation of coronary heart disease. Most focus either on increased myocardial oxygen supply or decreased myocardial work.[61]

In addition to the direct benefits in lowering coronary risk, individuals who exercise regularly are also more likely to have other healthy habits that lower coronary risk, such as eating moderately, coping more effectively with stress, and avoiding smoking. At the same time, a number of studies have demonstrated that regular exercise is associated with a lowering of other cardiovascular risk factors including hypertension, high serum triglyceride levels, and high serum cholesterol levels.[58,62-69]

Developing and initiating an exercise program as a coronary artery disease prevention strategy consists of several important steps. First, the individual should be encouraged to get a physical examination with special attention to the heart and lungs. Second, an activity must be chosen that best meets the needs of the individual in terms of goals (weight loss, endurance, conditioning, good health in general), time commitment, daily habits, cost of equipment, and so forth. Third, the individual must receive some type of motivational reinforcement to continue exercising. The average dropout rate for various exercise programs ranges from 30% to 70%.[70] Some of the factors that have been suggested as important to adherence to exercise include attitude, self-perception, feelings of health responsibility, injury, attitude of significant others, and attainment of exercise objectives.[71,72]

Stress

In 1978 the President's Commission on Mental Health estimated that one out of four Americans suffered from "severe emotional stress."[73] Inability to cope with stress is related, either directly or indirectly, to coronary heart disease, cancer, lung ailments, accidental injuries, cirrhosis of the liver and suicide—six of the leading causes of death in the United States.[74] In 1980, more than half of the worker's compensation cases filed in California were for stress-related disorders.[75]

Stress may be experienced by the individual in a variety of ways, including muscle tightness, stomach discomfort, feelings of tension and anxiety, tachycardia, and diaphoresis. A number of personal factors affect an individual's ability to cope with stress, including the sense of being in control of one's life, having a network of friends or family or a social support system, and such personality factors as flexibility and optimism.

The relationship of stress to the development or progression of cardiovascular disease is not well established. It is known that blood pressure rises in response to acute psychologic and physiologic stress, but there has been no consistent research support for the hypothesis that persistent elevation of blood pressure may occur in chronically stressed individuals.[76] The Type A behavior pattern and other psychosocial and behavioral precursors of coronary disease and their relationship to stress are described in Chapter 13. Stress is often an aggravating factor which contributes to a number of coronary risks. For example, some people smoke in response to stress, others abuse alcohol, while others overeat. Management of stress, on the other hand, can facilitate reduction of other risk factors, such as overweight, smoking, and high blood pressure.

The indirect approach to stress reduction includes such activities as exercise, listening to music, reading, and pet therapy. Almost every form of exercise performed regularly and rhythmically is useful in relieving the tension produced by stress.[77] Besides relieving the muscle spasms caused by job stress, exercise programs usually prevent the participants from thinking about their jobs and increase their feelings of well-being and self-esteem.

The direct approach for reducing stress includes physical massage, muscle tensing and relaxing exercises, biofeedback, self-hypnosis, rhythmic breathing, and time management, among others. Therapeutic relaxation has a variety of forms, including transcendental meditation (TM) and yoga. The "relaxation response," coined by cardiologist H. Benson, can be achieved just by following four simple steps: assume a comfortable position, close your eyes, concentrate on a single word, sound, or phrase, and cast off all other thoughts. Biofeedback teaches one to use technology to measure and regulate physiologic variables and restores a sense of self-control to the individual. Time management is a direct method of stress reduction that is commonly introduced in the work setting. It focuses on setting priorities, increasing functional time, and reducing perceptions of time urgency.[78]

Caffeine and Alcohol Intake

Although there is a great deal of literature discussing the deleterious effects of caffeine, the association between the use of caffeine and cardiovascular risk has not been established and the evidence is conflicting. Consumption of caffeine increases cardiac output and stroke volume and may precipitate cardiac rhythm disturbances.

The influence of alcohol on cardiovascular risk continues to be debated. Studies suggest that alcohol in small to moderate amounts may be protective. A 10-year study of 8060 patients of the Kaiser Permanente System in Oakland, California, revealed that individuals having two drinks or fewer daily had the lowest mortality from all causes. Nondrinkers and consumers of three to five drinks per day had similar mortality rates.[79] Mortality from coronary disease was highest among nondrinkers. When the records of past heavy drinkers were removed from the data, 3% of nondrinkers died of heart disease compared to 1.8% of moderate (two or fewer drinks per day) drinkers. When the data were analyzed for the effects of smoking, there was no difference between the heart disease rates of nondrinkers and moderate drinkers.

Other studies have reported similar associations between moderate alcohol consumption and lowered mortality from coronary heart disease. An inherent weakness of these studies is the failure to separate never-drinkers from former drinkers. A bias develops because individuals may cease drinking because of a health problem.

Consumption of alcohol increases HDL cholesterol levels in blood. Yet in a recent study moderate alcohol intake correlated positively with serum concentrations in *one* of the two major subclasses, HDL_3, (but not in the other, HDL_2).[80]

Multiple Risk Factor Prevention

Studies of multiple risk factors indicate that the reduction of one or more risk factors appears to lessen the incidence of coronary artery disease. In a series of studies[81,82] in Alameda County, California, findings showed substantial increases in the life spans of people who exercised regularly and vigorously, maintained normal weight, ate breakfast, did not snack between meals, avoided smoking, limited alcohol consumption, and slept at least 7 hours a night. A 45-year-old man who followed three or fewer of these seven behaviors could, on the average, expect to live to age 67. If he followed six or seven, he could expect to live to age 78.

The Oslo Heart Study, a multiple risk factor trial that attempted to control hypercholesterolemia and cigarette smoking, demonstrated successful alteration of both, with a concomitant reduction in coronary heart disease incidence.[83] The Multiple Risk Factor Intervention Trial (MRFIT) tested the effectiveness of intervention methods among 12,866 high-risk males on hypercholesterolemia, hypertension, and cigarette smoking. Reductions occurred in blood cholesterol, blood pressure, and smoking, with a 7.1% overall reduction (nonsignificant) in coronary heart disease mortality.[84]

Achieving change in life-style involves a process of sequential stages. First, the individual must become aware of the risk and accept that certain behaviors are harmful personally. This knowledge must be integrated into the person's self-image. Belief that change is possible and motivation to change must prevail. Effort must be made to change and apply the new knowledge in sustaining the behavior.[85] Finally, individuals must be supported in their efforts to maintain the new behavior. Green and associates[86] provide a list of recommended strategies for life-style change, including lectures, individual instruction, programmed learning, skill development, inquiry learning, peer-group discussions, modeling, behavior modification, simulations and games, audiovisual aids, educational television, social planning, and organizational change.

Summary

The most important primary prevention strategies for coronary artery disease are: (1) better nutrition, (2) increase in physical activity, (3) cessation of smoking, (4) weight reduction, (5) effective stress management, (6) moderate alcohol consumption (a limit of 50 grams or 2 to 3 average drinks per day), and (7) control of hypertension. Nearly one in five Americans has a genetic susceptibility to hypertension.[87] The best strategy is one that includes each of these goals, a comprehensive "life-style change" strategy.

PREVENTION IN THE COMMUNITY

Primary preventive strategies can be implemented singularly or in combination in a number of settings and through community and national health information programs. In general, health education programs aimed at providing information and altering the behavior of large groups of individuals are the most cost-effective.

Home

The importance of beginning preventive strategies in childhood cannot be overemphasized. Although many heart, lung, and blood diseases are not manifest until middle-age or later, their development begins during childhood and adolescence.[88-91] The fatty streaks and fibrous plaques that apparently result in end-stage cardiovascular disease have frequently been observed in children and youth.[92-94] It is also true that individuals with higher than average blood pressure as teenagers are more likely to have elevated blood pressure as adults.

The majority of unhealthy behaviors seen in adults are learned during childhood and have their origins in the home. Eating habits, exercise patterns, smoking, use of alcohol, attitudes that relate to self-confidence and to society, management of stress, involvement with others, and decision-making abilities are all first learned in the home.[95] Approximately one third of today's obese adults were overweight children.[96] Furthermore, an obese child is at least three times more likely than a normal-weight child to be an obese adult. Obesity, like other coronary risk factors, is more difficult to correct in adults than in children. A task force sponsored by the American Cancer Society concluded that teenagers are 50% more likely to smoke if adults with whom they associate smoke.[97] It has been demonstrated that children of parents who set examples conducive to health are more likely to assume a healthy lifestyle than if the opposite were true.[4] Primary prevention programs in the home must, therefore, involve both children and adults.

School

The evidence indicates that, for the most part, school health programs are of poor quality, provide students with insufficient information, and are usually unsuccessful in altering dietary behaviors. This is an important shortcoming in the U.S. educational system because, as already discussed, so many unhealthy behaviors start in children at very young ages, making prevention at the elementary school level of utmost importance. For example, since many children experiment with smoking before the age of 13, the existing antismoking education programs directed at preadolescents should be expanded. The same is true for educational programs devoted to other risk factors and multifactor approaches.

Health education programs in high schools also have a poor record. In fact, only 24 states require health education for graduation. On average, only 1% of classtime is devoted to health education in high schools across the country. By comparison, the average number of hours of English required accounts for 16.5% of available instructional time.[98]

The results are as expected. One study of students' knowledge of prevention of cardiovascular disease showed that such knowledge was largely superficial and composed of simple, factual information and that students lacked an understanding of functions, processes, and implications necessary for altering and maintaining healthy behavior patterns.[99] Health education is also not a recognized component of the Scholastic Aptitude Test (SAT) or the Graduate Record Examination (GRE), among others.[98]

Even when health education is provided in the schools, it receives minimum attention and is tacked on to other subjects such as biology or physical education. Indeed, one of the main reasons schools have been ineffective in health education programs is because very few teachers have had any specific health instruction as part of their own education and thus lack the understanding and skills necessary to develop and teach the appropriate courses.[41] Teacher training should include courses in health education, and in-service health education should be provided on a regular basis for elementary and secondary school teachers.

Some school-based prevention programs have met with success. "Great Sensations," a program aimed at changing the salt intake of elementary school students by changing their knowledge of and attitude toward snack foods is one such program.[100] Given that teenagers consume about 49% of their daily calories from snacks, many of which are high in salt, sugar, and saturated fat,[101] the impact of such programs could be wide-ranging. Analysis of the results of the program indicated that snack selection was significantly improved for up to 8 weeks after the completion of the program. The success of this program is especially important in light of the generally disappointing results of other school-based nutrition education programs.

Smoking intervention programs that use short videotapes to emphasize short-term and long-term benefits of not smoking and explain peer pressure and its influence on smoking behavior are also generally successful in adolescents, and they are much more successful than fear-arousal and impersonal, information-oriented approaches. In two studies use of relevant peer role models and active individual role-playing substantially reduced the incidence of smoking among seventh-grade students.[102] Similarly good results in reducing the number of new smokers were observed among eighth, ninth, and tenth-grade students who were given "life skills training", which focused on the key social and psychologic factors involved in the onset of smoking.[103]

The goals of coronary artery disease health education programs should be to increase students' understanding about disease, improve personal behaviors that influence health, provide skills necessary to establish and maintain healthful behaviors, help students maintain skills and health behaviors that will impact on their future families, and increase the skills necessary to maintain and improve the health of the communities and environments in which they will reside.[4] In addition to teaching healthy behaviors in the school, adults (such as teachers, principals, and school nurses) must act as role models by demonstrating healthy behaviors themselves, such as good dietary practices and refraining from smoking.

Since children spend most of their young lives under the influence of home and school, there should be an overlap between the two settings in contributing to the development of healthful behavior patterns in children.

Work Site

Industry has taken an increasing interest and played a growing role in health promotion and disease prevention among employees. In 1984 more than 400 major U.S. corporations had formal health/fitness programs and the number continues to grow at a steady pace.[104] The reasons are economic: employers now pay approximately one half of the nation's health care bill. Indeed, health benefits account for 10% of total compensation.[105] Indirect costs of unhealthy behaviors also play an important role in spurring corporate interest in prevention: in 1981, the most recent year for which data are available, businesses lost more than 338 million workdays because of illness-related absenteeism.

With 100 million adult Americans at work every day, the work site is an ideal setting for offering preventive health services and health education programs aimed at the prevention of coronary artery disease. Development of secondary prevention strategies is also important.

Prevention and promotion programs in the workplace are numerous and diverse. Johnson & Johnson and IBM have comprehensive health promotion programs for their employees that include health checkups, exercise, and "lifestyle" classes for smoking cessation and stress management. Ford Motor Company runs a cardiovascular risk reduction and intervention program at its world headquarters in Dearborn, Michigan, with testing, risk assessment, and group sessions to motivate employees to take steps to lower their risk factors. The Massachusetts Mutual Life Insurance Company carries out a program in which education, detection, and follow-up of hypertensives is carried out at the worksite and community physicians treat employees at the company's expense. General Foods has a fully-equipped gym with a staff of professional trainers at its headquarters in White Plains, New York.[106] The list of large corporations with fitness programs is extensive.

Work site health promotion programs have had varying degrees of success. Massachussetts Mutual Life has recouped more than one half the cost of its program in reduced absenteeism alone. Lockheed Missiles and Space Company reduced the rate of high blood pressure among one group of 7000 employees from 17% to 1.7% after it introduced an educational program aimed at improving diet and cutting stress and smoking. Tenneco Inc. employees who adhere to the company's exercise program have demonstrated higher job performance ratings than those who do not adhere to the program.[106]

With a few exceptions, notably the Campbell Soup Company, industry has yet to develop comprehensive dietary modification programs that include nutrition counseling aand measurement of dietary factors.[24] Worksite nutrition programs often consist of offering healthier foods in the cafeteria and vending machines.[107]

A recent study of a random sample of U.S. corporations showed that 15% offered workplace smoking cessation programs and 33% planned to expand their programs or to develop new ones.[108] Worksite smoking cessation programs can be categorized into educational/informational campaigns, workplace smoking restrictions, self-help programs, physician advice, incentive programs, and smoking cessation services.[109]

Community

During the past 20 years a number of community-wide health promotion demonstration programs have been undertaken, both in the United States and in other industrial nations. The Stanford Health Disease Prevention Program,[110,111] was originally a 2-year experimental program in three California communities whose major objective was to determine whether intensive educational efforts could reduce cigarette smoking, blood cholesterol levels, and high blood pressure. Two communities were exposed to a mass media campaign designed to influence adults to change their living habits in ways that could reduce the risk of heart attack and stroke. In one of these towns the media campaign was supplemented with intensive face-to-face instruction for people identified as being at high risk. A third community, which was relatively isolated from the media shared by the two communities, served as a control. After 2 years the overall risk of cardiovascular disease in the control community increased about 7%, while in the other two towns there was a substantial (15% to 20%) decrease in risk. In the community that had the media campaign plus personal instruction, the initial improvement was greater than in the other experimental town, and health education was more successful in reducing cigarette smoking. At the end of the second year the decrease in risk was roughly the same in both experimental communities. The program concluded that intensive face-to-face instruction and counseling seem important for changing such behaviors as smoking and inadequate diet; however, where resources are limited, mass media education campaigns are an effective influence in reducing the risk of cardiovascular disease.

The Five City Project is a major outgrowth of the original Stanford Heart Disease Project cities, designed to stimulate and maintain life-style changes that would result in reduction of cardiovascular disease risk in the community. The project recognized the need to reach persons who do not speak English and developed health promotion messages for Spanish radio stations. Field trials underway seek to determine the impact of educational programs in the community on changes in cardiovascular risk factors and morbidity and mortality.[112]

The North Karelia Project in Finland, begun in 1972, was the first major community-based cardiovascular disease prevention program. The program activities were primarily educational, aiming to teach the community how to adopt healthy life-styles and reduce cardiovascular risk.[113] Other strategies included development of a hypertension screening process and environmental changes such as smoking restrictions and introduction of low-fat food products. Follow-up surveys have indicated that health behaviors and risk factors did indeed change over a 5-year period, with a decreased risk of 17% for cardiovascular disease in men and 12% in women. In addition, approximately 17,000 hypertensives were recruited to the hypertension register as a result.[113]

Other community-based intervention trials have included the Interuniversity study on Nutrition and Health in Belgium, the Pawtucket Heart Health Project (Rhode Island), and the Minnesota Heart Health Program.[114,115,116]

Recently, many communities have passed local initiatives requiring all public places to restrict smoking to designated areas. Future research will demonstrate the comparative effect of community-wide behavioral restrictions versus educational efforts alone.

In general, effective community programs require a well-designed motivational media program in combination with follow-up that allows questions to be answered, ideas to be discussed, and experiences to be shared. Patient-education channels on cable television provide an excellent way to introduce health information into homes with an after-the-show phone call and personal follow-up.[117] Television is the mainstream culture in the United States. Americans spend more time watching TV than doing anything else, with the exception of sleeping. Television serves as the most common and pervasive source of health information for the less educated, low-income groups who have the poorest opportunity for health and are most in need of valid information.[118] One study indicated that more frequent viewers tended to be more complacent about eating, drinking, and exercise habits and relied more heavily on the physician for a cure than less frequent viewers.[118]

Since they reach into almost every home and are accessible at any hour, the media have a strong influence on the way Americans behave and perceive the world. In the nationwide anti-smoking advertising campaign between 1968 and 1970, cigarette consumption declined 14% per year.[40] The media not only promote attitudes and products, they also reflect community feelings, and they will transmit more health messages if they learn the community is interested.[119]

Different Cultures within the Community. There is often a specific need for community programs that address the unique needs of racial, ethnic, and cultural groups. In the San Antonio Heart Study, when health knowledge and behaviors related to the prevention and treatment of coronary heart disease between Mexican Americans and non-Hispanic Caucasians were compared, it was found that Mexican Americans at all socioeconomic levels had less knowledge about preventing heart disease. Furthermore, they had fewer "heart healthy" habits and less knowledge of heart attack symptoms. These ethnic differences persisted when compared within specific neighborhoods that were relatively homogeneous in socioeconomic status, suggesting that cultural factors may account for the differences.[120]

Despite their lack of knowledge regarding cardiovascular disease prevention, Mexican Americans, in a recent study, responded as well as whites to community-based health education campaigns.[121] Following a 3-year bilingual mass media health education program, all groups reported 20% to 40% decreases in dietary cholesterol and saturated fat. There was no difference in the decreases between groups of low and high socioeconomic status.

Preventive strategies for minority populations must take into account the influence of socioeconomic status, attitudes, belief systems and acculturation on individual life-style and potential for change in health habits. Research indicates that persons of lower socioeconomic status tend to adopt health innovations more slowly than those of upper socioeconomic status.[122] Decline in smoking and exercising regularly are behaviors more common to persons belonging to higher socioeconomic groups. Many minority groups have high percentages of persons classified as poor, a factor that needs to be considered in planning preventive strategies.

Perceptions of health and response to illness may be barriers to acquiring health habits or obtaining health care. For example, a belief system prevalent among certain Hispanic populations equates health with the ability to function normally, a robust, well-fleshed body, and the absence of pain.[123] Another common perception is that life is full of many difficulties that must be borne stoically. Signs or symptoms of illnesses (such as diabetes) may be ignored or tolerated until they interfere with one of the aforementioned criteria of health.[123] Often the decision to seek medical care and to undertake recommended treatment is made in consultation with family or friends. Simultaneous use of folk remedies with allopathic treatment is common.

Another perception of certain cultures is that the diagnosis of a symptom is validated only by successful treatment. Failure of treatment to effect cure may reduce patient compliance; conditions such as diabetes, hypertension or coronary heart disease may be neglected until late in the disease.

The degree of acculturation also influences risk and prevention. Language may serve as a barrier to accessing good health information. The acculturating power of Western dietary habits may contribute to the spread of common Western diseases such as diabetes and coronary heart disease.[124]

Clearly, there is need for more research within all population subgroups in order to understand the relationship between cultural and genetic influences and change in health habits and the reduction of risk of cardiovascular diseases.

NATIONAL PRIORITIES

Although the government has important responsibilities in national health education, since there is no established health policy governing life-style and behavior, the implementation and impact of government-sponsored programs is often disappointing. For example, the Department of Health and Human Services' National High Blood Pressure Education Program at the National Institutes of Health has increased awareness about hypertension among the population and may have influenced hypertensive people to seek medical care for their disease. Yet Medicare (also housed within the Department of Health and Human Services) does not provide reimbursement for the cost of the necessary drugs.[125] The National Clearinghouse on Smoking and Health has implemented a rigorous educational program for smoking cessation and the present Surgeon General has made reducing cigarette smoking a priority goal. However, the Department of Agriculture continues its unchallenged subsidization of tobacco crops.

One of the most important issues in the ambiguity of national policy concerning health promotion issues is that no single government agency has control. At the federal level, 12 departments, 17 independent agencies, and 3 quasi-official agencies have health-related responsibilities or functions. Food and nutrition programs are administered by the Department of Agriculture, occupational safety and health programs by the Department of Labor, environmental control programs by the Environmental Protection Agency, and so on.

This does not mean that effective health promotion programs have not emanated from the federal government. The National Conference on Health Promotion Programs in Occupational Settings (1979), the National Conference on Nutrition Education (1979), the National Conference on Physical Fitness and Sports for All (1980), Regional Forums on Community Health Promotion (1979), Pro-

moting Health through the Schools (1980), and the National Children and Youth Fitness Study (1985) are all examples of federally-sponsored health promotion efforts.[126,127] What is needed at this point is for public policy to be consistent, to be coordinated among the various bureaucracies and for some of the goals established in *Healthy People*[96] to be implemented at the policy level.

Policy as it relates to cigarette smoking can be used as an example. If the federal government is convinced that it is harmful to the health of Americans and truly wishes to change smoking behavior to improve disease risk, then a policy that restricts tobacco advertising (especially the kind that glamorizes smoking to young people), increases cigarette taxes, eliminates tobacco price supports, makes the purchase of cigarettes by children more difficult, and reduces taxes that feed into Medicare and Medicaid for non-smokers and raises them for smokers would be in order.

RESEARCH NEEDS IN HEALTH PROMOTION

A comprehensive approach to health promotion has been described as an essential part of a primary prevention program directed against the premature onset of coronary artery disease. Given the acceptance of disease prevention and health promotion by the American people, the scientific evidence upon which these concepts are based must be strengthened; program evaluation techniques must be refined; ways must be found to allocate resources fairly; the needs of special populations must be accommodated; new organizational structures must be developed—all these and many more issues must be carefully and intelligently considered for all levels of society.[95]

Preventive strategies must be tested through longitudinal, multidisciplinary, invasive studies of the intersection of high-risk groups and high-risk situations against control groups.[128] Research is also needed to identify the developmental determinants of unhealthful behavior during childhood and adolescence. For example, if it were possible to identify individuals whose genetic constitution makes them more susceptible to adapting unhealthy behavior, then efforts to change behavior could be focused on persons at greatest risk, rather than on society at large.[129] Genetic research is already making inroads in this regard, adding to the knowledge base information about the genes involved in heart disease, especially those responsible for the body's use and disposal of fats.[130] More studies on the impact of risk factor reduction on women, the elderly, and ethnic groups are also necessary.

Many ramifications of health education are still unknown. For example, what kinds of national education models will work most effectively on the heterogeneous U.S. population? Will benefits accrue rapidly or slowly? Will they be temporary or permanent? Will they occur in the general population or only in high-risk groups?[131] Unfortunately, there are major weaknesses in much of the evaluation of patient education: oversimplification of the behavior and causes of behavior that must be influenced by patient education; failure to make explicit the theoretic or assumed connection between educational interventions and behavioral or health results; and limited analyses of data, which leave many questions unanswered.[128] These issues are further complicated by the lack of reimbursement for patient education in the health care delivery system.

Clearly, successful health education programs offer great promise; consumers will assume more responsibility for adopting health practices that protect health and prevent illness or complications, and they will make more timely and appropriate use of health resources. Such changes should result in increased patient satisfaction, improved quality of life, better use of health care providers, fewer hospital admissions, and shorter hospital stays, thus helping to control rising health care costs.

REFERENCES

1. Leaf, A.: The biological constraints on human aging: implications for health policy—a national policy perspective. In Andreoli, K.G., Musser, L.A., and Reiser, S.J., editors: Health care for the elderly: regional responses to national policy issues, New York, The Haworth Press, Inc., 1986.
2. Opatz, J.P.: A primer of health promotion: creating healthy organizational cultures, Washington, D.C., 1985, Oryn Publications, Inc.
3. Arthur Andersen & Co. and The American College of Hospital Administrators: Health care in the 1990s: trends and strategies, New York, 1984, AHA, ACHA.
4. Kolbe, L.J., and Newman, I.M.: The role of school health education in preventing heart, lung, and blood diseases, School Health Res. 54(6):15, 1984.
5. Moriyama, I.M., Krueger, D.E., and Stamler, J.: Cardiovascular disease in the United States, Cambridge, Mass., 1971, Harvard University Press.
6. U.S. Department of Health and Human Services, Report of the Secretary's task force on black and minority health, vol. I: executive summary, GPO No. 017-090-00078-0, Bethesda, Md., 1985, U.S. DHHS.
7. Goldman, L., and Cook, E.F.: The decline in ischemic heart disease mortality rates—an analysis of the comparative effects of medical intervention and changes in life style, Ann. Intern. Med. 101:825, 1984.
8. Stern, M.P.: The recent decline in ischemic heart disease mortality, Ann. Intern. Med. 91:630, 1979.
9. Mann, J.I., and others: Risk factors for myocardial infarction in young women, Br. J. Prev. Soc. Med. 30:94, 1976.
10. Gotto, A.M., and Wittels, E.H.: Diet, serum cholesterol, lipoproteins, and coronary heart disease. In Kaplan, N.M., and Stamler, J., editors: Prevention of coronary heart disease: practical management of the risk factors, Philadelphia, 1983, W.B. Saunders Co.
11. Lipid Research Clinics: Coronary primary prevention trial results I: reduction in the incidence of coronary heart disease, JAMA 251:365, 1984.
12. Lipid Research Clinics: Coronary primary prevention trial results II: the relationship of reduction in incidence of coronary heart disease to cholesterol lowering, JAMA 251:365, 1984.
13. Hegsted, D.M.: What is a healthful diet? In Matarazzo, J.D., and others, editors: Behavioral health—a handbook of health enhancement and disease prevention, New York, 1984, John Wiley & Sons.
14. Gordon, D.J., and others: Habitual physical activity and high-density lipoprotein cholesterol in men with primary hypercholesterolemia: the Lipid Research Clinics Coronary Primary Prevention Trial, Circulation 67(3):512, 1983.
15. Morris, J.N., Marr, J.W., and Clayton, D.B.: Diet and heart: a postscript, Br. Med. J. 110:77, 1979.
16. Garcia-Palmieri, M.R., and others: Relationship of dietary intake to subsequent coronary heart disease incidence: the Puerto Rico Heart Health Program, Am. J. Clin. Nutr. 33:1818, 1980.
17. Kushi, L.H., and others: Diet and 20-year mortality from coronary heart disease: the Ireland-Boston diet-heart study, N. Engl. J. Med. 312:811, 1985.
18. Miller, G.J., and Miller, N.E.: Plasma-high-density lipoprotein concentration and development of ischaemic heart disease, Lancet. 1:16, 1975.
19. Levy, R.I., and Rifkind, B.M.: The structure, function and metabolism of high-density lipoproteins: a status report, Circulation 62(Suppl. 4):4, 1980.
20. Farquhar, J.W., and others: The American way of life need not be hazardous to your health, New York, 1978, W.W. Norton & Co., Inc.
21. Kuske, T.T.: Carbohydrate, fiber, and heart disease. In Feldman, E.B., editor: Nutrition and heart disease, New York, 1983, Churchill Livingstone.
22. Kromhout, D., Bosschieter, E.B., and Coulander, C.: Dietary fibre and 10-year mortality from coronary heart disease, cancer, and all causes, Lancet 2:518, 1982.
23. Arntzenius, A.C., and others: Diet, lipoproteins, and the progression of coronary atherosclerosis: the Leiden Intervention Trial, N. Engl. J. Med. 312:13, 1985.
24. Wadden, T.A., and Brownell, K.D.: The development and modification of dietary practices in individuals, groups, and large populations. In Matarazzo, J.D., and others, editors: Behavioral health—a handbook of health enhancement and disease prevention, New York, 1984, John Wiley & Sons.
25. Coronary Drug Project Research Group: Natural history of myocardial infarction in the Coronary Drug Project: long-term prognostic importance of serum lipid levels, Am. J. Cardiol. 42:489, 1978.
26. Select Committee on Nutrition and Human Needs, U.S. Senate: Dietary goals for the United States, ed. 2, Washington, D.C., 1977, U.S. Government Printing Office.
27. Fejfar, Z.: Prevention and treatment of coronary heart disease and its complications. In Levine, J., editor: Prevention and treatment of coronary heart disease and its complications: proceedings of the twenty-fifth International Congress of Therapeutics, Amsterdam, 1980, Excerpta Medica.
28. U.S. Department of Health and Human Services: The health consequences of smoking: cardiovascular diseases—a report of the Surgeon General, Washington, D.C., 1983, U.S. DHHS.
29. Aronow, W.S., and Kaplan, N.M.: Smoking. In Kaplan, N.M., and Stampler, J., editors: Prevention of coronary heart disease: practical management of the risk factors, Philadelphia, 1983, W.B. Saunders Co.
30. Institute of Medicine: Health and behavior: a research agenda interim report no. 1—smoking and behavior, Washington, D.C., 1980, Institute of Medicine.
31. American Cancer Society: Press release, February 7, 1985.
32. Fielding, J.: Smoking: Health effects and control, N. Engl. J. Med. 313:491, 1985.
33. Swingle, M.: The legal conflict between smokers and nonsmokers:

the majestic vice versus the right to clean air, Missouri Law Rev. **45**:444, 1980.

34. Ericksen, M.P.: Workplace smoking control: rationale and approaches: Advances in Health Education and Promotion, **1**, part A:65, 1986.

35. Levine, P.H.: An acute effect of cigarette smoking on platelet function: a possible link between smoking and arterial thrombosis, Circulation **48**:619, 1973.

36. DeBakey, M.E., and others: The living heart diet, New York, 1984, Raven Press/Simon & Schuster.

37. Mulcahy, R., and others: Factors influencing long-term prognosis in male patients surviving a first coronary attack, Br. Heart J. **37**:158, 1975.

38. Wilhelmsson, C., and others: Smoking and myocardial infarction, Lancet **1**:415, 1975.

39. Pyrola, K., and others, editors, in cooperation with members of the WHO: Secondary prevention of coronary heart disease, Stuttgart, West Germany, 1983, Georg Thieme.

40. U.S. Department of Health, Education, and Welfare: The smoking digest—progress report on a nation kicking the habit, Bethesda, Md., 1977, U.S. DHEW.

41. Orleans, C.: Health and behavior: a research agenda interim report no. 1, smoking and behavior, workshop presentation, Institute of Medicine, Washington, D.C., 1980, Institute of Medicine.

42. Puska, P., Bjorkqvist, S., and Koskela, K.: Nicotine-containing chewing gum in smoking cessation: a double-blind trial with half year follow-up, Addict. Behav. **4**:141, 1979.

43. Malcolm, R.E., and others: The use of nicotine chewing gum as an aid to stopping smoking, Psychopharm. **70**:295, 1980.

44. Jarvis, M.J., and others: Randomised controlled trial of nicotine chewing gum, Br. Med. J. **285**:537, 1982.

45. Schneider, N.G., and others: Nicotine gum in smoking cessation: a placebo-controlled, double-blind trial, Addict. Behav. **8**:253, 1983.

46. Norton, G.R., and Barske, B.: The role of aversion in the rapid smoking treatment procedure, Addict. Behav. **2**:21, 1977.

47. Elliott, C.H., and Denney, D.R.: A multiple-component treatment approach to smoking reduction, J. Consult. Clin. Psychol. **46**:1330, 1978.

48. Powell, D.R., and McCann, B.S.: The effects of a multiple treatment program and maintenance procedures on smoking cessation, Prev. Med. **10**:9, 1981.

49. Cohen, S.B.: Clinical confrontation: is hypnosis an effective deterrent to smoking, Med. Opinion and Rev. February:66, 1970.

50. Berkowitz, B., Ross-Townsend, A., and Kohberger, R.: Hypnotic treatment of smoking: the single-treatment method revisited, Am. J. Psychiatry **136**:83, 1979.

51. Stanton, H.E.: A one-session hypnotic approach to modifying smoking behavior, Int. J. Clin. Exp. Hypn. **26**(1):22, 1978.

52. Groblas, A.: Auricular acupuncture and the smoking habit, Nouvelle Presse Medicale **4**:980, 1970.

53. Kuller, L., and others: Control of cigarette smoking from a medical perspective, Annu. Rev. Public Health **3**:153, 1982.

54. Haskell, W.L.: The physical activity component of health promotion in occupational settings, Public Health Rep. **95**(2):109, 1980.

55. Paffenbarger, R.S., and others: A natural history of athleticism and cardiovascular health, JAMA **252**:491, 1984.

56. Morris, J.M., and others: Vigorous exercise in leisure-time: protection against coronary heart disease, Lancet **2**:1207, 1980.

57. Paffenbarger, R.S., and Hale, W.E.: Work activity and coronary heart mortality, N. Engl. J. Med. **292**:545, 1975.

58. Cooper, K.H., and others: Physical fitness levels vs. selected coronary risk factors, JAMA **236**:166, 1976.

59. Costas, R., and others: Relation of lipids, weight and physical activity to incidence of coronary heart disease: the Puerto Rico Heart Study, Am. J. Cardiol. **42**:653, 1978.

60. Salonen, J.T., Puska, P., and Tuonilehto, J.: Physical activity and risk of myocardial infarction, cerebral stroke and death: a longitudinal study in Eastern Finland, Am. J. Epidemiol. **115**:526, 1982.

61. Haskell, W.L.: Overview: health benefits of exercise. In Matarazzo, J.D., and others, editors: Behavioral health—a handbook of health enhancement and disease prevention, New York, 1984, John Wiley & Sons.

62. Kilbom, A., and others: Physical training in sedentary middle-aged and older men, Scan. J. Clin. Lab. Invest. **24**:315, 1979.

63. Miall, W., and Oldham, P.: Factors influencing arterial blood pressure in the general population, Clin. Sci. **17**:409, 1969.

64. Berkson, D., and others: Experience with long-term supervised ergometric exercise program for middle-aged sedentary American men (abstract), Circulation **36**(suppl. 2):67, 1967.

65. Wood, P., and others: The distribution of plasma lipoproteins in middle-aged male runners, Metabolism **25**:1249, 1976.

66. Holloszy, J., and others: Effects of a six month program of endurance exercise on the serum lipids of middle-aged men, Am. J. Card. **14**:743, 1975.

67. Lampman, R., and others: Comparative effects of physical training and diet in normalizing serum lipids in men with type IV hyperlipoproteinemia, Circulation **550**:652, 1977.

68. Rosenman, R.: The influence of different exercise patterns on the incidence of coronary heart disease in the Western Collaborative Group Study. In Brunnar, D., and Jokl, E., editors: Physical activity and aging, Baltimore, 1970, University Park Press.

69. Montoya, H., and others: Habitual physical activity and serum lipids: males, ages 16-64 in a total community, J. Chronic Dis. **29**:697, 1976.

70. Morgan, W.P.: Involvement in vigorous physical activity with special reference to adherence, Proceedings of the National College Physical Education Association National Conference, 1977.

71. Dishman, R.K.: Prediction of adherence to habitual physical activity. In Montoye, H.J., and Nagle, F.J., editors: Exercise in health and disease, Springfield, Ill., 1981, Charles C Thomas.

72. Cantu, R.C.: The exercising adult, Lexington, Mass., 1982, The Collamore Press.

73. President's Commission on Mental Health: Report of the President's Commission on Mental Health, Washington, D.C., 1978, U.S. Superintendent of Documents.

74. Wallis, C.: Stress: can we cope? As modern pressures take their toll, doctors preach relaxation, Time, p. 43, June 6, 1983.

75. Manuso, J.S.J.: Management of individual stressors. In O'Donnell, M.P., and Ainsworth, T.H., editors: Health promotion in the workplace, New York, 1984, John Wiley & Sons.

76. Harlan, W.R.: Rationale for intervention on blood pressure in childhood and adolescence. In Matarazzo, J.D., and others, editors: Behavioral health—a handbook of health enhancement and disease prevention, New York, 1984, John Wiley & Sons.

77. Maslow, A.H.: Eupsychian management, Homewood, Ill., 1965, Dorsey Press.

78. Everly, G.S.: Time management: a behavioral strategy for disease prevention and health enhancement. In Matarazzo, J.D., and others, editors: Behavioral health—a handbook of health enhancement and disease prevention, New York, 1984, John Wiley & Sons.

79. Klatsky, A.L., and others: Alcohol and mortality, Ann. Intern. Med. **95**:139, 1981.

80. Williams, P.T., and others: Association of diet and alcohol intake with high-density lipoprotein subclasses, Metabolism **34**:524, 1985.

81. Belloc, N.B., and Breslow, L.: Relationship of physical health status and health practices, Prev. Med. **1**:409, 1972.

82. Belloc, N.B.: Health practices and mortality, Prev. Med. **2**:67, 1973.

83. Hjermann, I., and others: Effect of diet and smoking intervention on the incidence of coronary heart disease, Lancet **2**:1303, 1982.

84. Multiple Risk Factor Intervention Trial Research Group: Multiple risk factor intervention trial: risk factor changes and mortality results, JAMA **248**:1465, 1982.

85. Milsum, J.H.: Health risk factor reduction and lifestyle change, Fam. Community Health **3**:2, 1982.

86. Green, L.W., and others: Health education planning: a diagnostic approach, Palo Alto, Calif., 1980, Mayfield Publishing Co.

87. O'Donnell, M.P., and Ainsworth, T.H., editors: Health promotion in the workplace, New York, 1984, John Wiley & Sons.

88. Inter-Society Commission for Heart Disease Resources, Atherosclerosis Study Group and Epidemiology Study Group: Primary prevention of the atherosclerotic diseases. In Wright, I., and Frederickson, D., editors: Cardiovascular diseases: guidelines for prevention and care, Washington, D.C., 1974, U.S. Government Printing Office.

89. Strong, J.: The pediatric aspects of atherosclerosis, J. Atherosclerosis Res. **9**:251, 1969.

90. Mitchell, S., editor: Symposium on prevention of atherosclerosis at the pediatric level, Am. J. Cardiol. **31**(5):539, 1973.

91. Mitchell, S., and Jesse, M.: Risk factors of coronary heart disease: their genesis and pediatric implications, Am. J. Cardiol. **31**:588, 1973.

92. Newman, W., and Strong, J.: Natural history, geographic pathology, and pediatric aspects of atherosclerosis. In Strong, W., editor: Atherosclerosis: its pediatric aspects, New York, 1978, Harcourt Brace Jovanovitch.

93. McMillan, G.: Development of arteriosclerosis, Am. J. Cardiol. **31**:542, 1973.

94. Stamler, J., and others: Hypertension: the problem and the challenge. In The hypertension book, West Point, Pa., 1974, Merck, Sharp, and Dohme.

95. Promoting health: a source book, regional forums on community health promotion, U.S. Office of Health Information and Health Promotion Pub. No. 282-78-0060, Washington, D.C., Spring, 1980, U.S. DHEW.

96. U.S. Department of Health, Education, and Welfare: Healthy people: the Surgeon General's report on health promotion and disease prevention, U.S. Public Health Service Pub. No. 79-55071, Washington, D.C., 1979, U.S. Government Printing Office.

97. American Cancer Society: Report on national task force on tobacco and cancer, Washington, D.C., 1976, American Cancer Society.

98. Gilbert, G.G. and Pruitt, B.E.: School health education in the United States, Hygie **3**:10, 1984.

99. Weinberg, A.D., Carbonari, J.P., and Laufman, L.: What high school students don't know about cardiovascular disease, J. Sch. Health **54**:112, 1984.

100. Simons-Morton, B.G., and others: Great sensations: a program to encourage heart healthy snacking by high school students, J. Sch. Health **54**:288, 1984.

101. Salt intake and eating patterns of infants and children in relation to blood pressure, American Academy of Pediatrics Committee on Nutrition, Pediatrics **53**:115, 1974.

102. Hurd, P.D., and others: Prevention of cigarette smoking in seventh-grade students, J. Behav. Med. **3**:15, 1980.

103. Botvin, G., Eng, A., and Williams, C.L.: Preventing the onset of cigarette smoking through life skills training, Prev. Med. **9**:135, 1980.

104. President's Council on Physical Fitness and Sports: Fitness in the workplace, Washington, D.C., 1983, Phillips Petroleum Company.

105. Brennan, A.J.: Wellness goes to work, Employee Serv. Manag., April 1985, p. 11.

106. Fitness, corporate style: companies are racing to invest in employee wellness, Newsweek, p. 96, Nov. 5, 1984.

107. Farnon, C.: Let's offer employees a healthier diet, J. Occ. Med. **23**:273, 1981.

108. National Interagency Council on Smoking and Health: Smoking and the workplace—a national survey, final report, New York, 1980, NICSH.

109. Orleans, C.S., and Shipley, R.H.: Worksite smoking cessation initiatives: review and recommendations, Addict. Behav. **7**:1, 1982.

110. Farquhar, J.W., and others: Community education for cardiovascular health, Lancet **1**:1192, 1977.

111. Maccoby, J., and others: Reducing the risk of cardiovascular disease: effects of a community-based campaign on knowledge and behavior, J. Community Health **3**:100, 1977.

112. Farquhar, J.W., and others: The Stanford Five City Project: an overview. In Matarazzo, J.D., and others, editors: Behavioral health—a handbook of health enhancement and disease prevention, New York, 1984, John Wiley & Sons.

113. Puska, P.: Community-based prevention of cardiovascular disease: the North Karelia Project. In Matarazzo, J.D., and others, editors: Behavioral health—a handbook of health enhancement and disease prevention, New York, 1984, John Wiley & Sons.

114. Kittel, F.: The Interuniversity Study on nutrition and health. In Matarazzo, J.D., and others, editors: Behavioral health—a handbook of health enhancement and disease prevention, New York, 1984, John Wiley & Sons.

115. Lasater, T., and others: Lay volunteer delivery of a community-based cardiovascular risk factor change program: the Pawtucket Experiment. In Matarazzo, J.D., and others, editors: Behavioral health—a handbook of health enhancement and disease prevention, New York, 1984, John Wiley & Sons.

116. Blackburn, H., and others: The Minnesota Heart Health Program: a research and demonstration project in cardiovascular disease prevention. In Matarazzo, J.D., and others, editors: Behavioral health—a handbook of health enhancement and disease prevention, New York, 1984, John Wiley & Sons.

117. Hecht, R.: Considerations on the use of media in patient education. In Squyres, W.D., editor: Patient education: an inquiry into the state of the art, vol. 4, New York, 1984, Springer Publishing Co.

118. Gerbner, G., and others: Special report: health and medicine on television, N. Engl. J. Med. **305**:901, 1981.

119. Levi, L.: Psychosocial factors in preventive medicine. In Healthy people: the Surgeon General's report on health promotion and disease prevention, Department of Health, Education, and Welfare, Public Health Service Pub. No. 79-55071A, Washington, D.C., 1979, U.S. Government Printing Office.

120. Hazuda, H.P., and others: Ethnic differences in health knowledge and behaviors related to the prevention and treatment of coronary heart disease, The San Antonio Heart Study, Am. J. Epidemiol. **117**:717, 1983.

121. Fortmann, S.P., and others: Does dietary health education reach only the privileged? The Stanford Three Community Study, Circulation **66**:77, 1982.

122. Stern, M.P., and Gaskill, S.P.: Secular trends in ischemic heart disease and stroke mortality from 1970 to 1976 in Spanish-surnamed and other White individuals in Bexar County, Texas, Circulation **58**:537, 1978.

123. Harwood, A.: Ethnicity and medical care. In Schreiber, J.M., and

Homiak, J.P., editors: Mexican Americans, London, 1981, Harvard University Press.

124. Freimer, N., Echenberg, D., and Kretchmer, N.: Cultural variation: nutritional and clinical implications in cross-cultural medicine, West J. Med. **139:**928, 1983.

125. Bauer, K.G.: Federal government policies and activities in health promotion. In Faber, M.M., and Reinhardt, A.M., editors: Promoting health through risk reduction, New York, 1982, Macmillan Publishing Co., Inc.

126. Faber, M.M., and Reinhardt, A.M.: Promoting health through risk reduction, New York, 1982, Macmillan Publishing Co., Inc.

127. Gilbert, G.G., Davis, R.L., and Damberg, C.L.: Current federal activities in school health education, Pub. Health Rep. **100:**499, 1985.

128. Task Force on Consumer Health Education, National Institutes of Health, American College of Preventive Medicine: Promoting health: consumer education and national policy, Germantown, Md., 1976, Aspen Systems Corp.

129. Institute of Medicine: Policy issues in the health sciences, Washington, D.C., 1977, National Academy of Sciences.

130. Bishop, J.E.: Probing the cell: scientists are learning how genes predispose some to heart disease, Wall Street Journal, February 6, 1986.

131. Green, L.W.: Evaluation and measurement: some dilemmas for health education, Am. J. Public Health **67:**155, 1977.

CHAPTER 4

Patient Assessment: History and Physical Examination

Debra Peeples
Virginia Kliner Fowkes
Kathleen Gainor Andreoli

People who have coronary artery disease enter the health care system at varying stages of disease progression. Thus to determine the individual goals of care and complementary management plans, a clinical data base must be generated. This information can be procured systematically through an interview with the patient and through a complete physical examination, plus pertinent laboratory and physiologic tests. This begins the process of identifying and solving patient problems, a process that continues throughout the therapeutic relationship. As plans are developed and implemented toward resolving each problem, subjective and objective data are collected to evaluate the success of the plan and determine the necessity of management revision.

The intent of this chapter is to focus on the data collection process as it pertains to the patient's cardiovascular status. It is important to remember, however, that other body systems may affect, or be affected by, cardiac disease, and other systems may be involved in disease processes that secondarily affect the heart. Consequently, any patient who develops a new problem should have a complete evaluation.

The discussion that follows includes the patient interview, physical examination, recording of data, assessment of common symptoms and risk factors, and the identification of medical and nursing diagnoses. This process of data gathering can be used to explore a patient's problem in an outpatient clinic, to develop a patient care plan in the coronary care unit, or to acquire further information about a new or acute problem.

CLINICIAN'S ABILITY IN ASSESSMENT

Patient assessment is a complicated, detailed, and orderly process that should incorporate physical, psychologic, and social dimensions. Its objective is to achieve a comprehensive view of the patient as a person in the context of his or her family, occupation, physical and psychologic health, and immediate needs to mobilize appropriate care interventions. Obviously, most clinicians have mastered the skills of simple data gathering and recording. What is more difficult in the often hurried clinical encounter is to absorb less obvious information, for example, about the patient's feelings.

Each examiner brings to the clinical encounter personal attitudes, beliefs, biases, and moods. These include such things as cultural experiences, personal limitations, and even (with other patients waiting to be seen) feeling pressed for time. Furthermore, settings such as the coronary care unit are replete with technologic equipment that may easily distract the clinician from focusing on the patient as a person. For example, the examiner may focus on the arterial line or monitoring equipment and miss the fact that the patient is frightened or in pain. Or, under pressure of time, the examiner may appear hurried, which may intimidate patients and make them refrain from sharing their worries or feelings.

The key to comprehensive assessment is to be wholly involved with the patient during the encounter. This means employing whatever tools one needs to relax, concentrate, and focus—perhaps taking the time to breathe deeply in the midst of a hurried schedule. It also entails maximizing for the moment one's skills in listening, touching, and observing quietly and carefully. In spite of the socioeconomic, intellectual, and language barriers that sometimes exist, the clinician must transmit and receive information. A willingness to learn and the ability to be sensitive to individual attitudes and needs enhances the quality of practitioner-patient interaction and of the information received.

PATIENT INTERVIEW

The patient interview, a powerful diagnostic tool, is the first step in the data collection process. It can be defined as a goal-directed method of communication—a medium for interaction between two persons. Its major purpose is to elicit pertinent information about the patient's present complaint or problem, health history, and family and social history. If the interaction between the clinician and the patient is marked by concern and sensitivity, the interview can help to establish a meaningful clinician-patient relationship. The accuracy and completeness of the subjective data gathered during the interaction depend on the clinician's ability to effectively communicate with others and elicit pertinent information and responses from them. Completeness depends also on the patient's ability to be a reliable historian. The clinician's responsibility includes recognizing when to validate the patient's history with the family or significant other (see Chapter 16 for interviewing skills adapted to elderly patients).

To facilitate the interview the clinician needs to remember some guidelines for establishing a good clinician-patient relationship.

Establishing a Clinician-Patient Relationship

1. Provide as much privacy as possible for the interview.
2. Introduce yourself.
3. Call the patient by his or her preferred name.
4. Tell the patient the purpose of the interview.
5. Sit at eye level, establish eye contact with the patient, and lean toward the patient.
6. Probe and listen for the patient's concerns and beliefs about his or her condition and health problems.
7. Show caring and concern for the patient as a human being.
8. Be nonjudgmental in your responses to the patient.
9. Use language that is appropriate for the patient's educational, cultural, and psychosocial background.
10. Observe the patient's nonverbal behavior such as facial grimacing or wringing of hands.

In addition to establishing a good clinician-patient relationship, it is important that the clinician be familiar with alternatives in guiding an interview and responding to patients. All too often the clinician uses only one or two alternatives. The use of the following techniques can help to structure the interview and facilitate more complete and accurate data collection.

Guiding the Interview

1. Use open-ended questions and statements ("Tell me about your chest pain").
2. Clarify words, phrases, or statements ("What do you mean by a little bit"?).
3. Summarize data during and after the interview to ensure accuracy.
4. Reflect words, phrases, statements, and feelings ("You've been having trouble sleeping").
5. Use silence to organize your thoughts and allow the patient time to answer questions.
6. Use supportive statements and gestures ("That must have been difficult—tell me more"). (Nod head yes.)
7. Focus the interview on the current topic(s) ("Let's talk some more about your chest pain").

Patient's Present Complaint or Problem

The patient's chief problem, whether it be chest pain, shortness of breath, or palpitations, among others, precipitates contact with the health care system. It is the chief concern and therefore the first subject of the interview. As the patient expresses perceived physical or mental changes, the interviewer should reorganize the patient's words into a clinical format to help identify the bodily or mental processes underlying each symptom. By asking the patient to identify dates and times, the relationship between symptoms and events can be more easily understood. In a seriously ill patient, priority must be given to those aspects of the history that appear more relevant to the immediate situation. This process is accomplished by employing seven basic characteristics or descriptors that differentiate symptoms of one disease from those of another (see box).

Patient's Health History

The patient's health history may contribute to defining the problem and planning interventions. The patient is asked about general health status and stability of weight. Allergies such as food, contact, or drug are noted. Additional queries are made about past infectious diseases, immunizations, surgical procedures, hospitalizations, injuries, major illnesses, obstetric history, and psychologic conditions.

The patient is asked specifically about previous heart problems, including heart enlargement, heart failure, murmurs, heart attacks, rheumatic heart disease, hypertension, elevated cholesterol or triglyceride levels, and diabetes. Information is recorded chronologically, with dates and other pertinent details.

Patient's Family History

The patient's family background and social profile also may contribute important information to the assessment. The age, sex, and health of parents, siblings, children, and spouse and the age and cause of death of deceased members are relevant. In addition, certain familial diseases that grandparents and close relatives may have had are pertinent. These include hypertension, coronary artery disease, rheumatic fever, stroke, kidney disease, diabetes, thyroid disease, cancer, blood disease, asthma, glaucoma, and gout.

Patient's Personal and Social History

This section of the data base provides information about the patient's life situation and lends perspective to an assessment of his or her ability to cope with the illness. This information is critical in planning care that considers home conditions and family resources. Knowledge of patient habits and life patterns aids in planning hospital routine.

Information is collected about the patient's place of birth, education, military affiliation, position in the family, and state of satisfaction with life situation. Inquiries about habits or patterns such as sleep, exercise, nutrition, alcohol consumption, use of tobacco, coffee or tea, and medications are important. When asking about medication and diet history, it is useful to ask the patient to pick a typical

---

DISEASE DESCRIPTORS

Location

Where did the symptom originate? Did it radiate? To what site? It is helpful if the patient indicates the location of the symptom and the radiation pattern with his or her hand.

Quality

How did the symptom feel to the patient? It may be described as being like something else. For example, the chest pain of myocardial infarction is often compared to "being squeezed in a vise." Other qualifiers include "choking," "burning," and "constricting."

Quantity

How intense is the symptom? Is it mild, moderate, severe, or unbearable?

Course

When did the symptom first occur? Was its onset sudden or gradual? How long did it last in terms of minutes, hours, or days? Over time, has the symptom stayed the same or become better or worse?

Setting

Describe the circumstances when the symptom first occurred. Look for associations between the symptom and the patient's physical activity, emotional status, and personal interactions.

Aggravating and alleviating factors

Are the symptoms influenced by certain activities or physiologic processes? What produces relief—resting, avoiding food, medication? What aggravates the problem—exertion, eating, body position, coughing?

Associated symptoms

Rarely is a disease process present with only one symptom. Therefore the presence or absence of symptoms commonly associated with cardiovascular conditions should be noted. The patient should be asked specifically about each of these, and affirmative responses should be characterized and described as stated in the six previous steps. Questions for eliciting this information should explore whether or not the patient is experiencing any of the following: (1) chest pain or discomfort, (2) unexplained weakness or fatigue, (3) weight loss or gain, (4) swelling of ankles *(edema)*, (5) shortness of breath on exertion *(dyspnea)*, (6) shortness of breath while sleeping that wakens the patient *(paroxysmal nocturnal dyspnea)*, (7) a need to sleep on more than one pillow to breathe comfortably *(orthopnea)*, (8) dizzy or fainting spells *(syncope)*, (9) coughing at night, (10) coughing up blood *(hemoptysis)*, (11) rapid heart beat or palpitations, (12) a need to get up several times during the night to urinate, and (13) pain or cramps in the legs while walking that is relieved by rest *(intermittent claudication)*. Finally, asking the patient generally about his daily activities and any self-imposed restrictions on these can provide clues as to the severity of the problem.

---

day and describe all drugs (physician- and self-prescribed) taken from morning until bedtime. This approach to diet is useful in giving the practitioner a complete picture of nutrition, including snacks which the patient may neglect to mention otherwise.

Medication history is particularly necessary with the elderly, who may see more than one health care provider and consume a series of drugs that have synergistic or mutually inhibitory effects.

Home conditions, nature of family relationships, economic resources, including source of income and insurance, satisfaction with sexual relationship, religious affiliation, and occupation are other areas important to assess.

REVIEW OF SYSTEMS

The review of systems is done as a part of the initial assessment and is a record of the patient's past and present health in each system. Content covered in the review of systems is detailed on page 30.

PHYSICAL EXAMINATION

The cardiovascular physical examination is performed to collect objective data about the patient's complaint, symptoms, or illness. The information that has been obtained from the patient interview is then correlated with the physical findings as the next step in the evaluation process. Often a sufficient and accurately obtained history estab-

REVIEW OF SYSTEMS

General

State of health, appetite, weight, fatigue

Skin

Temperature, rashes, growths, sun-sensitivity, itching, texture, change in pigment and color, excessive dryness or sweating

Head

Headaches, lumps, injury

Eyes

Diplopia, acuity, blurring, spots, lacrimation, itching, photophobia, pain, infection, discharge

Ears

Hearing, infections, earaches, discharge, tinnitus, vertigo

Nose

Discharge, obstruction, sinus, sense of smell, epistaxis

Mouth and throat

Sore throats, hoarseness, dysphagia, bleeding or sore gums

Neck

Pain, stiffness, lumps

Cardiopulmonary

Chest pain, dyspnea, palpitations, cough, hemoptysis, night sweats, edema, history of murmur, paroxysmal nocturnal dyspnea, orthopnea, wheezing, stridor, syncope, history of hypertension, past heart test

Gastrointestinal

Food intolerance, pyrosis, nausea, vomiting, abdominal pain, bloody stools or vomitus, diarrhea, constipation, melena, bowel habits (change in frequency, consistency, or color), jaundice, hemorrhoids

Genitourinary

Dysuria, polyuria, oliguria, urgency, frequency, hesitation, nocturia, hematuria, pyuria, urethral discharge, incontinence, sexual problems (decreased libido, chest pain or shortness of breath during intercourse), history of venereal disease

Male: prostate problems, impotence

Female: menarche, date of last menstrual period, usual menstrual period (duration, amount, and interval), dysmenorrhea, hypermenorrhea (amount), polymenorrhea (intermenstrual bleeding), menopause (date, if any), vaginal bleeding or discharge, pelvic inflammatory disease, birth control measures, gravida, para, abortions, complications of pregnancy, dyspareunia, last Pap smear

Musculoskeletal

Muscle pain or cramps, joint pain, swelling or stiffness of joints, back pain, or weakness, coldness, and discoloration of extremities

Nervous

Paresthesia, balance, numbness, paralysis, tremor, nervousness, depression (symptoms), hallucinations, therapy, memory

Hematopoietic

Easy bleeding or bruising, past transfusions and reactions

Endocrine

Temperature intolerance, polydipsia, thyroid problems, diabetes

Peripheral vascular

Varicose veins, thrombophlebitis, cramps

lishes the nature of the problem prior to the physical examination. The examination itself is conducted with sensitivity, gentleness, attention, and meticulous care. In an acute emergency situation an abbreviated examination should be conducted with deliberate speed.

The examiner evaluates the cardiovascular system in an orderly fashion, using the techniques of inspection, palpation, percussion, and auscultation as appropriate. An orderly and accurate physical examination requires effective motor and technical skills.

inspection Examining visually the parts of the system. It includes whatever the examiner can see, such as pulsations, deformities, color, manner of breathing, and so forth.

palpation Feeling or pressing with the fingers or hands to locate possible vibrations, thrills (blood flowing past an obstruction), impulses, grating sensations, and so on.

percussion Tapping the patient's body surface to determine, through touch and hearing, the relative amount of air or solid material underneath the skin.

auscultation Listening with or without the stethoscope to internally produced sounds. Such sounds include breath sounds, heart sounds, bruit (murmur over a peripheral vessel), friction rubs, and heart murmurs.

The physical examination actually begins when the patient meets the examiner. At this time the examiner makes general observations about the patient regarding apparent age versus stated age, grooming, speech, posture, gait, nutritional state, attitude, color, and degree of distress, if any. The collection of objective data begins with the recording of the patient's vital signs, including temperature, pulse, respiration, and blood pressure.

A temperature elevation above the normal level of 98.6° F or 37° C is common during the first few days following acute myocardial infarction. The fever is usually less than 101° F and is associated with necrosis of cardiac muscle. Prolonged, high, or late development of fever suggests other complications. Although fever may indicate the onset of infectious processes, it may also be the first sign of thrombophlebitis, pulmonary embolism, pericarditis, or atelectasis. Moreover, prolonged temperature elevation in the patient with a myocardial infarction may be harmful, since it causes a rise in the metabolic rate of body tissues and therefore a demand for increased circulation and oxygenation. This, in turn, increases the myocardial oxygen demands, a threatening situation in the face of infarction.

Temperature assessment is therefore a part of routine examination and daily monitoring activities for critically ill patients. The temperature is taken orally, rectally, or in the axilla for a period of 3 minutes. Rectal temperatures are the most accurate. In the past the taking of rectal temperatures was avoided in patients with myocardial infarctions as a precaution against undue vagal stimulation.

However, recent studies suggest that taking rectal temperatures is quite safe.

Temperature is measured on a Fahrenheit or centigrade scale. The formula for converting centigrade measurement to Fahrenheit and vice versa follows:

$$\text{Fahrenheit} = 1.8\ (^\circ C) + 32$$
$$\text{Centigrade} = \frac{^\circ F - 32}{1.8}$$

Pulse

Arterial Pulse. The arterial pulse is a propagated wave of arterial pressure resulting from left ventricular contraction. The pulse wave begins in the aorta with the opening of the aortic valve and the ejection of blood from the left ventricle (Fig. 4-1). The pressure in the aorta rises sharply, since blood enters the vessel more rapidly than it runs off to the peripheral vessels. A notch may appear during the sharp rise in the central arterial pressure curve. This is called the *anacrotic notch* and is generally absent from peripheral pulse recordings but may be prominent in valvular aortic stenosis. After peak pressure has been reached, aortic pressure decreases, ventricular ejection slows, and blood continues to flow to peripheral vessels. As the ventricles relax, there is a brief reversal of flow (from the central arteries back toward the ventricle) and the aortic valve closes. This produces the *dicrotic notch* on the peripheral pressure pulse tracing, corresponding to the *incisura* recorded centrally. Following this, aortic pressure increases slightly and then decreases as diastole continues and blood flows to the periphery, a result of energy imparted to the elastic tissue in the great vessels during systole. In the graphic recording of aortic pressure in Fig. 4-1 the peak of the pulse wave represents systolic pressure and the lowest point on the wave represents diastolic pressure.

The pulse wave changes in shape as it travels to the periphery. The height, or amplitude, of the wave (the systolic reading) increases as it moves from the aortic root to the peripheral arteries, with a slight decrease in the diastolic pressure. The ascending part of the wave becomes steeper and the peak becomes sharper.

The competency of the arterial system is assessed through blood pressure measurement, inspection of the carotid artery, palpation of the arteries, and auscultation of the arteries. Blood pressure is discussed in a subsequent section.

EXAMINATION. The arterial pulses are palpated to evaluate patency, heart rate and rhythm, and character of the pulse. This examination covers the carotid, brachial, radial, femoral, popliteal, dorsalis pedis, and posterior tibial pulses. These pulses can best be evaluated with the patient in a reclining position and the trunk of the body elevated about 30 degrees. If diffuse atherosclerosis in an elderly

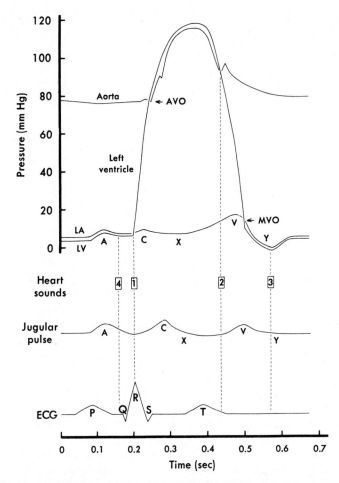

FIG. 4-1. Simultaneous ECG, pressures obtained from the left atrium, left ventricle, and aorta, and the jugular pulse during one cardiac cycle. For simplification, right-sided heart pressures have been omitted. Normal right atrial pressure closely parallels that of the left atrium, and right ventricular and pulmonary artery pressures time closely with their corresponding left-sided heart counterparts, only being reduced in magnitude. The normal mitral and aortic valve closure precedes tricuspid and pulmonic closure, respectively, whereas valve opening reverses this order. The jugular venous pulse lags behind the right atrial pressure.

During the course of one cardiac cycle, note that the electrical events *(ECG)* initiate and therefore precede the mechanical *(pressure)* events, and that the latter precede the auscultatory events *(heart sounds)* they themselves produce. Shortly after the P wave, the atria contract to produce the a wave; a fourth heart sound may succeed contraction. The QRS complex initiates ventricular systole, followed shortly by left ventricular contraction and the rapid buildup of left ventricular *(LV)* pressure. Almost immediately LV pressure exceeds left atrial *(LA)* pressure to close the mitral valve and produce the first heart sound. When LV pressure exceeds aortic pressure, the aortic valve opens *(AVO)*, and when aortic pressure is once again greater than LV pressure, the aortic valve closes to produce the second heart sound and terminate ventricular ejection. The decreasing LV pressure drops below LA pressure to open the mitral valve *(MVO)* and a period of rapid ventricular filling commences. During this time a third heart sound may be heard. The jugular pulse is explained under the discussion of the venous pulse. (Modified with permission from Hurst, J.W., and others: The heart: arteries and veins, ed. 6, New York, 1986, McGraw-Hill Book Co.)

patient has resulted in absence of the dorsalis pedis or posterior tibial pulse, this observation should be noted on initial examination so that the hospital staff do not interpret this finding as a new catastrophic event, such as arterial embolus, at a later time during the patient's hospitalization.

Although the radial pulse is commonly used in determining heart rate, the carotid pulse best correlates with central aortic pressure and reflects cardiac function more accurately than peripheral vessels. Furthermore, if the patient develops marked vasoconstriction, the radial pulse may be difficult to palpate. However, caution must be exercised in palpating the carotid pulse to avoid pressure on the carotid sinus, since palpating at that site may result in severe bradycardia.

The pulse is examined for *rate and rhythm, equality of corresponding pulses, contour,* and *amplitude.* The pulses should be palpated on both sides and simultaneously at the brachial and femoral arteries. To obtain information about *cardiac rate and rhythm,* the pulse should be palpated for 30 seconds in the presence of a regular rhythm and for 1 to 2 minutes in the face of an irregular rhythm. If an irregularity exists, an apical pulse should be recorded. The term *peripheral pulse deficit* indicates that the heart rate counted at the apex by auscultation exceeds the heart rate counted by palpation of the radial pulse. A deficit means that not every cardiac systole is forceful enough to produce a palpable radial pulse and may occur in the presence of premature extrasystoles or atrial tachyarrythmias, such as atrial fibrillation. Bilateral, simultaneous palpation of the radial and pedal pulses is helpful in determining whether the pulses arrive without delay and provides information about the peripheral arterial blood supply.

The *character of the arterial wall,* which normally feels soft and pliable, is noted by palpation. With significant atherosclerotic disease the vessel may be resistant to compression and feel much like a rope.

The pulse *contour* may be assessed by extending the patient's arm and palpating the radial or brachial pulse or the carotid pulse in the neck. The artery should be compressed lightly with a finger while the examiner ascertains the contour of the pulse wave. Variations in the contour of the arterial pulse are depicted in Fig. 4-2.

The *normal arterial pulse* (Fig. 4-2, *A*) has a pulse pressure of about 30 to 40 mm Hg; the systolic pressure measures the peaks of the waves, and the diastolic pressure measures the troughs. One can feel a sharp upstroke and a more gradual downstroke (the dicrotic notch of the descending slope of the wave is too weak to be palpable). The contour of the normal pulse is smooth and rounded.

With *large bounding pulses* (Fig. 4-2, *B*), the pulse pressure is increased and one feels a rapid upstroke, a brief peak, and a fast downstroke. This type of pulse wave is encountered most often in conditions termed *hyperkinetic*

circulatory states. These states include exercise, anxiety, fear, hyperthyroidism, anemia, patent ductus arteriosus, aortic regurgitation, and complete heart block with bradycardia and hypertension. It is also found as a result of generalized arteriosclerosis and rigidity of the arterial system in elderly people.

Small weak pulses (Fig. 4-2, *C*) are characterized by diminished pulse pressure and pulse contour that is felt as a slow gradual upstroke, a delayed systolic peak, and a prolonged downstroke. This pulse is found in severe cases of left ventricular failure as a result of decreased stroke volume and in moderate or severe cases of aortic stenosis as a result of slow ejection of blood through the narrowed orifice.

Pulsus alternans (Fig. 4-2, *D*) refers to a pulse pattern in which the heart beats with a *regular* rhythm, but the pulses alternate in size and intensity. When this alternation is present in lesser degrees, the difference may not be palpable, but it can be readily detected by measuring blood pressure by auscultation.

As the sphygmomanometer cuff is slowly deflated from a pressure above the systolic level, the sounds from the alternate beats are heard first. Then one hears the alternating loud and soft sounds or a sudden doubling of the rate as the cuff pressure declines. Pulsus alternans often accompanies left ventricular failure and can masquerade as a bigeminal pulse.

The *bigeminal pulse* (Fig. 4-2, *E*) is usually produced by a premature ventricular extrasystole that occurs regularly following a normally conducted beat. The stroke volume of the premature beat is less than that of the normal beat, since contraction occurs before complete ventricular filling. The rhythm is *irregular,* since the time between the normal beat and the premature beat is shorter than the time between the pairs. The irregularity may be consistent. Simultaneous arterial palpation and cardiac auscultation assist in diagnosing this cardiac irregularity.

The *amplitude* of pulses is categorized into levels in the following code and compared bilaterally:

0 = Not palpable	+3 = Full
+1 = Barely palpable	+4 = Bounding
+2 = Decreased	

In patients with significant vascular disease it is useful to draw a small stick figure and label the amplitude of pulses accordingly.

Pulsus paradoxus (Fig. 4-2, *F*) refers to the phenomenon in which the pulse diminishes perceptibly in amplitude during normal inspiration. Although the differences in pulse volume can be palpated, they can be more precisely demonstrated with sphygmomanometry. Under normal conditions of rest the systolic blood pressure ordinarily

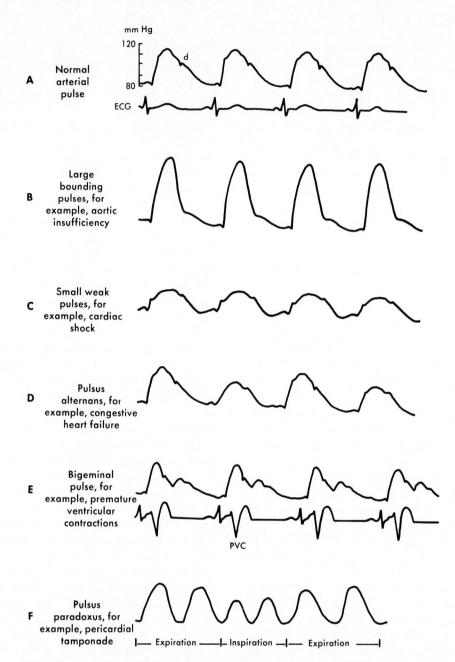

FIG. 4-2. Variations in contour of the arterial pulse with correlated ECGs for A, normal arterial pulses, and E, bigeminal pulse. See text for description.

decreases by 3 to 10 mm Hg. The procedure for detecting pulsus paradoxus is as follows:

1. Have the patient breathe *normally*.
2. Pump up the sphygmomanometer, then lower the pressure until the first sound (systolic) is heard.
3. Observe the patient's respirations. The systolic sound may disappear during normal inspiration.
4. Slowly deflate the cuff until all systolic sounds are heard, regardless of phase in the respiratory cycle.

The change (in millimeters of mercury) from the point at which systolic sounds were first heard to the point where they are heard during the entire respiratory cycle represents the millimeters of paradox observed. A paradox greater than 10 mm Hg is usually abnormal.

To be significant, a paradoxical pulse must occur during normal cardiac rhythm and with respirations of normal rhythm and depth. In short, it is an exaggeration of a

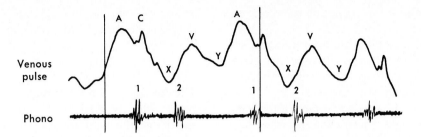

FIG. 4-3.   Relationship of jugular venous pulse to right atrial activity.

normal response during respiration. Pulsus paradoxus is found in cases of pericardial tamponade, adhesive pericarditis, severe lung disease, advanced heart failure, and other conditions.

AUSCULTATION OF ARTERIES. Arteries are normally silent when auscultated with the bell or diaphragm of the stethoscope, which is placed lightly over them. Occlusive arterial disease, such as arteriosclerosis, will interfere with normal blood flow through the artery, resulting in a blowing sound called a *bruit*. Auscultation of the carotid arteries should be done with the patient holding the breath so that the bruits can be distinguished from the sounds of respiration. Often these abnormal arterial vibrations can be felt as *thrills*. Auscultation is also done over the abdominal aorta and femoral arteries to detect the presence of bruits.

Venous Pulse. Examination of the neck veins provides diagnostic information about the dynamics of the right side of the heart. For this clinical evaluation, one must study the waveform of the venous pulsations, correlate them with the cardiac rhythm, and determine the venous pressure.

The character of the venous pulse is determined by four factors: (1) the rate at which blood is returned from the peripheral tissues to the venous system, (2) the amount of resistance to flow presented by the right atrium and ventricle during different phases of the cardiac cycle, (3) the pressure-volume properties of the segment of the vein, and (4) in part, the nature of the tissues overlying the veins at the focus of observation. Elevations in venous pressure occur with right ventricular failure, rapid blood flow due to exercise, fever, or hyperthyroidism, fluid overload, constriction of the heart from pericarditis, pericardial effusion or cardiac tamponade, and tricuspid valvular disease.

EXAMINATION. The examination begins with observation of the external and internal jugular veins on both sides of the neck as well as of the venous pulsations that may be present in the supraclavicular fossae or in the suprasternal notch. For accurate evaluation of the venous waveform the *right internal jugular vein* is usually selected, although one of the other veins may be preferred and is just

as revealing. If the venous pressure is relatively normal, the patient can assume a comfortable recumbent position with the head and trunk elevated to about a 30-degree angle without flexing the neck. If the venous pressure is greatly elevated, the pulses can be examined better with the patient in a completely upright position so that the pulsations appear at the jugular level.

The patient's head should be gently rotated away from the examiner. A light shined tangentially across the area being examined may help detect a slightly distended vein. A series of undulant waves that are more clearly seen than felt characterize the venous pulse, a graphic recording of which is shown in Fig. 4-3. These pulsations are evaluated in relation to the cardiac cycle and therefore the carotid pulse or heart sounds can be used for timing them.

a Wave. The a wave is produced by right atrial contraction and the retrograde transmission of the pressure pulse to the jugular veins. It occurs at the time of the fourth heart sound, preceding the first heart sound. The a wave can be easily identified by placing the index finger on the carotid pulse opposite the side being inspected. Because of the compliance of the great veins and the low pressures in the right side of the heart, the a wave will be seen to start just slightly before the carotid pulse is palpated in the neck. The a wave is absent during atrial fibrillation. Giant a waves reflect an elevated right atrial pressure and may be seen in such conditions as pulmonary hypertension and pulmonic and tricuspid stenosis. *Cannon a waves* are an exaggerated form of the giant a wave. In this situation the right atrium contracts during ventricular systole, when the tricuspid valve is closed, and the blood regurgitates into the neck veins. *Regular* cannon waves may occur during AV junctional (nodal) rhythm when the atria and ventricles contract almost simultaneously. *Irregular* cannon waves may occur during an AV dissociation of any cause and during ectopic beating.

c Wave. The c wave begins shortly after the first heart sound and may result from impact of the carotid artery on the adjacent jugular vein or from the retrograde transmission of a positive wave in the right atrium, generated by the bulging tricuspid valve during right ventricular systole.

The c wave is often difficult to visualize by inspecting the neck veins.

v Wave. Continued atrial filling during ventricular systole produces the v wave, which peaks just after the second heart sound, when the tricuspid valve opens. Tricuspid insufficiency causes a very large v wave.

x Descent. The x descent is the downslope of the a and c waves and results from right atrial diastole, plus the effects of the tricuspid valve being pulled downward during ventricular systole. Tricuspid insufficiency blunts or eliminates the x descent, whereas elevated right ventricular output and constrictive pericarditis may enhance it.

y Descent. The y descent represents the fall in the right atrial pressure from the peak of the v wave following tricuspid valve opening and occurs during the period of rapid atrial emptying in early diastole. Impedance to right atrial emptying, caused by tricuspid stenosis or atresia or by a right atrial myxoma, dampens the y descent. Constrictive pericarditis produces a speedy y descent and prominent trough, followed by a rapid y ascent as the ventricular, atrial, and venous pressures promptly rise when the non-distensible right ventricle becomes filled with blood.

• • •

Respiration alters the venous pulse. Deep inspiration lowers the level of the venous pressure pulsation (actual amplitude of the pulse waves may be increased) by a decrease in intrathoracic pressure. This increases venous return, reduces central venous pressure, and increases right-sided heart filling to lower the level of the venous pulse in the neck and collapse the neck veins. Expiration produces reversed effects. The *Valsalva maneuver,* that is, forced expiratory straining against a closed glottis, elevates the venous pressure by obstructing flow into the chest.

Kussmaul's sign is a paradoxical rise in venous pressure and neck vein distention during inspiration and is seen in the patient with severe right heart failure or pericardial constriction. The limited capacity of the right ventricle to receive the increased volume of venous return generated by inspiration results in a backing up of blood into the superior vena cava and distention of the neck veins.

Hepatojugular reflux is a sustained rise in the level of venous pressure during abdominal compression when the patient is breathing normally. As the liver or splanchnic vessels are compressed, the volume of venous blood returning to the right side of the heart is thought to increase. The normal heart accepts this extra load easily. During right-sided heart failure, constrictive pericarditis, or hypervolemia the venous pressure rises because the right ventricle is unable to accommodate the increased blood volume. The prominent v wave of tricuspid insufficiency may be exposed by this maneuver. Manual abdominal compression may cause discomfort resulting in muscular guarding.

This muscle tension may increase intraabdominal pressure (Valsalva maneuver) and give a falsely positive hepatojugular reflux.

Respiration

The rate and character of the patient's respiration should be carefully observed. Under normal conditions the adult should breathe comfortably about 16 to 20 times per minute. Variations in the normal rate and character of respirations include the following:

tachypnea Rapid shallow breathing that may indicate pain, cardiac insufficiency, anemia, fever, or pulmonary problems.

bradypnea Slow breathing as a result of opiates, coma, excessive alcohol, and increased intracranial pressure.

hyperventilation Simultaneous rapid, deep breathing found in extreme anxiety states, in diabetic acidosis, and after vigorous exercise.

Cheyne-Stokes respiration Periodic breathing with *hyperpnea* (increased depth of breathing) alternating with *apnea* (cessation of breathing), encountered in cardiac failure and central nervous system disease.

sighing respiration Normal respiratory rhythm interrupted by a deep inspiration, followed by a prolonged expiration accompanied by an audible sigh. This variation is often associated with emotional depression.

dyspnea Concious difficulty or effort in breathing. When the patient assumes an elevated position of the trunk at rest to breathe more comfortably, this is called *orthopnea.* Dyspnea is a cardinal sign of left ventricular failure and may also occur in certain lung disorders.

obstructive breathing (air trapping) In obstructive pulmonary diseases such as emphysema and asthma, it is easier for air to enter the lungs than for it to leave. During rapid respiration, sufficient time for full expiration is not available and air becomes trapped in the lungs. The patient's chest overexpands and his breathing becomes more shallow. Expiratory wheezes may be present. Further examination of lung function is discussed later in this chapter.

Blood Pressure

Arterial Blood Pressure. Cardiac contraction maintains blood pressure in both arteries and veins. The arterial blood pressure is an overall reflection of the function of the ventricles as pumps. Blood pressure in the arterial system is represented by the peak systolic and diastolic levels of the pressure pulse and is modified by cardiac output, peripheral arteriolar resistance, distensibility of the arteries, amount of blood in the system, and viscosity of the blood. Accordingly, changes in blood pressure reflect changes in these measurements. For example, the decrease in vessel distensibility in the elderly lowers diastolic pressure and increases systolic pressure to produce systolic hypertension. Increments in blood volume may raise both systolic and diastolic components.

Normal blood pressure in the aorta and large arteries,

such as the brachial artery, varies between 100 and 140 mm Hg systolic and between 60 and 90 mm Hg diastolic. Pressure in the smaller arteries is somewhat less, and in the arterioles, where the blood enters the capillaries, it is about 35 mm Hg. However, wide variation of normal blood pressure exists, and a value may fall outside the normal range in healthy adults. The normal range also varies with age, sex, and race. A pressure reading of 100/60 may be normal for one person but hypotensive for another.

Observing changes in blood pressure and in pulse pressure (the difference between systolic and diastolic pressures and normally 30 to 50 mm Hg) is important in the care of a patient with an acute myocardial infarction. A reduction in blood pressure from a prior level of 150/100 mm Hg to 115/70 after myocardial infarction may indicate impending cardiovascular decompensation, such as congestive heart failure or shock. Tachycardia and pericardial tamponade also may reduce arterial pressure and narrow pulse pressure.

MEASUREMENT. Arterial blood pressure can be measured directly or indirectly. The *indirect* method is performed with a sphygmomanometer. It is a simple procedure and accurate enough for most determinations. With this method systolic pressures may be slightly below and diastolic pressures slightly above directly obtained values. Rather than measuring one complete beat, the indirect method measures the systolic pressure of some beats and the diastolic pressure of other beats; it does not measure a mean pressure.

For routine indirect blood pressure measurements the patient may be either sitting or reclining. In some cases blood pressure may change with body position, and in this situation the pressure should be recorded with the patient in reclining, sitting, and standing positions. To obtain a realistic measurement the patient should have the opportunity to relax for a while.

The collapsed cuff should be affixed snugly and smoothly to the patient's arm, with the distal margin of the cuff at least 2.5 cm above the antecubital fossa. The cuff width should be 40% of the circumference of the arm. The patient's arm should be rested on a table or a bed at heart level and the examiner should palpate for the location of the brachial artery pulse. Pressure in the cuff is then rapidly increased to a level about 30 mm Hg above the point at which the palpable pulse disappears. As the cuff is deflated, observations may be made by either palpation or auscultation. The point at which the pulse can be felt is recorded from the manometer as the palpatory systolic pressure. The auscultatory method is usually preferred; with this method, vibrations from the artery under pressure, called *Korotkoff sounds,* are used as indicators.

For auscultatory blood pressure measurement the bell or diaphragm of the stethoscope is pressed lightly over the brachial artery while the cuff is slowly deflated, and pressure readings begin at the time the sounds first become audible. As the cuff is deflated further, the sounds become louder for a brief period, then they become muffled and finally disappear. The systolic blood pressure is the point at which at least two consecutive beats become audible, and the diastolic blood pressure is the point at which the sounds cease to be heard. If sounds continue to zero pressure, as they may at times in aortic regurgitation and thyrotoxicosis, three values may be recorded: the first value is the point of audibility of sounds; the second value is when sounds become muffled; and the third value is zero, when sounds disappear. The second value should be accepted as the diastolic pressure, since a diastolic pressure of zero is impossible.

Although the sounds may disappear at a certain reading on the sphygmomanometer, one should continue to listen at zero pressure to detect the possible presence of the *auscultatory gap.* In this situation the examiner may first detect systolic sounds at a high level, only to have them suddenly disappear and then reappear at a lower level. For example, sounds may be heard first at 180 mm Hg, disappear at 160 mm Hg, and then reappear at 120 mm Hg. This phenomenon is depicted in Fig. 4-4. One can appreciate the problem only by inflating the cuff to 150 mm Hg. In

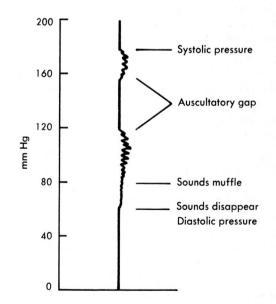

FIG. 4-4. Detection of auscultatory gap in blood pressure measurement. The systolic sounds are first heard at 180 mm Hg. They disappear at 160 mm Hg and reappear at 120 mm Hg; the silent interval is called the auscultatory gap. The Korotkoff sounds muffle at 80 mm Hg and disappear at 60 mm Hg. The blood pressure is recorded as 180/80/60 with auscultatory gap.

this instance the patient might be considered normotensive when actually he is hypertensive.

The patient's blood pressure should be checked in both arms, and any difference should be noted. A difference of 5 mm Hg may exist. If the patient has hypertension or reduced pulses in the lower extremities, blood pressure readings are also taken in the legs. In this situation the cuff is placed around the lower third of the thigh and the stethoscope is applied to the popliteal artery. In the event that the thigh is too thick for cuff placement the examiner may place the cuff around the calf and palpate the dorsalis pedis or posterior tibial pulse. The blood pressure in the leg should be equal to or slightly greater than that in the brachial artery. If the patient has hypertension, is taking medication that may affect blood pressure, or is just beginning to ambulate following a period of bed rest, it is also important to check the blood pressure in the standing, sitting, and supine positions.

Direct measurement of arterial pressure may be indicated for the patient in shock whose blood pressure is too low to be determined accurately by the cuff method. It also may be useful in managing patients who have a low blood volume or who are being treated with drugs for hypertension or hypotension. An arterial catheter, in addition to directly measuring blood pressure, provides continuous recording without disturbing the patient and allows frequent blood sampling to determine blood gas levels and arterial pH during the management of patients with cardiogenic shock or respiratory insufficiency and those using mechanical ventilators.

For direct measurement of arterial blood pressure, a needle or catheter is inserted into the brachial, radial, or femoral artery. A catheter may be advanced centrally into the aorta or even into the left ventricle. A catheter in the central aorta permits accurate assessment of the diastolic and mean aortic pressures and is very important for the patient who has a myocardial infarction because these pressures may significantly affect coronary blood flow. Catheters should not remain in the left ventricle or ascending arch of the aorta proximal to the origin of the cephalic arteries because of the risk of embolization. They may be maintained safely in the subclavian artery or the descending thoracic aorta for several hours or even several days with proper attention.

A plastic tube filled with heparinized saline solution connects the catheter to a pressure-sensitive device or a strain-gauge transducer. This device converts the mechanical energy that the blood exerts on the recording membrane into changes in electrical voltage or current that can be calibrated in millimeters of mercury. The electrical signal can then be transmitted to an electronic recorder and an oscilloscope, which continually record and display the pressure waves. The transducer and oscilloscope method is more accurate than the sphygmomanometer method and yields an electrically integrated mean pressure.

On the oscilloscopes, the arterial pressure waveforms for the brachial and radial arteries appear identical. The more distal the catheter is from the aorta, the higher the systolic pressure, resulting from the amplification effect in the arterial system during systole. The normal arterial waveform should be clearly discernible, reflecting a rapid upstroke to the peak of systolic pressure, followed by a more gradual downslope. Approximately at the end of ventricular systole, a secondary smaller upstroke, termed the *dicrotic notch* and caused by a rebound against the closing aortic valve, occurs (see Fig. 4-2, *A*). The accuracy of intraarterial pressure readings depends on accurate catheter placement, solid connections between the parts of the system, and arterial line patency. Further discussion of arterial monitoring can be found in Chapter 7.

Venous Blood Pressure. In addition to evaluating the contour of the jugular venous pulse, one can obtain further information about the right side of the heart by determining the level of venous pressure. Venous pressure refers to the pressure exerted within the venous system by the blood. It is highest in the venules of the extremities and lowest at the point where the vena cava enters the heart. Venous blood flow is continuous rather than pulsatory. In the arm, venous pressure normally ranges from 5 to 14 cm H_2O and in the inferior vena cava, from 6 to 8 cm H_2O. Blood volume, tone of the vessel wall, patency of veins, competence of venous valves, function of the right heart, respiratory function, and force of gravity all influence venous pressure. The veins most commonly used in this estimation are the hand and arm veins, the internal jugular veins, and the external jugular veins.

MEASUREMENT. When the examiner is using the veins on the dorsum of the hand to determine venous pressure, the patient should be sitting with his hand held sufficiently below the level of the heart to permit venous distention. As the arm is slowly raised, one can observe the level at which venous collapse occurs. Normally this occurs when the dorsum of the hand reaches a point just above the sternal notch. In cases of elevated venous pressure, the vertical distance above the sternal notch at which the veins collapse provides a rough estimate of the venous pressure.

The *external jugular vein* is commonly used because of its easy accessibility. It is considered less reliable in determining venous pressure than the internal jugular veins, since it is smaller and takes a less direct route to the superior vena cava. To evaluate the pressure in the external jugular vein, the examiner should have the patient recline with the trunk elevated at an angle of 30 to 60 degrees and the head rotated slightly away from the vein being examined. Slight elevation is important because the external jugular veins are normally collapsed above the level of the suprasternal notch when the person is upright. The examiner gradually elevates the head of the bed or table until venous distention is visible. The examiner then occludes the external jugular vein by pressing the neck just above and parallel to the clavicle. After waiting approximately 20 seconds for the vein to fill, the examiner quickly withdraws the finger and observes the height of the distended fluid column within the vein. If visible at all, the level will normally be less than 3 to 5 cm above the sternal angle of Louis (Fig. 4-5).

As previously mentioned, the *internal jugular vein* is the most reliable indicator of indirect venous pressure as well as venous pulse waveform. The patient's trunk should be elevated to the optimum angle for the observation of venous pulse. The highest point of visible pulsation of the internal jugular vein is determined and the vertical distance between this level and the level of the sternal angle of Louis is recorded. The angle of elevation of the patient should also be recorded.

It is important to note that the sternal angle is used as a bedside reference point for the sake of convenience. The ideal reference level for venous pressure measurement is the midpoint of the right atrium. This level is established by running an imaginary anteroposterior line from the

fourth interspace halfway to the back. A horizontal plane through this point is the zero level for the measurement of venous pressure. The vertical distance from this plane to the head of the blood column, or the meniscus, approximates the venous pressure (Fig. 4-6). Elevations of pressure above 10 cm H_2O are considered abnormal.

CENTRAL VENOUS PRESSURE. The direct measurement of central venous pressure (CVP) becomes important if there is a doubt about the value obtained by indirect measurement, or when monitoring a critically ill patient, a situation in which CVP is considered an important sign to follow.

The CVP indicates right arterial pressure, which primarily reflects alterations in right ventricular pressure and only secondarily reflects changes in the pulmonary venous pressure or the pressure in the left side of the heart. The CVP provides valuable information about blood volume and the adequacy of central venous return.

CVP can be obtained by inserting a polyethylene catheter into the external jugular, antecubital, or femoral vein and threading it into the vena cava. The medial antecubital veins are used more commonly than the others. The catheter offers a method of CVP measurement as well as an

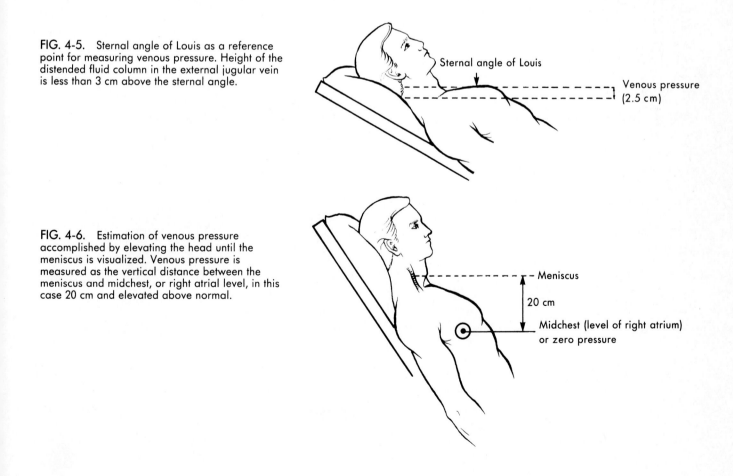

FIG. 4-5. Sternal angle of Louis as a reference point for measuring venous pressure. Height of the distended fluid column in the external jugular vein is less than 3 cm above the sternal angle.

Sternal angle of Louis

Venous pressure (2.5 cm)

FIG. 4-6. Estimation of venous pressure accomplished by elevating the head until the meniscus is visualized. Venous pressure is measured as the vertical distance between the meniscus and midchest, or right atrial level, in this case 20 cm and elevated above normal.

Meniscus

20 cm

Midchest (level of right atrium) or zero pressure

intravenous route for drawing blood samples, administering fluid or medications, performing phlebotomy, and possibly inserting a pacing catheter.

The procedure for setting up the CVP system is as follows:

1. Using a three-way stopcock, attach the catheter to a water manometer and an intravenous infusion line. When the venous pressure is not being read, the stopcock is adjusted so that the intravenous fluid will run through the catheter and keep it patent.
2. Mount the manometer on a pole by placing the zero marking at the level of the right atrium. The level of the right atrium can be determined by placing the patient flat and measuring 5 cm down from the top of the chest at the fourth interspace. Run a yardstick from the patient's chest to the baseline of the manometer.
3. Flush the line as necessary to maintain patency.
4. To prevent infection, place an antibiotic ointment and a 2 × 2 inch dressing over the catheter insertion site.

The procedure for measuring CVP is as follows:

1. Place the patient flat in bed and be certain that the zero point of the manometer is at the level of the right atrium.
2. Determine patency of the catheter by opening the intravenous infusion line briefly to a rapid flow rate.

3. Turn the stopcock to allow the intravenous solution to run into the manometer to a level of 10 to 20 cm above the expected pressure reading.
4. Turn the stopcock to allow the intravenous solution to flow from the manometer into the catheter. The fluid level in the manometer falls rapidly and fluctuates during respiration, decreasing with inspiration and increasing with expiration. Ventilatory assistance should be stopped during the measurement.
5. When the fluid level is constant, read the CVP. Some fluctuation occurs during respiration.
6. After the reading has been obtained, return the stopcock to the intravenous infusion position.

The normal CVP range is 4 to 10 cm H_2O. The CVP may be measured either in centimeters of water or in millimeters of mercury. The value in centimeters of water may be converted to millimeters of mercury by dividing the former by 1.36, since 1 mm Hg = 1.36 cm H_2O.

Abnormal CVPs must be interpreted according to the clinical situation and other considerations—urine output, skin turgor, temperature, systemic blood pressure, heart rate, and so on. An elevated CVP (above 10 cm H_2O) may indicate right ventricular failure secondary to left-sided heart failure, pulmonary disease such as pulmonary hypertension or embolism, or cardiac tamponade. A low CVP (below 4 cm H_2O) may indicate hypovolemia or peripheral blood pooling, as in septic shock. Taking a single CVP

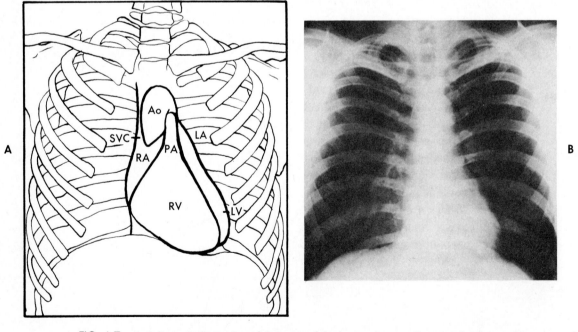

FIG. 4-7. **A,** Schematic illustration of the parts of the heart whose outlines can be detected in B. *Ao,* Aorta; *SVC,* superior vena cava; *RA,* right atrium; *PA,* pulmonary artery; *LA,* left atrium; *RV,* right ventricle; *LV,* left ventricle. **B,** Frontal projection x-ray film of the normal cardiac silhouette.

value is less useful than noting repeated measurements, particularly after administering a challenge volume load. Further discussion of this measurement appears in Chapter 7.

Inspection and Palpation of the Heart

The anterior part of the chest is inspected with the patient in a supine position and the trunk elevated to about a 30-degree angle. The patient's chest should be bared from the waist to the shoulders. The approach should be made from the patient's right side. Certain landmarks on the anterior chest wall are useful as points of reference in describing the location of the heart. The heart rests on the diaphragm and is located beneath and to the left of the sternum. The base of the heart is situated approximately at the level of the third rib; the apex of the heart lies approximately at the level of the fifth rib in the midclavicular line. The anterior surface of the heart proceeding from the examiner's left to right, facing the patient, is composed of the right atrium, right ventricle, and left ventricle (Fig. 4-7). The anterior surface of the chest closest to the heart and aorta is called the *precordium.*

Inspection begins by observing the precordium for abnormal pulsations. Tangential lighting may be helpful in detecting these pulsations. Any visible impulse medial to the apex and in the third, fourth, or fifth interspace generally originates in the right ventricle and is usually abnormal. The point of maximal impulse (PMI) may be normally visible between the fourth and sixth intercostal space just medial to the left midclavicular line. However, it is also normal not to see this impulse. In pronounced right ventricular enlargement, one can usually see the lower sternum heave with the heartbeat. It is important to determine when the movements occur by correlating them with the heart sounds or carotid artery pulsations.

Following inspection, palpation of the precordium is performed to confirm the findings of inspection and to locate further impulses and thrills. The palmar bases of the fingers are used, since this area is most sensitive to feeling vibrations. First palpate the areas where pulsations are visible, then feel specific areas of the precordium systematically (Fig. 4-8).

Aortic Area. The second interspace to the right of the sternum is felt for a pulsation, thrill, or vibration of aortic valve closure. Abnormal pulsations may be produced by dilatation of the ascending aorta. A vibratory thrill is associated with aortic stenosis, and an accentuated aortic valve closure is felt in patients with arterial hypertension. Thrills at the base can best be palpated with the patient sitting up and leaning forward.

Pulmonic Area. The second and third left interspaces are evaluated for abnormalities in the pulmonary artery or valve. A relatively slow, sustained, and forceful pulsation of the pulmonary artery may be felt in mitral stenosis and primary pulmonary hypertension. A palpable sustained pulse and a thrill are associated with pulmonary stenosis.

Right Ventricular Area. The lower left sternal border, incorporating the third, fourth, and fifth intercostal spaces, is palpated. Abnormal pulsations here are most commonly found in conditions associated with right ventricular enlargement. When the sternum can be felt to move anteriorly during systole, this movement is termed a *substernal heave* or *lift*. Furthermore, a thrill in this area may be palpated in patients who have a ventricular septal defect.

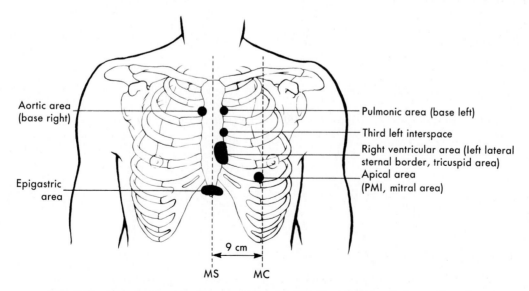

Aortic area (base right)

Pulmonic area (base left)

Third left interspace

Right ventricular area (left lateral sternal border, tricuspid area)

Apical area (PMI, mitral area)

Epigastric area

9 cm

MS   MC

FIG. 4-8. Palpation areas on the precordium for detecting normal and abnormal cardiac pulsations. See text for description.

Apical Area. The fifth intercostal space at or just medial to the left midclavicular line is palpated for the *point of maximum impulse* (PMI) and the thrills of mitral valve disease. The PMI is evaluated for its location, diameter, amplitude, and duration. In normal adults the PMI is located at or within the left midclavicular line in the fifth intercostal space (Fig. 4-8). The impulse is normally less than 2 cm in diameter and often is smaller. It is felt as a light tap, beginning approximately at the time of the first heart sound, and is sustained during the first one third and one half of systole.

When the PMI is displaced lateral to the midclavicular line, it indicates left ventricular enlargement. A weak PMI may be palpated and may indicate inadequate stroke volume or reduced left ventricular contraction. This finding is difficult to detect in a muscular or obese chest or in patients with emphysema. A sustained or forceful apical impulse usually indicates left ventricular enlargement, such as that associated with aortic stenosis or arterial hypertension. A diffuse systolic thrill may be found in patients with mitral regurgitation, whereas a localized diastolic thrill generally is associated with mitral stenosis. Thrills at the apex are best felt with the patient in the left lateral decubitus position. This maneuver helps one find the impulse, but since this position displaces the PMI, no assessment can be made about location.

Epigastric Area. The upper central region of the abdomen can have visible or palpable pulsations in some normal individuals. Abnormally large pulsations of the aorta may be produced by an aneurysm of the abdominal aorta or by aortic valvular regurgitation. In right ventric-

ular hypertrophy right ventricular pulsations may also be detected in this area, which may be the best location to palpate the apical impulse in a patient with a distended chest, as in emphysema. To distinguish aortic from right ventricular pulsations, the palm of the hand should be placed on the epigastric area, sliding the fingers up under the rib cage. The palmar surface feels the aorta pulsating as the fingertips feel the impulses of the right ventricle.

Auscultation of the Heart

Listening over the precordium with a stethoscope remains the most useful physical examination technique for providing information about heart function. Since the examiner depends on the stethoscope to register normal and abnormal sounds for interpretation, attention must be given to selection of the proper instrument. The stethoscope should have properly fitting earpieces, double tubes that are approximately 12 inches long and ⅛ inch in internal diameter, a bell, and a diaphragm. The bell accentuates the lower frequency sounds, such as diastolic gallops and the rumbling murmur of mitral stenosis, and filters out high-pitched notes. It should be placed very lightly on the skin, with just enough pressure to seal the edge of the unit. More pressure on the bell will cause the skin itself to act as a diaphragm, accentuating high-frequency sounds. Since the diaphragm brings out high-pitched sounds, it should be pressed very firmly against the skin. This will make high-frequency murmurs, such as the murmurs of aortic or mitral insufficiency, audible.

The environment and the patient's position also play important parts in the auscultation procedure. The room

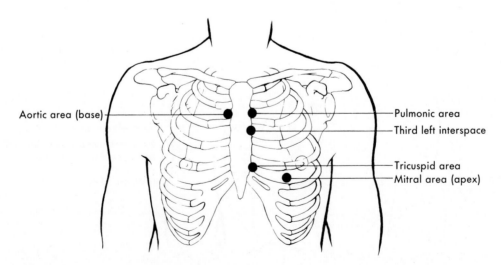

FIG. 4-9. Topographic areas on the precordium for cardiac auscultation. Auscultatory areas do not correspond to the anatomic locations of the valves but to the sites at which the particular valves are heard best. See text for description.

should be quiet and the patient should be on a table or bed that will accommodate him comfortably when he is asked to lie flat, sit up, or roll to one side.

Finally, auscultation of the heart should not be performed as an isolated event. The findings should be correlated with the other results of the physical examination, such as the arterial pulse contour, venous pulse waves, and precordial movements, to understand the altered cardiac physiology and anatomy.

Auscultation of the heart requires selective listening for each component of the cardiac cycle as the examiner inches the stethoscope over the five main topographic areas for cardiac auscultation (Fig. 4-9). Note that these auscultatory areas do not correspond to the anatomic locations of the valves, but rather to the sites at which the particular valve sounds are best heard. Accordingly, one listens with the stethoscope over the following areas:

1. *Aortic area* at the base of the heart in the second right intercostal space close to the sternum
2. *Pulmonic area* at the second left intercostal space close to the sternum
3. *Third left intercostal space* where murmurs of both aortic and pulmonic origin may be heard
4. *Tricuspid area* at the lower left sternal border
5. *Mitral area* at the apex of the heart in the fifth left intercostal space just medial to the midclavicular line

Auscultation is conducted in a systematic fashion. By beginning the process at the aortic area, one can determine the cardiac cycle time by identifying the first and second heart sounds. This will serve as a frame of reference as the examiner moves to other auscultatory areas of the precordium. The diaphragm of the stethoscope is used first to evaluate the high-pitched sounds, S_1 and S_2. The bell is used to detect lower-pitched sounds such as S_3 and S_4. At each site the procedure is as follows:

1. Listen to the first heart sound, noting its intensity and splitting.
2. Listen to the second heart sound, noting its intensity and splitting.
3. Note extra sounds in systole, identifying their timing, intensity, and pitch.
4. Note extra sounds in diastole, identifying their timing, intensity, and pitch.
5. Listen for systolic and diastolic murmurs, noting their timing, intensity, quality, pitch, location, and radiation.
6. Listen for extracardiac sounds, such as a pericardial friction rub.

If an abnormal sound is detected, the surrounding area is carefully explored to evaluate the distribution or radiation of the sound. The patient's position should be changed for better evaluation of abnormal sounds. For example, an aortic murmur may be heard best by having the patient sitting, leaning forward, exhaling, and holding the breath. Or an initial murmur or an S_3 may be heard by positioning the patient on his or her left side and listening to the apical area. Changes with respiration or during Valsalva maneuver may be important.

Changes in the intensity of heart sounds may be clinically significant. The intensity of valve sounds is probably related to the speed and force of the valve closure, the excursion of leaflets during closure, and the physical condition of the cusps. Intensity is modified by the proximity of the valve to the chest wall and by the nature of the tissues interposed between valve and stethoscope. Accordingly, the first sound heard at the mitral area (apex) may not only become softer at the aortic area (base), but may also seem shorter and have a different quality, which is caused by the dampening effect of the interposed soft tissues. Similarly, the second sound loses intensity as the stethoscope is moved toward the apex. The diagrams in Fig. 4-10 indicate the intensity and splitting of the first and second heart sounds, their relationship to the third and fourth heart sounds, and the auscultatory areas where these sounds can be heard best.

First Heart Sound (S_1). S_1 is associated with the closure of the mitral and tricuspid valves. It is synchronous with the apical impulse and corresponds to the onset of ventricular systole (Fig. 4-11). It is louder, longer, and lower pitched than the second sound at the apex (Fig. 4-10, *A*). As the ventricles begin to contract and pressure rises within, the tricuspid and mitral valves close. Valvular sounds of the left side slightly precede those of the right and are of higher intensity; the mitral valve closes from 0.02 to 0.03 second before the tricuspid valve. *Splitting* of the first sound may therefore be heard, particularly in the tricuspid area (Fig. 4-10, *B*). Tricuspid closure is normally inaudible to the examiner's ear. The intensity of S_1 relates to the relative position of atrial contraction with respect to ventricular contraction, that is, PR interval. When the PR interval is prolonged, the intensity of the first heart sound is decreased, and when the PR interval shortens up to a point, the S_1 is increased. During AV dissociation the intensity of the first sound varies as the PR interval varies.

As the pressure within the ventricles continues to rise and exceeds the pressure within the pulmonary artery and aorta, the pulmonic and aortic valves open. Opening of these valves is usually inaudible. If opening of the aortic valve is heard, this is called an aortic ejection sound or click. The same is true for the pulmonic valve. *Early systolic ejection clicks* occur shortly after S_1, as depicted in Fig. 4-11. Aortic ejection clicks are associated with aortic stenosis, dilatation of the aorta, and hypertension and are heard at both the base and the apex. Pulmonary ejection clicks are associated with pulmonary stenosis, dilatation of the pulmonary artery, and pulmonary hypertension and are heard

HEART SOUNDS   AREA HEARD BEST

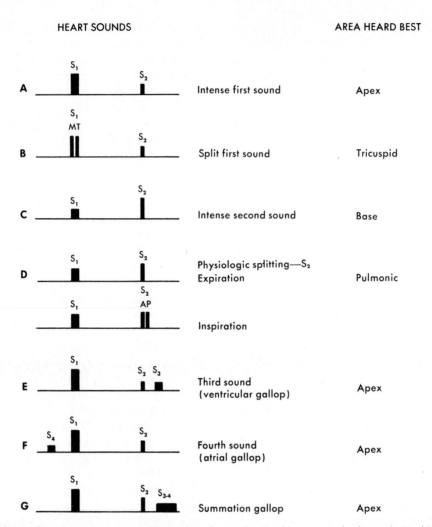

FIG. 4-10.   The intensity and splitting of the first and second heart sounds, their relationship to the third and fourth heart sounds, and the auscultatory areas where these sounds are heard best.

in the pulmonic area. A common syndrome is the single or multiple midsystolic click that imitates a late systolic murmur of mitral insufficiency, caused by prolapse of the mitral valve. The click in this instance is a nonejection click.

Second Heart Sound (S₂). S_2 is associated with the closure of the aortic and pulmonic valves. With the completion of ventricular contraction the pressure within the ventricles and great vessels decreases. The ventricular pressure decreases more rapidly than the pressures within the aorta and pulmonary arteries, causing the aortic and pulmonic valves to close. This is followed by the start of ventricular diastole. At the aortic area, or base, the second sound is almost always louder than the first sound (Fig. 4-10, C).

The aortic component is widely transmitted to the neck and over the precordium. It is, as a rule, entirely responsible

for the second sound at the apex. The pulmonary component is softer than the aortic and is normally heard only at and around the second left interspace (pulmonic area). Splitting of the second sound is therefore usually heard best in this region.

Again, events of the left side of the heart occur before those on the right, and aortic valve closure slightly precedes that of the pulmonic valve. Transient *splitting* of the second sound may be demonstrated in most normal people during inspiration. Closure of the aortic and pulmonary valves during expiration is synchronous or nearly so because right and left ventricular systoles are approximately equal in duration. With inspiration, venous blood rushes into the thorax from the large systemic venous reservoirs. This action increases venous return and prolongs right ventricular systole by temporarily increasing right ventricular stroke vol-

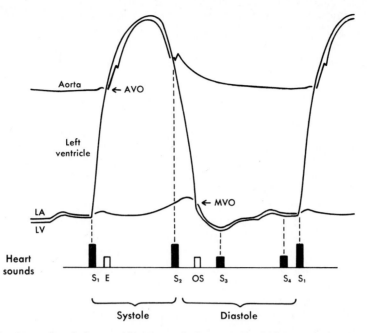

FIG. 4-11.   Normal and abnormal heart sounds during one complete cardiac cycle as correlated with left-sided heart pressure waves. Right-sided heart pressures have been omitted for simplification. At the onset of ventricular systole, left ventricular *(LV)* pressure exceeds left atrial *(LA)* pressure to close the mitral valve, producing S_1 (in association with tricuspid valve closure). When LV pressure exceeds aortic pressure, the aortic valve opens *(AVO)*. With valvular disease and hypertension, aortic valve opening may be audible and heard as an early ejection click *(E)*. When aortic pressure exceeds LV pressure, the aortic valve closes to produce S_2 in association with pulmonic valve closure. When LV pressure drops below LA pressure, the mitral valve opens *(MVO)*. With thickening of the mitral valve as a result of rheumatic heart disease an opening snap *(OS)* is produced in early diastole. During rapid ventricular filling an S_3, or ventricular gallop, is produced in patients with myocardial failure. Late in diastole an S_4, or atrial gallop, is produced in association with atrial contraction, owing to increased resistance to ventricular filling.

ume, which delays pulmonary valve closure. At the same time, venous return to the left heart diminishes because of the increased pulmonary capacity during inspiration, which decreases left ventricular stroke volume and shortens left ventricular systole. Thus the aortic valve tends to close earlier. These two factors combine to produce transient *physiologic splitting* of the second sound (Fig. 4-10, *D*).

As the pressure in the ventricles decreases below the pressure in the atria, the atrioventricular valves open. The opening of these valves is characteristically silent. However, when either the mitral or the tricuspid valve is thickened or otherwise altered, as by rheumatic heart disease, it produces an *opening snap* in early diastole (Fig. 4-11). The opening snap of the mitral valve is differentiated from a third heart sound at the apex because it occurs earlier, is sharper and higher pitched, and radiates more widely.

Third Heart Sound (S_3). S_3 occurs early in diastole during the phase of rapid ventricular filling, about 0.12 to 0.16 second after S_2 (Fig. 4-11). It is a low-pitched sound, heard best with the bell of the stethoscope pressed lightly over the apex and the patient in the left lateral decubitus

position (Fig. 4-10, *E*). When S_3 is heard in healthy children and young adults, it is called a *physiologic third heart sound* and usually disappears with age. When an S_3 is heard in an older person with heart disease, it usually indicates myocardial failure and is called a *ventricular gallop*. In patients with cardiac disease, one should search carefully for the presence of a ventricular gallop, since it is a key diagnostic sign for the presence of congestive heart failure from any cause.

Fourth Heart Sound (S_4). S_4 occurs late in diastole, prior to S_1, and is related to atrial contraction (Fig. 4-11). It is a low-pitched sound heard best at the apex with the bell (Fig. 4-10, *F*). It is uncommon to hear this sound in normal individuals. S_4, or *atrial gallop*, is associated with increased resistance to ventricular filling and is frequently heard in hypertensive cardiovascular disease, coronary artery disease, myocardiopathy, and aortic stenosis. It is a common finding in patients who have had a myocardial infarction. An S_4 may also be heard in patients with AV block where there is a delayed conduction between the atria and the ventricles.

Summation Gallop. In adults with severe myocardial disease and tachycardia, summation of S_3 and S_4 may occur, producing the so-called summation gallop (Fig. 4-10, *G*).

Murmurs. Although the physical principles governing the production of murmurs are complex, from a practical point of view murmurs are related to three main factors, which are as follows:

1. High rates of flow, either through normal or abnormal valves
2. Forward flow through a constricted or deformed valve or into a dilated vessel or chamber
3. Backward flow through a regurgitant valve

The identification of murmurs may contribute important information to the recognition and diagnosis of heart disease. Accordingly, murmurs should be carefully evaluated and described in a manner that provides maximum information. Murmurs are usually characterized in relation to the following criteria:

1. *Timing.* Does the murmur occur during systole, during diastole, or continuously through both? A murmur may be easily differentiated as systolic or diastolic by palpating the pulse. If the murmur occurs simultaneously with the pulse, it is systolic; if it does not, it is diastolic. If a murmur occupies all the time period measured, it is described as holosystolic (pansystolic) or holodiastolic (pandiastolic).
2. *Intensity.* How loud is the murmur? A graded point system is generally accepted to describe the intensity of murmurs, as follows:

   Grade 1: Softest audible murmur
   Grade 2: Murmur of medium intensity
   Grade 3: Loud murmur unaccompanied by thrill
   Grade 4: Murmur with thrill
   Grade 5: Loudest murmur that cannot be heard with the stethoscope off the chest, thrill associated
   Grade 6: Murmur audible with the stethoscope off the chest, thrill associated

3. *Quality.* What is the tonal characteristic of the murmur? Is it harsh? Musical? Blowing? Rumbling? The configuration or shape of a murmur further defines its quality. It may be a crescendo (increasing intensity), decrescendo (decreasing intensity), or crescendo-decrescendo (diamond-shaped) type. Fig. 4-12 depicts these configurations.
4. *Pitch.* What is the sound frequency of the murmur? Is it high? Medium? Low? If the murmur is heard best with the diaphragm of the stethoscope, it is high pitched. If it is heard best with the bell of the stethoscope it is low pitched. If it is heard equally well with either the bell or the diaphragm, it is medium pitched.
5. *Location.* Over what area on the precordium is the murmur heard best? The aortic area? The pulmonic area? The triscuspid area? The mitral area?
6. *Radiation.* Is there transmission of the murmur elsewhere in the body? Does it radiate across the chest? Into the axilla? Into the neck? Down the left sternal border?

In addition, each of these characteristics is further evaluated as it is influenced by the patient's position and respiration. Asking the patient to sit up, exhale, lean forward and hold his or her breath may make aortic murmurs easier to hear. The left lateral decubitus position makes mitral murmurs more easily heard. Certain other maneuvers may be used to define murmurs further, including Valsalva's maneuver, which decreases cardiac output and stroke volume during the strain and increases flow after release. Also, amyl nitrite can be administered, with resultant peripheral vasodilatation and increased cardiac output. Changes in the intensity and character of murmurs with these maneuvers aid in determining the type of lesion involved. For instance, with the administration of amyl nitrite, murmurs associated with stenotic lesions usually become louder, whereas regurgitant murmurs decrease in intensity.

SYSTOLIC MURMURS. Systolic murmurs are the most common murmurs and generally are either ejection or regurgitant murmurs. *Functional* or innocent systolic murmurs are commonly heard in young people and should be distinguished from those murmurs that represent valvular heart disease. Functional murmurs occur during ejection, are short (less than two thirds of systole), are grade 2 or less in intensity (they may become inaudible if the patient raises from a supine to a sitting position), and are heard best over the pulmonary outflow tract. It is important to remember that functional murmurs are intensified by fever, anxiety, anemia, and pregnancy. Therefore the patient should be reexamined under normal conditions.

MIDSYSTOLIC (EJECTION) MURMURS. *Aortic stenosis* and *pulmonic stenosis* produce systolic ejection murmurs that begin after the first sound, swell to a crescendo in midsystole, then decrease in intensity, and terminate before S_2, generated by closure of the appropriate valve (Fig. 4-12, *A*). The murmur may be harsh or musical and is usually high pitched because of the high velocity of blood flow. Aortic valve murmurs frequently radiate from the second right interspace to the cardiac apex and the carotid arteries. A systolic thrill may be present. Characteristically, pulmonic stenosis murmur is heard better at the second left interspace. Atrial septal defects increase pulmonary flow to produce a pulmonary ejection murmur.

HOLOSYSTOLIC (REGURGITANT) MURMURS. Holosystolic murmurs last throughout ventricular systole (Fig. 4-12, *B*) and no interval can be heard between S_1 and S_2. *Tricuspid* and *mitral regurgitation* and *ventricular septal defects* produce holosystolic murmurs owing to the backflow

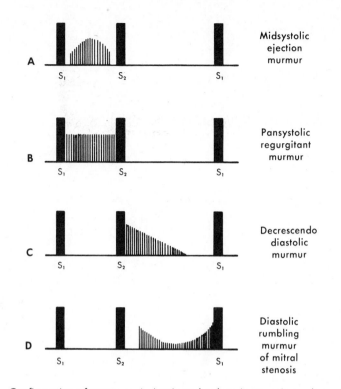

FIG. 4-12.   Configuration of murmurs. A, Aortic and pulmonic stenosis produce systolic ejection murmurs that begin after the S₁, swell to a crescendo in midsystole, then decrease in intensity (decrescendo), and terminate before the S₂. B, Tricuspid and mitral regurgitation and ventricular septal defects produce pansystolic (holosystolic) murmurs that last throughout ventricular systole; usually no interval can be heard between S₁ and S₂. C, Aortic and pulmonic regurgitation produce murmurs that begin early in diastole immediately after the S₂ and then diminish in intensity (decrescendo). D, Mitral and tricuspid stenosis produce murmurs that begin during early diastole, have a rumbling or rolling quality, and terminate in late diastole with a crescendo effect.

of blood from the ventricle (high pressure) to the atrium (low pressure) through an incompetent tricuspid or mitral valve or from a high-pressure ventricle (left) to a low-pressure ventricle (right). Unlike the production of ejection murmurs, when a holosystolic murmur is produced one chamber maintains a greater pressure than the other throughout *all* of systole, causing regurgitant blood flow (and the murmur) to last through the entire systolic period. Murmurs caused by ventricular septal defects may seem louder during early systole and those of mitral regurgitation louder during late systole. The murmurs may be blowing, musical, or harsh and are often high pitched. The tricuspid regurgitation murmur is best heard along the lower left sternal border, and the intensity commonly increases during inspiration. Mitral regurgitation is best heard at the apex with the patient lying on his left side and often radiates to the left axilla or back. Some forms of mitral regurgitation do not produce holosystolic murmurs. Ventricular septal defects are loudest at the third and fourth left interspaces along the sternal border; often a systolic thrill accompanies the murmur in that area.

During the acute phase of myocardial infarction the *interventricular septum* may *rupture*. Although uncommon, the resulting ventricular septal defect produces a loud systolic murmur, as described previously. The onset of this murmur is sudden, and it may be accompanied by a thrill and the features of left-sided and right-sided heart failure.

Myocardial infarction may also produce *papillary muscle rupture,* with subsequent mitral insufficiency and predominantly left-sided heart failure. The onset of the murmur is abrupt and may be difficult to distinguish from that of the perforated interventricular septum, since the features of both catastrophes overlap. Mitral valve dysfunction, without actual rupture of the papillary muscle or chordae tendineae, may establish less severe mitral insufficiency. Abnormalities of the chordae tendineae may produce clicking sounds that occur in the middle of ventricular systole and are referred to as *midsystolic clicks.* These may occur with or without a late systolic murmur. *Ventricular aneurysms* secondary to myocardial infarction may produce muffled heart sounds, gallop rhythms, and both systolic

TABLE 4-1. Characteristics of types of valvular heart disease

Time	Description of Murmurs				Other Signs	Condition	Causes
	Quality	Pitch (Frequency)	Location of Maximum Intensity	Radiation or Transmission			
Systolic (ejection)	Crescendo-decrescendo (diamond shaped) Harsh Rough	Variable pitch	Second interspace (aortic area)	Radiates to carotid arteries and apex	Slow rising "anacrotic" Sustained pulse Left ventricular lift Systolic thrill Ejection "click" Diminished aortic closing sound	Aortic stenosis (narrowing of valve)	Rheumatic Calcification Congenital
Diastolic	Blowing loudest just after S₂—diminishes during diastole decrescendo	High pitch	Second right interspace; third left interspace or along left sternal border with patient leaning forward and holding breath		Wide pulse pressure Left ventricular lift Brisk, quick pulses (water hammer) Tambour aortic closing sound	Aortic regurgitation (blood flows back from aorta into left ventricle)	Rheumatic Syphilitic Calcification Cystic medial necrosis
Diastolic	Rumbling, presystolic accentuation in sinus rhythm	Low pitch	Well localized to apex, best heard in left lateral decubitus position		Atrial fibrillation often develops Loud S₁ Opening snap	Mitral stenosis (narrowing of valve; blood flows through valve during diastole)	Rheumatic Congenital Tumor (myxoma)
Holosystolic	Blowing	High pitch	Apex, best heard in left lateral decubitus position	Axilla and back	S₃ common	Mitral regurgitation ("leaky" valve—blood reenters left atrium from left ventricle during systole)	Rheumatic Congenital Papillary muscle dysfunction/rupture Chordae tendineae dysfunction/rupture Heart failure associated with left ventricular dilation from any cause
Variable Late systolic can become holosystolic Decreased venous return (sitting, standing and Valsalva's maneuver) will cause murmur earlier in systole Increased venous return (squatting, lying down, elevating legs) causes murmur later in systole	Crescendo-decrescendo whooping, honking	High	Apex with patient in left lateral decubitus position		Loud mitral component of S₁, early midsystolic or late systolic nonejection click, intermittent atrial and ventricular arrhythmias	Mitral valve prolapse syndrome-billowing upward and backward of one or both valve leaflets into the left atrium during systole	Marfan's syndrome Rheumatic endocarditis Mitral valve surgery Trauma Lupus erythematosus Congestive cardiomyopathy

and diastolic murmurs; often a prominent systolic impulse may be palpated over the left precordium.

DIASTOLIC MURMURS. Diastolic murmurs generally can be classified into two types: the high-pitched decrescendo murmurs of aortic and pulmonic regurgitation and the lower-pitched mumurs of mitral and tricuspid stenosis.

Murmurs of aortic and pulmonic regurgitation begin early in diastole, immediately after the S_2, and then diminish in intensity (decrescendo), as shown in Fig. 4-12, *C*. They are high pitched and blowing and may vary in intensity roughly according to the size of the leak. The murmur of aortic regurgitation may be heard best at the second right or third left interspace along the left sternal border with the patient holding his breath in expiration while leaning forward. The murmur of pulmonic regurgitation is heard at the upper left border of the sternum and cannot be distinguished from its aortic counterpart by auscultation alone. The pitch, timing, quality, and location of these murmurs are similar, although the murmur of pulmonic regurgitation tends to be more localized in the pulmonic area.

Mitral stenosis characteristically produces a low-pitched, localized apical, diastolic rumble, which may be accentuated in late diastole (Fig. 4-12, *D*) when atrial systole causes increased flow across the narrowed mitral valve. A sharp mitral "opening snap" frequently imitates the murmur in early diastole. In addition, a loud, sharp S_1 and accentuation of the S_2 often accompany mitral stenosis. The murmur of mitral stenosis is usually confined to the apex and may be enhanced by mild exercise or by the patient's lying on his left side. The *tricuspid stenosis* murmur is heard near the tricuspid area and is often accentuated along the left sternal border by inspiration.

CONTINUOUS MURMURS. Murmurs audible in both systole and diastole are usually caused by connections between the arterial and venous or systemic and pulmonary circulations. A patent ductus arteriosus produces such a murmur. Table 4-1 summarizes the characteristics of the most common heart murmurs.

A benign sound heard at the lower border of the sternocleidomastoid muscle in some normal adults in the sitting position is called a *venous hum*. Although continuous, the venous hum is loudest in diastole and radiates to the first and second interspaces, with a soft to moderate intensity. It has a roaring quality, is low pitched, and can be obliterated by pressure on the jugular veins.

PERICARDIAL FRICTION RUB. An extracardiac sound that may be detected during the auscultation procedure is the pericardial friction rub. It is a sign of pericardial inflammation, and in its complete form it exhibits three components. One is associated with ventricular systole, the second with the phase of rapid ventricular filling early in diastole, and the third with atrial systole. If only the systolic component of the rub is present, it may be misinterpreted as a scratchy murmur. With the patient lying flat on his back the pericardial friction rub is best heard in the third or fourth interspace to the left of the sternum, although the location may be variable. There is little radiation, and the quality of the sound is a leathery, high-pitched, multiphasic, scratchy rub, which sounds like two pieces of sandpaper being rubbed together.

Examination of the Lungs

Disorders of the lungs may alter or be altered by cardiac conditions. Consequently, in assessing the cardiovascular status of a patient, one must also evaluate lung function. Examination of the anterior, lateral, and posterior aspects of the chest is best accomplished with the patient in the sitting position. This may be done immediately following or just prior to the cardiac examination, before the patient assumes the supine position.

Understanding the anatomy of the lungs is essential to conducting a proper examination, since each bronchopulmonary lobe must be evaluated. The schematic illustrations of the lung lobes in anterior, posterior, and right and left lateral views in Fig. 4-13 may be helpful.

The lungs rest in the thorax, with the apex of each lung rising about 2 to 4 cm above the inner one third of the clavicles. The inferior border of the lungs runs from approximately the sixth rib at the midclavicular line to the eighth rib at the midaxillary line anteriorly and along the level of the tenth thoracic spinous process posteriorly. The lungs are divided by fissures into lobes, the left lung into two lobes, the right lung into three lobes. The locations of the fissures are identified by corresponding surface sites. On the anterior chest wall the horizontal fissure of the right lung runs from the fifth rib at the midaxillary line to the level of the fourth rib. On the lateral chest wall the spinous process of the third thoracic vertebra and the sixth rib at the midclavicular line denote the direction of the right and left oblique fissures. When a patient holds up his arms, the oblique fissures are close to the vertebral borders of the scapulae on the posterior chest wall.

The following discussion briefly covers the physical findings gathered during inspection, palpation, percussion, and auscultation of the chest with reference to the lungs.

Inspection and Palpation. As discussed earlier in the chapter, the examiner observes the rate and pattern of respiration, the expansion of the chest with breathing, and the symmetry of the thorax. Normally the entire rib cage uniformly moves laterally and upward with respiration. Palpation refines assessment of the degree and symmetry of expansion in respiration, detects any areas of tenderness, and permits the examiner to feel *fremitus* (sound vibrations) when the patient speaks. Fremitus is most prominent over areas where the bronchi are relatively close to the chest

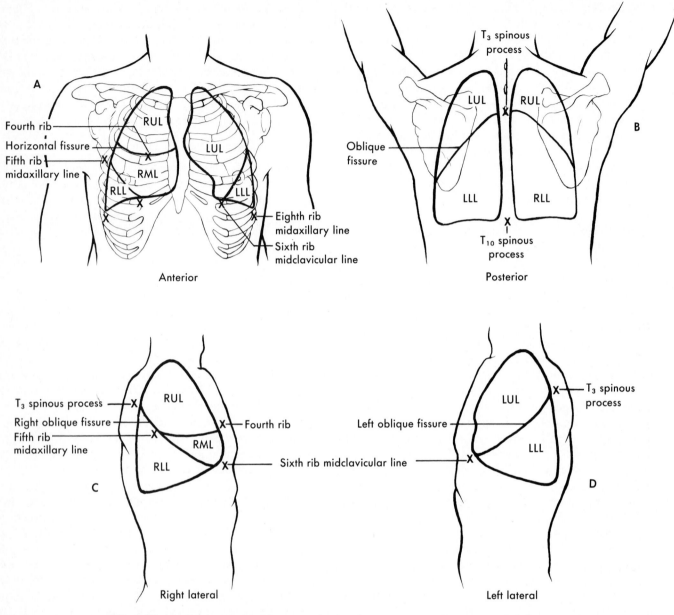

FIG. 4-13. Lung lobes and their anatomic landmarks in A, anterior, B, posterior, C, right lateral, and D, left lateral views. See text for description.

wall and can be elicited by asking the patient to repeat words such as "one-one-one" or "ninety-nine." Fremitus increases as the intensity of the voice increases and its pitch drops; conversely, it decreases as the intensity of the voice decreases and the pitch rises. Fremitus may also decrease or be absent with an obstructed bronchus, pneumothorax, or pleural effusion. If the chest wall is markedly thick, as in obesity, fremitus may be diminished. Increased fremitus is produced by consolidation of the lung in the presence of an intact airway.

Percussion. Percussion is performed to determine the relative amount of air or solid material in the underlying lung and to delineate the boundaries of organs or the portions of the lung that differ in structural density. The procedure of percussion involves placing the distal two phalanges of the middle finger of the right hand (for right-handed examiners) firmly against the patient's chest in the intercostal space parallel to the ribs. The palm and other fingers of the left hand should not touch the chest wall. Then with the tip of the middle finger of the right hand,

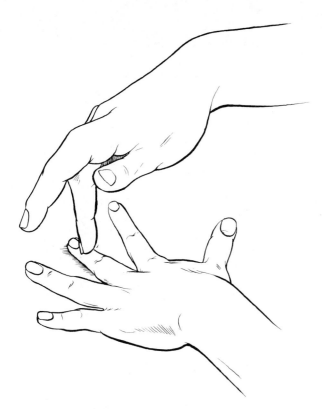

FIG. 4-14. Position of the hands in percussion. For a right-handed examiner the distal two phalanges of the middle finger of the left hand are placed firmly against the patient's chest in the intercostal space parallel to the ribs. The palm and other fingers of the left hand do not touch the chest wall. Then as shown here the examiner *quickly* strikes the distal phalanx of the stationary finger with the tip of the middle finger of the right hand.

quickly strike the distal phalanx of the stationary finger, as shown in Fig. 4-14. One or two rapid strikes in succession with a loose wrist action produces the desired percussion note. (To learn the technique of percussion, it may be helpful to percuss a wall in a room and note the difference in sound over the beams when compared with that over the hollows.)

The anterior and lateral chest walls are percussed in a top-to-bottom, side-to-side fashion while comparing the symmetry of sound and feeling. Similarly, the posterior lung fields are percussed, working down to the level of the diaphragm and comparing percussion notes.

The sounds produced by percussion should be evaluated with respect to four qualities:

1. *Resonance.* Resonance is the percussion note elicited over the normal lung. Although it may vary with the thickness of the chest wall, resonance projects a clear, low-pitched, and well-sustained note. A hyperresonant note, in general, is associated with hyperaeration of the lungs, as in pneumothorax or obstructive emphysema.

2. *Tympany.* The tympanic note is normally heard in the left upper quadrant of the abdomen over the air-filled stomach or over any hollow viscus. The note is loud, musical, and well sustained, with a high-pitched, clear, hollow, and drumlike quality.

3. *Dullness.* Dullness is produced when the air content of the underlying tissue is decreased and its solidity increased, as in pneumonia or pleural effusion. The dull sound is soft, short, and high pitched, with a thudding quality. It lacks the vibratory quality of the resonant note. A dull note is elicited normally over the heart or liver. Of particular importance is the phenomenon of shifting dullness, that is, a change in the site of abdominal percussion dullness with a change in posture, since it suggests free fluid in the pleural cavity.

4. *Flatness.* Flatness is produced when no air is present in the underlying tissue. It is absolute dullness. The flat note is short, high pitched, and feeble. Normally the flat sound is percussed over the muscles of the arm and thigh and over bone.

Diaphragmatic excursion can be measured by determining the distance between the levels of dullness on full expiration and full inspiration, normally about 5 cm. High levels of dullness over the posterior aspect of the chest are associated with pleural effusion, atelectasis, or an elevated diaphragm.

Auscultation. Auscultation of the lung fields permits the examiner to make determinations about the state of bronchial patency of various lung divisions, to assess the quality and intensity of breath sounds, and to note any abnormal sounds. The patient should be asked to breathe somewhat more deeply than usual, with the mouth open. Auscultation is then accomplished in a sequence similar to that of percussion, beginning with the upper lung fields; one side is listened to, then the other, and then both are compared down to the level of the diaphragm. All portions of the lung fields—posterior, anterior, and lateral—must be systematically auscultated. The examiner should first concentrate on normal breath sounds, then abnormal sounds.

NORMAL BREATH SOUNDS. Normal breath sounds can be categorized as vesicular, bronchial, and bronchovesicular. *Vesicular* breath sounds occur over most of the lungs and have a prominent inspiratory component and a brief expiratory phase. *Bronchial* breath sounds, also called tracheal breath sounds, are normally heard over the trachea and main bronchi. These sounds are hollow, tubular, and harsh and are heard best during expiration. *Bronchovesicular* breath sounds are heard over the main stem of the bronchi and represent an intermediate stage between bronchial and vesicular breathing.

ABNORMAL BREATH SOUNDS. Normal breath sounds in one area may be pathologic when heard somewhere else.

For example, bronchial and bronchovesicular breath sounds are heard over a consolidated, compressed, or fibrosed lung. Furthermore, diminished breath sounds occur with local or diffuse bronchial obstruction and with pleural disease associated with the presence of fluid, air, or scar tissue. With airways narrowed, the breath sounds are characteristically wheezing and whistling in nature, with a prolonged expiratory and a short inspiratory phase, as heard in patients with asthma.

Rales are abnormal sounds that occur when air passes through bronchi that contain fluid of any kind. They are subdivided into interrupted crackling sounds, termed *moist rales,* and continuous coarse sounds, called *rhonchi*. Rhonchi suggest a pathologic condition in the trachea or larger bronchi, whereas moist medium and fine rales imply bronchiolar and alveolar disease. *Fine rales* are short and high pitched and can be simulated by rubbing a strand of hair between the thumb and forefinger next to the ear. *Medium rales* are louder and lower pitched.

In left ventricular failure the presence of rales is one of the earliest physical findings. Rales occur as a result of the transudation of edema fluid into the pulmonary alveoli. At first the alveolar fluid is dependent in location, and rales are present at the base of the lungs. As the failure becomes increasingly severe, the rales become more generalized. The rales of left ventricular failure are typically fine and crepitant, but as failure progresses, they may become moist and coarse. The findings may be difficult to differentiate from those caused by pulmonary infiltrations of an inflammatory nature. Rales from left ventricular failure often develop first at the right lung base but are frequently bibasilar.

PLEURAL FRICTION RUB. Inflammation of the visceral and parietal pleurae may result in loss of lubricating fluid so that apposing pleural surfaces rub together, producing a low-pitched, coarse, grating sound with respiration. When the patient holds his breath the rub disappears.

Finally, one should be wary of the adventitious sounds produced when a stethoscope is not held firmly against the chest. Body hair can rub across the instrument during respiration and produce an annoying crackling sound.

ASSESSMENT OF COMMON SYMPTOMS AND SIGNS

A number of symptoms are commonly associated with heart disease. Most individuals with coronary heart disease or hypertension are asymptomatic. When symptoms or signs do appear, either they relate to complications from the disease, or the disease state is well advanced.

Patients who have heart disease should be queried specifically about the presence or absence of the following conditions. Each symptom, if present, should be evaluated and described carefully using the descriptors on p. 35 to p. 36.

1. *Dypsnea*. Dyspnea is labored or difficult breathing; it accompanies a number of cardiac conditions and is a manifestation of congestive heart failure. Commonly, this occurs with strain and may be affected by position. Dypsnea varies in degree. The amount of exertion required to cause it and the amount of rest necessary to relieve it should be quantitated carefully. *Paroxysmal nocturnal dypsnea* occurs at night; the patient awakens with a terrifying sensation of suffocating. The distress diminishes after sitting up for a few minutes. *Orthopnea* is associated with congestive heart failure; the patient has difficulty breathing when lying flat in bed and requires two or more pillows for sleep.
2. *Cardiac asthma*. Cardiac asthma refers to wheezing caused by pulmonary congestion.
3. *Palpitations*. Palpitations occur with premature beats or other rhythm disturbances and are perceived by the patient as abnormal sensations of the heartbeat, a skipped beat, or a flutter.
4. *Syncope*. Syncope is a temporary loss of consciousness due to inadequate oxygen supply to the brain. Heart block, cardiac asystole, severe sinus bradycardia or arrest, or ventricular tachyarrhythmias may be causes.
5. *Fatigue, mental confusion, failure to thrive*. These and other vague symptoms may be associated with coronary complications and are particularly common in elderly patients.
6. *Hemoptysis*. Hemoptysis, or coughing up blood, may be associated with pulmonary edema or pulmonary embolus.
7. *Edema*. Edema or fluid in the form of edema tends to accumulate in the dependent areas of the body: the hands and feet in the ambulatory patient and the sacral area of the bedridden patient. Edema accompanies rightsided heart failure. Edema is assessed by firmly indenting the skin with the fingertips. The degree of pitting that occurs should be quantitated and described with the following scale:

    0 = None present
    +1 = Trace—disappears rapidly
    +2 = Moderate—disappears in 10 to 15 seconds
    +3 = Deep—disappears in 1 to 2 minutes
    +4 = Very deep—present after 5 minutes[2]

    In examining the bedridden patient for edema it is important to press over the sacrum, buttocks, and posterior thighs. Sudden weight gain may be a sign of edema.
8. *Cyanosis*. Cyanosis is a bluish discoloration appearing in the extremities and lips caused by poor cir-

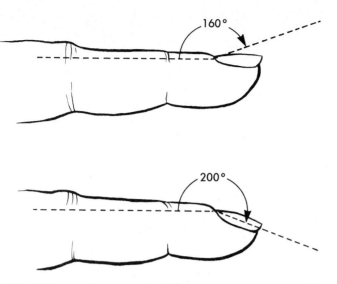

FIG. 4-15. Profile sign. Early clubbing is sometimes evidenced by nail-to-nailbed angle of more than 180 degrees. Top view is normal; bottom view is abnormal. (From Thompson, D.A.: Cardiovascular assessment: guide for nurses and other health professionals, St. Louis, 1981, The C.V. Mosby Co.)

culation. It is brought on by cold temperatures or some severe dysfunction, such as pulmonary disease or shock. The examiner should observe the color of earlobes, lips, fingernail beds, and mucous membranes. *Central cyanosis* occurs with low arterial oxygen saturation associated with congenital right-to-left shunts or pulmonary diseases such as pneumonia. It is observed in the mucous membranes such as the conjunctiva and the inside of the lips and cheeks. With *peripheral cyanosis* the arterial oxygen saturation may be normal, but the oxygen within the peripheral vascular bed is inadequate. This may occur with heart failure and shock.

9. *Clubbing* is a condition of the nail bed associated with certain pulmonary or cardiac diseases (Fig. 4-15).
10. *Hypoxemia (hypoxia)*. This is an insufficient supply of oxygen in the blood. Signs of hypoxia include increased pulse rate, irritability, restlessness, disorientation, and cyanosis.
11. *Chest pain*. Chest pain is a complaint associated with a reasonably large number of clinical problems, in addition to angina and acute myocardial infarction. To differentiate between myocardial ischemia and these other causes of chest pain requires a systematic evaluation of the patient's symptoms. The descriptors associated with angina and myocardial infarction are described in Chapter 7. Table 4-2 summarizes distinguishing features of other conditions commonly appearing in settings of cardiac care.

DIAGNOSIS

Diagnosis is defined as a statement or conclusion concerning the nature or cause of some phenomenon. Although the term *diagnosis* has most commonly been applied to the discipline of medicine, other professionals such as architects, scientists, and managers also collect and organize systematic data about a situation and form conclusions or judgments appropriate to their domain of expertise. In health care, data collected by the clinician are organized, analyzed, and interpreted to form a statement of the patient's problem: a diagnosis. A clinical diagnosis provides the tool for identifying the patient's health status clearly and concisely and leads to possible solutions to the problem. To formulate the diagnosis it is imperative that the clinician have as complete a data base as possible.

In the past all members of the health care team have developed the patient's plan of care from the medical diagnosis. The medical diagnosis labels a health problem/illness and provides a frame of reference to determine what to do and what to expect. This diagnosis describes medical pathology and focuses on the cellular response to the problem. The physician determines a medical diagnosis through a logical sequence of events.

All clinicians collect systematic data and draw conclusions appropriate to their particular expertise. As particular areas of concern become more defined, one's perception of patients and one's ability to help them resolve health problems will increase. The use of medical, nursing, and other diagnoses to direct the cardiac patient's plan of care can provide a comprehensive, humanistic view of the patient's needs in relation to his or her unique situation. Recognizing medical problems and responding appropriately to those problems ensures a more holistic approach to the care of the cardiac patient.

PROBLEM-ORIENTED PATIENT RECORD

The problem-oriented record is a method of organizing and recording the patient's health history, throughout which specific problems are defined, numbered, and referred to by number.

The problem-oriented record includes an *initial data base* consisting of the patient's health history, a complete physical examination, and laboratory data. The *problem list* consists of medical, social, and psychologic problems derived from the initial data base. The dates of onset and resolution of these problems (both active and inactive) are recorded and the problems numbered. Each problem retains its original number. The problem list usually is at the beginning of the record and serves as an index. Each problem has a plan that includes diagnostic measures, therapeutic approaches, and patient education.

This problem-oriented approach is useful in the process of nursing assessment and in the documentation of nursing

TABLE 4-2. Assessment of chest pain

Condition	Location	Quality	Severity	Course	Aggravating or Relieving Factors	Symptoms or Signs
Angina	Retrosternal region; radiates to neck, jaw, epigastrium, shoulders or arms—left common	Pressure, burning, squeezing, heaviness, indigestion	Moderate to severe	<10 minutes	Aggravated by exercise, cold weather, emotional stress, or after meals; relieved by rest or nitroglycerin; atypical (Prinzmetal's) angina may be unrelated to activity and caused by coronary artery spasm	S_4, paradoxical split S_2 during pain
Intermediate syndrome or coronary insufficiency	Same as angina	Same as angina	Increasingly severe	>10 minutes	Same as angina, with gradually decreasing tolerance for exertion	Same as angina
Myocardial infarction	Substernal, and may radiate like angina	Heaviness, pressure, burning, constriction	Severe, sometimes mild (in 25% of patients)	Sudden onset, 30 minutes or longer but variable; usually goes away in hours	Unrelieved	Shortness of breath, sweating, weakness, nausea, vomiting, severe anxiety
Pericarditis	Usually begins over sternum and may radiate to neck and down left upper extremity	Sharp, stabbing knifelike	Moderate to severe	Lasts many hours to days	Aggravated by deep breathing, rotating chest or supine position; relieved by sitting up and leaning forward	Pericardial friction rub, syncope, cardiac tamponade, pulsus paradoxus (Kussmaul sign)
Dissecting aortic aneurysm	Anterior chest; radiates to thoracic area of back; may be abdominal; pain shifts in chest	Tearing	Excruciating, tearing knifelike	Sudden onset, lasts for hours	Unrelated to anything	Lower blood pressure in one arm, absent pulses, paralysis, murmur of aortic insufficiency, pulsus paradoxus, stridor; myocardial infarction can occur
Mitral valve prolapse syndrome	Substernal; sometimes radiates to the left arm, back, jaw	Stabbing, sharp	Variable, generally mild, can become severe	Episodes are paroxysmal, may be prolonged	Not related to exertion, not relieved by nitroglycerin or rest	Variable palpitations dizziness, syncope, dyspnea

Condition	Location	Quality	Severity	Duration/Onset	Aggravating factors	Associated findings
Pulmonary embolism (most pulmonary emboli do not produce chest pain)	Substernal "anginal"	Not pleuritic unless infarction exists	Can be severe	Sudden onset; minutes to <hour	May be aggravated by breathing	Fever, tachypnea, tachycardia, hypotension, elevated jugular venous pressure, right ventricular lift, accentuated P_2, occasional murmur of tricuspid insufficiency and right ventricular S_4; with infarction usually in the presence of congestive heart failure, rales, pleural rub, hemoptysis, clinical phlebitis present in minority of cases
Pulmonary hypertension	Substernal	Pressure; oppressive	Variable		Aggravated by effort	Pain usually associated with dyspnea; right ventricular lift, accentuated P_2
Spontaneous pneumothorax	Unilateral	Sharp, well localized		Sudden onset, lasts many hours	Painful breathing	Dyspnea, hyperresonance, and decreased breath and voice sounds over involved lung
Pneumonia with pleurisy	Localized over area of consolidation	Pleuritic, well localized	Moderate		Painful breathing	Dyspnea, cough, fever, dull to flat percussion, bronchial breathing, rales, occasional pleural rub
Gastrointestinal disorders	Lower substernal area, epigastric, right or left upper quadrant	Burning, colic-like aching		Precipitated by recumbency or meals		Nausea, regurgitation, food intolerance, melena, hematemesis, jaundice
Musculoskeletal disorders	Variable	Aching		Short or long duration Prolonged period of time Unassociated with external events	Aggravated by movement, history of muscle exertion	Tender to pressure or movement
Neurologic disorders (herpes zoster)	Dermatomal in distribution					Rash appears in area of discomfort with herpes
Anxiety states	Usually localized to a point	Sharp burning, commonly location of pain moves from place to place	Mild to moderate	Varies; usually very brief	Situational anger	Sighing respirations, often chest wall tenderness

MEDICAL DIAGNOSIS DETERMINATION

Observation

Includes history, physical examination, and routine laboratory studies.

Description

Includes ordering these findings into logical clusters and eliminating irrelevant material.

Interpretation

Compares data with a known body of knowledge; that is, the information is synthesized into integrated concepts compatible with known diseases.

Verification

A course of action is determined and discussed with the patient. Differential diagnostic test results are analyzed and further patient observations are made.

Diagnosis

A final label, which is disease oriented, is determined. The most likely diagnosis that explains the present illness is recorded in descending order along with other active problems. Examples of medical diagnoses include angina pectoris, myocardial infarction, pulmonary edema, and congestive heart failure.

Action

A course of treatment based on the diagnosis is initiated.

NURSING DIAGNOSIS DETERMINATION

Just as medicine has identified diagnoses that reflect that discipline's area of concern, nursing has also begun to identify patient problems or concerns in which nurses are uniquely involved. These nursing diagnoses are statements of the patient's actual or potential health states that focus on human responses or reactions to that state. These human responses may be any observable manifestation, need, condition, concern, event, dilemma, occurrence, or fact within the target area of nursing practice. A nursing diagnosis is *not* a diagnostic test (e.g., cardiac catheterization), a piece of equipment (e.g., Swan-Ganz catheter), or a surgical procedure (e.g., pacemaker insertion). It is important that nursing diagnoses be derived from data collected by nurses. This nursing data base should describe the whole patient, not just medical problems. The nursing diagnosis consists of three components: the problem title, etiology, and signs and symptoms.

Problem title

The title or label gives a concise description of the health state of the patient. The title can be derived from the list from the North American Nursing Diagnosis Association (NANDA) or a new diagnostic category may be developed by the nurse. It may be described as actual, possible, or potential. A possible nursing diagnosis indicates that more data must be collected to be certain of the label. A potential diagnosis is a problem that may occur if the nurse does not initiate nursing measures to prevent it. Examples of problem titles are alteration in cardiac output, fear, and alteration in skin integrity.

Etiology

Etiology refers to the probable cause of the problem. It can be environmental, psychologic, spiritual, physiologic, sociocultural, or developmental. The term *related to* is used as the connecting link from the title to the etiology, for example, fear related to lack of knowledge concerning the cardiac catheterization procedure.

Signs and symptoms

These are the defining characteristics, derived from the assessment, that support the problem title and etiology. These signs and symptoms can be used to evaluate the patient's progress. For example, the patient states that he is fearful because he has never had a cardiac catheterization before and he does not know what to expect. Assessment indicates that the patient keeps asking patients and staff questions about the procedure; he is pacing his hospital room and has an increased heart rate. Nursing diagnoses help to define independent functions of the nurse and distinguish nursing from medicine. A nursing diagnosis describes a health state for which the nurse can legally provide primary assistance to the patient and may change more frequently than a medical diagnosis.

care and may be used to assess and describe the behavioral dimensions of care unique to the concern of nursing practice.

Patient assessment should be an orderly process whereby subjective and objective data are gathered and synthesized, assessment of the problem is made, and finally a plan is formulated for each problem identified.

Subjective information includes information obtained from the patient about the health history and present complaint, as well as the time interval since the last entry. Objective information includes information gathered by the health provider during the physical examination and laboratory studies. The assessment identifies one or more situations or problems and is stated in those terms until a firm diagnosis is made. The assessment includes the practitioner's analysis of the subjective and objective data relating to the etiology of the problem, the course of the problem, the patient's response to therapy and coping ability, the patient's participation in and reaction to the plans, and probable outcomes. A plan is formulated for each problem. The plan may include diagnostic studies, medication or other treatment, or health education, such as working with the patient to stop smoking.

Progress Notes

Progress notes include subjective (S), objective (O), assessment (A), and plan (P) components. The acronym SOAP refers to the format for recording progress notes.

S = subjective information from the patient's history
O = objective information including the physical examination and results of laboratory studies
A = assessment or analysis of the observations
P = plans for further treatment, diagnostic procedures or patient education

ASSESSMENT OF RISK FACTORS

Risk factors have been discussed in Chapters 2 and 3. The management of risk factors is an important clinical strategy in the care of patients who have coronary heart disease. It is therefore important to possess an orderly process of patient assessment to identify risk factors. The SOAP process can be applied as a reminder in completing a total risk assessment with the patient and planning interventions or modifications in life-style. The procedure for gathering and recording information is as follows:

1. *Subjective data* obtained from patient history, such as heredity, smoking, occupation, and exercise
2. *Objective data* obtained from physical examination and laboratory studies, such as age, sex, race, weight, blood pressure, cholesterol level, triglyceride level, and blood sugar level
3. *Assessment* of patient's risk
4. *Plan* or interventions

Using this process of health assessment gives the practitioner and patient a good perspective on quantitative and qualitative aspects of individual risk and facilitates planning for behavioral change.

SUGGESTED READINGS

Bates, B., and Hoekelman, R.A.: Physical examination, ed. 3, Philadelphia, 1983, J.B. Lippincott Co.

Carpenito, L.J.: Nursing diagnosis, Philadelphia, 1983, J.B. Lippincott Co.

DeGowin, E.L., and DeGowin, R.L.: Bedside diagnostic examination, ed. 4, New York, 1981, Macmillan Publishing Co.

Fowkes, W.C., and Hunn, V.K.: Clinical assessment for the nurse practitioner, St. Louis, 1973, The C.V. Mosby Co.

Fowler, N.O.: Inspection and palpation of venous and arterial pulses. Examination of the heart, part 2, New York, 1972, American Heart Association.

Guzzetta, C.E., and Dossey, B.M.: Cardiovascular nursing, St. Louis, 1984, The C.V. Mosby Co.

Harris, A., Sutton, G., and Towers, M., editors: Physiological and clinical aspects of cardiac auscultation, Philadelphia, 1976, J.B. Lippincott Co.

Hobson, L.B.: Examination of the patient, New York, 1975, McGraw-Hill Book Co.

Hurst, J.W., and others, editors: The heart, ed. 6, New York, 1986, McGraw-Hill Book Co.

Hurst, J.W., and Schlant, R.C.: Inspection and palpation of the anterior chest. Examination of the heart, part 3, New York, 1972, American Heart Association.

Jones, S.: Nursing diagnosis, Nursing (newsletter from Mount Sinai Medical Center) 7:1, 1985.

Judge, R.D., and Zuidema, G.D., editors: Methods of clinical examination: a physiologic approach, ed. 3, Boston, 1974, Little, Brown & Co.

Kritek, P.B.: Nursing diagnosis: theoretical foundations, Occupational Health Nursing 33:393, 1985.

Leatham, A.: Auscultation of the heart and phonocardiography, ed. 2, London, 1975, Churchill Livingstone.

Leonard, J.J., and Croetz, F.W.: Auscultation. Examination of the heart, part 4, New York, 1967, American Heart Association.

Lesser, L.M., and Wenger, N.K.: Carotid sinus syncope, Heart Lung 5:453, 1976.

Luckman, J., and Sorenson, K.C.: Medical surgical nursing, Philadelphia, 1980, W.B. Saunders Co.

Petersdorf, R.G., and others, editors: Harrison's principles of internal medicine, ed. 10, New York, 1983, McGraw-Hill Book Co.

Ravin, A., and others: Auscultation of the heart, ed. 3, Chicago, 1977, Year Book Medical Publishers, Inc.

Sanan, J., and Judge, D.: Physical appraisal methods in nursing practice, Boston, 1975, Little, Brown & Co.

Schroeder, J.P., and Daily, E.K.: Techniques in bedside hemodynamic monitoring, ed. 2, St. Louis, 1980, The C.V. Mosby Co.

Silverman, M.E.: The clinical history. Examination of the Heart, part 1, New York, 1975, American Heart Association.

Thompson, D.A.: Cardiovascular assessment: guide for nurses and other health professionals, St. Louis, 1981, The C.V. Mosby Co.

Walker, H.K.: The problem-oriented medical system, JAMA 236:2397, 1976.

Weed, L.: Medical records that guide and teach, N. Engl. J. Med. 278:593, 1968.

Winslow, E.H.: Visual inspection of the patient with cardiopulmonary disease, Heart Lung 4:421, 1975.

CHAPTER 5

Patient Assessment: Laboratory Studies

Gerald V. Naccarelli
Akira Nishikawa
Ruth A. Giebel

Noninvasive laboratory tests have become important diagnostic tools for evaluating patients with suspected cardiac disease. Exercise stress testing with or without nuclear imaging techniques often provides critical information about patients with coronary artery disease. Echocardiography and new advances in cardiac Doppler studies have improved the ability to study cardiac chamber and valvular abnormalities. In addition, long-term ECG recording (Holter monitoring) continues to be a useful tool for screening patients with arrhythmias and suspected ischemic heart disease. The purpose of this chapter is to review the use of the above laboratory studies and the use of invasive tests such as Swan-Ganz monitoring and cardiac catheterization.

EXERCISE STRESS TESTING

The treadmill exercise stress test is the most commonly used noninvasive technique to detect coronary artery disease. Physical or emotional stress typically precipitates myocardial ischemia in patients who have a fixed coronary obstruction. Exertional stress can induce ischemia by causing myocardial oxygen consumption to exceed available supply. During the exercise stress test, an attempt is made to provoke and electrocardiographically document exercise-induced myocardial ischemia and to correlate these electrocardiographic changes in with the patient's symptoms.

The treadmill stress test is performed as follows. A baseline ECG, heart rate, and blood pressure are obtained and these are monitored during exercise. An ECG is repeated following hyperventilation of the patient to screen for labile ST-T wave changes. Although stress testing may be performed with the patient supine or upright using a bicycle ergometer, it is usually performed in the upright position on a treadmill. The rate and incline at which the patient exercises on the treadmill are progressively increased, depending on the protocol, until the patient achieves a target heart rate. The target heart rate used is greater than 85% of the predicted maximum heart rate for the patient's age and sex, or in some situations it is greater than a predetermined heart rate. The exercise stress test is usually terminated before this target heart rate is achieved if there is the development of hypotension, malignant ventricular arrhythmias such as sustained or long runs of rapid nonsustained ventricular tachycardia, marked ST segment depression, or severe chest pain.[1]

A positive exercise stress test can be defined as being greater than 1 mm of horizontal or down-sloping ST segment depression occurring 80 msec after the J point (Fig. 5-1). Increasing the criteria to at least 2 mm of ST segment depression increases the specificity but decreases the sensitivity of the test. However, the pretest likelihood of coronary artery disease[2,3,4] (Fig. 5-2) affects the sensitivity and the specificity of stress testing significantly. The magnitude of ST segment depression and the level of exercise at which ST segment depression occurs provides an index of the severity of coronary artery disease.[5,6,7] For example, 3 mm of down-sloping ST depression developing at a heart rate of only 100 beats/minute would suggest multivessel coronary artery disease, severe proximal left anterior descending artery stenosis, or left main coronary artery stenosis. Prolonged persistence of ischemic changes in the recovery period also correlates with the severity of coronary disease.[6,7] The development of ventricular arrhythmias during exercise is a less specific marker of coronary artery disease than the development of ST segment abnormalities. Additional criteria for a positive stress test include the development of hypotension, inverted U waves, or anginal chest pain.[8]

The accompanying box lists accepted indications for stress testing.[9] The most frequent use of stress testing is to evaluate the patient who has chest pain that is suggestive of angina. In this setting an attempt is made to induce the patient's symptoms during exercise and to correlate these symptoms with electrocardiographic evidence of myocardial ischemia. Since the initial manifestation of coronary disease in many individuals is sudden death or acute myocardial infarction, the exercise stress test is often used as a

---

INDICATIONS FOR STRESS TESTING

Evaluation of chest pain
Evaluation of arrhythmias
Stratification of high-risk patients
Assessment of cardiac reserve and functional capacity

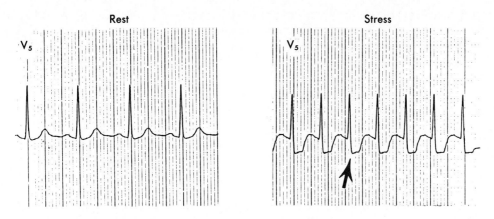

FIG. 5-1. Electrocardiographic lead V₅ demonstrating 4 mm horizontal ST segment depression *(arrow)* during exercise stress test.

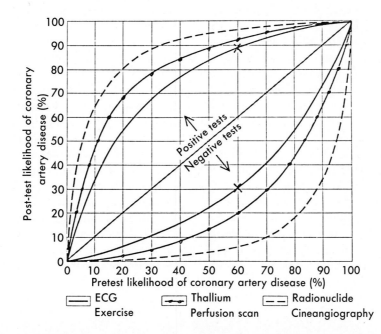

FIG. 5-2. Sensitivity and specificity curves for radionuclide cineangiography, thallium scan, and exercise stress tests. From Cohn, P.F.: Hosp. Pract. **18**:125, 1983.)

means of screening high-risk individuals in an attempt to make an earlier diagnosis of latent ischemic heart disease. Stress testing is also useful to evaluate the patients with known coronary artery disease such as those who have suffered myocardial infarction, angioplasty, or coronary artery bypass surgery. The exercise stress test is also useful for objectively evaluating an individual's overall physical condition and the New York Heart Association classification by measuring the maximal heart rate, blood pressure, and duration of exercise achieved.[10] This application of the stress test is especially important for the patient who has angina or valvular heart disease since the patient's functional status may determine the timing of surgical inter-

vention. Exercise testing is also used in conjunction with cardiac rehabilitation programs for the patient who has stable coronary artery disease or in serial assessment of the cardiovascular effects of exercise. The presence of angina, dyspnea, or exercise-aggravated arrhythmia at a certain reproducible workload can be useful in prescribing physical restrictions for the above patients.

A stress test is usually performed in patients with ventricular rhythm disturbances. Stress testing is more sensitive than the routine 12-lead electrocardiogram because of the longer sampling period and the induction of stress-related arrhythmias. The stress test is useful in screening for latent coronary disease or correlating ischemic ST segment changes with the occurrence of potentially malignant arrhythmias. In addition, it is useful in documenting exercise-aggravated or exercise-induced ventricular tachycardia.[11,12] In these patients the arrhythmia often responds to beta-blockers and the stress test can be performed serially during drug therapy to judge the efficacy of the treatment.[13] In patients in whom exercise-induced arrhythmia needs to be accurately quantitated, continuous electrocardiographic recording using a trendscriber has been found to be superior to intermittent recording.[13] Some investigators[14,15] feel that the loss of overt preexcitation at relatively slow exercise-induced heart rates may screen for patients with overt accessory connections that have longer refractory periods and are not capable of maintaining rapid rates during atrial fibrillation.

Stress testing is also useful in stratifying patients' risk after a myocardial infarction. Several studies have documented that the occurrence of angina, ventricular arrhythmia and diagnostic ST segment changes in the postmyocardial infarction period identifies patients at increased risk for developing future angina, myocardial infarction, and sudden death.[16,17] Patients found to be in high-risk categories with the above screening may need early cardiac catheterization with appropriate treatment to decrease this risk.[18] Since patients with normal stress tests and an ejection fraction greater than 30% have only a 1% to 3% incidence of sudden death, these patients may not be treated as aggressively as the high-risk patients.

The interpretation of ST segment shifts during exercise is difficult in patients with baseline ST segment abnormalities. Such patients include those taking digitalis, those with bundle branch block or left ventricular hypertrophy with associated ST-T changes, and those with the Wolff-Parkinson-White syndrome.[8] In addition, during stress testing many patients with mitral valve prolapse may have ST segment shifts that represent a false positive response.[8] In these patients thallium stress testing is more accurate.

RADIONUCLIDE TECHNIQUES
Thallium 201 Myocardial Imaging

Thallium 201 is a radionuclide whose biologic activity closely parallels that of potassium in normal myocardium. When thallium is injected into the bloodstream, it is concentrated in viable heart muscle in a ratio proportional to regional coronary blood flow. The major factors determining thallium uptake in myocardium are coronary blood flow and myocardial cellular viability.[19] Normal thallium images in the anterior and left anterior oblique projections (Fig. 5-3) appear in a horseshoe or doughnut configuration representing thallium uptake in the walls of the left ventricle.

Resting thallium imaging is useful in determining the location and extent of myocardial infarctions. Different areas of the myocardium for imaging with thallium are represented diagrammatically in (Fig. 5-4). However, thallium imaging cannot distinguish acute from previous myocardial injury.[20,21] Thallium scans are most accurate in diagnosing an acute myocardial infarction within 24 hours after the onset of symptoms.[22]

Myocardial imaging with thallium 201 is used primarily in conjunction with exercise stress testing. In response to exercise, coronary blood flow normally increases four to five times that of resting values. The presence of a significant coronary artery stenosis prevents this increase. Myocardial segments supplied by a stenotic coronary artery demonstrate a perfusion defect compared with normal seg-

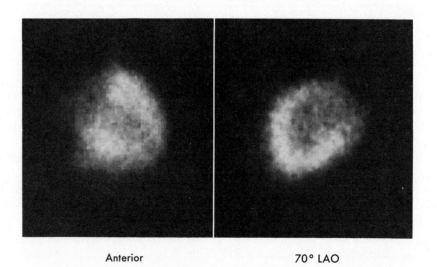

Anterior   70° LAO

FIG. 5-3. Normal thallium imaging in anterior and 70° LAO views.

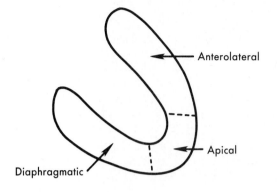

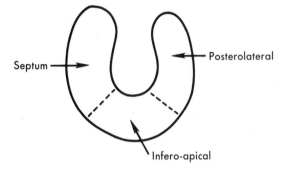

FIG. 5-4. Diagrammatic representation of the myocardium demonstrating regions that can be imaged in anterior and 60°-70° LAO view.

ments (Fig. 5-5). Since both coronary flow and tissue viability are necessary for myocardial uptake of thallium, either exercise-induced ischemia or previous myocardial infarction with nonviable scar could cause a perfusion defect. Because a single thallium myocardial perfusion image cannot reliably distinguish transient myocardial ischemia from previous myocardial infarction, a redistribution myocardial image is typically obtained 4 hours after the exercise.[23] During this time, ischemic viable myocardium demonstrates an increase in thallium content despite the presence of a severe coronary artery stenosis. This phenomenon occurs because there is a constant exchange of thallium between viable myocardium and the blood pool.[24] Therefore as blood flow in normal and stenotic coronary arteries becomes equivalent, regional myocardial uptake of thallium in normal and previously ischemic areas equilibrate. Therefore exercise-induced ischemia typically reduces transient perfusion defects (Fig. 5-5), whereas myocardial infarction, with resulting scar formation, results in a perfusion defect that remains during redistribution (Fig. 5-6).

Myocardial perfusion imaging combined with stress testing offers a number of advantages over the conventional exercise stress test. First, the sensitivity and specificity of thallium myocardial imaging during exercise in detecting significant coronary artery disease is 85% and 95% respectively compared with only a 65% sensitivity and 85% specificity with conventional treadmill exercise stress test.[25,26] Second, myocardial perfusion imaging provides a means of detecting ischemia in the patient in whom left bundle branch block, digitalis, or left ventricular hypertrophy may hamper interpretation of the electrocardiogram recorded during stress testing. Although myocardial perfusion imaging with stress testing cannot predict the num-

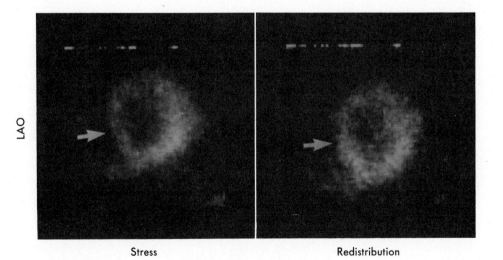

FIG. 5-5. Thallium images (LAO view) demonstrating septal *(arrow)* hypoperfusion during stress that redistributes with rest consistent with septal ischemia.

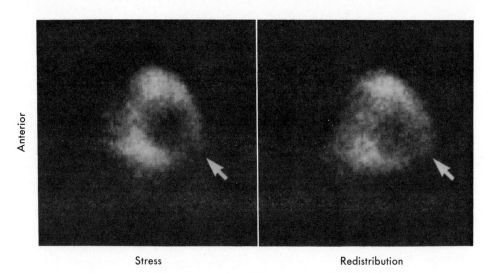

Anterior

Stress   Redistribution

FIG. 5-6. Anterior view of stress and redistributed thallium scan demonstrating persistent apical *(arrow)* hypoperfusion consistent with myocardial scar.

ber of diseased coronary vessels, it can be helpful in evaluating the functional and hemodynamic significance of a given coronary artery lesion. A recent study[27] using positron emission tomography and rubidium-82 has demonstrated that when combined with intravenous dipyridamole and handgrip stress, this new technique can provide a sensitive and specific diagnosis of flow reserve coronary in patients with coronary artery disease.

Myocardial Infarct Imaging

Technetium-99m pyrophosphate has been shown to concentrate in acutely necrotic myocardium because of the binding of the radiopharmaceutical to calcium within damaged myocardial cells.[28] This technique may be useful in a

clinical setting in which a diagnosis of acute myocardial infarction may be difficult to establish by electrocardiographic and serum enzyme methods. For example, the electrocardiographic recognition of acute myocardial infarction may be impossible in the patient who has a left bundle branch block or pacemaker rhythm. Similarly, the enzymatic criteria for acute myocardial infarction may be complicated by the presence of shock, cardioversion, or recent cardiac surgical procedures.

Technetium-99m pyrophosphate begins to accumulate in acutely necrotic myocardium about 12 to 16 hours after the onset of infarction; maximal uptake of radiotracer by infarcted myocardium occurs 24 to 72 hours after the onset of infarction (Fig. 5-7). Myocardial uptake of the tracer

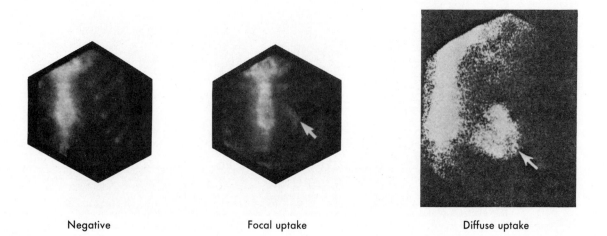

Negative   Focal uptake   Diffuse uptake

FIG. 5-7. Technetium-99 pyrophosphate scans in normal, focal abnormality, and diffuse doughnut abnormality.

becomes progressively less intense so that by 10 to 14 days after infarction, pyrophosphate imaging is typically negative. It is important to remember that technetium-99m pyrophosphate concentrates in bones and acutely infarcted myocardium but normal myocardium does not concentrate the tracer (Fig. 5-7). This contrasts with thallium perfusion imaging, in which normal myocardium concentrates the radionuclide although areas of infarction are indicated by decreased thallium activity. Positive pyrophosphate scans can demonstrate either a localized defect or the presence of a diffuse doughnutlike pattern (Fig. 5-7). This latter pattern is indicative of a large myocardial infarction often associated with a poor prognosis.

Technetium-99m pyrophosphate imaging has a sensitivity of about 90% and a specificity of about 85% in the detection of acute transmural myocardial infarction[29] if performed within 3 to 10 days of symptoms. However, false positive uptake of pyrophosphate can occur with multiple cardioversions, chest wall trauma, rib fractures, calcified valve structures, left ventricular aneurysm and cardiac tumors. Since the minimal myocardial infarction size that can be detected is 3 to 5 grams, small and subendocardial infarction may lead to a false negative image.

Radionuclide Angiocardiography

One of the most useful applications of nuclear medicine techniques for the patient who has coronary artery disease has been in the noninvasive evaluation of ventricular performance. Radionuclide angiography requires only an intravenous injection and is a reproducible method of assessing global and regional left ventricular performance.

Radionuclide angiocardiography measures overall left ventricular systolic pump performance in what is termed *ejection fraction*. Left ventricular ejection fraction is angiographically calculated from the following formula:[30]

Ejection fraction (%)
$$\frac{\text{End-diastolic volume}-\text{End-systolic volume}}{\text{End-diastolic volume}} \times 100$$

The numerator of the above equation is the stroke volume. With radionuclide techniques, the ejection fraction is calculated from changes in radioactive counts within a cardiac chamber rather than changes in volume (Figs. 5-8 and 5-9). A normal ejection fraction calculated by this technique is greater than 50%. Ejection fractions obtained by nuclear techniques correlate well with standard biplane angiographic measured ejection fractions (r = 0.92).[30]

The most commonly used radionuclide technique for assessing ventricular performance is gated cardiac blood pool imaging. With this technique the patient's red blood cells are labeled in vivo with technetium-99m. Changes in radioactive counts are therefore proportional to changes in blood volume within a cardiac chamber.[31] The patient's ECG provides a timing reference of when end-diastole and end-systole occur within the cardiac cycle. The RR interval on the patient's ECG is typically divided into 16 to 30 intervals by a computer, and the gamma camera records counts within the left or right ventricle during each of these intervals. This information is obtained over a period of several hundred heartbeats, and the individual beats are then added together and averaged to create a representative cycle of the patient's ventricular performance. In addition to measuring ejection fraction, gated cardiac blood pool imaging provides an excellent means of evaluating left ventricular regional wall motion.[32] Thus one can determine whether a wall of the left ventricle is hypokinetic or akinetic, or if a left ventricular aneurysm is present. Relative cardiac chamber size and dilatation of the aorta or pulmonary artery also can be qualitatively assessed with this technique.

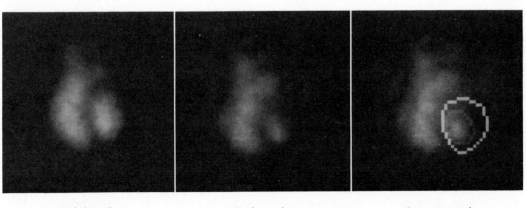

End-diastole   End-systole   Superimposed

FIG. 5-8. Gated nuclear ventriculogram demonstrating end-diastole, end-systole, and superimposed views of both in a normal patient with an ejection fraction of 53%.

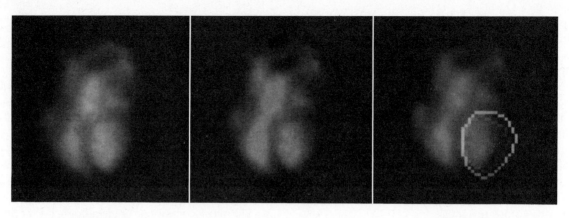

End-diastole   End-systole   Superimposed

FIG. 5-9. Gated nuclear ventriculogram demonstrating end-diastole, end-systole, and superimposed views of both in a patient with diffuse hypokinesis and an ejection fraction of 17%.

Radionuclide angiocardiography with gated cardiac blood pool imaging also can be used in conjunction with exercise stress testing. Normal patients demonstrate at least a 6% increase in left ventricular ejection fraction during exercise stress.[33] In contrast, most patients with coronary artery disease who develop ischemia during exercise either fail to increase ejection fraction or actually demonstrate a decrease in ejection fraction during exercise. In addition to an abnormal ejection fraction response, the patient with exercise-induced ischemia may also develop abnormalities in regional wall motion that can localize the site of exercise-induced ischemia. Therefore gated cardiac blood pool imaging with stress provides an alternative radionuclide technique for the detection of coronary artery disease and has a sensitivity comparable to myocardial perfusion imaging with thallium. Radionuclide angiocardiography is also useful as a noninvasive test for screening patients who might have left ventricular dysfunction postmyocardial infarction since patients with large infarctions and markedly diminished ejection fractions are at increased risk for sudden and nonsudden death.[34] In addition, it is important to quantify the presence or absence of left ventricular dysfunction in patients being evaluated for potentially lethal ventricular arrhythmias. The presence of left ventricular dysfunction in these patients is useful in defining patients at higher risk for sudden death and in assessing if antiarrhythmic drugs that have significant negative inotropic activity should be avoided. Radionuclide angiography is more accurate than echocardiography in quantifying left ventricular dysfunction. However, if the patient has atrial fibrillation with a rapid ventricular response, or frequent spontaneous premature complex and short runs of tachycardia, the gating of the heartbeats can be inaccurate and lead to gross errors in ejection fraction assessment.[30]

LONG-TERM ECG RECORDING

Long-term ECG recording has had widespread application as a noninvasive tool since Holter[35,36] originally demonstrated the use of this technique. Lightweight, battery-powered recorders, worn continuously for 24 hours or more can collect one- or two-lead ECG data for subsequent analysis. A two-lead system is preferred since the extra lead is more sensitive in documenting ST segment abnormalities, identifying aberrancy and screening out artifacts. Attached to a belt or shoulder strap, these recorders can be used in or out of the hospital. A clock on the recorder correlates electrocardiographic events with the patient's log of symptoms, activity, and medications.

Computer-based systems scan and analyze the record with the technician's input for interpretation. Data are reported by mounting representative printout strips of abnormalities (Fig. 5-10) or those corresponding with patient-log entries. An hourly quantitative analysis of the frequency of premature atrial or ventricular complexes, hourly heart rate, and any shifts in ST segment changes can be displayed either on a table or in graphic format. The physician must correlate data from long-term ECG reports with the total patient picture, since it is common for a 24-hour recording to show various abnormalities, even in patients with normal cardiac function. Marked sinus bradycardia, sinus pauses, premature atrial and ventricular complexes, transient AV block, and short runs of atrial tachycardia have been recorded in the normal population.[37,38]

The indications for long-term ECG recording are listed in the box on p. 65. The primary use of these recordings is the evaluation of cardiac rhythm disturbances. Since arrhythmias can be episodic, one must keep in mind that the detection of complex ventricular arrhythmias will vary log-

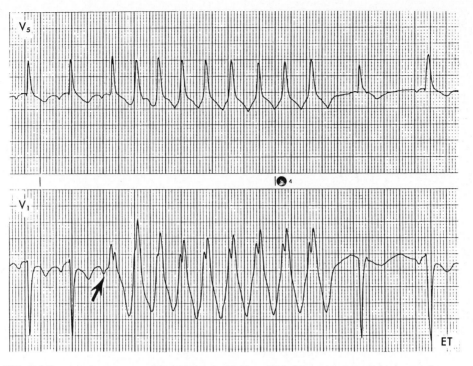

FIG. 5-10. Simultaneous modified Holter leads V₅ and V₁ demonstrating a 9-beat run of ventricular tachycardia in patient ET during diary-documented palpitations.

arithmically with the duration of the recording. The detection of the highest premature ventricular contraction (PVC) grade can usually be determined within 18 to 36 hours in 95% of the patients.

Long-term ECG recordings are used in a serial fashion to judge the efficacy of drug treatment. However, there are several limitations to this approach. First, there is a large amount of spontaneous variability in the occurrence of a patient's arrhythmia[39-42] (Fig. 5-11). Patients may have a low frequency of complex ventricular ectopic activity in between rare episodes of life-threatening arrhythmia. Serial comparisons of recordings during drug treatment are limited in patients with a low density of baseline arrhythmia on a control recording. In one study,[43] infrequent spontaneous ventricular ectopic activity was noted in 25% of patients with a history of sustained ventricular tachyarrhythmias. In patients with a low density of spontaneously occurring ventricular ectopic activity and a history of sustained ventricular tachyarrhythmias, invasive electrophysiologic studies should be used as part of the evaluation. In patients who have high-density ventricular ectopy noted on their Holter monitor, serial comparison of recordings has proved to be a reliable method of treating life-threatening ventricular arrhythmias in one study.[44]

Because of spontaneous variability, drug effect can be mimicked by a patient spontaneously having a low incidence of arrhythmias on a given day.[39] Although in an individual patient the definition of drug effect (statistical reduction in the number of arrhythmic events during arrhythmic drug treatment) may vary, pooled data suggest that an 83% reduction in the number of PVCs over a 24-hour period can define this endpoint ($p < .05$).[40,41] If longer recording periods are used before and after drug treatment, the spontaneous variability of the arrhythmia can be minimized and lower reduction of baseline arrhythmia can define a drug effect. It is important not to confuse drug effect with drug effectiveness, which is an endpoint following drug therapy that predicts no recurrence of life-threatening arrhythmia. Although no unequivocal criteria for drug effectiveness are known, in high-risk patients with high-density ventricular arrhythmia, elimination of spontaneously occurring runs of ventricular tachycardia, at least

---

INDICATIONS FOR LONG-TERM ECG RECORDINGS

Evaluation of patients with suspected or known cardiac rhythm disorders

Evaluation of symptoms suggestive of an arrhythmic disorder

Evaluation of clinical syndromes where arrhythmias may increase the risk of sudden death

Evaluation of pacemaker function

Evaluation of patients with chest pain

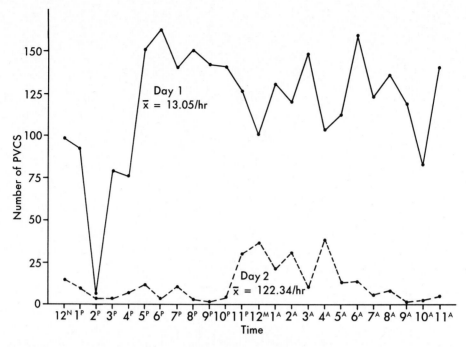

FIG. 5-11. Plot of number of PVCs per hour/day in patient undergoing 48 hours of consecutive Holter monitoring while off medication. Note the marked variability in the number of PVCs decreasing from a mean of 122/hour on day 1 to 13/hour on day 2.

a 90% reduction of ventricular couplets, and at least a 50% reduction of the number of PVCs every 24-hour period seems to be predictive of a favorable therapeutic response.[44] Whether the above criteria are useful in low-risk patients or in patients with less frequent spontaneous arrhythmias is not known. Limitations of the above endpoints were demonstrated in one study in patients who appeared to have drug effectiveness by long-term ECG recordings. Despite acceptable arrhythmia suppression documented by these recordings, 71% of patients still had ventricular tachycardia induced by programmed stimulation during drug therapy.[45] Longer recording periods may minimize some of these false negative responses.

Long-term ECG recording is also used for screening patients with symptoms such as syncope, possibly caused by a tachyarrhythmia, and in patients with suspected sinus node or AV node conduction abnormalities. Although these recordings are frequently used to correlate symptoms with the occurrence of arrhythmia, the test is more helpful in a negative correlative sense. A previous study[46] demonstrated that syncope or near-syncope occurred during a 24-hour recording in 46% of patients studied. In 14% the symptoms correlated with an ECG abnormality, and in 32% symptoms occurred without any arrhythmia. In the latter group of patients nonarrhythmic causes for symptoms need to be considered. In patients with syncope or suspected conduction disturbances, documenting an ar-

rhythmic abnormality correlating with symptoms prior to definitive therapy is critical.[47] Despite these limitations, long-term ECG recordings appear to be more sensitive than stress testing in identifying arrhythmic abnormalities in these patient groups.[48]

Although long-term ECG recordings can be useful in correlating episodes of chest pain with diagnostic ST-segment abnormalities, there are some limitations. First, since only 2 ECG leads usually are represented, significant ST-segment changes can occur during an episode of chest pain but ST-T wave changes from the area of the heart involved are not being recorded. Second, false positive ST-segment shifts with changes of position, hyperventilation, or heart rate can occur. A study[49] of 70 patients with normal resting ECGs and chest pain syndromes revealed that long-term ECG recording was less sensitive and less specific than stress testing in properly identifying patients with obstructive coronary artery disease. Despite this limitation in patients with typical effort angina, it is possible that these recordings may be more useful than stress testing for patients with suspected coronary artery spasm. These patients have frequent episodes of chest pain that cannot be induced routinely by stress testing. Long-term ECG recording can be useful in screening for ST segment elevation and arrhythmias that occur during spontaneous episodes of chest pain.[50]

Long-term ECG recordings can also be used to screen

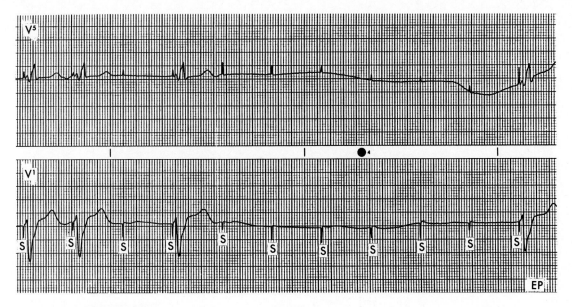

FIG. 5-12. Simultaneous modified Holter leads V$_5$ and V$_1$ in patient EP documenting multiple pacing stimuli *(S)* with failure to capture. Above findings occurred during diary-noted symptom of dizziness.

patients who have clinical syndromes associated with an increased risk of sudden death such as postmyocardial infarction,[51-53] ischemic heart disease syndrome,[54] dilated cardiomyopathy,[55] hypertrophic obstructive cardiomyopathy[56] and prolonged QT syndrome.[57] Long-term recordings have been found to be superior to treadmill testing in identifying arrhythmias in patients after myocardial infarction[58] and in patients with hypertrophic obstructive cardiomyopathy.[56] These recordings may also be useful in screening for arrhythmias in patients with mitral valve prolapse syndrome,[59,60] after coronary artery bypass grafting,[61] and in patients with Wolff-Parkinson-White syndrome.[14] However, in patients with bifascicular block, long-term ECG recordings have not been found to be very sensitive in identifying patients at high risk for complete AV block.[62]

Evaluation of suspected pacemaker malfunction can be accomplished through long-term recordings since intermittent failure of pacemaker sensing (Fig. 5-12) or oversensing problems may be difficult to document during short periods of observation.

Event Recorders

In patients with rare episodes of arrhythmias, noncontinuous forms of ambulatory recording are useful. These techniques include recorders tha can be intermittently activated by an event (for example, by bradycardia or tachycardia) or by the patient during symptoms. Some of these devices have the ability to telephonically transmit an ECG by recording and converting an ECG signal into an audiotone. This transmitted tone is then converted back to an elec-

trocardiographic signal by the receiving unit. New devices with memories can record and store up to 30 seconds of information. This may be particularly useful when the patient does not have access to a telephone because the information can be transmitted later. In addition to screening patients with infrequent symptoms, these devices can be used to document arrhythmia recurrences in treated patients[63,64] and to screen patients at high risk for arrhythmias, such as those who have recently suffered myocardial infarction.[65] Therefore event recorders may be more useful for patients with infrequent symptoms but are limited by short storage capabilities and by their dependence on the patient's perceiving an arrhythmia. These devices are also of limited use in patients who have syncopal spells with no prodrome because the device needs to be activated by a family member.

ECHOCARDIOGRAPHY

Echocardiography uses ultrasound to visualize cardiac structures. This technique can assess the motion and function of the cardiac valves and chambers noninvasively, thereby aiding in the diagnosis of a variety of cardiac abnormalities.

Techniques

Currently there are three techniques by which an echocardiogram can be obtained: M-mode echocardiography, two-dimensional or cross-sectional echocardiography, and Doppler echocardiography. All these techniques employ the transmission of high-frequency sound waves into the

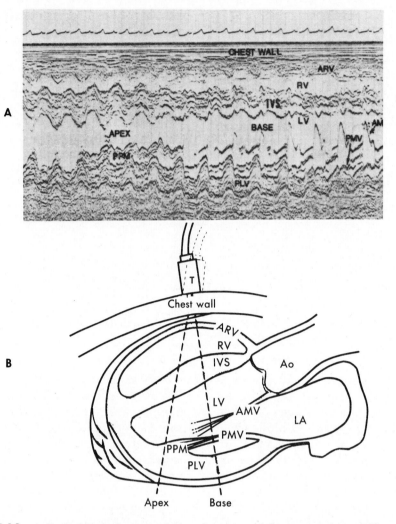

FIG. 5-13. A, Typical M-mode sweep. B, Two-dimensional left parasternal view of heart. From Corya, B.C., and others: Applications of echocardiography in acute myocardial infarction, Cardiovasc. Clin. 2:113, 1975.

chest. These sound waves are reflected to the transmitter, which also receives sound waves from the cardiac structures. The resultant signals are recorded either on a strip chart recorder or on videotape.

M-mode echocardiography uses a single ultrasound beam. This beam is swept across the cardiac structures, and the resulting time-motion information is displayed on a strip chart recording with the ECG of the patient (Fig. 5-13).

Two-dimensional or cross-sectional echocardiography uses a planar beam of ultrasound (Fig. 5-13) that can be transmitted by a single crystal that oscillates or rotates throughout a given plane or by a series of crystals with each crystal transmitting ultrasound through a different point on the chest. The resulting "echo" information is recorded on videotape for subsequent interpretation.

The M-mode and two-dimensional approaches to echo-

cardiography both have advantages and disadvantages, which will be discussed further. It is important to understand that although two-dimensional echocardiography is a more recent development, it cannot replace M-mode echocardiography. Two-dimensional echocardiography represents an additional technique to provide useful information that can be used in the diagnosis and care of the patient who has heart disease.

Applications

The Normal Heart. Figs. 5-14 and 5-15 show normal M-mode and two-dimensional echocardiograms in two different patients. Of importance is the relative size and position of the cardiac chambers and the motion of the cardiac valves during systole and diastole.

Cardiac Chamber Size and Functions. The size of the various cardiac chambers can be assessed by echocar-

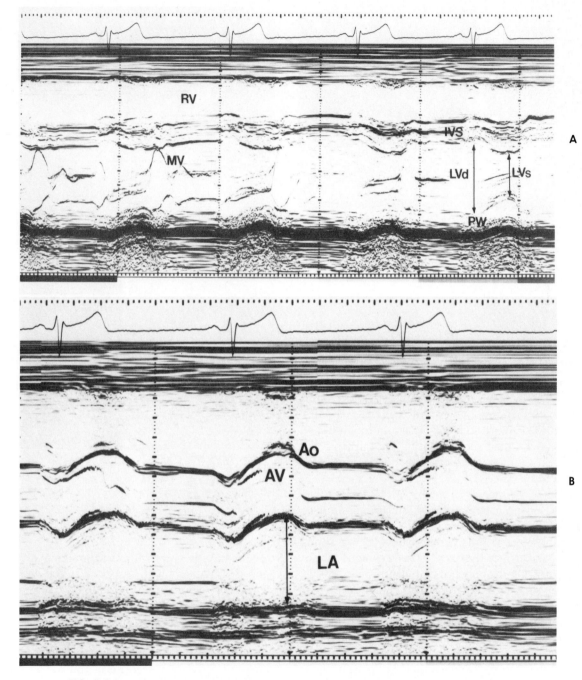

FIG. 5-14. A, Normal M-mode echocardiogram at the level of the ventricles and the mitral valve *(MV)* leaflet. B, Normal M-mode echocardiogram at the level of the aorta *(Ao)*, aortic valve *(AV)* leaflets, and left atrium *(LA)*.

Abbreviations: IVS -interventricular septum
                LVd -left ventricular diastolic dimension
                LVs -left ventricular systolic dimension
                PW -posterior wall
                RV   -right ventricle

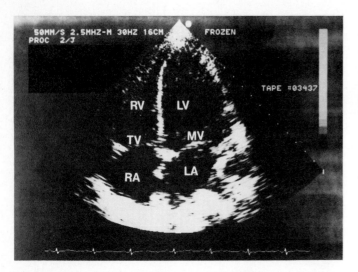

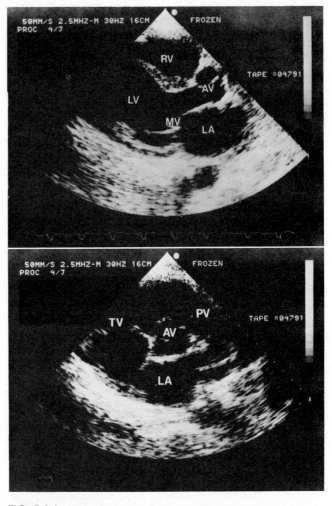

A

B

FIG. 5-15. Apical four-chamber two-dimensional echocardiographic view in a normal patient. Abbreviations as in Fig. 5-14.

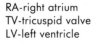

RA-right atrium
TV-tricuspid valve
LV-left ventricle

diography. The diameter of the left ventricle (Fig. 5-14, *A*), left atrium, and aortic root (Fig. 5-14, *B*) can be measured. Measurements of the right ventricle are less reliable because of its shape and the fact that it varies in size at various patient positions. Two-dimensional echocardiography allows a more accurate visualization of the cardiac chambers and their motion during the cardiac cycle (Fig. 5-16). In addition, the aorta, pulmonary artery, and vena cavae can be visualized.

Using the two-dimensional method, the anterior, inferior, septal, apical, lateral, inferior, and posterior segmental wall motion of the left ventricle can be assessed by applying various views.[66] Ischemic segments may show hypokinesis, akinesis, or dyskinesis. This technique is also useful in identifying the presence of mural thrombi,[67] ventricular aneurysm,[68] intracardiac masses,[69] and the existence and degree of left and right ventricular hypertrophy.

Hypertrophic cardiomyopathy is characterized by the presence of systolic anterior motion of the mitral valve, midsystolic closure of the aortic valve, and asymmetric hypertrophy of the septum.[70] Differentiation of patients with congestive cardiomyopathy from those with severe coronary artery disease is made by the presence of diffuse ventricular hypokinesis in the former, as opposed to regional wall motion abnormalities manifested in patients with coronary artery disease.

Valvular Functions. Echocardiography can be used to evaluate patients with various types of valvular heart dis-

FIG. 5-16. Two-dimensional echocardiographic view of A, Long-axis parasternal view—patient with dilated left ventricle and left atrium. B, short axis view. Abbreviations as in Figs. 5-14 and 5-15. *PV,* Pulmonic valve.

ease. Echocardiography is most commonly used in the diagnosis of patients with suspected mitral valve prolapse, stenosis or regurgitation, in addition to those with suspected aortic stenosis and regurgitation. Specific criteria for each of these are discussed below.

Mitral Valve. M-mode echocardiographic features of mitral stenosis include the presence of a thickened or calcified mitral valve, a decrease in the size of the valvular opening, a decrease in the EF slope of the valve, and the anterior motion of the posterior leaflet during diastole (Fig. 5-17).[71,72] Doming of the leaflets on two-dimensional echocardiography is also indicative of mitral stenosis. A decrease in the size of the mitral valve orifice can be measured using two-dimensional echocardiography because the size of the orifice can actually be measured directly

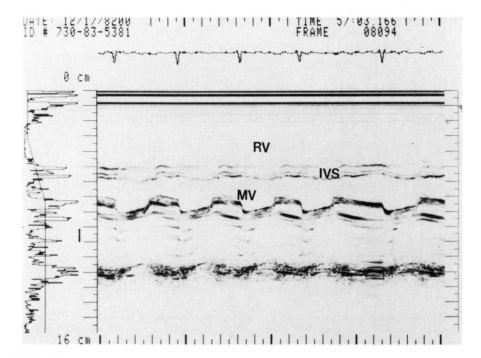

FIG. 5-17. M-mode echocardiogram demonstrating decreased amplitude, flattened EF slope, and anterior motion of the posterior mitral valve leaflet consistent with mitral stenosis.[71,72]

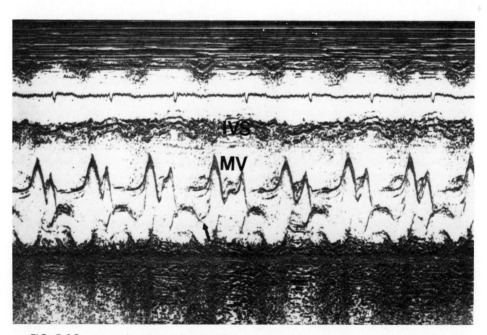

FIG. 5-18. M-mode echocardiogram demonstrating late systolic posterior displacement *(arrow)* of the posterior mitral valve *(MV)* leaflet consistent with mitral valve prolapse.

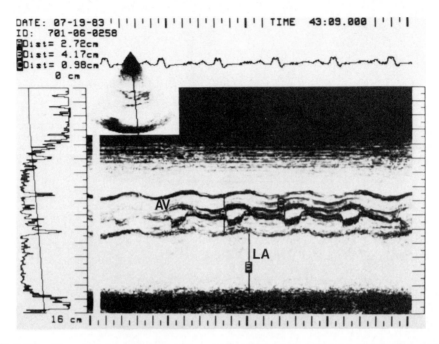

DATE: 07-19-83 ' | ' | ' | ' | ' | ' | ' | ' | TIME 43:09.000 | ' | ' |
ID: 701-06-0258
Dist= 2.72cm
Dist= 4.17cm
Dist= 0.98cm
0 cm
16 cm

FIG. 5-19. M-mode echocardiogram demonstrating thickened aortic valve *(AV)* leaflets and decreased aortic valve opening (c) consistent with aortic stenosis. Abbreviations as in Fig. 5-14.

from the image in the short-axis view. Moreover, changes in chamber size, such as the dilatation of the left atrium, can further suggest the severity of stenosis. Mitral valve regurgitation, on the other hand, is not directly assessed with echocardiography. Its presence may be suggested by increases in the size of the left ventricle and left atrium. Hemodynamic assessment of mitral stenosis and the semi-quantitative evaluation of mitral regurgitation are further discussed in the section on Doppler echocardiography.

Mitral valve prolapse can be reliably diagnosed with echocardiography by finding the abrupt posterior motion of the mitral valve apparatus in middle or late systole (Fig. 5-18).[73]

A flail mitral valve secondary to infective endocarditis or a ruptured chorda tendinea can be identified from the echocardiogram.[74] The flail leaflet may appear to displace posteriorly but to a much greater degree than mitral valve prolapse.[73] Also, the motion of the mitral valve leaflets may be in an irregular pattern. With two-dimensional echocardiography the leaflet may be seen to prolapse entirely into the left atrium during systole. By using M-mode echocardiography, various hemodynamic states, such as low cardiac output and decreased ventricular compliance, may be manifested by a diminished amplitude of the mitral valve opening or the presence of a B bump on the anterior mitral valve leaflet.

Aortic Valve. Echocardiography is useful in determining whether the aortic valve is tricuspid, bicuspid, thick-ened and/or calcified. In addition, the degree of pliability of each cusp can be determined.[75] Some echocardiographers think that the decreased and restricted opening of the valve is related to the severity of aortic stenosis (Fig. 5-19).[76] The indirect estimation of the severity of aortic stenosis can be estimated by measuring the extent of left ventricular hypertrophy.[77] However, the severity of aortic stenosis can be judged most accurately by Doppler echocardiography.

Aortic regurgitation cannot be directly assessed through echocardiography. Indirectly, fine fluttering of the anterior mitral valve leaflet during diastole caused by the regurgitant jet flowing into the left ventricle is indicative of aortic regurgitation.[78] Other indirect evidence of aortic valve regurgitation includes left ventricular dilatation, exaggerated motion activity of the interventricular septum, and premature mid-diastolic closure of the mitral valve. The latter finding is suggestive of severe, acute aortic regurgitation.[79]

Tricuspid and Pulmonic Valve. The tricuspid and pulmonic valves are not usually as well visualized as the mitral and aortic valves. Tricuspid valve stenosis is identified by noting abnormalities similar to those previously described with mitral stenosis. Tricuspid valve regurgitation manifests itself predominantly with signs of right ventricular overload,[80] such as right ventricular dilatation and paradoxical septal motion. Pulmonic valve stenosis appears as an early opening of the pulmonic valve caused by the right atrium contracting and ejecting blood into an overloaded

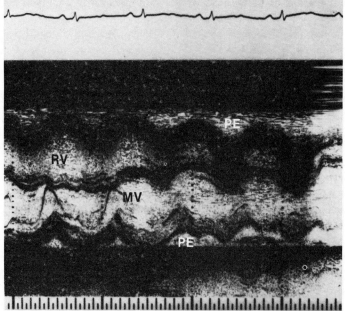

FIG. 5-20. M-mode echocardiogram demonstrating anterior and posterior pericardial effusion *(PE)* with diminished right ventricular dimension during inspiration. Abbreviations as in Fig. 5-14.

right ventricle.[81] The presence of pulmonary hypertension can be diagnosed by a change in the typical contour of the pulmonic valves on M-mode study with notching during systole and the loss of an "a" dip.

Pericardial Disease. Pericardial disease can be easily assessed with echocardiography. The existence of a pericardial effusion is determined by the presence of an echo-free space between the pericardium and the epicardium (Fig. 5-20). Furthermore, assessment of ventricular wall motion in the presence of pericardial effusion yields useful information regarding the possibility of cardiac tamponade. An echocardiogram with a moderately sized pericardial effusion and compression of the right ventricular free wall in early diastole suggests cardiac tamponade.[82] A collapse of the right atrial wall on the two-dimensional study may also be seen.[83] Constrictive pericarditis is indicated by a thickening of the pericardium and a flat diastolic slope of the posterior left ventricular wall.[84]

Other Applications. Echocardiography plays an important role in the assessment of congenital heart disease. The relative spatial arrangement of the cardiac structures as well as specific chamber abnormalities combine to provide useful information and identification of various congenital lesions. Intracardiac masses such as tumors and vegetations are frequently identified through echocardiography. Two-dimensional echocardiography is superior to M-mode study in this regard.

Doppler Echocardiography

The difference between reflected frequency and transmitted frequency is called a *Doppler shift*. By identifying this Doppler shift, the forward or backward velocity and the flow characteristics of blood can be determined. Doppler echocardiography provides information about the flow of blood within the heart, throughout its chambers, across the valves, and in the great vessels. It is a valuable adjunct to the conventional echocardiographic examination for a more complete noninvasive evaluation of cardiac function. Doppler echocardiography allows the quantitation of stenotic gradients, intracardiac pressures, and blood flow as well as a semiquantitative assessment of valvular regurgitation. Doppler echocardiography can allow the hemodynamic assessment of cardiac function which supplements the anatomic assessment obtained by the M-mode and two-dimensional echocardiography.

Two techniques of Doppler echocardiography are currently available: pulsed wave and continuous wave. Each technique can be used independently or in combination with simultaneously interrupted two-dimensional imaging capabilities. With the pulsed wave Doppler technique, one crystal emits short bursts of ultrasound and also receives the ultrasound reflected from moving red blood cells. The pulsed wave Doppler is combined simultaneously with two-dimensional echocardiography so that the exact location of the sample volume within the chamber can be visually displayed. Since this sample volume can be positioned in various cardiac chambers and vessels, it can be used to localize abnormal blood flow within cardiac structures. However, this technique has a disadvantage in that it measures velocity flow inaccurately. Continuous wave Doppler has one crystal that continuously emits the ultrasound signal and another that continuously receives the reflected signal. It also has the capability of detecting high velocity flow but cannot specify the location from which the flow is obtained.

Clinical Applications. Doppler echocardiography is used to evaluate five major cardiac conditions: valvular stenosis, valvular regurgitation, blood flow, intracardiac pressures, and intracardiac shunts.

Valvular Stenosis. The peak gradient and the valvular area across a stenotic valve can be obtained by measuring the peak velocity of blood flow across the valve by using Doppler techniques.[85,86] For example, a peak velocity in the ascending aorta in patients with aortic stenosis of 4 meters/second will produce a calculated peak pressure gradient of approximately 64 mmHg across the aortic valve by using the modified Bernoulli equation:

$$P = 4 \times V^2, \text{ where}$$
P: pressure gradient in mmHg
V: peak velocity in meters/second

Valvular Regurgitation. The presence of valvular regurgitation is detected as retrograde flow across the valve.

A "mapping" of the extent of regurgitant flow in the receiving cardiac chamber by the pulse mode allows semiquantitative assessment of severity.[87] For example, in patients with mild aortic insufficiency, a turbulent flow is detected in the upper left ventricle during diastole (Fig. 5-21). If this turbulence is detected at the level of the papillary muscle, the regurgitation is more severe than when it is detected only below the aortic valve. The further away from the aortic valve that turbulence is detected, the more severe the amount of regurgitation. Mitral regurgitation, tricuspid regurgitation, and pulmonic regurgitation all can be evaluated in the same way.

Blood Flow. Measurement of blood velocity, as well as the area through which blood flows, provides an estimate of volumetric blood flow. This estimate can be applied clinically as a noninvasive method of determining cardiac output, which can be calculated by measuring the mean velocity of the blood flow. The area can be calculated by measuring the diameter of either ascending aorta or pulmonary artery, and less accurately by measuring the inflow tract of the left ventricle. $CO = V \times A \times 60$, where CO: cardiac output, V: mean velocity of the blood flow, and A: the area of the cylinder where the blood flow is obtained.[88]

Intracardiac Pressures. In the presence of valvular regurgitation, the peak velocity of abnormal blood flow is proportional to the difference in pressure between the two cardiac chambers. Thus in tricuspid regurgitation if the

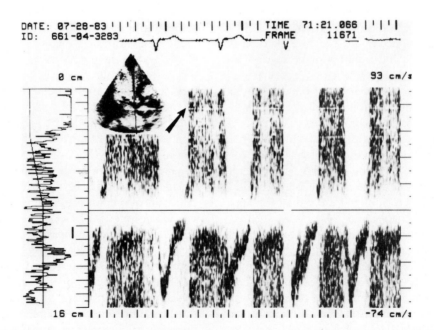

FIG. 5-21. Pulsed Doppler study demonstrating turbulent flow during diastole *(arrow)* with the sample volume being recorded from the left ventricular outflow tract. This is consistent with aortic regurgitation.

pressure in the right atrium is known by clinically estimating the jugular venous pressure, the pressure in the right ventricle can be derived. For example, if the regurgitant velocity of the tricuspid valve was 3 meters/sec and the jugular venous pressure was clinically estimated to be 10 mmHg, by adding these together, the systolic right ventricular and pulmonary artery pressure would be 46 mmHg, that is, 36 mmHg because of the pressure gradient $(4 \times V^2)$ and the addition of 10 mmHg. This calculation holds true as long as there is no obstruction in the right ventricular outflow tract.[89]

Intracardiac Shunts. The presence of an intracardiac shunt will result in abnormal velocity and patterns of blood flow on the lower pressure side of the shunt. In addition, by obtaining the amount of blood flow in the pulmonary artery and aorta, the ratio of the pulmonic versus systemic flow can be obtained noninvasively.

In summary, two-dimensional and M-mode electrocardiography along with Doppler echocardiography provide a sensitive, noninvasive means of assessing various cardiac conditions such as valvular heart disease, pericardial disease, congenital heart disease, cardiomyopathy, and coronary artery disease.

RIGHT-HEART CATHETERIZATION USING SWAN-GANZ TECHNIQUE

Right-sided heart catheterization can be performed at the bedside in the intensive care unit with the use of a Swan-Ganz thermodilution catheter. Continuous bedside hemodynamic monitoring provides a valuable adjunct to the assessment and management of a variety of cardiovascular disorders. The box below lists currently accepted indications for the use of Swan-Ganz catheter monitoring. In general, Swan-Ganz catheterization is indicated in any situation in which the obtained hemodynamic information substantially aids in choosing the best therapeutic modality for the patient.[90]

The Swan-Ganz technique involves inserting a balloon-tipped, flow-directed sterile catheter through a protective

sterile sheath or directly into an exposed vein. The catheter is advanced blindly while intracardiac pressure is monitored, until it is thought to be near the right atrium. The catheter balloon is then inflated and the catheter is advanced further, carried by the bloodstream across the tricuspid valve directly into the right ventricle. The catheter is then advanced across the pulmonic valve into the pulmonary artery until the balloon becomes wedged in an arterial branch. Pressure recordings should be obtained in each chamber as the catheter is being inserted, and pulmonary artery pressure should be recorded after the balloon has been deflated (Fig. 5-22).

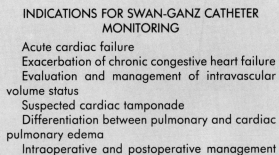

INDICATIONS FOR SWAN-GANZ CATHETER
MONITORING

Acute cardiac failure
Exacerbation of chronic congestive heart failure
Evaluation and management of intravascular volume status
Suspected cardiac tamponade
Differentiation between pulmonary and cardiac pulmonary edema
Intraoperative and postoperative management of high-risk surgical patients

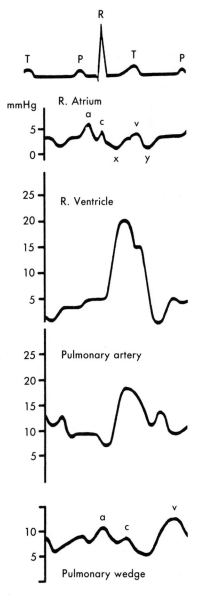

FIG. 5-22. Simultaneous normal right atrial ventricular, pulmonary artery, and pulmonary wedge tracings timed during cardiac cycle with surface electrocardiogram.

TABLE 5-1. Range of normal resting hemodynamic values (mm Hg)

Pressures	a Wave	v Wave	Mean	Systolic	End-diastolic
Right atrium	2-10	2-10	0-8		
Right ventricle				15-30	0-8
Pulmonary artery			9-16	15-30	3-12
Pulmonary capillary wedge (left atrium)	3-15	3-12	1-10		
Left ventricle				100-140	3-12
Systemic arteries			90-105	100-140	60-90

TABLE 5-2. Equations and normal values

	Equation	Normal values
Cardiac index (CI)	$CI = \dfrac{CO}{\text{Body surface area}}$	$2.5 - 4.2$ liter/min/M²
Stroke volume (SV)	$SV = \dfrac{CO}{\text{Heart rate}}$	
Stroke index (SI)	$SI = \dfrac{SV}{\text{Body surface area}}$	45 ± 13 ml/m²
Systemic vascular resistance (SVR)	$SVR = \dfrac{80\,(\overline{AO} - \overline{RA})}{Q_s}$ $\overline{AO}$: mean aortic pressure $\overline{RA}$: mean right atrial pressure Q_s: systemic blood flows	$770 - 1500$ dynes/sec/CM⁵
Pulmonary vascular resistance (PVR)	$PVR = \dfrac{80\,(\overline{PA} - \overline{LA})}{Q_p}$ $\overline{PA}$: mean pulmonary artery pressure $\overline{LA}$: mean left atrium pressure Q_p: pulmonary blood flow	$20 - 120$ dynes/sec/CM⁵

The Swan-Ganz catheter has two pressure lumens and one lumen for balloon inflation. The distal lumen located on the tip of the catheter is first used to record entry pressures and then to record the pulmonary artery and pulmonary capillary wedge pressure. The pressure obtained through the distal lumen when the balloon is wedged in the pulmonary artery is referred to as the *pulmonary capillary wedge pressure* and reflects the left ventricular end-diastolic pressure, provided there is no obstructive disease present in the pulmonary circulation or at the level of the mitral valve, which might affect the pressure readings. The proximal lumen, located 30 cm from the tip of the catheter, is used to record the right atrial pressure and is the injection port in the thermodilution cardiac output procedure. Normal pressure values for the anatomic sites mentioned above are shown in Table 5-1.

Cardiac output can be easily assessed after the Swan-Ganz thermodilution catheter is in position by using the thermodilution technique,[91] which involves the injection of a known volume of cold fluid into the proximal lumen.

A thermistor located near the catheter tip detects the change in temperature as the cold fluid flows through the pulmonary artery. The change in temperature is inversely proportional to cardiac output, that is, the greater the temperature change, the lower the cardiac output.

Once the right atrial (RA) pressure, pulmonary artery (PA) pressure, pulmonary capillary wedge pressure (PCWP), and cardiac output (CO) have been obtained, calculations of stroke volume (SV), systemic vascular resistance (SVR), and pulmonary vascular resistance (PVR) can be made using the equations shown in Table 5-2. These measures provide further information regarding the hemodynamic status of the patient.

CARDIAC CATHETERIZATION AND CARDIAC ANGIOGRAPHY

Cardiac catheterization and angiography are the definitive techniques for establishing the cause and severity of cardiac diseases. These techniques provide physiologic data regarding cardiovascular hemodynamics as well as the an-

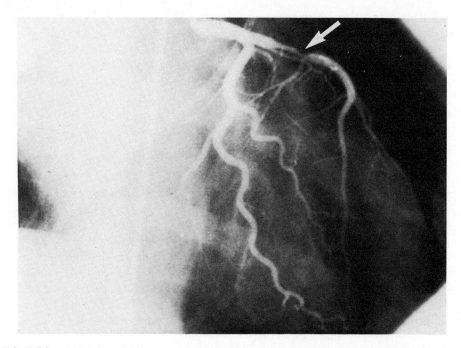

FIG. 5-23. RAO view of left coronary artery injection demonstrating high-grade stenosis of the left anterior descending artery *(arrow)* at the lead of the first septal perforator.

giographic evaluation of cardiac chambers and structures that can be visualized on X-ray film by the injection of radiopaque contrast media.

Cardiac catheterization involves passing a catheter through a vein or artery to the right or left cardiac chambers so that pressure and oxygen saturations within the chamber can be measured, and gradients across a stenotic cardiac valve can be determined. In addition, radiopaque contrast media can be injected to visualize the cardiac chambers, great vessels, and coronary arteries on fluoroscopy and X-ray film. Through these laboratory techniques the presence of regional wall motion abnormalities and the severity of valvular regurgitation can be accurately assessed. Complications of myocardial infarction, such as acquired ventricular septal defect with a left-to-right shunt, can be detected and quantitated through measurement of oxygen saturations in the right cardiac chambers.

The most commonly performed angiographic procedure in the patient who has known or suspected coronary artery disease is coronary arteriography. With this technique selective catheterization of the coronary arteries is performed either by a brachial arteriotomy (Sones technique) or by a percutaneous femoral puncture (Judkins technique). Coronary arteriography involves placing a specially designed catheter in the ostia of the left and right coronary arteries and injecting contrast media to visualize the coronary arterial circulation. Typically, several injections of both the left and right coronary arteries are per-

formed in multiple left and right caudal and cranial views to ensure adequate visualization of the proximal and distal portion of each vessel. A hemodynamically significant coronary artery stenosis is defined as a reduction in luminal diameter compared with that of a normal segment of the same vessel of greater than or equal to 50% in the left main coronary artery and 75% in the major branches, such as left anterior descending, circumflex, and right coronary artery (Fig. 5-23). However, quantitative coronary arteriography can be obtained more accurately by using a computerized analysis. By this method measurement of the exact area of the stenosis, percent reduction, and coronary flow reserve in the diameter or the area can be obtained for each stenotic lesion. In addition to atherosclerotic coronary artery lesions, conditions such as idiopathic hypertrophic subaortic stenosis or coronary artery spasm, which often mimic ischemic heart disease in their clinical presentations, can be diagnosed with cardiac catheterization and coronary arteriography.

Serious complications occur in approximately one in every 1000 cardiac catheterizations and include death, stroke, myocardial infarction, loss of peripheral pulse, and allergic reaction to contrast media.[92] The indications for cardiac catheterization and coronary arteriography vary slightly among institutions. Moreover, the indications for these procedures have changed as data about the natural history of coronary artery disease and valvular heart disease and the effects of interventional therapy on these lesions have become available. The measurement of valve areas or gradients and the assessment of indices of left ventricular performance such as end-diastolic pressure or cardiac output are often required to determine the optimal timing for surgical intervention.

Traditionally, coronary angiography has been performed in the patient who has classic angina in order to delineate the anatomic sites and the degree of coronary artery stenosis prior to considering aortocoronary bypass surgery or percutaneous transluminal coronary angioplasty (PTCA). For example, patients with left main coronary artery stenosis and stable angina have been shown to improve long-term survival with aortocoronary bypass surgery.[93] Coronary angiography can be performed in the setting of acute myocardial infarction or unstable angina to determine whether acute interventional therapeutic modalities are indicated. Intracoronary use of a thrombolytic agent such as streptokinase or tissue plasminogen activator (TPA) or PTCA with or without thrombolytic therapy, or coronary artery bypass surgery, are all therapeutic modalities that may be considered. Coronary angiography may be indicated for patients having atypical chest pain for whom noninvasive tests such as exercise with thallium imaging have been equivocal or nondiagnostic. For the patient who develops myocardial ischemia following aortocoronary bypass surgery or PTCA, coronary arteriography may be required to assess the patency of the graft or the status of the previously dilated lesions, or to determine if new coronary artery stenoses have developed in other vessels. Vasospastic angina such as Prinzmetal's variant angina may be diagnosed through the use of angiography in conjunction with the use of provocative agents such as ergonovine.[94]

In summary, coronary angiography and cardiac catheterization are the techniques best able to assist in the precise evaluation of the etiology and severity of cardiac diseases and in the determination of the prognosis and potential therapy for a given patient.

Serum Enzymes in Acute Myocardial Infarction

The diagnosis of acute myocardial infarction is typically confirmed by the patient's clinical history, electrocardiographic changes, and elevation of serum enzymes released from the heart muscle after myocardial injury. Necrosis can cause an increased permeability of cellular membranes, which allows these enzymes to leak into the bloodstream. There are three major enzymes that occur in abnormal levels in the serum following myocardial injury: creatinine phosphokinase (CPK), lactic dehydrogenase (LDH), and serum glutamic oxaloacetic transaminase (SGOT). The relative rates at which each enzyme appears in the serum following infarction is shown in Fig. 5-24. Creatinine phosphokinase (CPK) is present in cardiac and skeletal muscle and in the brain and gastrointestinal tract. Abnormal elevation in serum CPK begins to appear in the blood about 4 to 6 hours after the onset of acute myocardial infarction. Peak levels of this enzyme typically appear 16 to 30 hours after the onset of the infarction and return to normal within 3 to 4 days. However, the elevation of serum CPK is nonspecific for cardiac injury. For example, if the

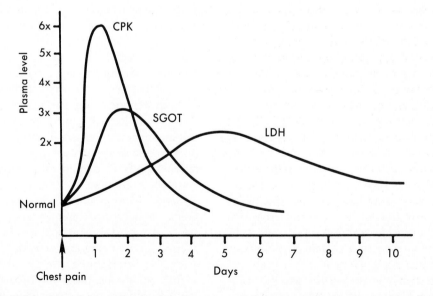

FIG. 5-24.   Plot of plasma levels of cardiac enzymes against time after chest pain. Note that CPK (creatine phosphokinase) and SGOT (serum glutamic-oxaloacetic transaminase) peak before LDH (lactate dehydrogenase).

patient had received an intramuscular injection of analgesic, this enzyme level also rises secondary to skeletal muscle necrosis. To determine the precise source of the elevated CPK, electrophoresis or radioimmunoassay can be used to separate CPK into three isoenzymes. The MM isoenzyme is found in skeletal muscle, and the BB isoenzyme appears to be uniquely present in brain tissue. The MB isoenzyme, like total serum CPK, appears in the serum about 4 hours after the onset of myocardial necrosis and peaks in about 18 to 20 hours.[95] However, if reperfusion occurs either spontaneously or with interventional therapy, such as with the use of a thrombolytic agent and/or PTCA, the peak value occurs sooner and is usually higher than without reperfusion.[96] Following acute interventions, peak levels are reached in about 6 to 8 hours for MB isoenzyme and in about 12 hours for the total CPK, presumably because of the rapid washout of the enzymes.

CPK levels in serum have also been used to estimate the size of myocardial infarctions.[97] Postmortem canine studies have shown a correlation between serum CPK levels drawn serially after myocardial infarction and the size of infarction. Although this technique appears to be less accurate in humans, some studies still claim close relationships in human subjects.

Another enzyme that is released after myocardial infarction is LDH, which appears in abnormal amounts in peripheral blood about 24 to 48 hours after the onset of infarction. Peak levels occur in 3 to 6 days, and the enzyme levels return to normal 7 to 10 days after infarction. LDH is widely distributed throughout such body organs as heart, kidney, skeletal muscle, lung, liver, and red blood cells. LDH can be separated into five isoenzymes. Cardiac muscle is particularly rich in the isoenzymes LDH_1; therefore after myocardial damage, the predominant isoenzyme found in the serum is LDH_1. If there are higher levels for LDH_1 than LDH_2 (known as LDH_1 *flip*[98]), or if the percentage of LDH_1 exceeds 40% of the total of LDH[99] values, it is considered sensitive for myocardial injury.

A third enzyme that appears in elevated levels in the serum is SGOT. Elevation of SGOT occurs about 12 to 18 hours after the onset of infarction, and peak levels occur about 24 to 48 hours after the onset of infarction. However, elevated levels of SGOT can also occur in patients who have pulmonary embolism, myocarditis, pericarditis, or skeletal muscle and hepatic disease. Since there are no specific isoenzymes of SGOT for myocardial tissue, this enzyme is not especially indicative of myocardial necrosis and the clinical usefulness of obtaining SGOT levels is debatable.[100]

If the patient is admitted within 24 hours of the onset of the suspected myocardial infarction, the total CPK and MB isoenzymes levels of the serum are considered to be the most informative laboratory test in detecting myocar-

dial cell injury. If those values do not rise in the first 24 hours it is highly indicative of the absence of myocardial necrosis. However, in rare cases, patients with myocardial infarctions may have small elevations in total CPK still within the normal range. In these patients the diagnosis can be confirmed by documenting an elevation in the MB isoenzyme.[101] If the patients are admitted more than 24 hours after the onset of the infarction or if the time of onset is not known, the evaluation of the total LDH and LDH_1 isoenzyme becomes important.

REFERENCES

1. Bruce, R.A.: Methods of exercise testing, Am. J. Cardiol. **33:**715, 1974.
2. Rifkin, R.D., and Hood, W.B.: Bayesian analysis of electrocardiographic exercise stress testing, N. Engl. J. Med. **297:**681, 1977.
3. Epstein, S.E.: Implications of probability analysis on the strategy used for noninvasive detection of coronary artery disease: role of single or combined use of exercise electrocardiographic testing, radionuclide cineangiography and myocardial perfusion imaging, Am. J. Cardiol. **46:**491, 1980.
4. Cohn, P.F.: Silent myocardial ischemia: to treat or not to treat? Hosp. Pract. **18:**125, 1983.
5. Kattus, A.A.: Exercise electrocardiography: recognition of the ischemic response, false positive and negative patterns, Am. J. Cardiol. **33:**721, 1974.
6. Goldschlager, N., Selzer, A., and Cohn, K.: Treadmill stress tests as indications of presence and severity of coronary artery disease, Ann. Intern. Med. **85:**277, 1976.
7. Goldman, S., Tselos, S., and Cohn, K.: Marked depth of ST-segment depression during treadmill exercise testing: indicator of severe coronary artery disease, Chest **69:**729, 1976.
8. Ellestad, M.H., Couke, B.M., and Greenberg, P.S.: Stress testing: clinical application and predictive capacity, Prog. Cardiovasc. Dis. **21:**431, 1979.
9. Council on Scientific Affairs: Indications and contraindications for exercise testing, JAMA **246:**1015, 1981.
10. Bruce, R.A.: Exercise testing for evaluation of ventricular function, N. Engl. J. Med. **296:**671, 1977.
11. Jelinek, M.V., and Lown, B.: Exercise stress testing for exposure of cardiac arrhythmia, Prog. Cardiovasc. Dis. **6:**497, 1974.
12. Woelfel, A., and others: Reproducibility and treatment of exercise-induced ventricular tachycardia, Am. J. Cardiol. **53:**751, 1984.
13. Antman, E., Graboys, T.B., and Lown, B.: Continuous monitoring for ventricular arrhythmias during exercise tests, JAMA **241:**2802, 1979.
14. Force, T., and Graboys, T.B.: Exercise testing and ambulatory monitoring in patients with preexcitation syndrome, Arch. Intern. Med. **141:**88, 1981.
15. Klein, G.J., and Gulamhusein, S.S.: Intermittent preexcitation in the Wolff-Parkinson-White Syndrome, Am. J. Cardiol. **52:**292, 1983.
16. Theroux, P., and others: Prognostic value of exercise testing soon after myocardial infarction, N. Engl. J. Med. **301:**341, 1979.
17. Cohn, P.F.: The role of noninvasive cardiac testing after an uncomplicated myocardial infarction, N. Engl. J. Med. **309:**90, 1983.
18. Epstein, S.E., Palmeri, S.T., and Patterson, R.E.: Evaluation of patients after acute myocardial infarction: indications for cardiac catheterization and surgical intervention, N. Engl. J. Med. **307:**1487, 1982.

19. DiCola, V.C., and others: Pathophysiologic correlates of thallium-201 myocardial uptake in experimental infarction, Cardiovasc. Res. **11**:141, 1977.

20. Hamilton, G.W., Trobaugh, G.B., Ritchie, J.J., and others: Myocardial imaging with intravenously injected thallium-201 in patients with suspected coronary artery disease: analysis of the technique and correlation with electrocardiographic, coronary anatomic and ventriculographic findings, Am. J. Cardiol. **39**:347, 1977.

21. Wackers, F.J., and others: Location and size of acute transmural infarction estimated from thallium-201 scintiscans: a clinicopathological study, Circulation **56**:72, 1977.

22. Wackers, F.J., and others: Value and limitations of thallium-201: scintigraphy in the acute phase of myocardial infarction, N. Engl. J. Med. **295**:1, 1976.

23. Pohost, G.M., and others: Differentiation of transiently ischemic from infarcted myocardium by serial imaging after a single dose of thallium 201, Circulation **55**:294, 1977.

24. Beller, G.A., and Pohost, G.M.: Mechanism for thallium 201 redistribution after transient myocardial ischemia (abstract), Circulation **56**(3):141, 1977.

25. Okada, R.D., and others: Exercise radionuclide imaging approaches to coronary artery disease, Am. J. Cardiol. **46**:1188, 1980.

26. Ritchie, J.L., and others: Myocardial imaging with thallium 201 at and during exercise, Circulation **56**:66, 1977.

27. Gould, K.L., and others: Noninvasive assessment of coronary stenoses by myocardial perfusion imaging during pharmacologic coronary vasodilation: VIII clinical feasibility of positron cardiac imaging without a cyclotron using generator-produced Rubidium 82, J. Am. Coll. Cardiol. **7**:775, 1986.

28. Buja, L.M., and others: Pathophysiology of thallium 201 scintigraphy of acute anterior myocardial infarcts in dogs, J. Clin. Invest. **57**:1508, 1976.

29. Holman, B.L., Tanaka, T.T., and Lesch, M.: Evaluation of radiopharmaceuticals for the detection of acute myocardial infarction in man, Radiology **121**:427, 1976.

30. Pitt, B., and Strauss, W.H.: Evaluation of ventricular function by radioisotope techniques, N. Engl. J. Med. **296**:1097, 1977.

31. Wackers, F.J.Th., and others: Multiple-gated cardiac blood pool imaging for left ventricular ejection fraction: validation of the technique and assessment of variability, Am. J. Cardiol. **43**:1166, 1979.

32. Okada, R.D., and others: Observer variance in the qualitative evaluation of left ventricular wall motion and the quantitation of left ventricular ejection fraction using rest and exercise multigated blood pool imaging, Circulation **61**:128, 1980.

33. Borer, J.S., and others: Real-time radionuclide cineangiography in the noninvasive evaluation of global and regional left ventricular function and rest and during exercise in patients with coronary artery disease, N. Engl. J. Med. **296**:839, 1977.

34. The Multicenter Postinfarction Research Group: Risk stratification and survival after myocardial infarction, N. Engl. J. Med. **309**:331, 1983.

35. Holter, N.J.: Radioelectrocardiography: a new technique for cardiovascular studies, Ann. N.Y. Acad. Sci. **65**:913, 1957.

36. Holter, N.J.: New method for heart studies, Science **134**:1214, 1961.

37. Kennedy, H.L., and Underhill, S.J.: Frequent or complex ventricular ectopy in apparently healthy subjects, Am. J. Cardiol. **38**:141, 1976.

38. Brodsky, M., and others: Arrhythmias documented by 24-hour continuous electrocardiographic monitoring in 50 male medical students without apparent heart disease, Am. J. Cardiol. **39**:390, 1977.

39. Winkle, R.A.: Antiarrhythmic drug effect mimicked by spontaneous variability of ventricular ectopy, Circulation **57**:1116, 1978.

40. Morganroth, J., and others: Limitations of routine long-term electrocardiographic monitoring to assess ventricular ectopic frequency, Circulation **58**:408, 1978.

41. Michelson, E.L., and Morganroth, J.: Spontaneous variability of complex ventricular arrhythmias detected by long-term electrocardiographic recording, Circulation **61**:690, 1980.

42. Pratt, C.M., and others: Analysis of the spontaneous variability of ventricular arrhythmias: consecutive ambulatory electrocardiographic recordings of ventricular tachycardia, Am. J. Cardiol. **56**:67, 1985.

43. Sokoloff, N., and others: Utility of ambulatory electrocardiographic monitoring for predicting recurrence of sustained ventricular tachyarrhythmias in patients receiving amiodarone, J. Am. Coll. Cardiol. **7**:938, 1986.

44. Graboys, T.B., and others: Long-term survival of patients with malignant ventricular arrhythmia treated with antiarrhythmic drugs, Am. J. Cardiol. **50**:437, 1982.

45. Heger, J.J., and others: Comparison between results obtained from electrocardiographic testing, exercise testing, and ambulatory ECG recordings. In Wenger, N.K., Mock, M.B., and Ringquist, I., editors: Ambulatory electrocardiographic recording, Chicago, 1981, Year Book Medical Publishers, Inc.

46. Zeldis, S.M., and others: Cardiovascular complaints: correlation with cardiac arrhythmias on 24-hour electrocardiographic monitoring, Chest **78**:456, 1980.

47. Clark, P.A., Glasser, S.P., and Spoto, E.: Arrhythmias detected by ambulatory monitoring: lack of correlation with symptoms of dizziness and syncope, Chest **77**:722, 1980.

48. Boudoulos, H.B., School, S.F., and Lewis, R.P.: Superiority of 24-hour outpatient monitoring over multi-stage exercise testing for the evaluation of syncope, J. Electrocardiol. **12**:103, 1979.

49. Crawford, M.A., and others: Limitations of continuous ambulatory electrocardiogram monitoring for detecting coronary artery disease, Ann. Intern. Med. **89**:1, 1978.

50. Guazzi, M., and others: Continous electrocardiographic recording in Prinzmetal's variant angina pectoris: a report of 4 cases, Br. Heart J. **32**:611, 1970.

51. Vismara, L.A., and others: Identification of sudden death risk factor in acute and chronic coronary artery disease, Am. J. Cardiol. **39**:821, 1979.

52. Kotler, M.N., and others: Prognostic significance of ventricular ectopic beats with respect to sudden death in the late post-infarction period, Circulation **49**:959, 1973.

53. Anderson, K.P., DeCamilla, J., and Moss, A.J.: Clinical significance of ventricular tachycardia (3 beats or longer) detected during ambulatory monitoring after myocardial infarction, Circulation **57**:890, 1978.

54. Ryan, M., Lown, B., and Horn, H.: Comparison of ventricular ectopic activity during 24-hour monitoring and exercise testing in patients with coronary heart disease, N. Engl. J. Med. **292**:224, 1975.

55. Follansbee, W.P., Michelson, E.L., and Morganroth, J.: Nonsustained ventricular tachycardia in ambulatory patients: characteristics and association with sudden cardiac death, Ann. Intern. Med. **92**:741, 1980.

56. McKenna, W.J., and others: Exercise electrocardiographic and 48-hour ambulatory electrocardiographic monitor assessment of arrhythmia on and off beta blocker therapy in hypertrophic cardiomyopathy, Am. J. Cardiol. **43**:420, 1979.

57. Schwartz, P.J., Periti, M., and Malliani, A.: The long QT syndrome, Am. Heart J. **89**:378, 1975.

58. DeBusk, R.F., and others: Serial ambulatory electrocardiography and treadmill testing after uncomplicated myocardial infarction, Am. J. Cardiol. **45**:547, 1980.

59. Winkle, R.A., and others: Arrhythmias in patients with mitral valve prolapse, Circulation **52**:73, 1975.
60. DeMaria, A.N., Amsterdam, E.A., and Vismara, L.A.: Arrhythmias in the mitral valve prolapse syndrome: prevalence, nature, and frequency, Ann. Intern. Med. **84**:656, 1976.
61. Price, J.E., and others: Evaluation of ventricular arrhythmias postcoronary bypass surgery: decreased prevalence following hospital discharge determined by ambulatory ECG-monitoring, Am. J. Cardiol. **39**:269, 1977.
62. McAnulty, J.N., Rahimtoola, S.H., and Murphy, E.S.: A prospective study of sudden death in "high-risk" bundle branch block, N. Engl. J. Med. **299**:209, 1978.
63. Pritchett, E.L.C., and others: Electrocardiogram recording by telephone in antiarrhythmic drug trials, Chest **81**:473, 1982.
64. Hasin, Y., David, D., and Rogel, S.: Transtelephonic adjustment of antiarrhythmic therapy in ambulatory patients, Cardiology **63**:243, 1978.
65. Tuttle, W.B., and Schoenfeld, C.D.: ECG phone monitoring of the convalescing MI patients, Prim. Cardiol. Clin. **1**:13, 1984.
66. Moynihan, P.F., Parisi, A.F., and Feldman, C.L.: Quantitative detection of regional left ventricular contraction abnormalities by two-dimensional echocardiography, Circulation **63**:752, 1981.
67. Reeder, G.S., Tajik, A.J., and Seward, J.B.: Left ventricular mural thrombus: two-dimensional echocardiographic diagnosis, Mayo Clin. Proc. **56**:82, 1981.
68. Barrett, M.J., Charuzi, Y., and Corday, E.: Ventricular aneurysm: cross-sectional echocardiographic approach, Am. J. Cardiol. **46**:1133, 1980.
69. Perry, L.S., and others: Two-dimensional echocardiography in the diagnosis of left atrial myxoma, Br. Heart J. **45**:667, 1981.
70. Shah, P.M., and others: Role of echocardiography in diagnosis and hemodynamic assessment of hypertrophic subaortic stenosis, Circulation **44**:891, 1971.
71. Joiner, C.R., Reid, J.M., and Bond, J.P.: Reflected ultrasound in the assessment of mitral valve disease, Circulation **27**:506, 1963.
72. Feigenbaum, H.: Echocardiography, ed. 3, Philadelphia, 1981, Lea & Febiger.
73. DeMaria, A.N., and others: The variable spectrum of echocardiographic manifestations of the mitral valve prolapse syndrome, Circulation **50**:33, 1974.
74. Sweatman, T., and others: Echocardiographic diagnosis of mitral valve regurgitation due to ruptured chordae tendineae, Circulation **46**:580, 1972.
75. Gramiak, R., and Shah, P.M.: Echocardiography of the normal and diseased aortic valve, Radiology **96**:1, 1970.
76. Weyman, A.E., and others: Cross-sectional echocardiography in assessing the severity of valvular aortic stenosis, Circulation **52**:828, 1975.
77. Reichek, N., and Devereux, R.B.: Reliable estimation of peak left ventricular systolic pressure by M-mode echocardiographic-determined end-diastolic relative wall thickness: identification of severe valvular aortic stenosis in adult patients, Am. Heart J. **103**:202, 1982.
78. Dillon, J.C., and others: Significance of mitral fluttering in patients with aortic insufficiency (abstract), Clin. Res. **18**:304, 1970.
79. Botuirick, E.H., and others: Echocardiographic demonstration of early mitral valve closure in severe aortic insufficiency: its clinical implications, Circulation **51**:836, 1975.
80. Popp, R.L., and others: Estimation of the right and left ventricular size by ultrasound: a study of echoes from the interventricular septum, Am. J. Cardiol. **24**:253, 1969.
81. Weyman, A.E., and others: Echocardiographic patterns of pulmonic valve motion in pulmonic stenosis, Am. J. Cardiol. **34**:644, 1974.
82. Armstrong, W.F., and others: Diastolic collapse of the right ventricle with cardiac tamponade: an echocardiographic study, Circulation **65**:1491, 1982.
83. Gillam, L.D., and others: Hydrodynamic compression of the right atrial free wall, a new highly-sensitive echocardiographic sign of cardiac tamponade, Am. J. Cardiol. **49**:1010, 1982.
84. Voelkel, A.G., and others: Echocardiographic features of constrictive pericarditis, Circulation **58**:871, 1978.
85. Holen, J., and others: Determination of pressure gradient in mitral stenosis with a non-invasive ultrasound Doppler technique, Acta. Med. Scand. **199**:455, 1976.
86. Hatle, L., Angelsen, B., and Tromsdal, A.: Noninvasive assessment of atrioventricular pressure half-time by Doppler ultrasound, Circulation **60**:1096, 1979.
87. Abbasi, A.S., and others: Detection and estimation of the degree of mitral regurgitation by range-gated pulsed Doppler echocardiography, Circulation **61**:143, 1980.
88. Huntsman, L.L., and others: Noninvasive Doppler determination of cardiac output in man: clinical validation, Circulation **67**:593, 1983.
89. Yock, P.G., and Popp, R.L.: Noninvasive estimation of right ventricular systolic pressure by Doppler ultrasound in patients with tricuspid regurgitation, Circulation **70**:657, 1984.
90. Swan, H.J.C.: The role of hemodynamic monitoring in the management of the critically ill, Crit. Care Med. **3**:83, 1975.
91. Forrester, J.S., and others: Thermodilution cardiac output determination with a single flow-directed catheter, Am. Heart J. **83**:306, 1972.
92. Grossman, W.: Complication of cardiac catheterization: incidence, causes and prevention. In Grossman, W., editor: Cardiac catheterization and angiography, ed. 2, Philadelphia, 1980, Lea & Febiger.
93. Zeft, J.H., Manley, J.C., and Huston, J.H.: Left main coronary artery stenosis results of coronary bypass surgery, Circulation **49**:68, 1974.
94. Ricci, D.R., and others: Reduction of coronary blood flow during coronary artery spasm occurring spontaneously and after provocation by ergonovine maleate, Circulation **57**:137, 1978.
95. Irvin, R.G., Cobb, F.R., and Roe, C.R.: Acute myocardial infarction and MB creatinine phosphokinase: relationship between onset of symptoms of infarction and appearance and disappearance of enzymes, Arch. Intern. Med. **140**:329, 1980.
96. Neuhaus, K.L., and others: High-dose intravenous streptokinase infusion in acute myocardial infarction, Z. Kardiol. **70**:791, 1981.
97. Shell, W.E., Kjekshus, J.K., and Sobel, B.E.: Quantitative assessment of the extent of myocardial infarction in the conscious dog by means of analysis of serial change in serum creatinine phosphokinase activity, J. Clin. Invest. **50**:2614, 1971.
98. Leung, E.Y., and Henderson, A.R.: Thin-layer agarose electrophoresis of lactate dehydrogenase isoenzymes in serum: a note on the method of reporting and on the lactate dehydrogenase isoenzyme-1/isoenzyme-2 ratio in acute myocardial infarction, Clin. Chem. **25**:209, 1979.
99. Weidner, N.: Laboratory diagnosis of acute myocardial infarct: usefulness of determination of lactate dehydrogenase (LDH)-1 level and of ratio LDH-1 to LDH, Arch. Pathol. Lab. Med. **106**:375, 1982.
100. Fisher, M.C., and others: Routine serum enzyme tests in the diagnosis of acute myocardial infarction: cost effectiveness, Arch. Intern. Med. **143**:1541, 1983.
101. McQueen, M.J., Holder, D., and El-Maraghi, N.R.H.: Assessment of the accuracy of serial electrocardiograms in the diagnosis of myocardial infarction, Am. Heart J. **105**:258, 1983.

CHAPTER 6

Introduction to Electrocardiography

Douglas P. Zipes
Kathleen Gainor Andreoli

This chapter explains some basic principles of electrocardiography, describes the use of the normal ECG, and introduces certain abnormalities commonly encountered in patients who have cardiac disease manifesting electrocardiographic changes. Additional electrocardiographic disorders are presented in Chapter 8.

BASIC CONSIDERATIONS

An ECG is a graphic tracing of the electrical forces produced by the heart. For patients who have heart disease this test is a frequently used and highly important diagnostic procedure. The ECG, however, has limitations, so it is important to evaluate it in conjunction with a clinical examination of the patient. For example, electrocardiographic abnormalities may occur in healthy persons, and conversely, structural heart disease may occur in patients who have normal electrocardiographic patterns. Premature ventricular complexes found in the ECG of a young patient with no heart disease and complaints of palpitations raise different diagnostic considerations than do premature ventricular complexes found in the ECG of a middle-aged patient who has had a myocardial infarction and syncope. Thus the nature and the effect of the rhythm disturbance on the individual patient influence the clinical importance of the findings.

It is important to remember that the health care professional evaluates the patient who has an ECG abnormality, not the ECG in isolation. Some rhythm disturbances, for example, are hazardous to a patient regardless of the clinical setting, but others are hazardous only because of the clinical setting.

Numerous extrinsic factors not related to the heart per se such as drugs, metabolic changes, and electrolyte imbalances may alter the final ECG recording. Technical factors such as inadequate skin preparation to reduce skin resistance, muscle tremor, 60-Hz cycle interference, and incorrectly applied electrodes also must be considered.

STANDARDIZATION

The ECG comprises a series of horizontal and vertical lines that measure amplitude and duration of the various deflections, segments, and intervals. The horizontal lines are 1 mm apart and are used to measure the *amplitude* of the ECG deflections. The vertical lines are also 1 mm apart and are used to measure the time or *duration* of the ECG events. Each fifth horizontal and vertical line is darker than the others, forming a large square that incorporates 25 smaller squares.

Conventionally, the ECG is *standardized* so that the amplitude of a 1 millivolt (mV) impulse causes a deflection

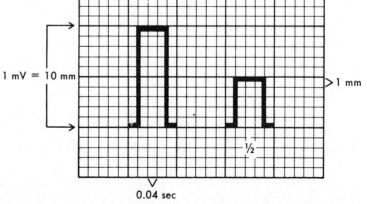

FIG. 6-1. Normal standardization of the ECG. One millivolt (mV) causes a deflection of 10 millimeters (mm). For large ECG deflections the standard must be halved so that 1 mV = 5 mm. For small ECG deflections the standard may be doubled so that 1 mV = 20 mm. Any changes in standardization must be noted on the ECG recording.

of 10 mm that is two large squares (Fig. 6-1). Therefore each 1-mm deflection equals 0.1 mV. If the amplitude of the deflection recorded from the heart is too large for the ECG paper, the standardization must be halved so that 1 mV results in a deflection of 5 mm (one large square). If the standardization is halved, it must be noted on the ECG paper. The standardization may also be doubled so that 1 mV equals 20 mm.

The usual paper speed for recording is 25 mm/second, and therefore each vertical line separated by 1 mm equals 0.04 sec (40 msec). At twice the normal recording speed (50 mm/second), each small box equals 0.02 second (20 msec).

DEFLECTIONS

Any wave or complex recorded in the ECG is inscribed as a *positive* (above the base line) or *negative* (below the base line) deflection. When a deflection is partly above the base line and partly below it, and the positive and negative components are approximately equal, the complex is called *diphasic* or *biphasic*. As previously mentioned, the amplitude of deflections is recorded in millimeters or millivolts. Measurement of positive deflections is made from the upper edge of the base line to the peak of the wave; negative deflections are measured from the lower edge of the base line to the lowest point of the wave. Deflections also have *duration,* recorded in seconds or milliseconds (msec).

The six major deflections of the normal ECG are designated by the letters P, Q, R, S, T, and U (Fig. 6-2). These waves are produced by the electrical energy caused by the movement of charged particles across the membranes of myocardial cells (depolarization and repolarization).

ELECTROPHYSIOLOGIC PRINCIPLES

The membrane surrounding a cell is a semipermeable two-layered lipid envelope that maintains a high concentration of potassium (K^+) and a low concentration of sodium (Na^+) inside the cell and a high concentration of Na^+ and a low concentration of K^+ outside the cell. The voltage inside a resting (polarized) cardiac cell is negative with respect to the outside of the cell, in large part because of the cell membrane's relative permeability to K^+ and impermeability to Na^+ during diastole. The ratio of extracellular to intracellular potassium concentrations primarily determines the resting potential of the cell; when the cell becomes depolarized the cell membrane alters its permeability so that it becomes more permeable to Na^+ and less permeable to K^+. Na^+ rushes into the cell, making the voltage inside the cell positive with respect to the voltage outside the cell. These events occur in atrial and ventricular muscle and the His-Purkinje system. In the normal sinus and AV nodes, and possibly in other fibers if they become damaged and lose membrane potential, calcium appears to play a prominent role in the depolarization process. Calcium (and possibly sodium in some instances) enters the cell through the "slow channel," producing the *slow response*. It is called the slow response because the time to activate and inactivate the channel (in essence, turn it on and off) is slow, compared to the sodium or "fast channel,"

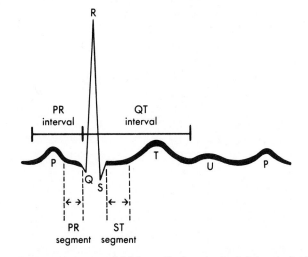

FIG. 6-2.   The deflections in a normal ECG are the P wave (atrial depolarization), QRS complex (ventricular depolarization), and T wave (ventricular repolarization). The U wave is sometimes present and follows the T wave. The PR segment is the interval between the end of the P wave and the beginning of the QRS complex. The ST segment is the interval between the end of the QRS complex and the beginning of the T wave. Sometimes atrial repolarization, the Ta wave, can be recorded (see Fig. 6-6). The PR interval is from the onset of the P wave to the onset of the QRS complex. The QT interval is from the onset of the QRS complex to the end of the T wave.

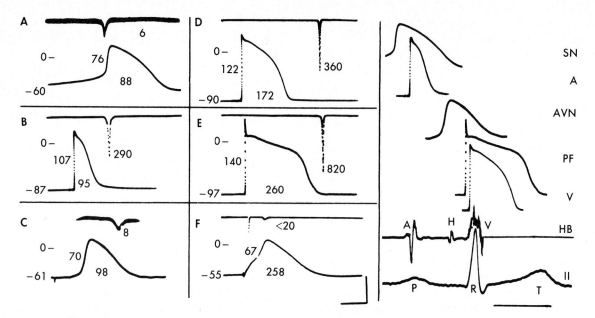

FIG. 6-3. Action potentials recorded from different tissues in the heart *(left),* remounted with a His bundle recording and scalar ECG from a patient *(right)* to illustrate the timing during a single cardiac cycle. In A to F the top tracing is dV/dt of phase 0 and the second tracing is the action potential. For each panel the numbers *(from left to right)* indicate maximum diastolic potential (mV), action potential amplitude (mV), action potential duration at 90 percent of repolarization (msec), and Vmax (maximum rate of rise in volts/second of cardiac action potential) of phase 0 (V/sec). Zero potential is indicated by the short horizontal line next to the zero on the upper left of each action potential. A, Rabbit sinoatrial node; B, canine atrial muscle; C, rabbit atrioventricular node; D, canine ventricular muscle; E, canine Purkinje fiber; F, diseased human ventricle. Note that the action potentials recorded in A, C, and F have reduced resting membrane potentials, amplitudes, and Vmax compared to the other action potentials. In right panel, *SN* = sinus nodal potential; *A* = atrial muscle potential; *AVN* = atrioventricular nodal potential; *PF* = Purkinje fiber potential; *V* = ventricular muscle potential; *HB* = His bundle recording; *II* = lead II. Horizontal calibration on left: 50 msec for A and C, 100 msec for B, D, E, and F. Vertical calibration on left: 50 mV. Horizontal calibration on right: 200 msec. (From Gilmour, R.F., Jr., and Zipes, D.P.: Basic electrophysiology of the slow inward current. In Antman, E., and Stone, P.H., editors: Calcium blocking agents in the treatment of cardiovascular disorders, Mt. Kisco, NY, 1983, Futura Publishing Co., Inc.)

which is active in muscle and in His-Purkinje fibers (Fig. 6-3).

Understanding these ionic mechanisms is clinically important because of the development of drugs such as verapamil that *fairly* specifically block the slow channel. These drugs are often called "calcium channel or calcium entry blockers."

The cell in a resting, *polarized* state can be represented by negative and positive charges lining, respectively, the inside and outside of the cell membrane (Fig. 6-4, *A*). If an electrode of an ECG machine (galvanometer) were attached to this polarized cell, no electrical potential would be registered because no net change in ionic composition would occur. Hence, there would be no voltage shift and no deviation from the isoelectric base line (Fig. 6-4, *A*).

When a cell or, more likely, a group of cells is stimulated, and the change in membrane permeability permits sodium ions to migrate rapidly into the cell making the inside

positive with respect to the outside *(depolarization)*, an electrical field is generated between the depolarized and polarized areas of myocardium. The P *wave* represents *atrial depolarization,* and the *QRS* complex represents *ventricular depolarization* (Fig. 6-4, *B* to *D*).

A slower movement of ions across the membrane restoring the cell to the polarized state is termed *repolarization.* Movement of potassium ions out of myocardial cells primarily accounts for repolarization. In late diastole, after most of the repolarization has occurred, potassium and sodium reverse positions to restore ionic concentrations to the polarized state. The *Ta wave,* representing *atrial repolarization,* generally lies buried in the QRS complex and ST segment. The ST segment is an isoelectric line extending from the end of the QRS complex to the beginning of the T wave, during which early ventricular repolarization is beginning very slowly (Fig. 6-4, *E*). The *T wave* represents *ventricular repolarization* (Fig. 6-4, *F*).

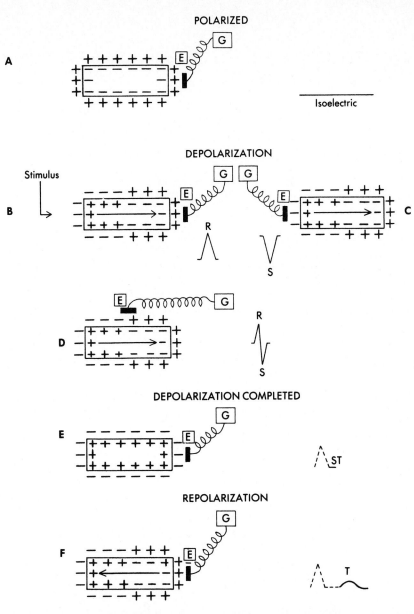

FIG. 6-4. A, A schematic illustration of a polarized (resting) myocardial muscle cell maintaining a negative charge on the inside of the cell membrane and a positive charge on the outside of the membrane. An electrode *(E)* facing the right side of the polarized cell and attached to an ECG machine (*G,* galvanometer) will record no current, and an isoelectric line results. B, The cell is stimulated from the left, and depolarization proceeds from left to right in the direction of the arrow. The depolarized left end of the cell becomes electrically negative, whereas the right end of the cell is still polarized and electrically positive. There now exists a difference of electrical potentials (negative and positive ions), and an electric current is flowing. The electrode facing the positive side of this current and attached to an ECG machine will record a positive deflection, and in the case of ventricular depolarization, this deflection is called an R wave. C, The same myocardial cell is stimulated again from the left; however, the electrode is facing the negative side of the current, and will therefore record a negative deflection. In the case of ventricular depolarization, this deflection is called an S wave. D, Once again the cell is activated from the left. The electrode facing the center of the cell will first write a positive and then a negative deflection. In the case of ventricular depolarization, this deflection is called an RS complex. E, With the completion of depolarization, the outer surface of the myocardial cell becomes electrically negative; the flow of electric current ceases, and the R wave returns to the isoelectric line. The short period following complete ventricular depolarization is recorded as the ST segment. F, In the previous illustration, the myocardial muscle cell was depolarized from left to right. Now the cell returns to the resting state, repolarization, in the opposite direction, from right to left. The right end of the cell becomes positive first and an electrode facing this site will inscribe a positive deflection. In the case of ventricular repolarization, this deflection is termed a T wave.

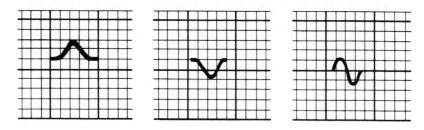

FIG. 6-5. The P wave is gently rounded in contour, may be normally positive, negative, or diphasic in different ECG leads, and should not exceed 2 or 3 mm.

WAVES AND COMPLEXES
P Wave

As previously mentioned, the P wave represents atrial depolarization, and begins as soon as the impulse leaves the sinus node (sinoatrial, or SA, node) and initiates atrial depolarization. Since the sinus node is situated in the right atrium, right atrial activation begins first and is followed shortly thereafter by left atrial activation. As left atrial activation begins, before the end of right atrial activation, the two processes overlap. This close overlap of the forces results in a gently rounded P wave. As will be discussed later in this chapter, the P wave normally may be positive, negative, or diphasic, depending on which lead of the ECG is recorded. Whatever the case, the amplitude of the P wave should not exceed 2 or 3 mm in any lead (Fig. 6-5).

Although usually not visible on the ECG, the Ta wave of atrial repolarization occurs in a direction opposite to that of the P wave and is recorded after the first portion of the P wave and continues through the PR interval. It is usually not identified unless the P wave occurs independently of the QRS, as in complete AV block (see Chapter 8). When the P wave is large, the Ta wave is also generally large and may be seen to extend beyond the QRS complex, resulting in a distortion of the initial portion of the ST segment. This may cause a depression of the ST segment that may be mistaken as having a pathologic significance.

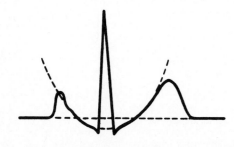

FIG. 6-6. Atrial repolarization as a cause of ST segment deviation. Note that the PQ (PR) and ST segments can be connected by a smooth curve, and that the direction of the deviation is opposite in direction to the P wave. (Adapted from Hurst, J.W., and others: The heart: arteries and veins, ed. 6, New York, 1984, McGraw-Hill Book Co.)

To make a correct interpretation in the setting of a depressed ST segment, one must (1) observe the configuration of the atrial repolarization wave (smooth curve with upward concavity), (2) recognize a similar deviation of the base line before the QRS is recorded, and (3) recognize a large P wave (Fig. 6-6).

QRS Complex

The QRS complex representing ventricular depolarization may have various components, depending on which lead of the ECG is recorded. These components are illustrated in Fig. 6-7 and described as follows:

R wave: The first positive deflection
Q wave: The initial negative deflection preceding an R wave
S wave: The negative deflection following an R wave
R' wave: The second positive deflection
S' wave: The negative deflection following the R' wave
QS wave: The totally negative deflection

The QRS complexes should be examined for the following:
1. The *duration* of the complex (see Chapter 8 discussion of QRS interval)
2. The *amplitude* of the components
3. The general *configuration* of the complex, including the presence and location of any slurred component (see Chapter 8 discussion of bundle branch block and Wolff-Parkinson-White syndrome)
4. The presence of abnormal Q *waves* (discussed under myocardial infarction in this chapter)
5. The timing of the *intrinsicoid deflections* in precordial leads V_1 to V_6

Amplitude. The *amplitude* of the QRS complex has wide normal limits; however, it is generally agreed that if the total amplitude (above and below the base line) is 5 mm or less in all three standard leads, it is abnormally low. Such low voltage may be seen in patients who have cardiac failure, diffuse coronary disease, pericardial effusion, myxedema, primary amyloidosis, or any other conditions producing widespread myocardial damage. Furthermore, it may be found in patients who have emphysema, generalized edema, and obesity. The minimal normal QRS amplitude in precordial leads varies from right to left across

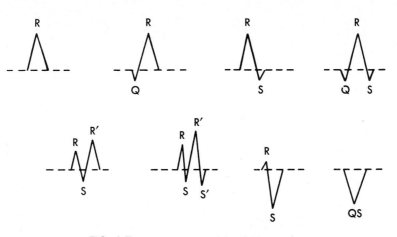

FIG. 6-7.   Components of the QRS complex.

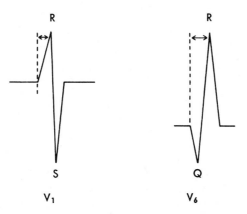

FIG. 6-8.   The time of onset of the intrinsicoid deflection is measured from the beginning of the QRS complex to the peak of the R wave.

the chest, being generally accepted as 5 mm in V_1 and V_6, 7 mm in V_2 and V_5 and 9 mm in V_3 and V_4.

Upper limits for normal QRS voltage (amplitude) have been difficult to set. Diagnostic evaluation is important when QRS amplitudes reach the following upper limits: V_1 an R wave of 5 mm; V_1, V_2 an S wave of 30 mm; V_5, V_6 an R wave of 30 mm; and in the limb leads an R or S wave of 20 mm.

Intrinsicoid Deflection. Ventricular activation time is the interval between the beginning of the QRS complex and the onset of the intrinsicoid deflection. The time of onset of the intrinsicoid deflection is measured from the beginning of the QRS complex to the peak of the R wave, and it is measured in the precordial leads (Fig. 6-8). In right-sided precordial leads (V_1 or V_2) the time of onset for the intrinsicoid deflection is normally 0.03 second or less. In left-sided precordial leads (V_5 or V_6) the time of onset is normally 0.05 second or less in adults. If the time of onset for the intrinsicoid deflection exceeds 0.03 or 0.05

second in right- and left-sided leads respectively, it is taken to indicate that the impulse arrived late at the epicardial surface of the ventricle under the electrode. Such delay may be caused by thickening or dilatation of the ventricular wall or a block in the conducting system to the ventricle involved (bundle branch block).

ST Segment

The interval that occurs between the end of the QRS complex and the beginning of the T wave is called the ST segment. It represents the time during which the ventricles have been completely depolarized and are beginning ventricular repolarization. Usually, the ST segment is isoelectric (see Fig. 6-2), but it may normally deviate between -0.5 and $+1.0$ mm from the base line in the standard and unipolar leads (ECG leads are presented in the next section). In some instances, upward displacement of 2 or 3 mm may be normal, provided that the ST segment is concave upward and the succeeding T wave is tall and

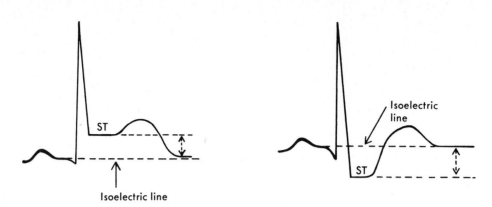

FIG. 6-9. Elevation of the ST segment is measured from the upper edge of the isoelectric line to the upper edge of the ST segment; depression is measured from the lower edge of the isoelectric line to the lower edge of the ST segment.

upright. This is called *early repolarization*. Downward displacement in excess of 0.5 mm generally is abnormal. In all situations, depression caused by a depressed PR segment must be considered. More important are ST segments, elevated or depressed, that vary temporarily (see discussions of myocardial infarction, pericarditis). Correlation with the clinical condition of the patient is often necessary to determine the significance of ST segment displacement.

Elevation of the ST segment is measured from the upper edge of the isoelectric line to the upper edge of the ST segment; depression is measured from the lower edge of the isoelectric line to the lower edge of the ST segment (Fig. 6-9).

T Wave

The T wave, normally slightly rounded and slightly asymmetric, represents the electrical recovery period (repolarization) of the ventricles. Upright T waves are measured from the upper level of the base line to the summit of the T wave, whereas inverted T waves are measured from the lower level of the base line to the lowest point of the T wave. Diphasic T waves are measured by adding the amplitudes above and below the base line. T waves normally do not exceed 5 mm in any standard lead or 10 mm in any precordial lead. T wave contour is often very labile and, as with the ST segment, correlation with the clinical status of the patient, often in serially repeated ECGs, is necessary for correct interpretation.

U Wave

The U wave is a small wave of low voltage sometimes observed following a T wave and in the same direction as its preceding T wave; that is, when the T wave is upright, the U wave normally will be upright. It is best observed in the chest leads, although it is present, but barely detectable, in the limb leads.

Relatively little is known about the U wave. Although the cause and clinical significance of the U wave are uncertain, the appearance of U waves or an increase in their magnitude is seen in certain disorders (see Chapter 8 discussion of hypokalemia). The U wave is generally upright in the precordial leads. A negative U wave may occur in patients who have left ventricular hypertrophy, hypertension, or coronary artery disease. An upright (positive) U wave that becomes inverted (negative) during an exercise stress test often indicates the presence of significant coronary artery obstruction in the main left or left anterior descending coronary artery.

ELECTROCARDIOGRAM LEADS

As previously mentioned, the deflections on the ECG are produced by the electrical energy caused by the movement of charged ions across the membranes of myocardial cells (depolarization and repolarization). This movement of charged particles results in a flow of electrical current. The pressure behind the flow of electrical current is called *electrical potential,* and it creates an electrical field. This electrical field extends to the body surface, where the electrical potential can be measured by the ECG.

By convention 12 lead recordings comprise the ECG. Each lead has a positive and negative pole (electrode), and the location of these poles determines the *polarity* of the lead. A hypothetic line joining the poles of a lead is known as the *axis* of the lead. Moreover, every lead axis is oriented in a certain direction, depending on the location of the positive and negative electrodes.

Six of the twelve ECG leads measure cardiac forces in the *frontal plane* (the standard limb leads and the augmented leads I, II, III, aV_R, aV_L, and aV_F); the remaining six leads (V_1 to V_6) measure the cardiac forces in the *horizontal plane*.

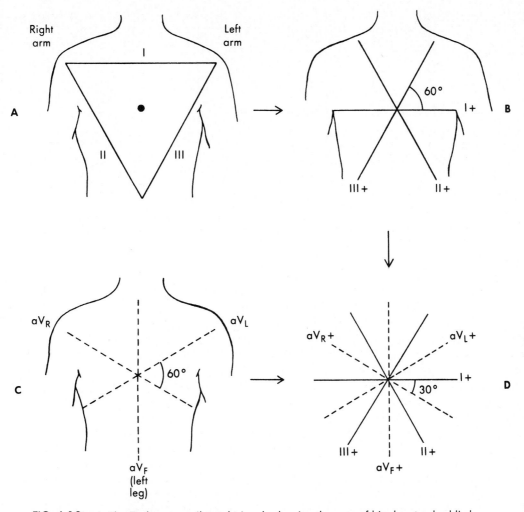

FIG. 6-10.   A, The Einthoven equilateral triangle showing the axes of bipolar standard limb leads I, II, and III. The heart is at the center or zero point. B, The axes of the standard limb leads are shifted to the center of the triangle (zero point of the electrical field), forming a triaxial figure. C, The axes of the unipolar augmented leads. D, The axes of the standard and augmented limb leads are combined to form a hexaxial figure. Each lead is labeled at its positive pole.

Standard (Bipolar) Limb Leads (I, II, III)

The standard limb leads, designated leads I, II, and III, were developed by Willem Einthoven (1860-1927), physiologist and inventor of the string galvanometer. Using the principle that the heart is situated in the center of the electrical field it generates, Einthoven placed the electrodes of the three standard leads as far away from the heart as possible, that is, on the extremities—the right arm, left arm, and left leg.* These three electrodes, therefore, are considered to be electrically equidistant from the heart. Consequently, the heart may be viewed as a point source in the center of an equilateral triangle, whose apices are

the right arm, left arm, and left leg. This is called Einthoven's triangle (Fig. 6-10, *A*).

The standard bipolar limb leads measure the *difference* between two recording sites. The actual potential under either of the electrodes is not known as it is for the unipolar leads. For lead I, the negative electrode is placed on the right arm and the positive electrode on the left arm. For lead II, the negative electrode is on the right arm and the positive electrode on the left leg. For lead III, the left arm electrode is negative, and the left leg electrode is positive (Fig. 6-10, *A*). This is summarized as follows:

Lead	Location
I	Right arm (−) to left arm (+)
II	Right arm (−) to left leg (+)
III	Left arm (−) to left leg (+)

*The right leg serves as a ground electrode, thereby providing a pathway of least resistance for electrical interference in the body. Actually, the ground electrode can be placed at any location on the body.

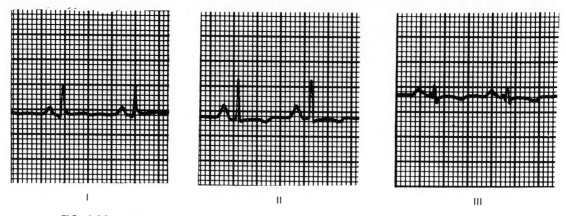

FIG. 6-11. Einthoven's law states: Lead I + Lead III = Lead II. The deflections in the ECG leads demonstrate this law.

Because of the established relationship of the standard limb leads to each other, at any given instant during the cardiac cycle the sum of the electrical potentials recorded in leads I and III equals the electrical potential recorded in lead II. This is *Einthoven's law,* and it applies to a triangle of any shape. Stated mathematically, the law is as follows:

$$\text{Lead I} + \text{Lead III} = \text{Lead II}$$

Einthoven's law may be used to detect errors in electrode placement. Furthermore, it may clarify perplexing findings in one or another lead. If, for example, the deflections of lead II are obscured by muscular or electrical interference or by a wandering base line, the characteristics of the other two leads may be used to determine the presence of a Q wave or ST segment deviation in lead II. Einthoven's law also is helpful in evaluating serial tracings. For example, if in a given tracing the T wave in lead I appears to be more negative than in the previous tracing, changes must be present in the T waves of the other two limb leads as well, so that $T_1 + T_3 = T_2$ (Fig. 6-11).

To prevent confusion about polarities the ECG machine records a positive deflection in the bipolar leads when in lead I the left arm is in the positive portion of the electrical field, in lead II the left leg is in the positive portion of the electrical field, and in lead III the left leg is in the positive portion of the electrical field.

Triaxial Reference Figure. The three lead axes of the equilateral triangle can be shifted without changing their direction so that their midpoints intersect at the same point. Thus the *triaxial reference figure* is formed with each of the lead axes separated from one another by 60 degrees (Fig. 6-10, *B*).

Augmented (Unipolar) Leads (aV_R, aV_L, aV_F)

All unipolar leads are called V leads and consist of extremity (limb) leads and precordial (chest) leads. The augmented leads aV_R, aV_L, and aV_F use the same electrode locations as the standard limb leads. Therefore the positive electrode is attached to the right arm (aV_R), left arm (aV_L), or left leg (aV_F). The negative electrode, however, is formed by combining leads I, II, and III, whose algebraic sum is zero. Since the electrical center of the heart is at zero potential, the augmented leads measure the difference in potential between the limbs and the center of the heart.

The axis for each augmented lead is a line drawn from the extremity, where the positive electrode is placed, to the zero point of the electrical field of the heart, which is at the center of the equilateral triangle (Fig. 6-10, *C*). These three unipolar lead axes also form a triaxial reference system with the axes 60 degrees apart.

Hexaxial Reference Figure. When the triaxial figure of the standard leads and the triaxial figure of the augmented leads are combined, they form a *hexaxial reference figure* in which each augmented lead is perpendicular to a standard limb lead (Fig. 6-10, *D*). The hexaxial figure is a useful reference for plotting mean cardiac forces in the frontal plane.

Precordial (Unipolar) Leads (V₁ to V₆)

In the horizontal plane, precordial leads are used to determine how far anteriorly or posteriorly from the frontal plane the electrical forces of the heart are directed. The standard precordial ECG consists of six unipolar leads, V_1 through V_6. In Fig. 6-12, *A*, the V leads are shown with reference to their electrode positions on the anterior chest wall. These chest electrodes represent a positive pole (unipolar). Any electrical force traveling toward one of these leads will produce a positive deflection; traveling away from it will produce a negative deflection. For descriptive purposes, leads V_1 and V_2 are called right-sided precordial leads; leads V_3 and V_4, midprecordial leads; and leads V_5 and V_6, left-sided precordial leads.

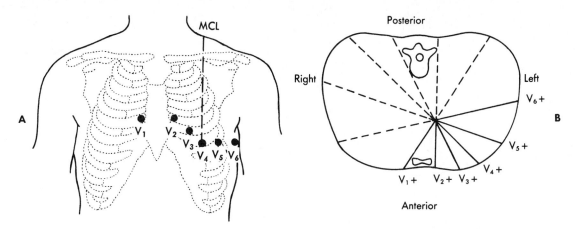

FIG. 6-12.   A, Electrode positions of the precordial leads: V_1, fourth intercostal space at the right sternal border; V_2, fourth intercostal space at the left sternal border; V_3, halfway between V_2 and V_4; V_4, fifth intercostal space at the midclavicular line; V_5, anterior axillary line directly lateral to V_4; V_6, midaxillary line directly lateral to V_5. B, The precordial reference figure. Leads V_1 and V_2 are called right-sided precordial leads; leads V_3 and V_4, mid-precordial leads; and leads V_5 and V_6, left-sided precordial leads.

Precordial Reference Figure. A transverse representation of the chest wall and the V leads results in the precordial reference figure (Fig. 6-12, *B*). This figure is a useful reference for plotting mean cardiac forces in the horizontal plane.

THE VECTOR APPROACH TO ELECTROCARDIOGRAPHY

The electrical potentials generated during the cardiac cycle can be described and measured. To adequately characterize such an electrical potential or force, both the magnitude and the direction of the force must be specified; this can be done by a *vector*. Briefly stated, a vector is a quantity of electrical force that has a known magnitude and direction. A vector may be illustrated graphically by an *arrow*, the length of the arrow representing the *magnitude* of the force and the direction of the arrow indicating the *direction* of the force. The *arrowhead* depicts the location of the positive field.

Representing electrical forces of the heart by vectors more easily explains the relationship between the electrical activity generated by the heart and the recording of this electrical activity by a specific lead. When an electrical force (and therefore the vector that represents it) establishes a direction *parallel* to the lead that records it, this electrical force causes the *largest deflection* to be inscribed by that lead. An electrical force perpendicular to the recording lead produces no deflection in that lead. Forces in between these extremes generate deflections according to their directions: the more nearly parallel the force (and vector) to the recording lead, the larger the deflection produced in that lead; the more nearly perpendicular the force to the recording lead, the smaller the deflection. When the positive

and negative forces on a lead are equal, the net area of the deflection is zero. This results in a biphasic or transitional deflection (Fig. 6-13).

Sequence of Electrical Events in the Heart

In the normal heart, depolarization of the ventricle is a sequential process. The process can be represented by *instantaneous vectors,* each of which corresponds to all the heart's electrical forces at a given moment in time. A diagram of successive instantaneous vectors depicting ventricular depolarization is shown in Fig. 6-14, *A*. Initial depolarization passes from left to right across the interventricular septum. During the second phase, depolarization of subendocardial muscle occurs near the apex. The last phase of depolarization occurs in the posterior free wall of the left ventricle.

The deflection recorded by any given lead results from the projection of the cardiac vector generated during depolarization onto the axis of the lead. Thus arrow 1 (Fig. 6-14, *B*), depicting depolarization of the septum, usually causes a small negative deflection in lead I, resulting in a Q wave and a larger positive deflection in lead III, resulting in an R wave. Arrow 2, illustrating depolarization of the apical region of the heart, usually produces a very small positive deflection (R wave) in lead I because of its leftward orientation and an R wave in lead III. Late depolarization of the heart, being from right to left in the posterior free wall of the left ventricle, causes a large positive deflection in lead I (the major part of the R wave) and an S wave in lead III. Following the completion of depolarization of ventricles, the electrical wave returns to the base line. Therefore the three arrows have generated a small initial Q wave followed by a large R wave in lead I and an R

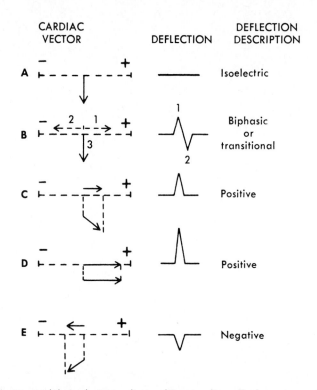

FIG. 6-13.   Vectors and their electrocardiographic recordings. Each arrow represents the vector generated by an electrical force. This force produces an electrocardiographic deflection, shown on the right. A, Because the vector is perpendicular to the axis of the recording lead, no projection appears on that lead. The absence of a deflection establishes an uninterrupted isoelectric line. B, The mean vector (number 3) is perpendicular to the axis of the recording lead when the positive and negative forces are equal (the net area of the deflection is zero). A biphasic or transitional deflection is recorded because the initial forces moved rightward (vector 1) at the same distance that the later forces moved leftward (vector 2). The instantaneous vectors have equal magnitude but opposite direction. C, The vector projects on the positive side of the axis of the recording lead to inscribe a small positive deflection. D, When the vector is parallel with the lead axis, the projection onto the recording lead has its maximum magnitude. E, The vector projects on the negative side of the lead axis, and a small negative deflection is recorded.

wave followed by an S wave in lead III (Fig. 6-14, C and D).

As previously discussed, each ECG lead has a different orientation to the heart. Therefore the instantaneous vectors of ventricular depolarization will produce a different deflection in each lead. This is also true of ventricular repolarization and atrial depolarization.

In this chapter, detailed consideration is given to the vectors of the QRS complex. However, the positions of the P wave and T wave in the frontal plane are also important. Normally the P wave is upright in leads I and II and may be biphasic, flat, or inverted in lead III; inverted in lead aV_R; upright, biphasic, or inverted in lead aV_L; and upright in lead aV_F.

Normally the T wave is upright in leads I and II, flat, biphasic, or inverted in lead III, and inverted in lead aV_R. In lead aV_L, the T wave may be upright, flattened, or biphasic, according the the QRS pattern. It may also be

inverted, provided that the T wave in lead aV_R is also inverted. In lead aV_F the T wave is usually upright; however, it can be normally flattened, biphasic, or inverted, provided that the T wave in lead aV_R is also inverted.

In the horizontal plane the P wave is normally upright in all precordial leads, but it may be inverted in V_1 and V_2 without being abnormal. The normal QRS complex is transitional at some point between V_3 and V_4. The precordial transition zone is characterized by the transition from the RS complexes recorded by the leads oriented to the right ventricle to the QR complexes recorded by the leads oriented to the left ventricle (Fig. 6-15). The normal T wave is upright in leads V_2 through V_6. The T wave may be flat or inverted in V_1 and still be normal.

Mean Cardiac Vector

The mean cardiac vector, which is the average of all the instantaneous vectors, can be expressed accurately on the

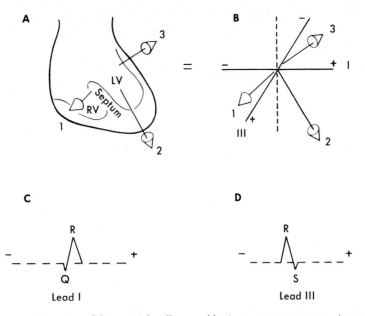

FIG. 6-14. Depolarization of the ventricles illustrated by instantaneous vectors. Arrow 1 depicts depolarization of the septum from left to right and is directed to the right and somewhat anteriorly. Arrow 2 illustrates depolarization of the apical region of the heart and is directed to the left and inferiorly. Arrow 3 represents depolarization of the posterior aspect of the left ventricle and is directed to the left and posteriorly. B, The instantaneous vectors representing ventricular depolarization are inscribed on lead I and lead III. C and D, Arrow 1 causes a small negative deflection in lead I, resulting in a Q wave, and a larger positive deflection in lead III, resulting in an R wave. Arrow 2 produces a small positive deflection (R wave) in lead I and an R wave in lead III. Arrow 3 causes a large R wave in lead I and S wave in lead III.

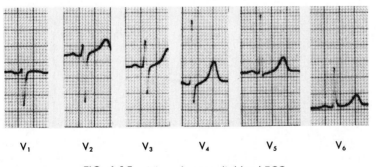

FIG. 6-15. Normal precordial lead ECG.

hexaxial reference figure. Furthermore, since the hexaxial reference system divides the frontal plane into 30-degree intervals, the leads have been classified as follows: all degrees in the upper hemisphere of the hexaxial figure are labeled as negative degrees, and all degrees in the lower hemisphere are labeled as positive degrees. Accordingly, commencing at the positive end of the standard lead I axis (labeled 0 degrees and progressing counterclockwise), the leads are successively at −30, −60, −90, −120, −150, and −180 degrees. Progressing clockwise, the leads are successively at +30, +60, +90, +120, +150, and +180 degrees* (Fig. 6-16).

The position of the mean cardiac vector provides information about the electrical "position" of the heart, also expressed as the mean electrical axis, and is influenced by the anatomic position of the heart within the chest, the anatomy of the heart itself, and the pathway traveled by

*The conventional labeling of the hexaxial reference figure as positive and negative units should not be confused with the positive and negative poles of the lead axes.

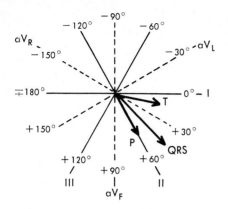

FIG. 6-16. The hexaxial reference system divides the frontal plane into 30-degree intervals. All degrees in the upper hemisphere are labeled as negative degrees, and all degrees in the lower hemisphere are labeled as positive degrees. The mean P vector normally lies along the +60-degree axis. The mean QRS vector normally lies anywhere between 0 and +90 degrees; in the figure the mean QRS vector lies on the +45-degree axis. The mean T vector normally lies between −10 and +75 degrees. In the figure the mean T vector lies on the +15-degree axis. The mean frontal plane QRS axis and T wave axis are usually similarly detected, and the angle between them normally does not exceed 60 degrees.

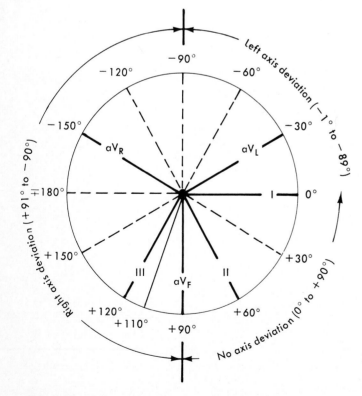

FIG. 6-17. Flexaxial reference figure indicating values for no axis deviation, left axis deviation, and right axis deviation.

the depolarizing wave. If the P vector is projected on the hexaxial figure, the mean electrical axis of the P in the frontal plane lies approximately along the +60-degree axis (Fig. 6-16). The mean QRS vector lies normally between 0 and +90 degrees, whereas the mean electrical axis of the T wave lies between −10 and +75 degrees. The mean frontal plane QRS axis and T wave axis are usually similarly directed, and the angle between them normally does not exceed 60 degrees (Fig. 6-16).

Mean QRS Axis

The remainder of this section discusses the significance and determination of the mean QRS axis. The principles also may be applied to the mean P and T vectors.

Deviations in the mean electrical axis, even without other ECG abnormalities, may assist in the diagnosis of cardiac disease. As indicated in Fig. 6-17, the mean QRS vector normally lies between 0 and +90 degrees. Right axis deviation occurs when the mean QRS vector lies between +90 and −90 degrees. Right axis deviation with a mean QRS vector between +90 and +110 degrees may be abnormal, as in patients who have block in the posterior division of the left bundle branch (Chapter 8), but is frequently normal, as seen in young adults or asthenic individuals. This vector is illustrated in Fig. 6-18, *A. Abnormal right axis deviation* is present when the mean QRS vector lies between +110 and −90 degrees. This usually implies either delayed activation of the right ventricle as seen in right bundle branch block (Chapter 8) or right ventricular enlargement.

"Normal" left axis deviation is present when the mean QRS vector lies between 0 and −30 degrees. For example, this situation can occur in patients who have ascites or abdominal tumors, are pregnant, or are obese. *Abnormal left axis deviation,* however, is present when the mean QRS vector lies between −30 and −90 degrees. This vector is illustrated in Fig. 6-18, *B.* It may indicate delayed activation of the left ventricle as seen in left anterior hemiblock (Chapter 8) or left ventricular enlargement.

Occasionally the electrical position of the heart is described as horizontal, semihorizontal, intermediate, semivertical, or vertical. It has been convenient to refer to a heart with an axis in the range of 0 to −30 degrees as a *horizontal heart,* and to one with an axis between +60 and +90 degrees as a *vertical heart.* Semihorizontal and semivertical positions are halfway stations between the intermediate position and the horizontal and vertical extremes and are not very useful terms.

Determination of the Frontal Plane Projection of the Mean QRS Vector. First, recall the following principles: an electrical force perpendicular to a lead axis will record a small or biphasic complex in the ECG lead. An electrical force parallel to a given lead axis will record its

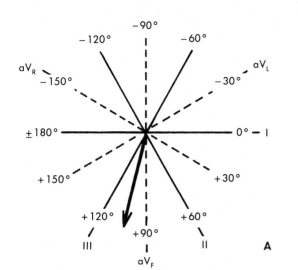

largest deflection in that ECG lead. With this in mind, follow the procedure below by referring to Fig. 6-18, *A*.

1. Examine the six frontal plane leads and identify the lead with the smallest or most diphasic deflection.
2. In Fig. 6-18, *A*, this is lead I.
3. The electrical axis must be near perpendicular to lead I, and it must run near parallel to the lead that intersects lead I at right angles. Perpendicular to lead I is aV_F.
4. The deflection in lead aV_F, therefore, must be largest in the frontal plane.
5. Since the deflection in lead aV_F is positive, the vector must be directed toward the positive pole of that lead.

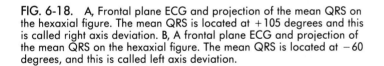

FIG. 6-18.   A, Frontal plane ECG and projection of the mean QRS on the hexaxial figure. The mean QRS is located at +105 degrees and this is called right axis deviation. B, A frontal plane ECG and projection of the mean QRS on the hexaxial figure. The mean QRS is located at −60 degrees, and this is called left axis deviation.

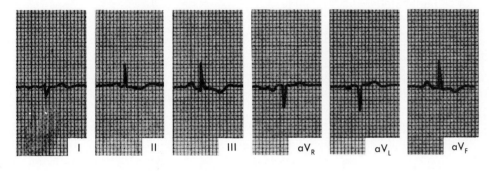

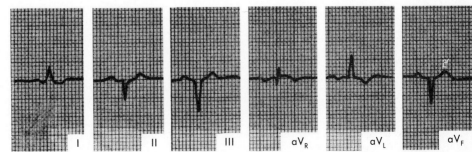

6. Examine the six frontal plane leads to see if any other lead deflections are as large as lead aV_F. If the QRS complex is equal in amplitude in two leads, the mean QRS vector is directed halfway between the axes of these leads.

7. In this case the deflection in lead III is equal to that in lead aV_F.

8. The mean electrical axis of the QRS, therefore, lies between lead aV_F and lead III and is located at +105 degrees (right axis deviation).

In the example just given, if the deflection in lead aV_F had been greater than that in lead III, then the mean QRS vector would have been more parallel to lead aV_F, that is, at +100 or even +95 degrees, depending on how much larger the deflection in lead aV_F was compared with lead III.

Another example in which this procedure can be followed is shown in Fig. 6-18, *B*.

1. The smallest, or in this case the diphasic, deflection is seen in lead aV_R.

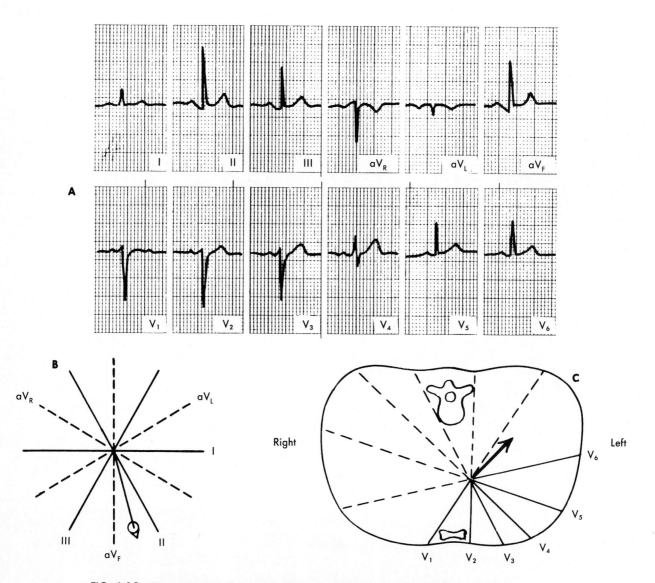

FIG. 6-19.   Determination of the mean QRS vector in the frontal and horizontal planes. A, Twelve-lead ECG. B, The mean QRS vector in the frontal plane is located at +70 degrees. The arrowhead indicates that the mean QRS vector points posteriorly in the horizontal plane. C, The horizontal plane projection of the mean QRS is drawn in a posterior direction on the precordial reference figure. This calculation gives information for the direction of the arrowhead in the frontal plane (B).

2. The mean QRS vector thus runs perpendicular to lead aV_R.
3. Since lead III runs perpendicular to lead aV_R, the deflection in lead III must be the largest.
4. The deflection in lead III is negative; therefore the mean axis is directed toward the negative pole of lead III.
5. The mean QRS vector in this figure is located at −60 degrees (left axis deviation).

Determination of the Horizontal Plane Projection of the Mean QRS Vector

1. Identify the precordial lead with the transitional QRS deflection in Fig. 6-19, *A*.
2. Lead V_4 is transitional.
3. The QRS vector is perpendicular to the transitional lead (V_4).
4. The vector should be directed toward the positive sides of the leads with positive deflections, and on the negative sides of the leads with negative deflections, as shown in Fig. 6-19, *C*.
5. When the horizontal plane direction of the mean QRS is noted, an arrowhead may be placed on the mean QRS frontal plane vector to indicate the vector's anterior or posterior direction, as shown in Fig. 6-19, *B*.

It should be noted that the transitional QRS deflection may appear early, that is, between V_1 and V_2 or late, that is, between V_5 and V_6. One explanation for this is that the heart has rotated on its longitudinal axis. In describing the rotation about this axis, one must consider a view of the heart from under the diaphragm. From this viewpoint, if the front of the heart rotates toward the left, this is called *clockwise rotation*. If the front of the heart rotates toward the right, this is called *counterclockwise rotation*. With a counterclockwise rotation the transitional zone will move toward the right (V_1, V_2). With the clockwise rotation the transitional zone will shift to the left (V_5, V_6). Such rotations may be normal or abnormal.

LEFT VENTRICULAR ENLARGEMENT

It is not usually possible in the ECG to differentiate ventricular dilatation and hypertrophy. The term *hypertrophy* is commonly used; however, this presentation will use *enlargement*, since it includes both dilatation and hypertrophy.

Hypertension, aortic valvular disease, mitral insufficiency, coronary artery disease, and congenital heart disease (for example, patent ductus arteriosus and coarctation of the aorta) commonly produce left ventricular enlargement. Under these circumstances the wall of the left ventricle is thicker or more dilated than normal. Furthermore, this increase in muscle mass results in increased voltage of those QRS deflections that represent left ventricular potentials. Accordingly, the QRS interval may increase in duration to the upper limits of normal; the intrinsicoid deflection may be somewhat delayed over the left ventricle; and the voltage of the QRS complex will increase—producing deeper S waves over the right ventricle (leads V_1 and V_2) and taller R waves over the left ventricle (leads V_5, V_6, I, aV_L).

Leads oriented to the left ventricle may also demonstrate a *strain* pattern, that is, depressed ST segments and inverted T waves. "Strain" is a useful, noncommittal term and its mechanism is not understood. It is known, however, to develop in patients who have long-standing left ventricular enlargement, and the pattern intensifies when dilatation and failure set in. Myocardial ischemia and slowing of intraventricular conduction are some of the important factors that probably contribute to the pattern.

In general, the voltage criteria proposed for the diagnosis of left ventricular enlargement are unreliable. However, the best approach so far is the Estes scoring system, which is as follows (compare with Fig. 6-20):

1. R wave or S wave in limb lead = 20 mm or more; or S wave in V_1, V_2, or V_3 = 30 mm or more; or R wave in V_4, V_5, or V_6 = 30 mm or more
2. Any ST segment shift opposite to mean QRS vector (without digitalis). Typical "strain" segments T wave (with digitalis).
3. Left axis deviation: −30 degrees or more
4. QRS interval: 0.09 second or more
   Intrinsicoid deflection in V_{5-6}: 0.05 second or more
5. Left atrial enlargement

Definite left ventricular enlargement is present with a *point score of 5 or more. Probable left ventricular enlargement* is present if the *point score is 4.*

It should be noted that left ventricular enlargement may be present without concomitant left axis deviation. Left axis deviation supports the diagnosis of left ventricular enlargement only when the voltage criteria are fulfilled. The voltage criteria just listed, however, include a small percentage of both false positive and false negative diagnoses. Therefore, in making an electrocardiographic diagnosis of left ventricular enlargement, it is wise to evaluate such factors as body build, the thickness of the chest wall, and the presence of complicating disease. Echocardiography has eliminated many uncertainties about the presence of ventricular enlargement.

LEFT ATRIAL ENLARGEMENT

Left atrial abnormality occurs frequently in left ventricular enlargement, but this is not always the case. For example, left atrial enlargement caused by mitral stenosis is not associated with left ventricular enlargement unless there is mitral insufficiency or concomitant aortic valvular disease.

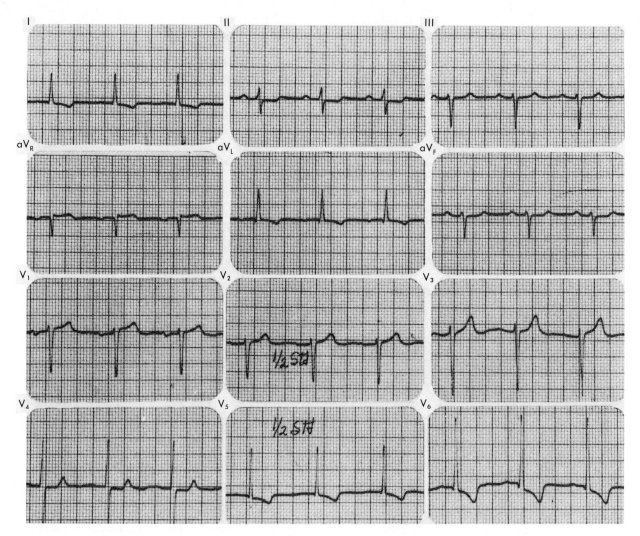

FIG. 6-20. Left ventricular enlargement. This tracing illustrates left ventricular hypertrophy using the Estes criteria: S wave in V₂ and R wave in V₅ and V₆ (note half standard in V₂ and V₅) exceed 30 mm (3 points); ST segment depression in the absence of digitalis (3 points); terminal negativity of P wave in V₁ (1 point). A score of 5 or more points is interpreted as indicating left ventricular hypertrophy. The "score" for this ECG is 7 points.

The following criteria are used in the ECG diagnosis of left atrial enlargement (Fig. 6-21):

1. The duration of the P wave is often widened to 0.12 second or more. (Normal P wave duration is 0.11 second.)

2. The contour of the P wave is *notched* and slurred in leads I and II *(P mitrale)*. (Notching per se is not abnormal unless the P wave shows increased voltage or duration or both, or the summits are more than 0.03 second apart.)

3. The right precordial leads (V₁, V₂) reflect diphasic P waves with a wide, deep, negative terminal component. The duration (in seconds) and amplitude (in millimeters) of the terminal component are mea-sured and the algebraic product determined. A more negative value than −0.03 second is considered abnormal.

4. The mean electrical axis of the P wave may be shifted left, to between +45 and −30 degrees.

RIGHT VENTRICULAR ENLARGEMENT

Right ventricular enlargement is commonly seen with mitral stenosis, some forms of congenital heart disease, and chronic diffuse pulmonary disease such as pulmonary hypertension, emphysema, and bronchiectasis. For right ventricular enlargement in the adult to become evident electrocardiographically, however, the right ventricle must enlarge considerably, since the normal adult ECG reflects left

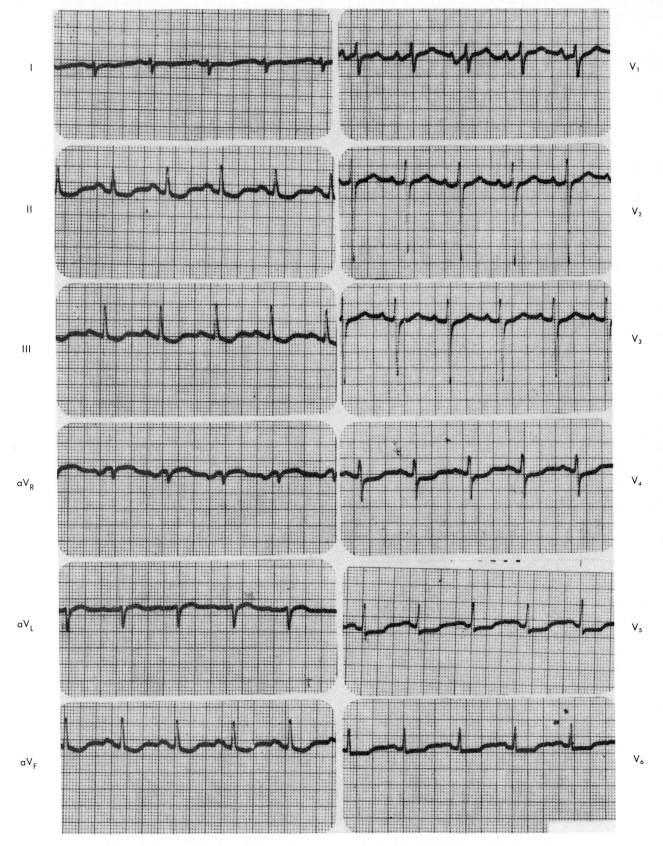

FIG. 6-21.   Left atrial enlargement. In this example, left atrial enlargement may be diagnosed by the P terminal force abnormality seen in V_1. The negative portion of the diphasic P wave is approximately 0.04 second in duration and 1 mm in amplitude. The M-shaped broad contour seen prominently in leads I, II, III, and a V_F and the lateral precordial leads are also found in left atrial enlargement. In addition, right axis deviation of approximately +110 degrees exists in this patient with mitral stenosis.

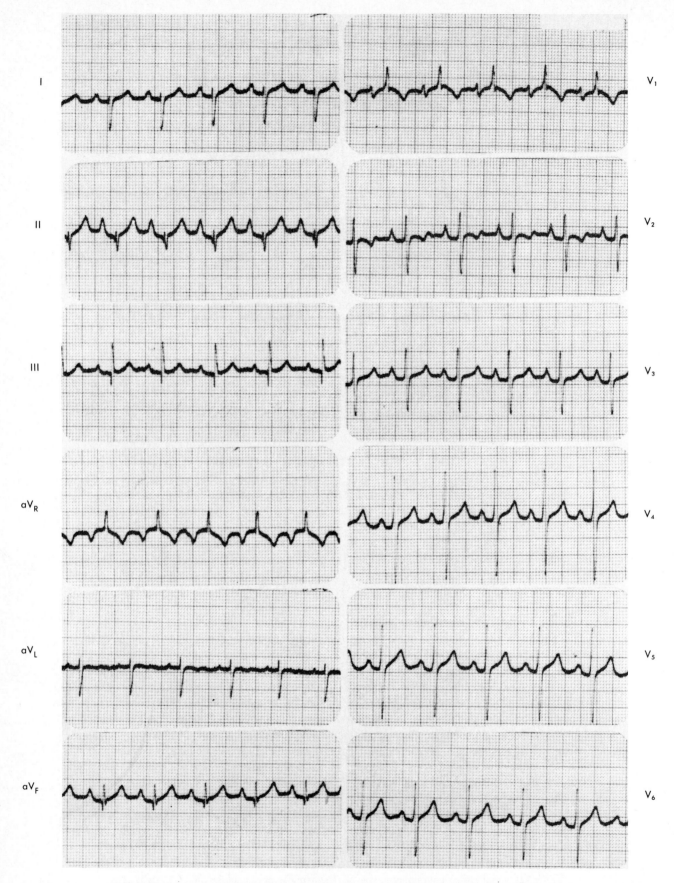

FIG. 6-22. Right ventricular enlargement. The presence of right axis deviation (approximately +160 degrees), an R wave in V_1 that exceeds 5 mm, and an R:S ratio in V_1 that exceeds 1.0 are all diagnostic of right ventricular hypertrophy. In addition, the totally upright R wave in V_1 suggests that the pressure in the right ventricle equals or almost equals the pressure in the left ventricle. The P waves suggest right atrial enlargement.

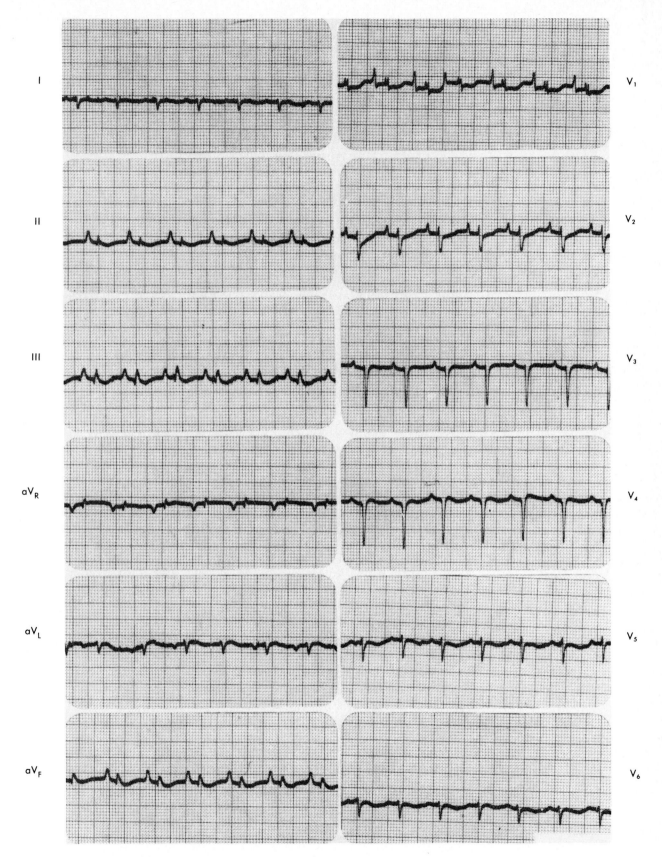

FIG. 6-23. Right atrial enlargement. The large peaked P waves in leads II, III, aV_F, and V₁, with an amplitude that exceeds 2.5 mm in leads II and III, characterize right atrial enlargement. The mean P axis is more positive than +60 degrees, another criterion for right atrial enlargement. The patient has pulmonic stenosis.

ventricular predominance. This accounts for the relative frequency of a normal ECG in the presence of right ventricular enlargement.

Most of the criteria for diagnosing right ventricular enlargement focus on the QRS pattern in the right precordial leads. As the right ventricle enlarges, the height of the right precordial R waves increases, with a concomitant decrease in the depth of the S wave. When right ventricular enlargement becomes fully developed, the normal precordial pattern is completely reversed so that tall R waves (QR or RS) are recorded in V_1 with deep S waves (RS) in V_6.

Prolongation of the QRS interval does not develop unless an intraventriular conduction defect develops with the enlarged right ventricle. The time of onset of the intrinsicoid deflection, however, may be delayed in the right precordial leads because the vectors representing activation of the right ventricle usually occur later in the QRS interval than they do normally and are of increased magnitude.

Right axis deviation is the most common sign of right ventricular enlargement. The diagnosis of right ventricular enlargement, however, should not be made on this finding alone unless other causes for right axis deviation have been ruled out. Furthermore, right ventricular enlargement may occur without abnormal right axis deviation.

A right ventricular strain pattern is manifested in ST and T wave alterations, with T wave changes similar to those seen in left ventricular enlargement. The ST segment is depressed and the T wave is inverted in the right-sided precordial leads and often in leads II, III, and aV_F, as well. This is a nonspecific abnormality.

Right bundle branch block is seen in right ventricular enlargement, especially of the volume-overload variety. In the younger person, right ventricular enlargement is commonly associated with right bundle branch block, either complete or incomplete. In the older age group (40 years and up) coronary artery disease is the most common cause. The surface ECG is less useful than the vectorcardiogram in the assessment of the degree of right ventricular enlargement in cases of incomplete or complete right bundle branch block. Further elaboration on the vectorcardiogram is beyond the scope of this presentation; therefore the reader is encouraged to refer to other textbooks on this subject. See Chapter 8 for a discussion of right bundle branch block.

A summary of the features of right ventricular enlargement is given here; these should be compared with the example in Fig. 6-22.

1. Reversal of precordial lead pattern with tall R waves over the right precordium (V_1, V_2), and deep S waves over the left precordium (V_5, V_6); the R to S ratio in V_1 becomes greater than 1.0
2. Duration of QRS interval within normal limits (if no right bundle branch block)

3. Late intrinsicoid deflection in V_1, V_2
4. Right axis deviation
5. Typical strain ST segment T wave patterns in V_1, V_2, and in leads II, III, and aV_F

RIGHT ATRIAL ENLARGEMENT

In the presence of right ventricular enlargement, it is not unusual to find an enlarged right atrium. Moreover, right atrial enlargement is often an indirect sign of right ventricular enlargement.

The following criteria are used in the ECG diagnosis of right atrial enlargement (Fig. 6-23):

1. The duration of the P wave is 0.11 second or less.
2. The contour of the P wave is tall, *peaked (P pulmonale)*, and measures 2.5 mm or more in amplitude in leads II, III, and aV_F.
3. The right precordial leads reflect diphasic P waves, often with increased voltage of the initial component.
4. The mean electrical axis of the P wave may be shifted right to +70 degrees or more.

It should be noted that abnormal P waves may occur in healthy patients. For example, acceleration of the heart rate alone may cause peaking and increased voltage of the P wave. Conversely, normal P waves may be identified in the presence of atrial disease.

MYOCARDIAL INFARCTION

To diagnose myocardial infarction, the ECG should be used to confirm the clinical impression. Because the ECG may not be diagnostic in many instances, if a patient is suspected clinically of having experienced a myocardial infarction, he should be treated accordingly, regardless of what the ECG shows.

Only Q wave changes (necrosis) are diagnostic of infarction, but changes in the ST segments (injury) and T waves (ischemia) may be suspicious and provide presumptive evidence. These changes are illustrated in Fig. 6-24.

Q Wave

The Q wave is one of the most important, and sometimes most difficult to interpret, assessors of myocardial infarction on the ECG. For example, with normal intraventricular conduction, small Q waves are present in leads V_5, V_6, aV_L, and I, particularly with a horizontal heart position or left axis deviation. Furthermore, with a vertical heart position or right axis deviation, small Q waves may be present in leads II, III, and aV_F. Finally, deep wide Q waves or QS complexes are normally present in aV_R and may be present in lead V_1.

Major importance is placed on the development of *new* Q waves in ECG leads where they previously were not present.

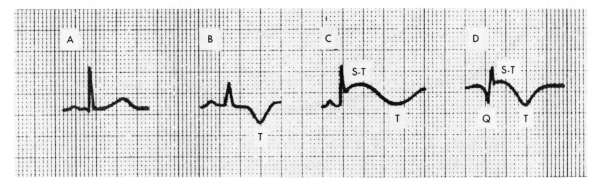

FIG. 6-24.   ECG wave changes indicative of ischemia, injury, and necrosis of the myocardium. A, Normal left ventricular wave pattern. B, Ischemia indicated by inversion of the T wave. C, Ischemia and current of injury indicated by T wave inversion and ST segment elevation. The ST segment may be elevated above or depressed below the baseline, depending on whether or not the tracing is from a lead facing toward or away from the infarcted area and depending on whether epicardial or endocardial injury occurs. Epicardial injury causes ST segment elevation in leads facing the epicardium. D, Ischemia, injury, and myocardial necrosis. The Q wave indicates necrosis of the myocardium.

Accordingly, the *appearance* of abnormal Q waves must be considered in light of the overall picture, considering that pathologic Q waves have the following features:
1. Q waves are 0.04 second or longer in *duration*.
2. Q waves are usually greater than 4 mm in *depth*.
3. Q waves appear in *leads* that do not normally have deep, wide Q waves. V_1 and aV_R normally record Q waves. Pathologic Q waves are usually present in several leads that are oriented in similar directions (e.g., II, III, and aV_F; or I, aV_L).

Vector Abnormalities

In acute myocardial infarction, electrical and anatomic death of the myocardium occurs in the region of the infarct; hence the initial forces of depolarization tend to point away from the infarcted area, producing Q waves in the ECG leads facing the involved site. The mean T vector also tends to point away from the site of infarction, presumably because of electrical ischemia in the tissues surrounding the infarct. The ST vector represents the effect of injury current. When the injury current is in the epicardial layers of the myocardium, as in myocardial infarction and pericarditis, the ST segment is elevated in leads facing the injury and the ST vector points toward the injured area. When the injury current is located in the subendocardial layers, as in angina pectoris, coronary insufficiency, and subendocardial infarction, The ST segment is depressed in leads facing the injury, and the ST vector points away from the site of injury (see Fig. 6-34). The ST displacement in subendocardial infarction persists longer than that of angina pectoris and coronary insufficiency.

Thus with an acute myocardial infarction the ST vector is opposite in direction to the Q vector and the mean T vector, resulting in ST segment elevation in those leads that have Q waves and inverted T waves. The relationship of these three vectors to one another is diagrammed in Fig. 6-25, *B*.

From animal studies, loss of resting membrane potential in the ischemic cells occurs first and is responsible for T-Q segment depression in the scalar ECG. Reduction in action potential duration and amplitude follows and causes ST segment elevation. Delayed repolarization in the ischemic area results in T wave inversion.

Localization of Infarction

Localization of infarcts may be important for several reasons, including prognosis. Localization is based on the principle that diagnostic ECG signs of myocardial infarction (Fig. 6-24) occur in leads whose positive terminals face the damaged surface of the heart. To facilitate localization, the left ventricle has been divided into four topographic regions where infarctions may occur (Fig. 6-25, *A*). Although these locations represent electrical rather than anatomic sites of infarction, anatomic correlations occur with reasonable frequency, particularly for the first myocardial infarction.

An *anterior infarction* produces characteristic changes in leads V_1, V_2, and V_3; a *diaphragmatic* or *inferior infarction* affects leads II, III, and aV_F; a *lateral infarction* involves leads I, aV_L, V_5, and V_6. In strictly *posterior infarction*, there are no leads whose positive terminals are directly over the infarct. However, the changes of the electrical field produced by any infarction still apply; hence in purely posterior infarction the initial forces of the QRS complex and the T wave point anteriorly away from the site of the infarct, and the ST segment is directed posteriorly. This is

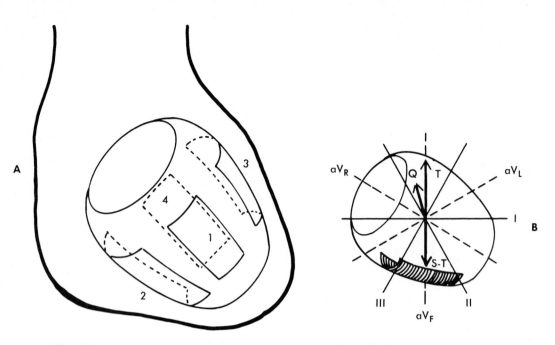

FIG. 6-25. A, Lie of the left ventricle in the chest as viewed frontally. The left ventricle has been divided into four topographic regions where infarctions may occur: (1) anterior, (2) diaphragmatic or inferior, (3) lateral, and (4) posterior (pure). B, Vectors of a diaphragmatic myocardial infarction. Hexaxial reference figure is superimposed on the left ventricle as viewed in B. The mean vector for the initial 0.04 second of the QRS complex points *away* from the infarcted area and indicates the dead zone. This produces Q waves in the leads "looking at" the infarction. The mean T vector indicates the ischemic zone surrounding the infarct and points *away* from the infarcted area. The ST vector indicates the injury zone and in the event of myocardial infarction, the ST vector points *toward* the injured area. In this example of a diaphragmatic myocardial infarction, leads II, III, and aV$_F$ will exhibit the Q waves, ST segment elevation, and T wave inversion shown in Fig. 6-24, D.

recognized in the ECG as tall broad initial R waves, ST segment depression, and tall upright T waves in leads V$_1$ and V$_2$. In other words, a mirror image of the typical infarction pattern of an anterior myocardial infarction is recorded. Stated another way, infarction of the true posterior surface of the heart must be inferred from reciprocal (opposite) changes occurring in the anterior leads. These locations are summarized in Table 6-1.

It should be noted that although diagnostic signs of myocardial infarction appear in leads facing the infarcted heart surface, *reciprocal changes* occur concomitantly in leads facing the diametrically opposed surface of the heart. These changes include absence of a Q wave, some increase of the R wave, depressed ST segment, and upright tall T wave.

Reciprocal changes, therefore, in an anterior infarction will occur in leads II, III, and aV$_F$. In a diaphragmatic or inferior infarction, reciprocal changes occur in leads I, aV$_L$, and some of the precordial leads. In lateral wall infarction, lead V$_1$ may show reciprocal changes.

Frequently the localization of an infarction is not as strict as just described. If the anterior and lateral walls of the left ventricle are both involved in the process, it is called an *anterolateral infarction*. If the limb leads indicate an inferior infarction and diagnostic changes are also present in leads V$_5$ and V$_6$, then it is called an inferior infarction with lateral extension or an *inferolateral infarction*, and so on.

Text continued on p. 110.

TABLE 6-1. Location of myocardial infarction

Area of Infarction	Leads Showing Wave Changes
Anterior	V$_1$, V$_2$, V$_3$
Diaphragmatic or inferior	II, III, aV$_F$
Lateral	I, aV$_L$, V$_5$, V$_6$
Posterior (pure)	V$_1$ and V$_2$: tall broad initial R wave, ST segment depression, and tall upright T wave

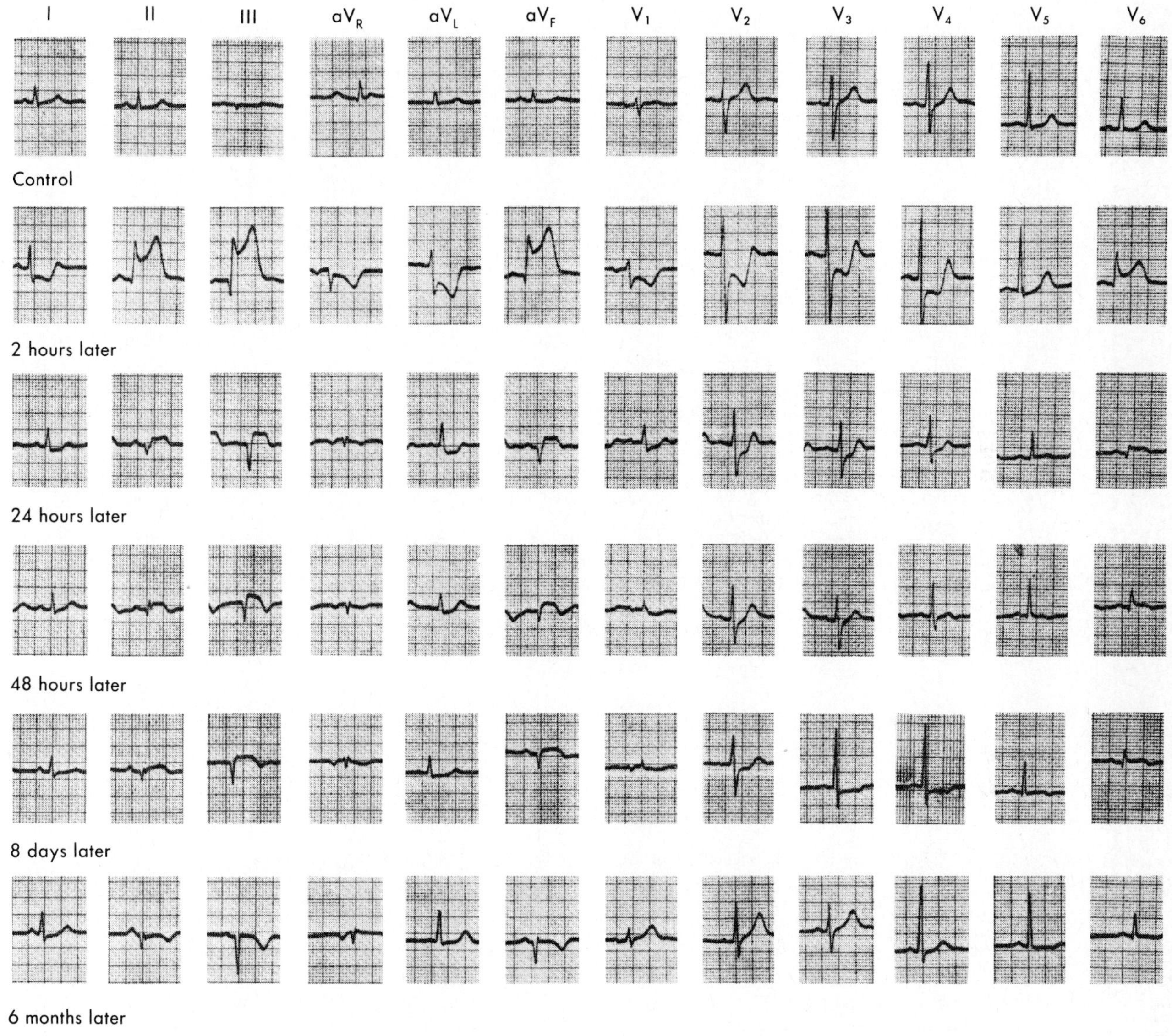

FIG. 6-26. Evolutionary changes in a posteroinferior myocardial infarction. *Control tracing* is normal. The tracing recorded *2 hours* after onset of chest pain demonstrates development of early Q waves, marked ST segment elevation, and hyperacute T waves in leads II, III, and aV$_F$. In addition, a larger R wave, ST segment depression, and negative T waves have developed in leads V$_1$ to V$_2$. These are early changes indicating acute posteroinferior myocardial infarction. The *24-hour* tracing demonstrates evolutionary changes. In leads II, III, and aV$_F$ the Q wave is larger, the ST segments have almost returned to baseline, and the T wave has begun to invert. In leads V$_1$ to V$_2$ the duration of the R wave now exceeds 0.04 second, the ST segment is depressed, and the T wave is upright. (In this classic example, ECG changes of true posterior involvement extend past V$_2$; ordinarily only V$_1$ and V$_2$ may be involved.) Only minor further changes occur through the *8-day* tracing. Finally, *6 months later* the ECG illustrates large Q waves, isoelectric ST segments, and inverted T waves in leads II, III, and aV$_F$, large R waves, isoelectric ST segments, and upright T waves in V$_1$ and V$_2$ indicative of an "old" posteroinferior myocardial infarction.

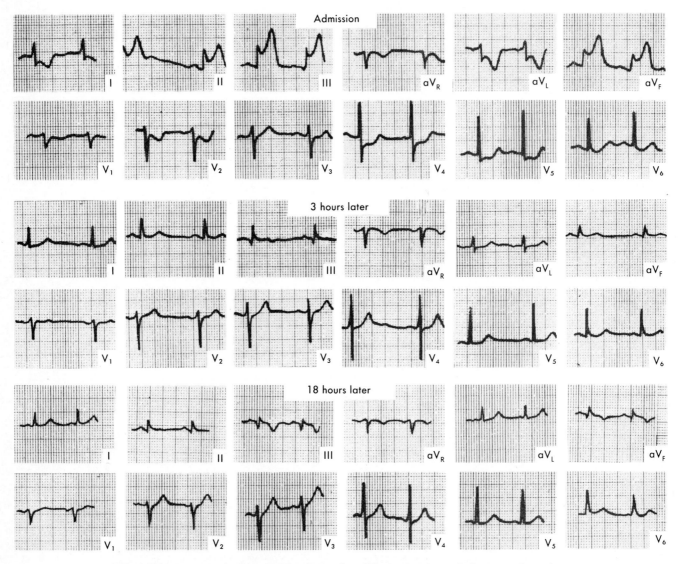

FIG. 6-27. These three 12-lead ECGs obtained at different time intervals from a patient who had an unequivocal myocardial infarction demonstrate that at one point during the electrocardiographic evolution of a myocardial infarction, the ECG may appear almost normal. Note the hyperacute T wave changes and unquestionable injury current portrayed in the admission ECG. Hyperacute T wave changes are normally upright; these enlarged T waves can occur very early after infarction, preceding the more characteristic T wave inversion. Three hours later, the ST segment has returned almost completely to the baseline, significant Q waves have not yet appeared, and the T waves remain fairly normal. This ECG is at most "nonspecifically" abnormal. Eighteen hours after admission, classic changes in an acute diaphragmatic myocardial infarction have evolved. This illustration serves to deemphasize the value of a single ECG in diagnosing an acute myocardial infarction. The patient quite possibly would have been sent home if the determination for admission to the CCU had been based solely on a single ECG, that is, the second tracing.

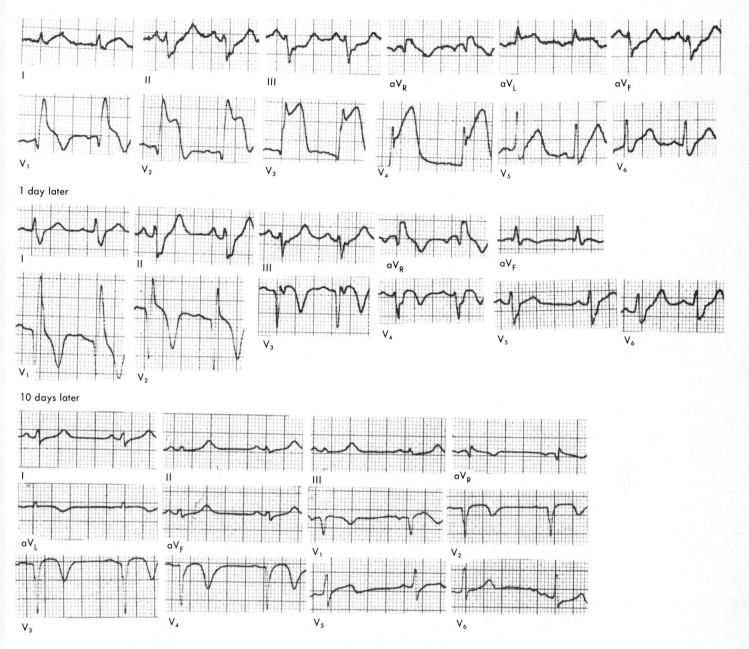

1 day later

10 days later

FIG. 6-28. Serial tracings on a patient with an acute anterior myocardial infarction. On admission patient's ECG showed left axis deviation (left anterior hemiblock) and right bundle branch block, thus supporting the presence of bifascicular block (see Chapter 8). Terminal T wave inversion in V_1 to V_2 and profound ST segment elevation are present in V_1 to V_5. These changes are not masked by the presence of the right bundle branch block. One day later the ST segments have returned toward the baseline, the Q waves in the anterior precordial leads have enlarged greatly, and there is now T wave inversion in these leads. Left anterior hemiblock and right bundle branch block are still present. In the tracing recorded 10 days later the right bundle branch block and left anterior hemiblock have disappeared, leaving the electrocardiographic changes of an anteroseptal myocardial infarction with Q waves in V_1 to V_3 and T wave inversion in V_1 to V_4.

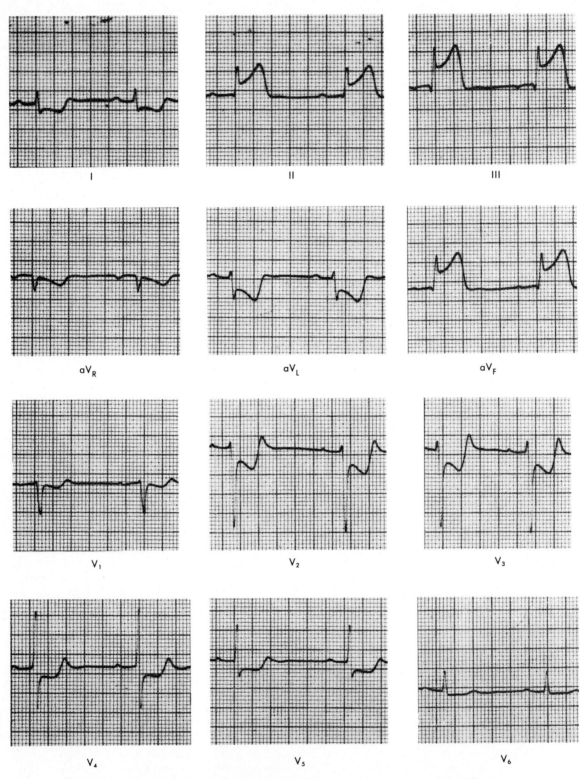

FIG. 6-29. Inferior (diaphragmatic) myocardial infarction, hyperacute stage. Note ST segment elevation in leads II, III, and aV$_F$ with reciprocal ST depression in the anterior precordial leads. The T waves in leads II, III, and aV$_F$ are still upright and pointed and indicate the hyperacute stage of myocardial infarction. Note the development of only very small Q waves in leads II, III, and aV$_F$. Subsequent evolution of this ECG will demonstrate the progressive development of significant (greater than 0.04 second) Q waves and T wave inversion in leads II, III, and aV$_F$; the ST segment will return to an isoelectric position.

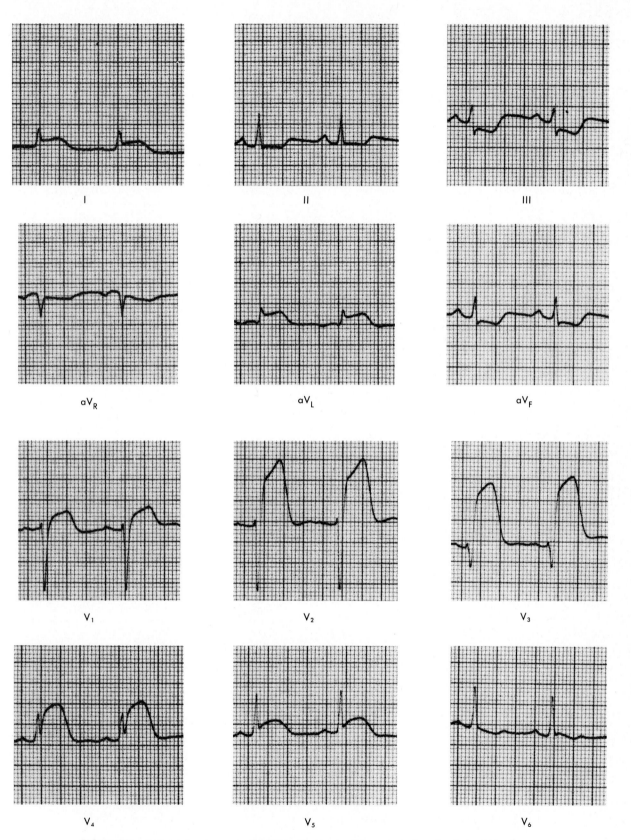

FIG. 6-30. Anterolateral myocardial infarction, acute. ST segment elevation in leads I, aV_L, and V_1 to V_5 indicate an acute anterolateral myocardial infarction. During the evolution of this tracing, one would expect the development of Q waves and T wave inversion in leads I and aV_L and the precordial leads, with the ST segment returning to baseline.

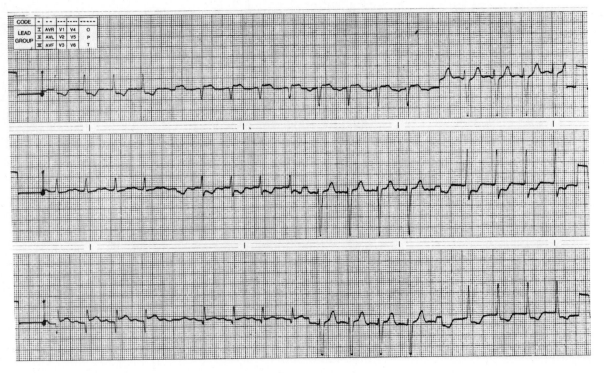

FIG. 6-31. Sinus tachycardia. Q waves in III and aV_F, along with ST segment elevation, suggesting evolving inferior myocardial infarction.

Evolution of a Myocardial Infarction

The evolution of a myocardial infarction is a sequential process, and it is important to record the time relationships in the diagnosis. Within the first few hours after infarction, sometimes referred to as the hyperacute state, elevated ST segments and tall (hyperacute) upright T waves appear in those leads facing the infarction. Q waves may appear early or may not develop for several days. Within several days of the infarct the ST segment begins to return to base line, whereas the T waves develop progressively deeper inversion. After weeks or months the T waves become shallower and may finally return to normal. The Q waves are most likely to remain as a permanent record of the myocardial scar (Fig. 6-26). Persistent ST segment elevation (beyond 6 weeks) suggests the possibility of ventricular aneurysm (Table 6-2). The different locations of myocardial infarction in different stages of clinical evolution are shown in Fig. 6-27 to 6-34.

TABLE 6-2. Time relationships in the evolution and resolution of a myocardial infarction

ECG Abnormality	Onset	Disappearance
ST segment elevation	Immediately	1 to 6 weeks
Q waves >0.04 second	Immediately or in several days	Years to never
T wave inversion	6 to 24 hours	Months to years

FIG. 6-32. Anterolateral myocardial infarction, acute. The 12-lead ECG on admission, A, demonstrates ST segment elevation in leads I, aV_L, and V_1 to V_6, indicating the anterolateral injury current of an acute anterolateral myocardial infarction. B, Seven hours later. The patient has developed right bundle branch block with abnormal Q waves in leads I, aV_L, and V_2 to V_5. C, Twenty-six hours later. In addition to the right bundle branch block, the patient has now developed left anterior hemiblock. D, Three months later. The left anterior hemiblock and right bundle branch block are still present. The Q waves in leads I and aV_L are not as prominent as the Q waves in V_1 to V_5. Persistent ST segment elevation for a duration greater than 6 weeks after the myocardial infarction raises the possibility of a left ventricular aneurysm.

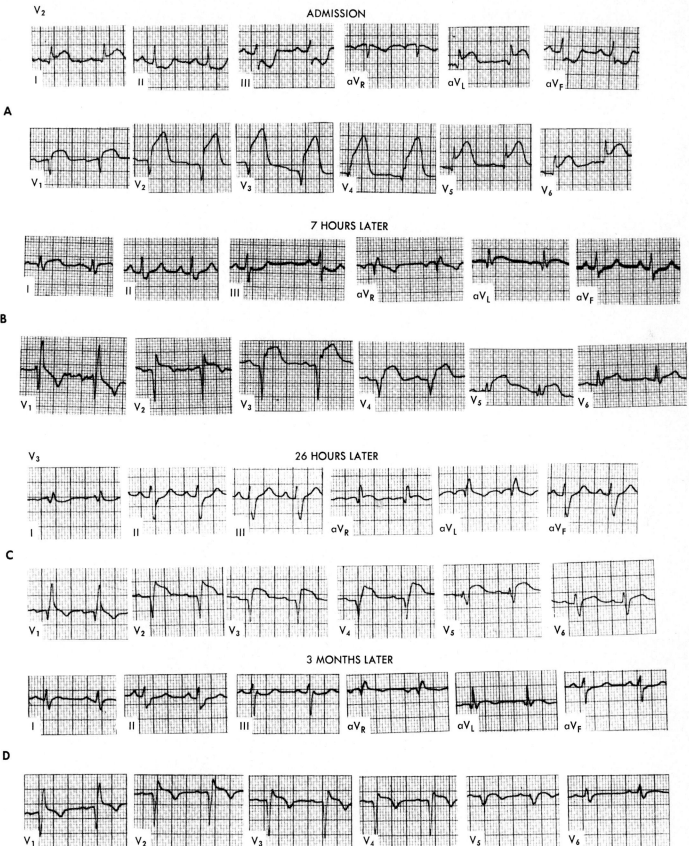

ADMISSION

7 HOURS LATER

26 HOURS LATER

3 MONTHS LATER

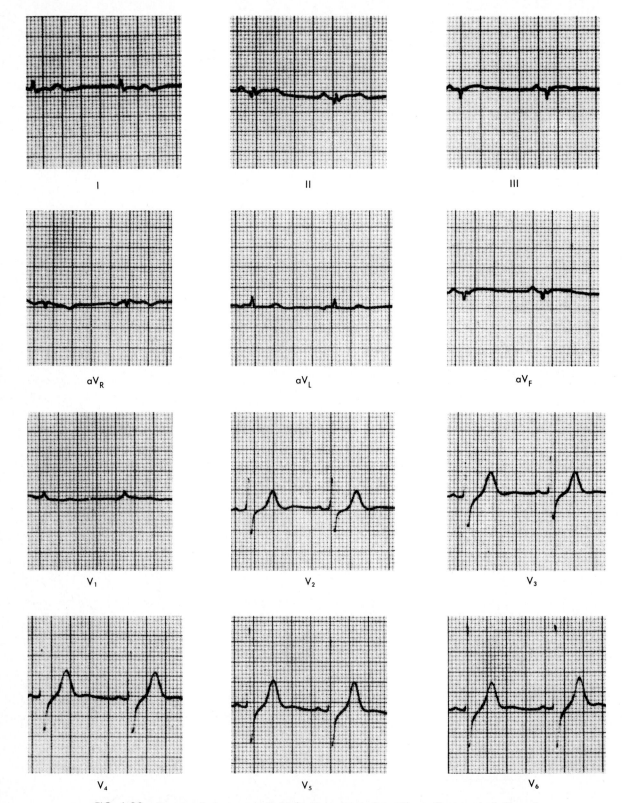

FIG. 6-33.   Posteroinferior myocardial infarction, date indeterminant. Q waves in II, III, and aV$_F$ are consistent with an old inferior myocardial infarction. The large R wave in V$_1$ signifies true posterior infarction as well. Compare with Fig. 6-26 at 6 months.

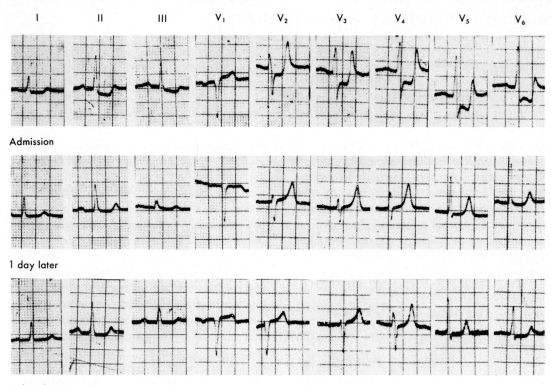

FIG. 6-34. Subendocardial myocardial infarction. Note slight ST segment depression in leads I, II, and III with marked ST segment depression in leads V_2 to V_6 on admission. One day later the ST segments have returned to normal and there is diminution of the height of the R wave in the precordial leads but no other changes. The tracing 4 days later is essentially unchanged. Note failure to develop the classic Q waves of a transmural myocardial infarction. The patient died and at autopsy had an extensive subendocardial myocardial infarction.

SUGGESTED READINGS

Beckwith, J.R.: Grant's clinical electrocardiography; the spatial vector approach, New York, 1970, McGraw-Hill Book Co.

Braunwald, E., editor: Heart disease, a textbook of cardiovascular medicine, ed. 2, Philadelphia, 1984, W.B. Saunders Co.

Chung, E.K.: Electrocardiography: practical applications with vectorial principles, Hagerstown, Md., 1980, Harper & Row Publishers, Inc.

Hurst, J.W., and others: editors: The heart, ed. 6, New York, 1986, McGraw-Hill Book Co.

Kennedy, H.L. and others: Long-term follow-up of asymptomatic healthy subjects with frequent and complex ventricular ectopy, N. Engl. J. Med. **312:**193, 1985.

Ruberman, W., and others: Ventricular premature complexes and sudden death after myocardial infarction, Circulation **64:**297, 1981.

Schamroth, L.: Diagnostic pointers in clinical electrocardiology, vol. 2, Bowie, Md., 1979, Charles Press.

CHAPTER 7

Complications of Coronary Artery Disease

Paula Hindle
Andrew G. Wallace

To accomplish its task of pumping blood to all organs and tissues of the body, heart muscle requires a substantial flow of blood that can increase appropriately when demands on the heart increase with physical or emotional activity. The function of heart muscle is hindered when coronary artery disease compromises the supply of coronary blood flow.

During normal activity the heart extracts approximately 75% of the oxygen in arterial blood. Other organs usually extract a maximum of 25% to 30%. Thus the oxygen reserve available to the heart when it is stressed is very limited. Under these circumstances an increase in coronary blood flow is the only means by which increased myocardial needs can be met. If the coronary blood flow fails to satisfy the myocardial need for oxygen, ischemia results.[1]

The rate of blood flow in most arteries is determined by the mean arterial pressure. The rate of coronary blood flow, in contrast, is determined mainly by the diastolic arterial blood pressure. During ventricular systole the high stress within the myocardial wall causes the heart muscle to constrict the transmural coronary blood vessels. In diastole, wall stress drops precipitously and flow through the coronary arteries reaches its maximal velocity.

Under any given set of conditions, coronary blood flow is determined by a complex interaction between hydraulic factors (wall stress, arterial pressure, and heart rate) and local metabolic factors. Both of these in turn are modulated by the activity of the autonomic nervous system. When these controls operate normally, the supply of coronary blood flow closely matches the metabolic requirements of heart muscle. When a hydraulically significant obstruction develops within a coronary artery, the flow and the distribution of flow are compromised and ischemia develops. The functional significance of any given coronary artery stenosis depends in part on the demands placed on the myocardium and in part on the extent of collateral vessels, which provide an alternative source of perfusion to the muscle.

CLINICAL PRESENTATIONS: AN OVERVIEW

Deficits in myocardial perfusion may be manifested in the following clinical syndromes.

1. *Angina pectoris.* Pathophysiologically this syndrome is a state of transient myocardial ischemia without clinically recognizable cell death. It is characterized by chest discomfort that is usually precipitated by activities or events that increase the metabolic demand for oxygen. At the time of the patient's first episode of anginal pain, the coronary artery obstruction is usually well developed. As the disease progresses, the anginal pain may change from its stable, predictable nature to "unstable" angina in which pain may be present at rest and relief may be inconsistent despite aggressive medical therapy.

2. *Myocardial infarction.* This condition is defined as myocardial ischemia of sufficient intensity and duration to produce recognizable death (necrosis) of tissue. The most common symptom is severe, persistent pain that may be accompanied by intense anxiety, nausea, vomiting, dyspnea, and diaphoresis. Ancillary clinical and laboratory tests show evidence of dead heart muscle. The patient may or may not be able to cite a precipitating factor, although approximately two thirds have premonitory symptoms. Rupture of a plaque or thrombosis on the surface of a plaque is thought to account for most episodes of acute infarction.

3. *Heart failure.* When cardiac output fails to meet metabolic demands, heart failure ensues. It may involve either ventricle initially, but since they work in series, one ventricle does not fail for long without affecting the other. Pulmonary edema is a medical emergency caused by severe left heart failure (Table 7-1). Cardiogenic shock, referred to as *pump failure,* is frequently caused by massive myocardial damage, which leaves the ventricle so disabled that it cannot generate an adequate contraction or adequate cardiac output. Such profound failure is usually irreversible.

4. *Cardiomegaly.* Cardiomegaly is enlargement of the heart that may result from either dilatation or hypertrophy or both. Patients with long-standing angina or with recurrent infarctions demonstrate multiple scars and areas of replacement fibrosis in the heart; the heart appears to adapt to these changes by dilatation. In part because of dilatation and in part because the work load on the heart muscle shifts from areas of damage to residual healthy muscle, the remaining normal components undergo hypertrophy. As a result, heart size seen by x-ray examination, heart dimensions measured by angiography, and heart mass all increase.

5. *Abnormal electrocardiogram.* Certain changes on the ECG may strongly indicate coronary insufficiency in an

TABLE 7-1. Treatment of acute pulmonary edema

Therapeutic Goal	Therapy	Principle	Precaution
Improve gaseous exchange	Morphine sulfate, 8-15 mg IV	Morphine decreases anxiety, reduces venous return, and decreases musculoskeletal and respiratory activity	Monitor vital signs; hypoxic depression of respiratory system seriously aggravated by morphine; morphine antagonist nalorphine (Nalline) and respiratory stimulants should be available.
	Intermittent positive pressure breathing (IPPB) apparatus delivering 100% O_2 via well-fitted nonrebreathing face mask, using airway pressure of 4-9 cm H_2O	IPPB decreases alveolar fluid, reduces ventilatory rate, increases arterial oxygen, facilitates uniformity of ventilation in all lung segments	Oxygen always administered with humidification to avoid airway drying and inspissation of bronchial secretions; antifoaming agents (20%-50% alcohol) may be used; remember that face mask is frightening to "suffocating" patient
	Aminophylline, IV at rate of about 20 mg/min, to total dose of 240-280 mg*	Aminophylline dilates bronchioles; also increases cardiac output, lowers venous pressure by relaxing smooth muscles of blood vessels	This drug injected slowly IV; otherwise headache, palpitation, dizziness, nausea, and fall in blood pressure occur; sedation required to relax anxious patient; cardiac arrhythmias may also occur
	Arterial line inserted for arterial blood gas determination	Normal blood gas values: pH: 7.38-7.42; Po_2: 90-100 mm Hg; Pco_2: 35-45 mm Hg; $\%O_2$ saturation: 95%-100%	Keep arterial line open with heparin flush
Decrease intravascular volume	Diuretic therapy selecting one of the following: Furosemide (Lasix), 40-120 mg IV Ethacrynic acid (Edecrin), 50 mg IV	These rapidly acting diuretics given IV begin work within minutes; decrease in intravascular volume improves ability of lungs to exchange gases and decreases cardiac work	Monitor blood pressure and intake and output; given in excessive amounts these diuretics can lead to a profound diuresis with volume and electrolyte depletion; local infiltration of ethacrynic acid
	Phlebotomy of 300-500 ml	See preceding	If pulmonary edema has already precipitated circulatory collapse, phlebotomy will aggravate shock
Improve cardiac performance	All of the preceding Digitalis, IV administration of rapidly acting preparation	See preceding Increase force of contraction and efficiency of heart	See preceding Monitor for arrhythmias; in presence of hypoxia in an acutely dilated heart, digitalis-induced arrhythmias likely to occur
Decrease venous return	Sitting (Fowler's) position	Sitting up increases lung volume and vital capacity, decreases venous return and work of breathing	In presence of hypotension, Fowler's position avoided or used cautiously
	IPPB	IPPB effectively reduces venous return by replacing normal negative intrathoracic pressure of spontaneous inspiration with positive pressure, varied as needed and impeding venous flow; reduces work of breathing to a degree	High pressure settings avoided, since excessive reduction of peripheral venous return can cause circulatory collapse; also see preceding
	Tourniquets applied to three extremities with greater pressure than that of estimated venous pressure, but below arterial diastolic pressure; peripheral arterial pulses maintained at all times; tourniquets rotated so that each extremity is free, in sequence for 15 min†	Pooling of blood in the extremities retards venous return, reduces capillary-alveolar transudation, decreases cardiac work	Prolonged constriction of extremities causes pain and loss of function; resultant dramatic edema of extremities may be upsetting to patient; at conclusion of acute phase, tourniquets released one at a time, at 15-min intervals, to avoid flooding pulmonary circulation

*Aminophylline in suppository form has been used effectively for this stage of pulmonary edema and may be safer than IV administration.
†Rotating tourniquets are generally used if other measures are unavailable or when all of the measures above have been tried without success.

asymptomatic patient. On the other hand, the resting ECG may be normal in a patient with serious coronary artery disease. To establish evidence of coronary insufficiency, it is helpful to obtain an ECG during and after stress (exercise). The most significant change on the ECG is the development of ST segment depression, seen more frequently in the lateral precordial leads (V4, V5, and V6) and less often in leads V2, II, III, and AVF. Frequently, a patient suffering an anginal attack will also show these changes. When the pain has subsided, the ST segments will return to normal. Prinzmetal's angina, also called *atypical angina* or *variant angina*, is characterized electrocardiographically by ST elevation, may occur unrelated to exertion and is usually relieved by nitroglycerin. In most instances transient coronary artery spasm is thought to play a role in Prinzmetal's angina.

6. *Arrhythmias.* Disorders of impulse formation or abnormal conduction, or both, frequently signal the presence of coronary artery disease and may be caused by inadequate oxygenation, areas of scar formation, or acute infarction. The patient having arrhythmias may complain of palpitations, dizziness, fatigue, or syncope. (See Chapter 8.)

7. *Sudden death.* In this text sudden death is defined as death occurring within 1 hour of the onset of symptoms. In patients without obvious preexisting disease, sudden death is usually ascribed to ventricular fibrillation and may also occur without infarction. Most sudden deaths occur before the patient reaches the hospital. (See Chapter 9.)

8. *Mitral insufficiency.* The normal competence of the mitral valve depends on a structurally and functionally intact mitral apparatus, including the posterior left atrial wall, the anulus, the leaflets, the chordae tendineae, and the papillary muscles and their base of support within the left ventricular wall. The most common cause of mitral insufficiency is probably coronary artery disease. Ischemic injury to the papillary muscle and its base of support or frank rupture of the papillary muscle or its chordae also may lead to mitral insufficiency. Murmurs caused by mitral insufficiency may develop during an angina attack or may be a stable consequence of the fibrotic changes that follow an old infarction. Mitral insufficiency may develop acutely in the setting of myocardial infarction and may contribute to or cause acute left heart failure and pulmonary edema.

9. *Ventricular aneurysm.* With transmural myocardial infarction the hydraulic stress on the necrotic portion of the ventricular wall may cause it to bulge during systole and to become extremely thin as the necrotic material is absorbed. If this occurs before a substantial scar has formed, the resulting scar may develop as an outward balloon or bulge that communicates with the ventricular chamber through a "neck." Ventricular aneurysms usually develop during the weeks that follow acute infarction. Their hemodynamic consequence can be related to their size, to the amount of residual normal muscle, and to their location, which sometimes involves the papillary muscles. For reasons that are not completely apparent, patients with ventricular aneurysms are particularly prone to recurrent ventricular tachyarrhythmias. Once a scar has developed, aneurysms seldom rupture. Hence they are detected either by x-ray examination, radionuclide angiograms, typical ECG changes, echocardiography, or during angiography.

10. *Ventricular rupture.* Hydraulic stresses on necrotic myocardium may rarely produce myocardial rupture.[2] When rupture of the heart occurs, it usually develops within 10 days after the onset of symptoms of infarction. The ventricle may rupture to the outside, producing acute cardiac tamponade or, more often, it may rupture internally through necrotic muscle near the apical end of the interventricular septum. A holosystolic murmur at the apex and left sternal border in a patient with acute infarction should always suggest the possibility of rupture. Heart failure usually develops or is worsened concurrently with this event. Treatment consists of hemodynamic stabilization with drug therapy and intraaortic balloon counterpulsation and immediate surgery to repair the septum.

Ventricular rupture can be diagnosed by relatively simple, even bedside, catheter techniques. With the pulmonary artery line, right atrial, right ventricular, and pulmonary artery blood samples are obtained. These samples are analyzed for their oxygen content. A step up in oxygen content in either the right ventricle or the pulmonary artery would indicate a left-to-right shunt. M-mode Doppler echocardiography can also detect left-to-right shunting associated with ventricular septal rupture. Two-dimensional echocardiography visualized the rupture in only 7 of 11 patients but assessed the size and location of the associated aneurysm in 10 of 11 patients.[3]

11. *Cardiogenic shock*—Signs of impaired tissue perfusion and a systolic blood pressure of less than 90 mm Hg or at least 30 mm Hg lower than the prior basal level in a patient with acute myocardial infarction is generally a result of severe cardiac dysfunction. The diagnosis of cardiogenic shock should not be made, however, until other precipitating factors, such as cardiac arrhythymias, hypovolemia, hypoxemia, and acidosis, are corrected. Once the diagnosis is made, the goal is to improve cardiac output and tissue perfusion. (See last section of this chapter.)

Angina Pectoris

The diagnosis of angina pectoris is usually made from a characteristic history because frequently there are few abnormalities found through physical examination and the ECG may be normal at rest. It is best to allow patients to describe what they have been feeling without the use of suggestive terms. Time and patience are necessary to explore the patient's life-style, habits, and emotions to obtain a clear picture of the pain and the extent of incapacitation.

Although the term *angina pectoris* literally means chest pain, perhaps it should be referred to as discomfort because many patients may deny experiencing chest pain. Rather, they often refer to vague sensations, feelings, or aches. These unpleasant feelings have been described in a variety of ways, including a sense of pressure or burning, squeezing, heaviness, smothering, and very frequently as "indigestion." Since the discomfort of angina is usually located in the retrosternal region, patients will often illustrate the nature and location of their symptoms by placing a clenched fist against their sternum. Often angina pectoris is not confined to the chest but may radiate to the neck, jaw, epigastrium, shoulders, or arms. Most often it radiates to the left shoulder and left arm. Occasionally, angina may produce discomfort in an area of radiation without affecting the retrosternal region.

Attacks of exertional angina are typically preceded by an elevation of blood pressure or heart rate or both. During the attack, pulse rate and blood pressure usually increase further, presumably as a consequence of anxiety and as a physiologic response to pain. In some instances, however, blood pressure and pulse may fall dramatically as a result of vagally mediated reflexes analogous to vasodepressor syncope or fainting. The patient may remain motionless; some experience feelings of impending doom. More important than the location is the duration of the pain and the circumstances under which it occurs. Angina pectoris lasts usually only a few minutes if the precipitating factor is relieved. Attacks are often induced by effort and *during* rather than after exertion. Exertion during cold weather or following meals is particularly likely to produce pain. Anxiety, smoking, stressful situations, worry, anger, hurry, and excitement are common precipitating factors. Patients have described the following situations as producing chest pain: running to catch a bus, driving in heavy traffic, nightmares, painful stimuli, sexual intercourse, and straining at stool.

Angina typically lasts from 1 to several minutes and usually no more than 3 to 5 minutes. It is relieved by rest, by nitroglycerin, or by any influence that will drop arterial pressure or heart rate and equalize the supply of blood and nutrients with the demand.

Various types of anginal pain occur. During "walk-through" angina the patient is able to continue activity until the pain gradually disappears. Angina decubitus is chest pain occurring when the patient is at rest in the supine position. Nocturnal angina may awaken a patient from sleep (usually caused by dreams) with the same sensation experienced during exertion.

Prinzmetal's or "variant" angina[4] produces symptoms similar to typical angina but is believed to be caused by coronary artery spasm. This form of angina frequently occurs at rest and can be difficult to induce by exercise testing. It is cyclic in nature, frequently happening at the same time each day. ECG tracings show ST segment elevation that usually returns to baseline with relief of the pain. In order to document the presence of variant angina, ergonovine maleate[5] can be injected into the coronary artery during cardiac catheterization to induce spasm. Atherosclerotic lesions may or may not be present at the site of spasm. Treatment for spasm[6] consists of rest, nitroglycerin, and longer-acting nitrates. Calcium-blocking agents have been found especially effective.[7-9]

Medical Management. The first principle in the medical management of angina pectoris is to minimize the discrepancy between the demand of the heart muscle for oxygen and the ability of the coronary circulation to meet this demand. Accordingly, patients must learn to pace themselves so that physical activity is kept below the threshold of discomfort. Moderate exercise performed below the angina threshold should be encouraged. Additional measures include adopting a diet designed to achieve the individual's ideal weight and the cessation of smoking. Hypertension, if present, should be treated.

Pharmacologic treatment is directed at two objectives: first, relief from symptoms when they occur and, second, prevention of angina. For the first objective, nitroglycerin taken sublingually is the treatment of choice. For prevention, beta-adrenergic blocking agents are prescribed to slow the heart rate and attenuate the contractile response to physical or emotional activity. Longer-acting nitrates such as isosorbide dinitrate (Isordil) or nitrol paste exert an action for 2 to 4 hours and are very effective. Reichek and others[10] have found that transdermal nitroglycerin patches did not offer 24 hours of stable antianginal protection. During sustained transdermal treatment, patients develop tolerance to nitroglycerin, and antianginal efficacy was diminished.

Recent reports indicate that vasodilators acting principally on the arterial system (e.g., hydralazine or prazosin) may attenuate the hypertensive response to exertion and aid in preventing angina. Calcium-blocking agents[11-13] (e.g., nifedipine, verapamil, and diltiazem) are another group of potent vasodilators for coronary and peripheral arteries that also have the ability to decrease afterload and myocardial contractility. The combination of nitrate therapy and calcium blockers has been extremely effective.[14] Other investigators have demonstrated improved LV function, improved exercise tolerance, and delayed onset of chest pain with combination therapy consisting of nitrates, beta-adrenoreceptor-blocker therapy and calcium antagonists.[15]

Other general measures for the management of angina include sedation, relief of anxiety, and supervised exercise programs designed to enhance physical condition and thereby reduce the blood pressure and heart rate response to exercise.[16,17]

When a patient first has angina, significant stenosis of at least one coronary artery is usually present. Electrocardiographic evidence of ischemia at low heart rates during exercise, a large area or more than one area of reduced coronary perfusion during thallium 201 scanning, and known risk factors such as smoking and hypercholesterolemia each increase the probability of disease involving more than one coronary artery. Coronary arteriography is presently the only definitive way to assess the severity and extent of coronary artery disease. If the probability of multivessel disease is high or if symptoms fail to respond significantly to medical management, arteriography should be entertained. At the present time either angioplasty or coronary bypass surgery provides good relief of symptoms and prolongs life in selected subgroups of patients with angina. Criteria for and results of angioplasty and surgical intervention are discussed in Chapter 15.

Acute Myocardial Infarction

Chest pain is the presenting symptom in most patients with acute myocardial infarction. The pain is frequently severe, but there may be minimal discomfort and, on occasion, none. It is usually substernal and may radiate to the epigastric region, the jaw, shoulders, elbows, or forearms. The pain is usually described as a heaviness, tightness, or constriction but occasionally as indigestion or a burning sensation. It usually persists for 30 minutes or longer, often until potent analgesics have been administered. In its classic presentation the symptoms of myocardial infarction are more severe than typical angina. On the other hand, the symptoms of infarction may be subtle, and very often severity and duration of pain do not distinguish between prolonged angina, coronary insufficiency (prolonged ischemia), and myocardial infarction.

In addition to chest pain, patients with myocardial infarction may experience shortness of breath, sweating, weakness or extreme fatigue, nausea, vomiting, and severe anxiety. On physical examination they may show evidence of overactivity of the sympathetic nervous system, including tachycardia, sweating, and hypertension. Alternatively, evidence of vagal hyperactivity may predominate with bradycardia and hypotension. Many patients look surprisingly normal. Hypotension with tachycardia and peripheral cyanosis suggests a markedly reduced cardiac output and shock. In some patients normal blood pressure is maintained, but an S_3 gallop and pulmonary rales indicate acute left ventricular failure. Murmurs related to mitral insufficiency or a ruptured interventricular septum may develop and a pericardial friction rub may be heard. Heart sounds are usually diminished in intensity, and particularly with anterior infarction a paradoxical parasternal systolic lift can be felt inside the apex region.

The diagnosis of myocardial infarction is initially made on the basis of the patient's history and ECG tracings and finally confirmed with cardiac enzymes. Ancillary but nonspecific findings of infarction include low grade fever, elevation of the white blood cell count, and elevation of the erythrocyte sedimentation rate. The ECG may show typical findings of infarction or nonspecific changes of the ST segment or T wave. Rarely, if ever, are serial ECGs normal in a patient with documented infarction.

With necrosis of heart muscle, enzymes that are normally confined within the myocardial cell leak out and appear in peripheral blood; serum glutamic-oxaloacetic transaminase (SGOT), lactate dehydrogenase (LDH), and creatine phosphokinase (CPK) are the enzymes measured most frequently. LDH and CPK appear in more than one form and are referred to as isoenzymes. The isoenzymes of LDH and CPK are distributed differently in different tissues so that elevations of the "heart" isoenzymes are more specific evidence of heart muscle necrosis than elevation of either the total CPK or LDH. Elevations of CPK-MB and of LDH-1 (the predominant heart isoenzymes) are typically observed in myocardial infarction.[18,19]

In the past 10 years, the use of imaging to confirm the diagnosis of myocardial infarction has received considerable attention. These imaging methods include thallium 201 scintigraphy and technitium-99M pyrophosphate imaging.[20-23] Myocardial uptake of thallium 201 is dependent on blood flow; with decreased blood flow an area of diminished activity is visualized. Because a single study cannot differentiate between ischemic and necrotic myocardium, serial studies are necessary and the first thallium 201 study should be done within 6 hours after the onset of symptoms. In conjunction with other findings noted above, serial thallium 201 images can be used to diagnose a myocardial infarction as well as to estimate the location and extent of decreased coronary perfusion and resulting necrosis.

Dipyridamole-thallium 201 scintigraphy has been useful in identifying subsets of patients at high risk for future cardiac events after a myocardial infarction. Dipyridamole is a potent coronary vasodilator. When used in conjunction with thallium 201, it simulates an exercise thallium 201 test.[24,25] In studies with 51 patients, Leppo and others,[26,27] found that dipyridamole-thallium scintigraphy had 93% sensitivity and 80% specificity for coronary artery disease and was a useful predictor of postmyocardial infarction events.

The radionuclide imaging test using technetium 99M pyrophosphate is regarded as a fairly sensitive technique for confirming myocardial damage. The isotope is taken up by necrotic cells within 12 to 18 hours after the onset of infarction; uptake persists for 4 to 5 days and then typically decays. Even small areas of infarction can be identified by appropriate scanning equipment from the "hot spot" produced on the scintigram. For optimal results the test should be done between 48 and 72 hours after the onset of infarction.

Because wall motion abnormalities and wall thinning correlate with ischemia and infarction, two-dimensional echocardiography may be used to assess the ischemic heart. Systolic wall thickening is normally seen. Systolic wall thinning is seen when the infarct involves more than 20% of the transmural thickness. Although echocardiographic wall motion abnormalities seem to consistently overestimate infarct size, echocardiography can give a reasonable estimatae of overall left ventricular function. Echocardiography is also useful in determining acute and chronic mechanical complications of infarction. The acute complications easily defined include a ruptured mitral valve, papillary muscle dysfunction, papillary muscle rupture, ventricular septal rupture, cardiac rupture, and pericardial effusion. The chronic complications consist of aneurysm formation and intracavitary clot formation.[28-31]

The mortality of patients with acute myocardial infarction is approximately 20% to 25%. A substantial number of these deaths occur suddenly and before hospitalization. Mortality among patients who survive to reach the hospital is approximately 20%, and most of these deaths occur within the first 3 or 4 days. Since the 1950s, the age-adjusted mortality attributable to myocardial infarction has decreased.[32] This overall decline in mortality has been associated with a decrease in the incidence of coronary artery disease and a decrease in the case fatality rate. These marked improvements are attributed in part to the development of cardiac care units, new drugs, and new diagnostic and treatment procedures and, more importantly, to primary prevention.[33,34]

It is useful to distinguish between patients with complicated and uncomplicated acute myocardial infarction, since nearly all deaths occur in the former group, whereas those patients in the latter group have an excellent prognosis and are candidates for early mobilization and discharge. The conditions that identify the complicated group include the following:

1. *Persistent Pain.* Pain that persists or recurs is frequently associated with unusually high enzyme elevations or secondary rises and suggests that ischemia persists and infarction is in a process of evolution.

2. *Serious Arrhythmia.* Nearly all patients with acute infarction experience some transient alterations of rhythm. The alterations considered serious include ventricular fibrillation or ventricular tachycardia, second or third degree heart block, and new atrial flutter or fibrillation.[35] In addition, sinus tachycardia (≥ 100 beats/minute) that persists for more than 24 to 48 hours in the absence of fever should alert those caring for the patient to the possibility of heart failure.[36]

3. *Pulmonary Edema.* Pulmonary edema produces a sense of breathlessness, wet rales on examination, and typical changes on the chest x-ray film. It is nearly always accompanied by a significant rise in pulmonary artery and wedge pressure and indicates acute left ventricular failure.

4. *Persistent Hypotension.* The arterial systolic blood pressure may drop below 90 mmHg without accompanying signs of shock. Often this is an early and transient finding associated with bradycardia and other signs of vagal overactivity. Alternatively, it may reflect an inadequate blood volume. When hypotension persists despite an adequate heart rate and central venous pressure, it usually signifies a markedly reduced cardiac output.

In a study of 500 patients with acute myocardial infarction, the sample was classified on the basis of the presence or absence of complications during the first 4 days of hospitalization.[37] Among the group who were *not* free of complications through the fourth day, most either died subsequently in the hospital or suffered a serious late complication. Patients who were free of complications for the first 4 days appeared to be candidates for early mobilization and early discharge. Among patients without complications discharged on the seventh hospital day, there were no serious complications or deaths at home during early follow-up. DeBusk and associates demonstrated a similar low complication rate among patients discharged early after uncomplicated myocardial infarctions.[38]

Myocardial infarction patients can be further classified according to whether they had nontransmural or transmural infarcts. In the past patients with nontransmural infarcts were thought to follow an uncomplicated course. Evidence suggests that patients with nontransmural infarctions are actually at higher risk for complications and sudden death after discharge from the hospital.[39] In view of these findings, survivors of nontransmural infarction are especially appropriate candidates for early functional assessment and arteriography.

Low level exercise testing before discharge has proven to be of value in predicting patients at high risk for subsequent complications. Evidence indicates that patients who develop either ST segment abnormalities, angina pectoris, or abnormal blood pressure responses during low level exercise testing are at higher risk of developing cardiac complications.[40,41] Nishimura and associates found that wall motion studies using two-dimensional echocardiography may be helpful in identifying subsets of patients at high risk for complications.[42]

Medical Management. In the early stages of acute myocardial infarction, pain, anxiety, and alterations of rhythm dominate the clinical picture. After establishing a route for intravenous therapy and ECG monitoring, morphine should be given in doses that eliminate or greatly reduce chest pain and relieve anxiety. Excessive bradycardia with a pulse rate below 50 to 55 beats/minute, particularly if accompanied by hypotension and ectopic beats, should be treated with atropine.[43] (See Chapter 10.)

The greatest threat to life in the early hours after myocardial infarction is ventricular fibrillation. In approximately 50% of patients episodes of ventricular fibrillation are preceded by ventricular premature beats. The high prevalence of premature beats and the fact that fibrillation is sometimes not heralded by these changes has led in recent years to the use of prophylactic antiarrhythmic therapy in some centers. Lidocaine is given as an initial bolus (75 to 100 mg), followed by a continuous intravenous infusion.[44]

Since a decrease in arterial PO_2 caused by ventilation perfusion inequalities is common, oxygen is administered to all patients. Most physicians also advocate giving routine low-dose subcutaneous heparin to reduce the possibility of thromboembolic complications.[45]

In patients who have persistent or recurrent pain despite therapy, efforts are made to balance the oxygen supply and demand and hence to diminish ischemia. For example, if sinus tachycardia persists and signs of left ventricular failure are absent, propranolol in doses of 0.05 to 0.10 mg/kg can be given to reduce heart rate. Although this treatment has been shown to eliminate pain and reduce ST segment elevation, the hemodynamic response needs to be monitored closely.[46] Other patients with persistent or recurrent pain have elevated arterial blood pressure. Reducing blood pressure with propranolol or nitroprusside has a favorable effect in these patients. Finally, in patients with left ventricular failure and elevated pulmonary artery and wedge pressures, vasodilators such as nitroprusside or IV nitroglycerin will "unload" the ventricle and often reduce pain and ST segment elevation.

Intravenous nitroglycerin has been demonstrated to be efficacious in limiting complications (pump failure, chest pain) of an acute myocardial infarction. Nitroglycerin is an excellent coronary vasodilator, whereas sodium nitroprusside may have deleterious effects on the ischemic heart. Nitroprusside dilates the intramyocardial resistance arteries supplying the normal myocardium. Since resistance vessels supplying the ischemic areas are already presumably maximally dilated, dilating other resistance vessels further would shunt blood from the ischemic areas to normal areas, resulting in a "coronary steal" phenomenon. Consequently, intravenous nitroglycerin is the preferred drug.[47,48]

Myocardial infarction is a dynamic process in which the ultimate fate of ischemic but still viable heart muscle is not determined until several hours or perhaps days after the onset of symptoms. Acute and late complications of infarction are determined at least in part by the ultimate size of the infarction. These considerations and the recognition that the balance between oxygen supply and demand can be influenced have led to considerable efforts to protect

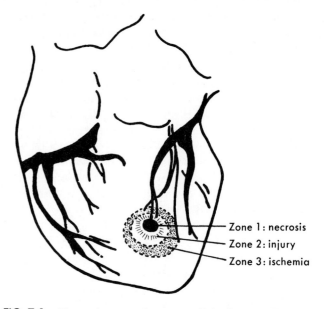

FIG. 7-1. Tissue damage after myocardial infarction. *Zone 1,* Necrotic tissue; *zone 2,* injured tissue; *zone 3,* ischemic tissue.

ischemic muscle and to reduce infarct size (Fig. 7-1). These efforts have been hampered by the lack of a reliable and quantifiable index of the volume of ischemic muscle in patients. Despite this problem, favorable clinical results, directionally appropriate changes in indices of muscle death, and even a reduction in anticipated mortality have been reported with therapy directed at reducing infarct size. Most of the early interest in this area focused on the use of hyaluronidase or solutions containing glucose-insulin-potassium, propranolol, or vasodilators.[49-52] The first reports of restoring coronary artery perfusion with intracoronary streptokinase in the setting of acute infarction appeared in the early 1980s. Several trials have now been reported.[53] Efficacy in terms of patency was evident in 70% to 90% of patients. Improvement of ventricular function and presumed reduction of infarct size was evident in those in whom patency could be reestablished in less than 4 hours. Effects on survival were not statistically impressive, and early reocclusion was common.

The National Heart, Lung and Blood Institute established the Thrombolysis in Myocardial Infarction trial, which involved the use of intravenous rather than intracoronary thrombolytic agents, including tissue-type plasminogen activator (TPA). Open coronary arteries were observed in 66% of TPA-treated patients and 30% of streptokinase-treated patients after infusion.[53] Based upon these observations, the current approach to infarct reduction involves early intravenous thrombolytic therapy, followed in most cases by angioplasty. Effects of this aggressive approach on long-term coronary artery patency, ventricular function, and survival are being evaluated. (See Chapter 15 for details of thrombolytic therapy and angioplasty in acute infarction.)

A pericardial rub is heard in about 25% of patients with transmural infarction, usually on the third to fifth day. Within 1 to 4 weeks after infarction, pericarditis with effusion and fever develops in about 2% to 5% of patients. This is Dressler's syndrome, which is thought to result from an autoimmune response. Pericarditis, early or late, is generally treated symptomatically. Use of aspirin, indomethacin, or even steroids may be required; anticoagulation should be discontinued unless there is an overriding reason to continue its use, such as an overt pulmonary embolus. Pulsus paradoxus is evaluated to detect early signs of potential cardiac tamponade.

Prolongation of the PR interval and Wenckebach cycles are common after posterior and inferior infarctions. They usually regress or can be treated with atropine. Third degree AV block and conditions associated with a high incidence of progression to complete block, for example, Mobitz type II second degree block or new bifascicular bundle branch block, especially associated with PR prolongation, are regarded as indications for insertion of a temporary transvenous pacemaker. Use of the pacemaker is then determined primarily by the ventricular rate and the patient's hemodynamic response. (See Chapter 11.)

Heart Failure

Heart failure may be defined as a state in which the cardiac output is insufficient to meet the metabolic needs of the body. It can occur when the cardiac output is normal, increased, or decreased. In most cases, patients with heart failure have a decreased cardiac output. Congestive failure is manifested by retention of fluid and the formation of edema.[54] Low output failure occurs when the heart is unable to supply the tissues with adequate perfusion. The basis for the inadequate perfusion lies in the inability of the failing heart to meet the metabolic demands of tissues, even if they are normal. A number of cardiac disorders can result in low output failure. For example, myocardial infarction affecting a large area of the left ventricle or stenosis or insufficiency of the cardiac valves can impair the heart's ability to pump. Constrictive pericarditis or pericardial effusion can restrict the ability of the heart to fill and empty.

Less commonly, heart failure occurs when peripheral demands exceed even the capacity of a normal heart to adequately perfuse the tissues. This is called *high output failure* and can occur in severe anemia, sepsis, thyrotoxicosis, and in patients who have arteriovenous fistulas.

The usual defect in heart failure is a decrease in the pumping capacity of the heart. Patients with early or mild heart disease may show no significant abnormalities at rest because of reserve in cardiac function. Despite a normal cardiac output at rest, cardiac output with exercise will be subnormal, the patient demonstrating decreased exercise tolerance.

As the heart begins to fail, a large number of compensatory mechanisms are set in motion in an effort to maintain cardiac output at a level that is adequate to meet the metabolic needs of the body. Most of these adaptations employ mechanisms that are the same as those used by normal persons during exercise or during periods of increased stress. The principal initial adjustments are a reflex increase in sympathetic nerve discharge and a decrease in parasympathetic activity. These autonomic alterations, affecting the heart, arteries and veins, result in maintenance of arterial pressure despite a decrease in stroke volume. Venous tone increases, which in turn increases venous pressure and helps maintain venous return. The resulting increase in end-diastolic volume helps to maintain stroke volume.

An increase in heart rate (tachycardia) by itself may increase cardiac output when mechanisms to improve stroke volume are exhausted. Above a certain rate, however, cardiac output may actually begin to decrease. This rate is about 170 to 180 beats/minute for most normal young individuals. In trained athletes the rate may be 200 to 220, whereas in patients with myocardial disease the rate limit may be 120 to 140. A decrease in cardiac output above a certain heart rate is caused by a shortening of diastole, which limits the time for adequate filling of the ventricles and for coronary blood flow. Slow heart rates allow more complete diastolic filling.

When cardiac output falls for whatever reason, the kidney retains salt and water as an early compensatory mechanism. This is caused in part by sympathetic stimulation, which produces renal vasoconstriction and a reduction in renal blood flow. Sympathetically mediated activation of the renin-angiotensin system triggers aldosterone release and further promotes sodium retention. Expansion of the intravascular blood volume results in increases in the end-diastolic volume and pressure and ultimately in transudation of fluid from the vascular bed and edema formation (Table 7-2) by raising systemic venous and capillary pressures.

A major long-term hemodynamic adjustment to heart failure is ventricular hypertrophy. This is presumably caused by a chronic increase in the systolic force or tension developed by the myocardial fibers. Although the contractility of hypertrophied myocardium is lower than normal for each unit of muscle and is associated with an imbalance between energy production and energy usage, the hypertrophied myocardium may maintain compensation because the total mass of myocardium is increased. If the pumping capacity of the ventricle is restored by hypertrophy, tachycardia and edema may no longer be present.

TABLE 7-2. Edema formation

Organ	Edema	Description
Skin	Dependent edema, pitting type	Increased venous pressure forces fluid through capillary walls into subcutaneous tissues; in ambulatory patients edema localized in dependent parts of body (hands and feet); patients in bed may lose edema of legs and feet, have it only in presacral region
Liver	Hepatomegaly	Increased pressure in hepatic veins causes accumulation of fluid in liver, which becomes enlarged and tender
Pleural cavity	Pleural effusion; hydrothorax	Venous congestion forces fluid into pleural cavity
Pericardial cavity	Pericardial effusion	Fluid accumulation in pericardial cavity

Left Ventricular Failure

The heart is really comprised of two pumps in series, the right ventricle and the left ventricle. Certain events may alter the function of one of these pumps without significant initial impairment to the other. In acute myocardial infarction, for example, the primary insult is usually to the performance of the left ventricle. When the ability of the left ventricle to pump blood is compromised without compromise to the right ventricle, a temporary imbalance in the output of the two sides of the heart results. The right side of the heart continues to pump blood into the lungs. At the same time, the left side of the heart is unable to move the blood adequately into the systemic circulation. This results in accumulation of blood in the lungs and increases the pressure in all the pulmonary vessels. Consequently, one of the cardinal symptoms associated with acute left ventricular failure is dyspnea. If dyspnea occurs when the patient is recumbent, it is called orthopnea and is usually relieved by sitting up. Dyspnea is the symptomatic manifestation of increased work of breathing consequent to pulmonary venous engorgement and an expanded pulmonary blood volume.

Paroxysmal nocturnal dyspnea, which represents a form of acute pulmonary edema, is almost a specific sign of left ventricular failure. The patient awakens suddenly at night, extremely breathless, and seeks relief by sitting up or running to an open window for fresh air. When the patient goes to sleep, the metabolic needs of the body may decrease. As a result, the cardiac output that had previously been inadequate may now be adequate to supply the body needs. Fluid that had been pocketed away is mobilized into the vascular system, thus increasing the blood volume. The expanded blood volume and a redistribution of this volume to the lungs resulting from the recumbent position are major factors in precipitating nocturnal dyspnea.

As the heart's compensatory mechanisms fail, the already-elevated diastolic filling pressure continues to increase, but stroke volume does not, so that left atrial pressure necessarily increases. To maintain flow, the pressure in the pulmonary veins and capillaries exceeds the intravascular osmotic pressure (approximately 30 mm Hg), and fluid rapidly leaks into the interstitial regions of the lung tissue. Pulmonary edema greatly reduces the amount of lung tissue available for the exchange of gases and consequently results in a dramatic clinical presentation characterized by extreme dyspnea, cyanosis, and severe anxiety. This is called acute pulmonary edema.

In the early stages of pulmonary edema, the patient appears anxious, restless, or vaguely uneasy. Wheezing, orthopnea, diaphoresis, and pallor appear as left ventricle failure progresses. A third heart sound may be heard as the distensibility of the ventricle decreases. Sinus tachycardia and increased systemic arterial pressure are common as neural reflexes attempt to correct the imbalance. If these physiologic compensations fail, hypotension occurs, rales develop from alveolar edema, and copious blood-tinged, frothy sputum is expectorated. As the accumulation of pulmonary interstitial and intra-alveolar fluid progresses, arterial hypoxemia and cyanosis occur in varying degrees. Arterial blood gases document the presence of hypoxia with a drop in the PO_2. The chest x-ray typically shows mottling from the hilar regions, which may cover both lung fields. With the elevation of the pulmonary venous pressure diffuse interstitial edema results and is seen as cloudy lung fields. In severe pulmonary edema Kerley-B lines appear and possibly a total "white out" of the lung fields. This deterioration in pulmonary function is reflected in the patient's mental status. Anxiety progresses to mental confusion and eventually to stupor and coma. The patient is literally drowning in his own secretions.

Right Ventricular Failure

Usually right ventricular failure follows left ventricular failure. Right heart failure without left heart failure may be caused by pulmonary hypertension secondary to lung disease or recurrent pulmonary emboli and is referred to as *cor pulmonale*. In either case, pulmonary hypertension presents an increased resistance to right ventricular ejection and a resulting increase of right ventricular end-diastolic and right atrial pressures. This impedes venous return.

Clinical manifestations include: (1) distention of the neck veins, which appear full even when the head is raised (normally these empty when the head is elevated to a 45-degree angle), (2) a distended and often tender liver, and (3) peripheral edema (Table 7-2). When the accumulation of fluid becomes extensive and generalized, the patient is said to have anasarca. Other consequences of congestive heart failure include pleural effusions, ascites jaundice due to hepatic engorgement, and ultimately cardiac cachexia.

Treatment of Heart Failure. Treatment of patients with heart failure requires an understanding of the condition(s) that lead to this clinical state and of the mechanisms that produce congestion regardless of the primary cardiac problem.

When heart failure results from certain specific mechanical problems such as aortic or mitral valve stenosis or insufficiency, persistent uncontrolled arrhythmias, severe anemia, hypertension, or a congenital cardiac lesion, therapy is directed at correcting the cause. It is important to recognize that regardless of cause of heart disease, infections, arrhythmias, anemia, thyrotoxicosis, and pregnancy may each place a sufficient added burden on the heart to precipitate heart failure. Thus, appropriate treatment of these conditions may convert a patient with heart disease from a decompensated to a compensated state.

Heart failure has previously been defined as a condition in which the cardiac output is not sufficient to meet the metabolic demands of the body. Essentially all of the situations that aggravate heart failure do so by increasing the metabolic demands on a heart that is not capable of responding with an adequate output. A favorable response in patients with heart failure often can be obtained by rest. Defining the level of physical activity that a patient can tolerate without precipitating failure is a major objective of subsequent follow-up and treatment.

In addition to prescribing rest and defining the level of physical activity a patient can tolerate, a second focus of therapy is improving cardiac performance and cardiac output. Obviously if tight aortic stenosis or another structural defect is present, surgery is indicated. On the other hand, digitalis, which increases the contractility of heart muscle, has a favorable effect on cardiac performance and output. In most instances of heart failure it is used routinely with beneficial results. In acute myocardial infarction with heart failure, the evidence of benefit from digitalis is minimal. Furthermore, because of a potentially increased sensitivity to toxic manifestations of digitalis excess, its use in this situation is still controversial.

In patients with a severely decompensated congestive heart, the renin-angiotensin system is activated, resulting in the maintenance of elevated systemic vascular resistance. Captopril inhibits this renin-angiotensin mechanism, reducing afterload and resulting in clinical improvement of congestive heart failure.[55,56] Vasodilator agents are an important addition to the treatment of heart failure. This class of agents includes nitrates, nitroprusside, hydralazine, minoxidil, and prazosin.[57-63] Some are designed for intravenous use and some for oral use. Some act predominantly on the arterial system, and others exert significant actions on veins as well. The principle behind the use of these agents is to reduce arterial resistance, which is accompanied by an increase in cardiac output, a decrease in left atrial and pulmonary venous pressure, and a decrease in left ventricular end-diastolic volume and pressure. These agents have proven very useful in the treatment of acute heart failure in myocardial infarction, in heart failure associated with severe mitral insufficiency, and in chronic heart failure caused by myocardial disease. The benefits of vasodilator therapy are greatest when left atrial and pulmonary pressures are elevated. Vasodilators lack utility and may even be detrimental in patients with a normal or reduced left ventricular filling pressure.

Two additional agents used in the treatment of congestive heart failure are melrinone and amrinone. These are nonadrenergic, nonglycoside agents with combined positive inotropic and vasodilating properties. Intravenous amrinone causes an increase in cardiac output and a decrease in the pulmonary capillary wedge pressure, right atrial pressure, and systemic vascular resistance. Subsequently, the myocardial oxygen consumption rate is also decreased. No major change in the blood pressure or heart rate is observed. Amrinone has been comparable to dobutamine and dopamine as inotropic therapy in heart failure.[64-66] Melrinone has shown similar results in the treatment of congestive heart failure.[67]

The third focus in the treatment of patients with heart failure is achieving and maintaining an appropriate blood volume. As noted before, several compensatory mechanisms invoked when cardiac output is insufficient affect sodium and water balance by the kidney. The net effect of these influences is sodium (and water) retention and a diminished ability to excrete a sodium load. A normal sodium intake of 5 g to 8 g/day cannot be tolerated by most patients with heart failure and should be reduced to 2 g/day or even less. Diuretics promote the excretion of sodium and hence water by the kidneys through one or more of several specific actions. Thiazide diuretics inhibit sodium transport primarily in the distal or cortical segment of the nephron. Loop diuretics such as ethacrynic acid and furosemide are very potent and act on both the cortical and medullary segments of the nephron. Spironolactone is a diuretic that specifically antagonizes the effect of aldosterone on the collecting duct. Triamterene has an action on sodium transport identical to spironolactone, but its action is not dependent on blocking aldosterone. In general thiazides and loop diuretics also cause potassium loss, whereas spironolactone and triamterene do not. These agents vary in potency but with appropriate selection and dosage can promote a diuresis in patients with edema due to heart failure and with chronic use can diminish the tendency of patients with heart failure to retain salt and water.

Mild to moderate heart failure in patients with acute infarction is usually managed successfully with bed rest, morphine, careful attention to fluid balance with optimization of pulmonary artery wedge pressure, and the use of vasodilators and diuretics when indicated.

Cardiogenic Shock

When oxygen and other nutrients become unavailable to the cells of the body, shock may occur. Shock is a descriptive term denoting a clinical picture that develops in the presence of inadequate tissue perfusion. It occurs in about 15% of patients hospitalized with acute myocardial infarction. The clinical picture is characterized by (1) a systolic blood pressure of less than 90 mm Hg or at least 30 mm Hg lower than the prior basal level and (2) signs of impaired tissue perfusion such as pallor, cyanosis of varying degrees, cool clammy skin, mental confusion or obtundation, and a urine output of less than 20 ml/hr. Shock may be caused by a variety of conditions unrelated to myocardial infarction. Before treating shock, it is essential that its cause be determined.

For the purposes of this discussion, cardiogenic shock is present when the above clinical characteristics are seen in a patient with acute myocardial infarction. Patients with hypotension related to pain or with vasovagal reactions responsive to atropine are specifically excluded from the group defined as having cardiogenic shock. Although cardiac arrhythmias such as excessive tachycardia or bradycardia can cause the picture of shock, the following remarks are intended to describe abnormalities noted in patients in whom these rhythm disturbances either are not present or have been corrected and the picture of shock persists.

Hemodynamic Assessment. Most coronary care units have developed means of measuring hemodynamic status by the bedside without increasing risk or discomfort for the patient. With the aid of fluoroscopy or a pressure recorder or both, a balloon-tipped, flow-directed catheter is inserted into the subclavian or brachial vein and directed into the right ventricle and pulmonary artery (Fig. 7-2, *A* and *B*). This catheter provides a guide for more precise management of heart failure and especially cardiogenic shock by furnishing a means to measure the pulmonary artery end-diastolic pressure (PAEDP) and pulmonary capillary wedge pressure (PCWP). Since there is a direct relationship between the PAEDP, the PCWP and the pressure in the left ventricle immediately before systole (LVEDP), an elevated PAEDP or PCWP reflects the elevated LVEDP that occurs when left ventricular contractility is impaired sufficiently to prevent normal emptying.

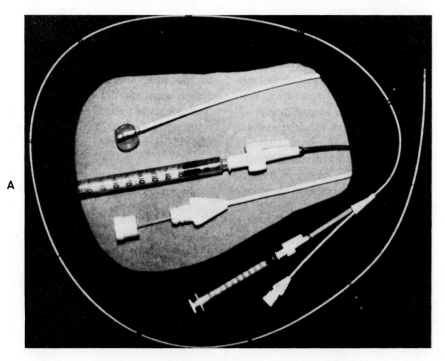

A

FIG. 7-2.   A, The Swan-Ganz flow-directed catheter.

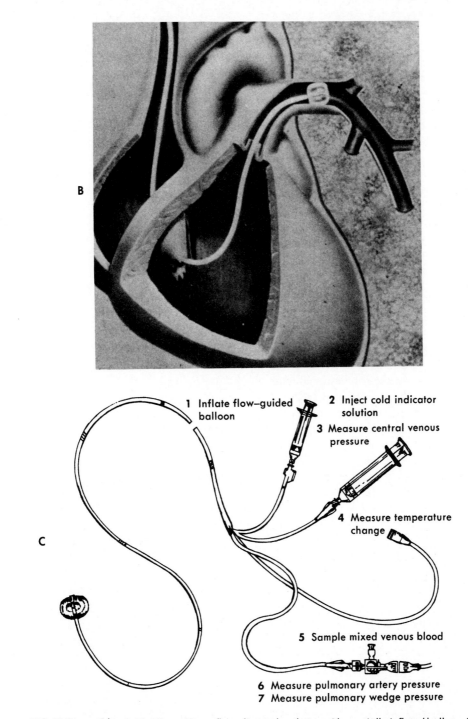

1 Inflate flow–guided balloon

2 Inject cold indicator solution

3 Measure central venous pressure

4 Measure temperature change

5 Sample mixed venous blood

6 Measure pulmonary artery pressure
7 Measure pulmonary wedge pressure

FIG. 7-2, cont'd.   B, The Swan-Ganz flow-directed catheter with *partially inflated* balloon is passed through the superior vena cava and into the right atrium, where the balloon is then inflated to its maximum recommended capacity. Continued catheter advancement propels the balloon-tipped catheter into the right ventricle, pulmonary artery, and finally into the wedged position that is evidenced by a characteristic change in pressure waveform. C, The Swan-Ganz flow-directed thermodilution catheter (A and C with permission of Edwards Laboratories, Division of American Hospital Supply Corp., Santa Ana, Calif.)

A PAEDP or PCWP measurement of greater than 12 mm Hg is considered abnormal. The balloon-tipped catheter may also aid in establishing the cause of heart failure or shock, as well as in evaluating the effectiveness of the therapy. For example, in a state of hypotension caused by hypovolemia, infusing normal saline, whole blood, or low weight molecular dextran elevates the systemic pressure. In this case the PAEDP and PCWP, initially low, will return to normal when the blood volume has been restored. If the PAEDP is elevated because of heart failure, effective therapy should lower the pressure readings that were initially elevated.[68,69]

The use of the central venous pressure (CVP) to measure right atrial pressure (RAP) is no longer considered sufficiently accurate because the relationship between the RAP and LVEDP is inconsistent. Therefore PAEDP and PCWP, rather than CVP, should be used as major guides in the treatment of heart failure and shock.

As the clinical features of heart failure worsen, they are usually accompanied by an elevation of the PAEDP and PCWP, a drop in cardiac output, a drop in arterial and right atrial oxygen saturations, and a widening of the oxygen difference between arterial and venous blood samples, commonly referred to as the A-V oxygen difference. The drop in arterial oxygen tension is a sign of abnormal lung function and is thought to result, at least in part, from elevation of left atrial pressure. Changes in pulmonary function include (1) abnormalities of diffusion, particularly of oxygen, (2) a redistribution of pulmonary blood flow into the less well-ventilated upper lobes, and (3) intrapulmonary shunting. Not only is the arterial oxygen tension reduced in patients with acute infarction and shock, but it also fails to increase to expected values with the administration of oxygen, until pulmonary congestion has cleared.[70]

When right atrial oxygen saturation is reduced, a widened A-V oxygen difference and a low cardiac output can be suspected. If arterial oxygen saturation remains at normal levels, reduced right atrial oxygen saturation reflects increased extraction of oxygen during the passage of blood from the arterial to the venous circulation. A widened A-V oxygen difference reflects this increased extraction and indicates a reduced cardiac output. Right atrial or pulmonary artery oxygen saturation can be useful indices of circulatory failure in patients with acute infarction. In addition to the bedside techniques for measuring pulmonary artery and pulmonary capillary wedge pressure, the simple test of determining whether the right atrial or pulmonary artery oxygen saturation is above or below 65% is a useful guide to therapy. The use of this variable is based on the Fick equation for measuring cardiac output.

$$\text{Cardiac output} = \frac{\text{Oxygen consumption}}{\text{A-V oxygen difference}}$$

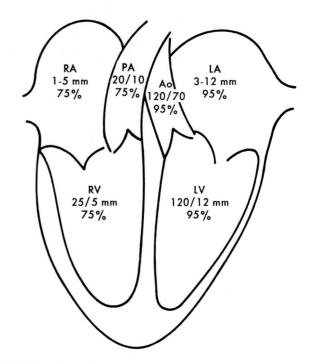

FIG. 7-3. Normal average cardiac pressures (mm Hg) and normal oxygen content (%) in each chamber.

A specially designed pulmonary artery catheter with a thermistor (temperature) electrode has been used to measure cardiac output using the principle of thermodilution. The procedure involves the injection of cold or room temperature solution into the right atrium or superior vena cava.[71,72] The temperature change is perceived by the thermistor electrode in the pulmonary artery. Cardiac output is inversely proportional to the temperature change, that is, the greater the cardiac output the less the temperature change. The use of such a catheter facilitates measurement of the cardiac output and eliminates the need for a systemic arterial blood sample to determine cardiac output (Fig. 7-2, *C*). Normal cardiac chamber oxygen values are found in Fig. 7-3.

Treatment of Shock. The current term to describe the problem of patients in cardiogenic shock with or without congestive heart failure is *pump failure*. Most studies indicate a mortality rate of at least 80% in cardiogenic shock during the course of acute myocardial infarction; unfortunately, current therapeutic measures have not affected these figures.

Although the primary therapeutic goals are to increase cardiac contractility and to maintain renal blood flow, there is no clear-cut regimen for the treatment of cardiogenic shock that can be applied to all patients since therapy depends on the specific findings in the individual patient. Therefore for the physician to direct treatment intelligently, as much clinical and hemodynamic information as possible should be available.

Therapy, as well as the natural evolution of the shock state, may change these values; therefore measurements should be repeated as often as necessary. Clinical management of the patient in cardiogenic shock is divided into general and specific measures as follows:

A. General therapeutic measures
1. Have patient assume a supine position with a pillow. Trendelenburg position is not recommended for treating cardiogenic shock.
2. Relieve pain with intravenous morphine doses (5 to 10 mg initially) just sufficient to be effective. Large doses of morphine sulfate should be avoided if possible. Observe for lowering of arterial pressure.
3. Insert a Foley catheter to measure hourly urine output as an index of kidney function. Maintain urine output at a minimum of 20 ml/hour to prevent renal failure.
4. Insert an intra-arterial needle or catheter to monitor arterial blood pressure, blood gases, pH, cardiac output, A-V oxygen difference, and peripheral resistance.
5. Insert a balloon-tipped, flow-directed catheter to monitor PAEDP and PCWP as a reflection of left ventricular performance.

B. Specific therapeutic goals
1. Correct arrhythmias and establish appropriate heart rate. If the heart rate is above normal but not in the abnormal tachycardia range, no special therapy is necessary. If the rate is abnormally slow, the use of atropine in patients with myocardial infarction may be considered. For the symptomatic (ventricular ectopic systoles, hypotension, and so forth) patient with sinus bradycardia, atropine is clearly indicated. Also Isuprel in a continuous infusion may be indicated to increase heart rate. However, Isuprel may increase myocardial oxygen consumption. For the asymptomatic patient with sinus bradycardia, it would appear best not to administer atropine, but to monitor closely. When atropine is indicated, initial doses should be in the range of 0.4 to 0.6 mg IV, repeating with 0.2 to 0.4 mg if the initial dose does not produce the desired effect. If atropine does not raise the heart rate sufficiently to eliminate the symptoms accompanying the slower rate or if the cause of the low heart rate is complete heart block, then AV sequential pacing should be considered.
2. Correct hypovolemia. Elderly patients with myocardial infarction are prime candidates for relative hypovolemia, especially if they have been receiving diuretics or are on a low sodium diet. The acute stages of acute myocardial infarction are associated with a reduced fluid intake due to pain, resulting from analgesic therapy, nausea, and vomiting. Further routes of fluid loss are profuse sweating, diarrhea secondary to medication, vigorous treatment with diuretics, and phlebotomy. Consequently, patients showing evidence of low cardiac output with hypotension and oliguria may be given a trial of fluid loading particularly if PAEDP and PCWP are low. Patients with evidence of severe pulmonary congestion are not suitable for this therapy. With low PAEDP and PCWP values, normal saline, blood products, or low molecular dextran may be infused until the PCWP reaches 15 to 18 mm Hg. Current experience indicates that PCWP should be kept slightly elevated in patients with cardiogenic shock.
3. Correct hypoxemia. Hypoxia with P_{O_2} values below the level of 70 to 75 mm Hg while the patient is receiving nasal oxygen indicates that the patient should probably be intubated and given positive pressure or volume assistance and 100% oxygen.
4. Correct acidosis. When circulatory impairment exists, the metabolic activity of the perfused cells of the body changes, and lactic acid and other metabolic products are released into the vascular system and ineffectively metabolized as a result of which systemic acidosis develops. This state contributes to poor tissue perfusion and is indicated by the blood pH. The complication is treated with intravenous sodium bicarbonate, taking precautions not to produce sodium overload.
5. Improve cardiac contractility. Use of digitalis in the management of cardiogenic shock is not well supported by existing data. Recent experimental studies show that the positive inotropic effect of digitalis preparations improves contractility but significantly increases myocardial oxygen demand.[73,74] Other agents that enhance the state of cardiac contractility have been employed in cardiogenic shock. In patients with adequate filling pressures and normal or increased peripheral resistance, dopamine hydrochloride, dobutamine, or amrinone can cause a significant increase in cardiac output. Dopamine has a strong inotropic effect causing renal vasodilatation. Dobutamine has less effect on the blood pressure and cardiac output than dopamine.[75-77] Amrinone has no effect on blood pressure or heart rate but will decrease PCWP, systemic resistance, and MVO2.
6. Improve circulation. Clinical estimates of the degree of increased peripheral resistance usually pres-

ent in the shock syndrome can be made from the degree of increased venous pressure, the amount of decrease in pulse pressure, the decrease in cutaneous blood flow with cold and cyanotic extremities, the poorly palpable peripheral pulses in spite of bounding pulsations, urine flow, and the clinical appearance of the patient. If these findings persist, a dangerously inappropriate prolonged period of peripheral vasoconstriction may exist. If the patient exhibits signs of the shock syndrome with a low or normal calculated peripheral resistance, an infusion of a drug with combined alpha and beta adrenergic properties may be considered. Norepinephrine (Levarterenol, Levophed) is used to increase arterial blood pressures and improve perfusion of ischemic areas of myocardium that are functionally depressed. The elevated pressure may open existing or latent coronary collateral channels, which require a relatively high pressure to maintain blood flow through them, bypassing concomitant areas of arterial atherosclerosis. Consequently this drug improves myocardial function and increases cardiac output. However, at the same time, it increases cardiac afterload (resistance against which the ventricle pumps) and thus myocardial oxygen consumption. Therefore the use of this agent should be aimed at producing the desired balance between coronary perfusion and afterload.

Several groups of investigators are evaluating agents that produce vasodilatation and decrease peripheral resistance, thereby increasing cardiac output, for use in patients who exhibit clinical signs of shock with an increased peripheral resistance. Such agents include nitroprusside and intravenous nitroglycerin. Current studies of these drugs show promise in patients with an increased pulmonary capillary wedge pressure and signs of left ventricular failure. They should not be used if arterial pressure is below 90 mm Hg unless they are used in conjunction with dopamine to maintain an adequate blood pressure.

A technique currently receiving growing recognition in the management of cardiogenic shock is mechanical circulatory assistance in the form of intra-aortic balloon counterpulsation. The balloon is inserted percutaneously into the femoral artery and connected to a console that controls the inflation of the balloon with helium. Timing and inflation and deflation of the balloon are correlated with the ECG. The intra-aortic balloon is deflated during ventricular systole and thus partially empties the aorta. The effect is to potentiate forward stroke volume but to reduce developed ventricular pressure and hence enhance myocardial oxygen consumption. In diastole the balloon is inflated, restoring arterial pressure and coronary perfusion. In patients counterpulsation improves cardiac output, reduces

evidence of myocardial ischemia, and frequently relieves pain and reduces ST-segment elevation. Patients with shock usually demonstrate a favorable hemodynamic and systemic metabolic response to balloon pumping. A minority of patients can be weaned off the pump. Most revert to the picture of shock when pumping is stopped. Thus balloon pumping per se has a minimal effect on mortality associated with shock, despite its temporary utility. However, several groups have reported that when patients in shock are pumped and then in 12 to 24 hours are taken to a catheterization laboratory and studied to define surgical candidates, significant numbers can be saved.[78,79,80] In one report 35 patients were pumped and studied by catheterization. Of these, 28 were felt to be surgical candidates (80%) and of these 21 were discharged alive after surgery (55%). Others have reported survival ranging from 40% to 50% with balloon pumping and surgery in shock patients. This should be compared with a mortality of 80% to 90% in comparable patients treated only medically. Thus balloon pumping as a support device while diagnostic and subsequent surgical therapy are contemplated has a much more favorable outcome than pumping alone. Based on these data, counterpulsation probably is indicated for the treatment of shock at institutions where an experienced pump team, catheterization laboratory, and coronary surgery program are established.

Other indications for intra-aortic balloon counterpulsation include severe congestive heart failure, medically refractory ischemia, ventricular septal defects, and left main coronary stenosis. In most instances, the intra-aortic balloon pump provides additional protection for the myocardium until surgery can be done.

Hagemeijer and associates studied the effectiveness of intra-aortic balloon pumping in patients with severe congestive heart failure associated with a recent MI and without subsequent surgery. Of 25 patients, 20 were successfully weaned from the pump; 13 of these patients lived for more than 1 year; 12 patients improved their functional class and returned to work.[81]

Intra-aortic balloon counterpulsation is not without risk. The most common serious complication associated with it is limb ischemia, which occurs in approximately 14% of patients. Other less common complications include dissection of the aorta, septicemia, localized groin sepsis, and thrombocytopenia. The least serious common complication is catheter injury of the atherosclerotic aortic wall, which requires subsequent thrombectomies.[82-84]

REFERENCES

1. Harrison, T.R., and Reeves, T.J.: Principles and problems of ischemic heart disease, Chicago, 1968, Year Book Medical Publishers, Inc.
2. Matsui, K., and others: Ventricular septal rupture secondary to myo-

cardial infarction: clinical approach and surgical results, JAMA **245**:1537, 1981.

3. Recusani, E., and others: Ventricular septal rupture after myocardial infarction: diagnosis by two dimensional and pulsed Doppler echocardiography, Am. J. Cardiol. **54**:277, 1984.

4. Prinzmetal, M., and others: Angina pectoris. I. A variant form of angina pectoris: a preliminary report, Am. J. Med. **27**:35, 1959.

5. Schroeder, J.S., and others: Provocation of coronary spasm with ergonovine maleate: new test results with 57 patients undergoing coronary arteriography, Am. J. Cardiol. **40**:487, 1977.

6. Schroeder, J.S., and others: Medical therapy of Prinzmetal's variant angina, Chest **78**(suppl.):231, 1980.

7. Schroeder, J.S., and others: Multiclinic controlled trial of diltiazem for Prinzmetal's angina, Am. J. Med. **72**:227, 1982.

8. Antman, E., and others: Nifedipine therapy for coronary artery spasm, N. Engl. J. Med. **302**:1269, 1980.

9. Bertrand, M.E., and others: Treatment of Prinzmetal's variant angina: role of medical treatment with nifedipine and coronary revascularization combined with plexectomy, Am. J. Cardiol. **47**:174, 1981.

10. Reichek, N., and others: Antianginal effects of nitroglycerin patches, Am. J. Cardiol. **54**:1, 1984.

11. Stone, P.H., and others: Calcium channel blocking agents in the treatment of cardiovascular disorders. Part 2, Hemodynamic effects and clinical applications, Ann. Intern. Med. **93**:886, 1980.

12. Check, W.: Calcium antagonists: long awaited new therapy for heart disease, JAMA **245**:807, 1981.

13. Galle, J.: Clinical use of calcium channel blockers, Conn. Med. **47**:605, 1983.

14. Mukharji, J., and others: Early positive exercise test and extensive coronary disease: effect of antianginal therapy, Am. J. Cardiol. **55**:267, 1985.

15. Ho, S.W.C., and others: Effect of beta adrenergic blockade in results of exercise testing related to extent of coronary artery disease, Am. J. Cardiol. **55**:258, 1985.

16. Hoekenga, D., and Abrams, J.: Rational medical therapy for stable angina pectoris, Am. J. Med. **76**:309, 1984.

17. Flaherty, J.: Unstable angina: rational approach to management, Am. J. Med. **76**:52, 1984.

18. Romhilt, D.W., and Fowler, N.O.: Physical signs in acute myocardial infarction, Heart Lung **2**:74, 1973.

19. Harvey, W.P.: Some pertinent physical findings in the clinical evaluation of acute myocardial infarction, Circulation **39**(suppl. 4):175, 1969.

20. Pitt, B.: Clinical application of myocardial imaging with radioisotopes in the evaluation and management of patients with coronary artery disease, Adv. Cardiol. **26**:30, 1980.

21. Wackers, F.J.T.: Current status of radionuclide imaging in the management and evaluation of patients with cardiovascular disease, Adv. Cardiol. **27**:40, 1980.

22. Wackers, F.J.T.: Radionuclide evaluation of patients in the CCU, Adv. Cardiol. **27**:105, 1980.

23. Willerson, J.T., and others: Radionuclide imaging in acute myocardial infarction, Cardiovasc. Med. **3**:69, 1978.

24. Held, A.C.: Dipyridamole-thallium imaging, Arch. Intern. Med. **145**:1927, 1985.

25. Riesman, S.: Dipyridamole thallium testing: an alternative form of stress testing in patients unable to exercise, Chest **88**:321, 1985.

26. Leppo, J.A., and others: Dipyridamole-thallium-201 scintigraphy in the prediction of future cardiac events after acute myocardial infarction, N. Engl. J. Med. **310**:1014, 1984.

27. Leppo, J.A., and others: Serial thallium 201 myocardial imaging after dipyridamole infusion: diagnostic utility in detecting coronary stenoses and relationship to regional wall motion, Circulation **66**:649, 1982.

28. Tennant, R., and Wiggers, C.J.: The effect of coronary occlusion on myocardial contraction, Am. J. Physiol. **112**:351, 1935.

29. Lieberman, A.N., and others: Two dimensional echocardiography and infarct size: relationship of regional wall motion and thickening to the extent of myocardial infarction in the dog, Circulation **63**:739, 1981.

30. Kisslo, J., and others: Serial wall changes after acute myocardial infarction by two dimensional echo, Circulation **60**(suppl. 11):151, 1979.

31. Pandian, N., and Kerber, R.: Two dimensional echocardiographic assessment of wall thinning and its relation to perfusion during graded coronary stenosis, Am. J. Cardiol. **47**:1384, 1981.

32. Feinlieb, M.: The magnitude and nature of the decrease in coronary heart disease mortality rate, Am. J. Cardiol. **54**:2C, 1984.

33. Gillum, R.F., Folsom, A.R., and Blackburn, H.: Decline in coronary heart disease mortality: old questions and new facts, Am. J. Med. **76**:1055, 1984.

34. Lerey, R.: Causes of the decrease in cardiovascular mortality, Am. J. Cardiol. **54**:7C, 1984.

35. Waugh, R.A.: Immediate and remote prognostic implications of fascicular block during acute myocardial infarction, Circulation **47**:765, 1973.

36. Crimm, A., and others: Prognostic significance of isolated sinus tachycardia during first 3 days of acute myocardial infarction, Am. J. Med. **76**:983, 1984.

37. McNeer, J.F., and others: Hospital discharge the week after acute myocardial infarction, N. Engl. J. Med. **298**:229, 1978.

38. DeBusk, R.F., and others: Medically directed at-home rehabilitation soon after clinically uncomplicated acute myocardial infarction: a new model for patient care, Am. J. Cardiol. **55**:251, 1985.

39. Cannon, D.S., and others: The short and long term prognosis of patients with transmural and nontransmural infarction, Am. J. Med. **61**:452, 1976.

40. Haskell, N., and DeBusk, R.: Cardiovascular response to repeated treadmill exercise testing soon after myocardial infarction, Circulation **60**:1247, 1978.

41. Starling, M.R., and others: Exercise testing early after myocardial infarction: predictive value for subsequent unstable angina and death, Am. J. Cardiol. **46**:909, 1980.

42. Nishimura, R.A., and others: Prognostic value of predischarged 2-dimensional echocardiogram after acute myocardial infarction, Am. J. Cardiol. **53**:429, 1984.

43. Rackley, E., and others: Modern approach to myocardial infarction: determination of prognosis and therapy, Am. Heart J. **101**:75, 1981.

44. Resnekov, L.: Management of acute myocardial infarction, Cardiovasc. Med. **2**:949, 1977.

45. Ewy, G.A.: Anticoagulation in patients with acute myocardial infarction, Pract. Cardiol. **4**:25, 1978.

46. Mueller, H., and Ayers, S.: Propranolol in the treatment of acute myocardial infarction, Circulation **49**:1078, 1974.

47. Cohn, J.N., and others: Effect of short term infusion of sodium nitroprusside on mortality rate in acute myocardial infarction complicated by left ventricular failure, N. Engl. J. Med. **306**:1129, 1982.

48. Chiarello, M., and others: Comparison between the effects of nitroprusside and nitroglycerin on ischemic injury during acute myocardial infarction, Circulation **54**:766, 1976.

49. Braunwald, E., and Maroko, P.R.: The reduction of infarct size: an idea whose time (for testing) has come, Circulation **50**:206, 1974.

50. Maroko, P.R., and others: Infarct size reduction: a critical review, Adv. Cardiol. **27**:127, 1980.

51. Rogers, W.J., and others: Reduction of hospital mortality rate of

acute myocardial infarction with glucose-insulin-potassium infusion, Am. Heart J. **92:**441, 1976.

52. McEwan, M.P., and others: Effect of intravenous and intracoronary nitroglycerin in left ventricular wall motion and perfusion in patients with coronary artery disease, Am. J. Cardiol. **47:**201, 1981.

53. Passamani, E.: Thrombolytic therapy in patients with acute myocardial infarction. In Califf, R.M., and Wagner, G.S., editors: Acute coronary care, Boston, 1986, Martinus Nijhoff Publishing.

54. Hanlan, N.R., and others: Chronic congestive heart failure in coronary artery disease: clinical criteria, Ann. Intern. Med. **87:**133, 1977.

55. Dzau, V.J., and others: Relation of renin-angiotensin-aldosterone system to clinical state in congestive heart failure, Circulation **63:**645, 1981.

56. Dzau, V.J., and others: Sustained effectiveness of converting enzyme inhibition in patients with severe congestive heart failure, N. Engl. J. Med. **302**(25):1371, 1980.

57. Chatterjee, J., and Parmley, W.W.: The role of vasodilator therapy in heart failure, Prog. Cardiovasc. Dis. **19:**301, 1977.

58. Cohn, J.N.: Choice and rationale for vasodilators treatment of hypertension or relief of heart failure, Cardiovasc. Rev. Rep. **1:**686, 1980.

59. Mason, D.T., and others: Treatment of acute and chronic congestive heart failure by vasodilator-afterload reduction, Arch. Intern. Med. **140:**1577, 1980.

60. Massia, B., and others: Long term vasodilator therapy for heart failure: clinical responses and its relationship to hemodynamic measurements, Circulation **63:**269, 1981.

61. Parmley, W.: Pathophysiology of congestive heart failure, Am. J. Cardiol. **56:**7A, 1985.

62. Franciosa, J.A., and others: Hemodynamic improvement after oral hydralazine in left ventricular failure, Ann. Intern. Med. **86:**388, 1977.

63. Franciosa, J.A., and Cohn, J.N.: Effects of minoxidil on hemodynamics with congestive heart failure, Circulation **63:**652, 1980.

64. Mancini, D., LeJentel, T., and Sonnenblack, E.: Intravenous use of amrinone for the treatment of the failing heart, Am. J. Cardiol. **56:**8P, 1985.

65. Benotti, J., and others: Comparative inotropic therapy in heart failure, Circulation **68**(suppl. 3):128, 1983.

66. Taylor, S.H., and others: Intravenous amrinone in left ventricular failure complicated by acute myocardial infarction, Am. J. Cardiol. **56:**29B, 1985.

67. Simonton, C.A., and others: Melrinone in congestive heart failure: acute and chronic hemodynamic and clinical evaluation, J. Am. Coll. Cardiol. **6:**453, 1985.

68. The Pathfinder family of Swan-Ganz flow-directed right heart catheters, Santa Anna, Calif., 1973, Edwards Laboratories, Division of American Hospital Supply Corp.

69. Ratshin, R.A., and others: Hemodynamic elevation of left ventricular function in shock complicating myocardia infarction, Circulation **45:**127, 1972.

70. Rotman, M., and others: Pulmonary artery diastolic pressure in acute myocardial infarction, Am. J. Cardiol. **33:**357, 1974.

71. Larson, C.A., and Woods, S.L.: Effect of injectate volume and temperature on thermodilution cardiac output measurements in acutely ill adults (abstract), Circulation **66**(suppl. 2):98, 1982.

72. Vennex, C.V., Nelson, D.H., and Pierpont, D.L.: Thermodilution cardiac output in critically ill patients: comparison room-temperature and iced injectate, Heart Lung **13:**574, 1984.

73. Shubin, H., and Weil, M.H.: Practical considerations in the management of shock complicating acute myocardial infarction: a summary of current practice, Am. J. Cardiol. **26:**603, 1970.

74. Loeb, H.S., and Gunnau, R.M.: Treatment of pump failure in acute myocardial infarction, JAMA **245:**2093, 1981.

75. Holzer, J., and others: Effectiveness of dopamine in patients with cardiogenic shock, Am. J. Cardiol. **32:**79, 1973.

76. Loeb, H.S., and others: Acute hemodynamic effects of dopamine in patients with shock, Circulation **44:**163, 1971.

77. Keung, E.C.H., and others: Dubotamine therapy in myocardial infarction, JAMA **245:**13, 1971.

78. Lamberti, J.J., and others: Mechanical circulatory assistance for the treatment of complications of coronary artery disease, Surg. Clin. North Am. **56:**83, 1976.

79. Ehrich, D.A., and others: The hemodynamic response to intra-aortic balloon counterpulsation in patients with cardiogenic shock complicating acute myocardial infarction, Am. Heart J. **93:**274, 1977.

80. Mueller, H., and Ayers, S.: The effects of intra-aortic balloon counterpulsation on cardiac performance and metabolism in shock associated with acute myocardial infarction, J. Clin. Invest. **50:**1885, 1971.

81. Hagemeijer, F., and others: Effectiveness of intra-aortic balloon pumping without cardiac surgery for patients with severe heart failure secondary to a recent myocardial infarction, Am. J. Cardiol. **40:**951, 1977.

82. Berger, R.L., and others: Applications of intra-aortic balloon counterpulsation, Isr. J. Med. Sci. **11:**231, 1975.

83. Beckman, C.B., and others: Results and complications of intra-aortic balloon counterpulsation, Ann. Thorac. Surg. **24:**550, 1977.

84. McCabe, J.C., and others: Complications of intra-aortic balloon insertion and counterpulsation, Circulation **57:**769, 1978.

Douglas P. Zipes
Lori B. Maloy

NORMAL CARDIAC CYCLE

Before discussing electrocardiographic interpretation of cardiac arrhythmias, a review of the normal electrical events that occur during a cardiac cycle, as well as a discussion of basic electrophysiologic principles is necessary[1] (see also Chapters 1 and 6). During normal sinus rhythm the cardiac impulse originates in the sinus node and then travels to right and left atria. Sinus node discharge and conduction from the sinus node to the atria are not recorded from the body surface, and therefore these events are not present in the ECG. In response to the sinus node impulse, the atria depolarize and generate the P wave; atrial repolarization (Ta wave) is generally obscured by the QRS complex and is therefore not usually seen. Atrial conduction probably proceeds through both atria in a more or less radial fashion (like spreading ripples caused by a rock thrown into still water), eventually reaching the AV node and His bundle. Some data suggest that conduction through the atria travels preferentially through loosely connected bundles of atrial muscle called the anterior, middle, and posterior internodal pathways, which, it is argued, provide specialized pathways of conduction from the sinus node to the left atrium (via Bachmann's bundle, a division of the anterior internodal pathway) and to the AV node. However, the functional importance of these pathways in providing specialized tracts for conduction is unsettled. Most experts agree that these pathways are *not* analogous to the specialized conducting pathways in the ventricles, e.g., the bundle branches and Purkinje fibers, which are discrete histologically identifiable tracts of tissue. However, preferential internodal conduction (more rapid conduction velocity between nodes in some parts of atrium compared with other parts) probably does exist and may be caused by fiber orientation, size, geometry or other factors, rather than by specialized tracts located between the nodes.

The speed at which the impulse travels (conduction velocity) becomes reduced as the impulse traverses the AV node but once again accelerates through the His bundle, bundle branches, and Purkinje fibers. The Purkinje fibers distribute the impulse rapidly and uniformly over the ventricular endocardium, finally depolarizing the ventricular myocardium (Fig. 8-1). It is important to remember that the surface ECG records only ventricular muscle depolarization (QRS) and repolarization (T wave), atrial depolarization (P wave), and sometimes repolarization (Ta wave). Activity from the SA and AV nodes, His bundle, bundle branches, and Purkinje fibers is not recorded in the ECG. Special intracardiac electrodes can be employed to record activity from some of these structures and are discussed briefly later in this chapter.

It has been postulated that the bundle branches are really composed of three divisions, called fascicles,[2] that are formed by the right bundle branch and two divisions of the left bundle branch, the anterosuperior division, and the posteroinferior division. The term *hemiblock* has been used to describe block in one of these fascicles.[2] A more accurate term is *fascicular block*. Although a number of careful anatomic and pathologic studies of human hearts have failed to substantiate the anatomic separation of the left bundle branch into two distinct and specific divisions, the fascicular block concept has been useful to explain observed electrocardiographic and clinical entities (see discussion of bundle branch block).

The electrical activity of the heart is recorded by an ECG machine onto ECG paper. This graph paper is divided into a series of vertical lines measuring time and horizontal lines measuring voltage (Fig. 8-2). The electrical pattern of a typical cardiac cycle is displayed in Fig. 8-3 and is discussed in Table 8-1. (See also Chapter 6.)

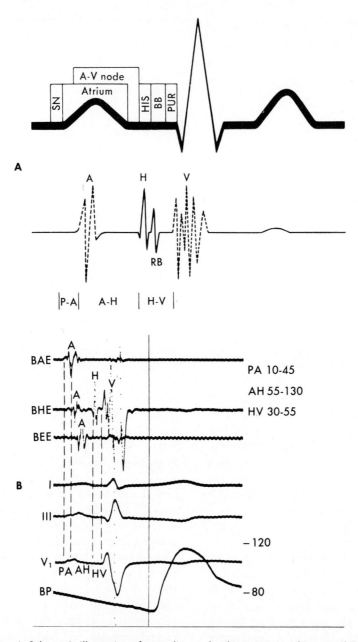

FIG. 8-1. A, Schematic illustration of a cardiac cycle, demonstrating the normal ECG *(top)* and an intracardiac recording *(bottom)*. The diagram illustrates the approximate time of activation of various structures in the specialized conduction system. It is important to emphasize that conduction has already reached the Purkinje fibers just before the onset of the QRS complex. *SN,* Sinus node; *HIS,* bundle of His; *BB,* bundle branches; *PUR,* Purkinje fibers; *A,* low right atrial deflection; *H,* His bundle deflection; *RB,* right bundle branch deflection; *V,* ventricular septal muscle depoloarization; *P-A,* interval from the onset of the P wave in the surface tracing to the onset of the low right atrial deflection, serving as a measure of intraatrial conduction; *A-H,* measurement of conduction across the AV node; *H-V* measurement of conduction through the His bundle distal to the recording electrode, the bundle branches, and the Purkinje system up to the point of ventricular activation. (Top panel modified from Hoffman, B.F., and Singer, D.H.: Prog. Cardiovasc. Dis. 7:226, 1964.) B, Electrophysiologic and blood pressure recordings during one cardiac cycle. *BAE,* Bipolar high right atrial electrogram; *BHE,* bipolar His electrogram; *BEE,* bipolar esphageal electrogram. Normal intervals in milliseconds to the right.

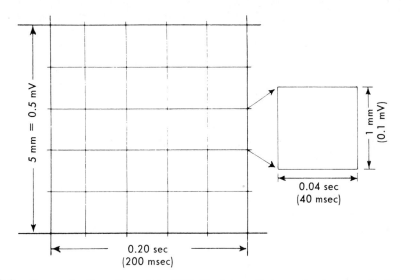

FIG. 8-2.   Time and voltage lines of the ECG. The interval between two heavy vertical lines is 0.20 second (200 msec) and between each light line 0.04 second (40 msec). The voltage between each heavy horizontal line is 0.5 mV.

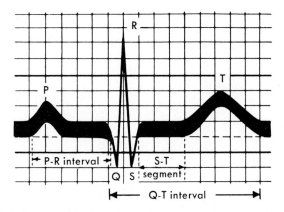

FIG. 8-3.   Electrical pattern of cardiac cycle. (Refer to Table 8-1.)

TABLE 8-1. Definition and significance of ECG intervals*

Description	Duration	Significance of disturbance
PR interval: from beginning of P wave to beginning of QRS complex; represents time taken for impulse to spread through the atria, AV node and His bundle, the bundle branches and Purkinje fibers, to a point immediately preceding ventricular activation	0.12 to 0.20 second	Disturbance in conduction usually in AV node, His bundle, or bundle branches but can be in atria as well
QRS interval: from beginning to end of QRS complex; represents time taken for depolarization of both ventricles	0.06 to 0.10 second	Disturbance in conduction in bundle branches and/ or in ventricles
QT interval: from beginning of QRS to end of T wave; represents time taken for entire electrical depolarization and repolarization of the ventricles	0.36 to 0.44 second	Disturbances usually affecting repolarization more than depolarization such as drug effects, electrolyte disturbances, and rate changes

*Heart rate influences the duration of these intervals, especially that of the PR and QT intervals.

Several methods are available for determining the heart rate from an ECG recording. The atrial rate (P-P interval) in beats per minute may be determined by dividing the time interval between regularly occurring consecutive P waves into 60. The ventricular rate (R-R interval) is determined in the same fashion by dividing the time interval between regularly occurring consecutive R waves into 60. The rate can be more rapidly determined by dividing the number of large (0.20 second) squares between two consecutive complexes into 300 or small (0.04 second) squares into 1500. Any of these methods will be accurate for de-

termining the heart rate of a regular rhythm (Fig. 8-4). Table 8-2 can be used to calculate the rate of a regular rhythm. For irregular rhythms, the rate must be averaged over a longer interval; for example, the number of large divisions separating four QRS complexes (three complete cardiac cycles) may be divided into 900, or the number of P waves (atrial rate) or R waves (ventricular rate) occurring in a 6-second interval (30 large boxes) may be multiplied by 10 (Fig. 8-5). Most ECG paper has markers across the top at either 1 or 3 second intervals; these markers facilitate the latter method.

TABLE 8-2. Determination of heart rate from the ECG

Time (Second)	No. of Small Squares	Rate (Beats per Minute)	Time (Second)	No. of Small Squares	Rate (Beats per Minute)
0.10	2.5	600	0.60	15.00	100
0.12	3.0	500	0.64	16.00	94
0.15	3.75	400	0.70	17.50	86
0.16	4.0	375	0.72	18.00	83
0.20	5.0	300	0.76	19.00	79
0.24	6.0	250	0.80	20.00	75
0.26	6.5	230	0.84	21.00	71
0.28	7.0	214	0.88	22.00	68
0.30	7.5	200	0.92	23.00	65
0.32	8.0	188	0.96	24.00	63
0.34	8.5	176	1.00	25.00	60
0.36	9.0	167	1.08	27.00	56
0.38	9.5	158	1.14	28.50	53
0.40	10.0	150	1.20	30.00	50
0.42	10.5	143	1.40	35.00	43
0.44	11.0	136	1.50	37.50	40
0.46	11.5	130	1.60	40.00	38
0.48	12.0	125	1.80	45.00	33
0.50	12.5	120	2.00	50.00	30
0.52	13.0	115	2.50	62.50	25
0.56	14.0	107	3.00	75.00	20

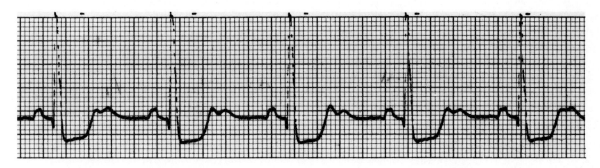

FIG. 8-4. Calculation of atrial and ventricular rates. Heart rate is almost 60 beats/minute, determined by dividing time interval between consecutive P waves and/or consecutive R waves by 1 second; by dividing 5 large squares into 300 or 25 small squares into 1500; or by multiplying the number of complexes occurring in a 6-second strip by 10. See Table 8-2.

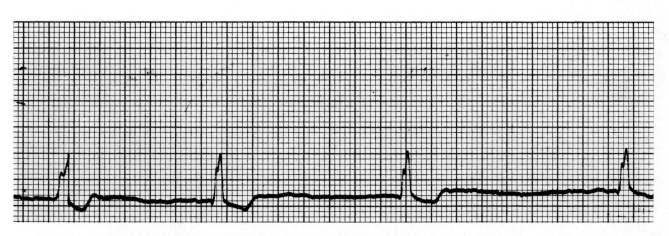

FIG. 8-5. Calculation of the rate of an irregular rhythm. Heart rate is 40 beats/minute, determined by dividing 22 (the number of large divisions separating 4 QRS complexes) into 900 or by multiplying 4 (number of R waves occurring in a 6-second strip) by 10.

ELECTROPHYSIOLOGIC PRINCIPLES

Certain specialized cells, such as those in the sinus node, some parts of the atria, AV node, and His-Purkinje system, are able to discharge spontaneously; they do not require an external or propagated stimulus to fire. This property, known as *automaticity* (also called diastolic depolarization), creates the potential for these cells to depolarize the rest of the heart. Normally the sinus node rules as the pacemaker, since it spontaneously discharges at a rate of 60 to 100 times/minute, which is faster than these other latent pacemakers.

Should a latent pacemaker possessing the property of automaticity discharge more rapidly than the sinus node, it may depolarize atria, ventricles, or both. This may occur in two ways. If the SA node discharges more slowly than the discharge rate of the latent pacemaker (see Fig. 8-13), or if the sinus impulse is blocked before reaching the latent pacemaker site (see Fig. 8-13), the latent pacemaker may passively *escape* sinus domination and discharge automatically at its own intrinsic rate. Such escape beats are slower than normal, since the AV junction and bundle branch–Purkinje system (two probable escape focus sites) generally beat at 40 to 60 times/minute and 30 to 40 times/minute, respectively. However, should a latent pacemaker abnormally accelerate its discharge rate and actively *usurp* control of the heartbeat from the sinus node, a premature beat results. This may happen in the atria, ventricles, or AV junction. A series of these premature beats in a row produces a tachycardia. A shift in the normal manner of atrial or ventricular activation, such as might be produced by a shift in pacemaker focus, is reflected by a change in P or QRS contour.

Automatic discharge of a pacemaker focus is not sufficient to depolarize a cardiac chamber; the impulse must also be conducted from its site of origin to surrounding myocardium. The heart possesses the property of *excitability,* which is a characteristic enabling it to be depolarized by a stimulus; this is an integral part of the propagation or conduction of the impulse from one fiber to the next. Many factors may influence the level of excitability but the most important, in the normal state, is how long after depolarization the heart is restimulated. Cardiac tissue requires a recovery period following depolarization. If a stimulus occurs too early, the heart has had insufficient time to recover, and it will not respond to the stimulus no matter how intense it is (absolute refractory period, excitability zero). A slightly later stimulus allows more time for recovery (relative refractory period, excitability improving), and a still later stimulus finds the heart completely recovered (no longer refractory, full excitability).

If conduction becomes unevenly depressed, with block in some areas and not in others, some regions of the myocardium (unblocked areas) must necessarily be activated (and recover) earlier than others. Under appropriate circumstances, when the block is in only one direction (unidirectional), this uneven conduction may allow the initial impulse to *reenter* areas previously inexcitable but that have now recovered. Should the reentering impulse then be able to depolarize the entire atria and/or ventricles, a corresponding premature extrasystole results; maintenance of the *reentrant excitation* establishes a tachycardia. A special form of reentry may produce echo or reciprocal beats (see Fig. 8-54, *D*).

Thus disorders of impulse *formation* (automaticity) or *conduction* (unidirectional block and reentry) or, at times, combinations of both may initiate arrhythmias.

Only indirect evidence exists to enable a clinical classification of arrhythmias according to electrophysiologic mechanisms. In addition, an arrhythmia may be initiated and perpetuated by different mechanisms. For example, spontaneous diastolic depolarization (automaticity) may trigger a premature atrial or ventricular systole that initiates an arrhythmia caused by reentry. Also, recent studies on parasystole,[3] a type of automaticity, and reflection,[4] a form of reentry, is causing us to rethink many of our clinical definitions (Table 8-3). Thus the clinical classification of

---

TABLE 8-3. Probable electrophysiologic mechanism responsible for various cardiac arrhythmias

Automaticity	Reentry	Automaticity or Reentry
Escape beats—atrial, junctional, or ventricular	AV nodal reentry	Premature systoles—atrial, junctional, or ventricular
Atrial rhythm	AV reciprocating tachycardia using an accessory (WPW) pathway	Flutter and fibrillation
Atrial tachycardia with or without AV block	Atrial flutter	Ventricular tachycardia
Junctional rhythm	Atrial fibrillation	
Nonparoxysmal AV junctional tachycardia	Ventricular tachycardia	
Accelerated idioventricular rhythm	Ventricular flutter	
Parasystole	Ventricular fibrillation	

arrhythmias according to mechanism remains speculative. Antiarrhythmic agents specifically indicated to treat one mechanism or the other do not yet exist.[5]

Depolarization of cells in the atria, ventricles, and His-Purkinje system depends on a rapid movement of sodium into the cell. Such an event is called the *fast response*. In the sinus and AV nodes depolarization depends primarily on intracellular movement of calcium and is called the *slow response*.[6] The slow response may play a role in the genesis of certain cardiac arrhythmias and is affected by a specific class of drugs called calcium entry blockers such as verapamil, diltiazem and nifedipine.[7]

TABLE 8-4. Classification of normal and abnormal cardiac rhythms

Rhythms originating in the sinus node	**Rhythms originating in the ventricles**
Sinus rhythm	Ventricular escape complexes
Sinus tachycardia	Premature ventricular complex
Sinus bradycardia	Ventricular tachycardia
Sinus arrhythmia	Idioventricular tachycardia (accelerated idioventricular rhythm)
Sinus arrest	Ventricular flutter
Sinus exit block	Ventricular fibrillation
Sinus nodal reentry	
Rhythms originating in the atria	**AV block**
Wandering pacemaker between sinus node and atrium or AV junction	First-degree
Premature atrial complex	Second-degree
Intraatrial reentry	Type I (Wenckebach)
Atrial flutter	Type II
Atrial fibrillation	Third-degree (complete)
Atrial tachycardia (with or without block)	**Bundle branch block**
Multifocal atrial tachycardia	Right
	Left
Rhythms originating in the AV junction (AV node–His bundle)	Fascicular blocks (hemiblocks)
Premature AV junctional complex	**Parasystole**
AV junctional escape complexes	Atrial
AV junctional rhythm	Junctional
AV nodal reentry	Ventricular
AV reciprocating tachycardia using an accessory (WPW) pathway	

From reference 8.

ARRHYTHMIA ANALYSIS (Table 8-4)

For proper analysis, each arrhythmia must be approached in a systematic manner. A suggested guide follows:

1. What is the rate? Is it too fast or too slow? Are P waves present? Are atrial and ventricular rates the same?
2. Are the PP and RR intervals regular or irregular? If irregular, is it a consistent, repeating irregularity?
3. Is there a P wave (and therefore atrial activity) related to each ventricular complex? Does the P wave precede or follow the QRS complex? Is the PR or RP interval constant?
4. Are all P waves and QRS complexes identical and normal in contour? To determine the significance of changes in P or QRS contour or amplitude, one must know the lead being recorded.
5. Are the PR, QRS and QT intervals normal?
6. Are premature complexes present? If so, are they atrial, junctional, or ventricular? Is there a constant coupling interval between the premature complex and the normal complex? Is there a constant interval between premature complexes?
7. Are escape beats present? If so, are they atrial, junctional, or ventricular in origin?
8. What is the dominant rhythm?
9. Considering the clinical setting, what is the significance of the arrhythmia?
10. How should the arrhythmia be treated?

THERAPY OF ARRHYTHMIAS (Table 8-5)
General Therapeutic Concepts[9,10,11]

Initial Assessment. The therapeutic approach to a patient who has a cardiac arrhythmia begins with an accurate electrocardiographic *interpretation* of the arrhythmia and continues with determination of the *cause* of the arrhythmia (if possible), the nature of the underlying *heart disease* (if any), and the *consequences* of the arrhythmia for the individual patient. Thus one cannot treat arrhythmias as isolated events without having knowledge of the clinical situation; *patients* who have arrhythmias, not arrhythmias themselves, are treated.

Electrophysiologic and Hemodynamic Consequences. The ventricular rate and duration of an arrhythmia, its site of origin, and the cardiovascular status of the patient primarily determine the electrophysiologic and hemodynamic consequences of a particular rhythm disturbance. Electrophysiologic consequences, often influenced by the presence of underlying heart disease such as acute myocardial infarction, include the development of serious arrhythmias as a result of rapid (and slow) rates, initiation of sustained arrhythmias by premature complexes, or the degeneration of rhythms like ventricular tachycardia into ventricular fibrillation. Hemodynamic performance of the heart and circulation may be altered by extremes of heart rate or by loss of atrial contribution to ventricular filling. Rapid rates greatly shorten the diastolic filling time, and, particularly in diseased hearts, the increased heart rate may fail to compensate for the reduced stroke output; blood pressure, along with cardiac output, declines. Arrhythmias such as nonparoxysmal AV junctional tachycardia (Fig. 8-51) that prevent sequential AV contraction mitigate the hemodynamic benefits of the atrial booster pump, whereas atrial fibrillation causes complete loss of atrial contraction and may reduce cardiac output.

Slowing the Ventricular Rate. When a patient develops a tachyarrhythmia, slowing the ventricular rate is the initial and frequently the most important therapeutic maneuver. Since medical therapy frequently involves a time-consuming and potentially dangerous biologic titration of drugs such as digitalis or quinidine, electrical direct current (DC) cardioversion may be preferable, depending on the clinical situation. Therapy may differ radically for the very same arrhythmia in two different patients because the consequences of the tachycardia on the individual patients differ. For example, a supraventricular tachycardia at 200 beats/minute may produce little or no symptoms in a healthy young adult and therefore require little or no

TABLE 8-5. Cardiac arrhythmias*

Type of Arrhythmia	P Waves			QRS Complexes		
	Rate	Rhythm	Contour	Rate	Rhythm	Contour
Sinus rhythm	60 to 100	Regular†	Normal	60 to 100	Regular	Normal
Sinus bradycardia	<60	Regular	Normal	<60	Regular	Normal
Sinus tachycardia	100 to 180	Regular	May be peaked	100 to 180	Regular	Normal
AV nodal reentry	150 to 250	Very regular except at onset and termination	Retrograde; difficult to see; lost in QRS complex	150 to 250	Very regular except at onset and termination	Normal
Atrial flutter	250 to 350	Regular	Sawtooth	75 to 175	Generally regular in absence of drugs or disease	Normal
Atrial fibrillation	400 to 600	Grossly irregular	Base line undulations; no P waves	100 to 160	Grossly irregular	Normal

*In an effort to summarize these arrhythmias in a tabular form, generalizations have to be made, especially under therapy. Particularly, acute therapy to terminate a tachycardia may be different from chronic therapy to prevent a recurrence. Some of the exceptions are indicated by the footnotes, but the reader is referred to the text for a complete discussion.
†P waves initiated by sinus node discharge may not be precisely regular because of sinus arrhythmia.
‡Often, carotid sinus massage fails to slow a sinus tachycardia.

therapy; the very same arrhythmia may precipitate pulmonary edema in a patient with mitral stenosis, syncope in a patient with aortic stenosis, shock in a patient with an acute myocardial infarction, or hemiparesis in a patient with cerebrovascular disease. In these situations the tachycardia requires prompt electrical conversion.

Etiology. The etiology of the arrhythmia may influence therapy markedly. Electrolyte imbalance (potassium, magnesium, calcium), acidosis or alkalosis, hypoxemia, and many drugs may produce arrhythmias. Because heart failure may cause arrhythmias, digitalis may effectively suppress arrhythmias during heart failure when all other agents are unsuccessful or prevent more severe arrhythmias by reversing early congestive heart failure. Similarly, an arrhythmia secondary to hypotension may respond to leg elevation or vasopressor therapy. Mild sedation or reassurance may be successful in treating some arrhythmias related to emotional stress. Precipitating or contributing disease states such as infection, hypovolemia, anemia, and thyroid disorders should be sought and treated. Aggressive management of premature atrial or ventricular complexes that often presage or precipitate the occurrence of sustained tachyarrhythmias may prevent later occurrence of more serious tachyarrhythmias.

Risks of Therapy. Since therapy always involves some risk, one must decide, particularly as the therapeutic regimen escalates, if the risks of not treating the arrhythmia continue to outweigh the risks of the therapy. The antiarrhythmic agents[7,10-12] lidocaine, procainamide, quinidine, propranolol, disopyramide, and phenytoin exert negative inotropic effects on the myocardium, and when given parenterally, they may produce hypotension. Antiarrhythmic agents may slow conduction velocity, depress the activity of normal (sinus) as well as abnormal (ectopic) pacemaker sites, and cause arrhythmias. It should be remembered that doses of all drugs may need to be adjusted according to the size of the patient, routes of excretion or degradation, presence of impaired organ function (heart, liver, kidney), degree of absorption (if given orally), adverse side effects, interaction with other drugs, electrolyte imbalance, hypoxemia, and the like.

The remainder of this chapter will be devoted to a discussion of cardiac arrhythmias (see Tables 8-4 and 8-5). An analysis similar to that presented in the discussion of arrhythmia analysis will be employed.

Ventricular Response to Carotid Sinus Massage	Physical Examination			Treatment
	Intensity of S_1	Splitting of S_2	A Waves	
Gradual slowing and return to former rate	Constant	Normal	Normal	None
Gradual slowing and return to former rate	Constant	Normal	Normal	None, unless symptomatic; atropine, isoproterenol
Gradual slowing‡ and return to former rate	Constant	Normal	Normal	None, unless symptomatic; treat underlying disease
Abrupt slowing caused by termination of tachycardia, or no effect†	Constant	Normal	Constant cannon A waves	Vagal stimulation, verapamil, digitalis, propranolol, DC shock, pacing
Abrupt slowing and return to former rate; flutter remains	Constant; variable if AV block changing	Normal	Flutter waves	DC shock, digitalis, quinidine, propranolol, verapamil, pacing
Slowing; gross irregularity remains	Variable	Normal	No A waves	Digitalis, quinidine, DC shock, verapamil, propranolol

§Any independent atrial arrhythmia may exist or the atria may be captured retrogradely.
‖Constant if atria captured retrogradely.
¶Atrial rhythm and rate may vary, depending on whether sinus bradycardia or tachycardia, atrial tachycardia, or something else is the atrial mechanism.
**Regular or constant if block is unchanging.

Continued.

TABLE 8-5. Cardiac arrhythmias—cont'd

Type of Arrhythmia	P Waves			QRS Complexes		
	Rate	Rhythm	Contour	Rate	Rhythm	Contour
Atrial tachycardia with block	150 to 250	Regular; may be irregular	Abnormal	75 to 200	Generally regular in absence of drugs or disease	Normal
AV junctional rhythm	40 to 100§	Regular	Normal	40 to 60	Fairly regular	Normal
Reciprocating tachycardia using an accessory (WPW) pathway	150 to 250	Very regular except at onset and termination	Retrograde; difficult to see; follows the QRS complex	150 to 250	Very regular except at onset and termination	Normal
Nonparoxysmal AV junctional tachycardia	60 to 100§	Regular	Normal	70 to 130	Fairly regular	Normal
Ventricular tachycardia	60 to 100§	Regular	Normal	110 to 250	Fairly regular; may be irregular	Abnormal, >0.12 second
Accelerated idioventricular rhythm	60 to 100§	Regular	Normal	50 to 110	Fairly regular; may be irregular	Abnormal, >0.12 second
Ventricular flutter	60 to 100§	Regular	Normal; difficult to see	150 to 300	Regular	Sine wave
Ventricular fibrillation	60 to 100§	Regular	Normal; difficult to see	400 to 600	Grossly irregular	Base line undulations; no QRS complexes
First-degree AV block	60 to 100¶	Regular	Normal	60 to 100	Regular	Normal
Type I second-degree AV block	60 to 100¶	Regular	Normal	30 to 100	Irregular**	Normal
Type II-second-degree AV block	60 to 100¶	Regular	Normal	30 to 100	Irregular**	Abnormal, >0.12 second
Complete AV block	60 to 100§	Regular	Normal	<40	Fairly regular	Abnormal, >0.12 second
Right bundle branch block	60 to 100	Regular	Normal	60 to 100	Regular	Abnormal, >0.12 second
Left bundle branch block	60 to 100	Regular	Normal	60 to 100	Regular	Abnormal, >0.12 second

Ventricular Response to Carotid Sinus Massage	Physical Examination			Treatment
	Intensity of S_1	Splitting of S_2	A Waves	
Abrupt slowing and return to former rate; tachycardia remains	Constant; variable if AV block changing	Normal	More A waves than CV waves	Stop digitalis if toxic; digitalis, if not toxic; possibly verapamil, quinidine
None; may be slight slowing	Variable‖	Normal	Intermittent cannon waves‖	None, unless symptomatic; atropine
Abrupt slowing caused by termination of tachycardia, or no effect	Constant but decreased	Normal	Constant cannon waves	See paroxysmal supraventricular tachycardia above
None; may be slight slowing	Variable‖	Normal	Intermittent cannon waves‖	None, unless symptomatic; stop digitalis if toxic
None	Variable‖	Abnormal	Intermittent cannon waves‖	Lidocaine, procainamide, DC shock, quinidine
None	Variable‖	Abnormal	Intermittent cannon waves‖	None, unless symptomatic; lidocaine, atropine
None	None	None	Cannon waves	DC shock
None	None	None	Cannon waves	DC shock
Gradual slowing caused by sinus slowing	Constant, diminished	Normal	Normal	None
Slowing caused by sinus slowing and an increase in AV block	Cyclic decrease and then increase after pause	Normal	Normal; increasing AC interval; A waves without C waves	None, unless symptomatic; atropine
Gradual slowing caused by sinus slowing	Constant	Abnormal	Normal; constant AC interval; A waves without C waves	Pacemaker
None	Variable‖	Abnormal	Intermittent cannon waves‖	Pacemaker
Gradual slowing and return to former rate	Constant	Wide	Normal	None
Gradual slowing and return to former rate	Constant	Paradoxical	Normal	None

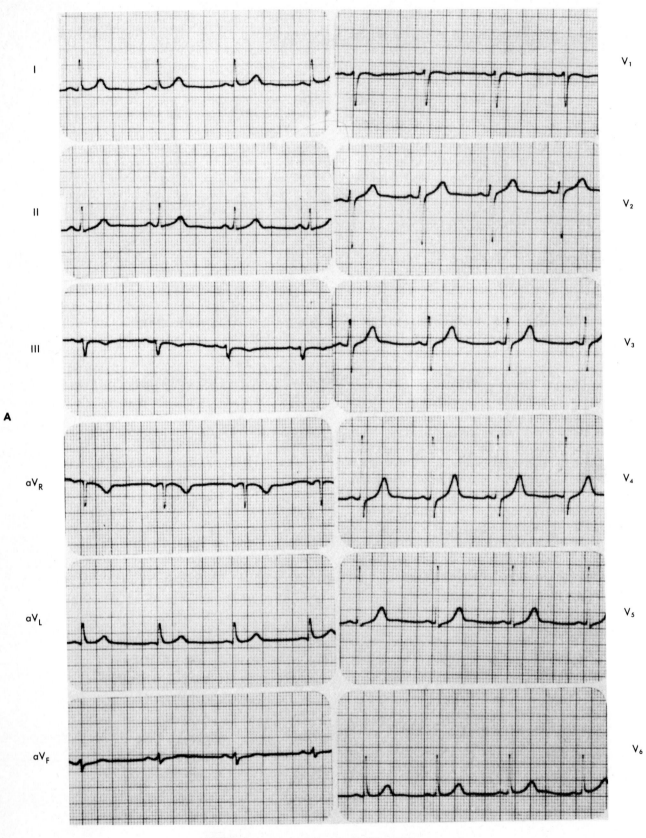

FIG. 8-6. A, Normal sinus rhythm. The ECG is normal.

NORMAL SINUS RHYTHM (Fig. 8-6)

Normal sinus rhythm is arbitrarily limited to rates of 60 to 100 beats/minute. The P wave is upright in leads I and II and negative in lead aV$_R$ with a vector in the frontal plane between 0 and +90 degrees. In the horizontal plane the P vector is directed anteriorly and slightly leftward and may therefore be negative in V$_1$ and V$_2$ but is positive in V$_3$. The PP interval characteristically varies slightly but by less than 0.16 second per cycle. The PR interval is between 0.12 and 2.0 seconds and may vary slightly with rate. The QRS duration is 0.06 to 0.20 second, and the QT duration is 0.36 to 0.44 second. The sinus node responds readily to autonomic stimuli; parasympathetic (cholinergic) stimuli slow and sympathetic (adrenergic) stimuli speed the rate of discharge. The resulting rate depends on the net effect of these two opposing forces.

SINUS TACHYCARDIA (Figs. 8-7 and 8-8)

The conduction pathway in sinus tachycardia is the same as that in normal sinus rhythm but, because of enhanced discharge of the sinus node from vagal inhibition or sympathetic stimulation (or both), the sinus rate is between 100 and 180 beats/minute. It may be higher with extreme exertion and in infants. It has a gradual onset and termination, and the PP interval may vary slightly from cycle to cycle. P waves have a normal contour but may develop a larger amplitude and become peaked. Carotid sinus massage and Valsalva or other vagal maneuvers gradually slow a sinus tachycardia, which then accelerates to its previous rate. More rapid sinus rates may fail to slow in response to a vagal maneuver.

Significance. Sinus tachycardia is the normal reaction to a variety of physiologic stresses such as fever, hypotension, thyrotoxicosis, anemia, anxiety, exertion, hypovolemia, pulmonary emboli, myocardial ischemia, congestive

heart failure, or shock. Inflammation such as pericarditis may produce sinus tachycardia. Sinus tachycardia is usually of no physiologic significance; however, in patients with organic myocardial disease, reduced cardiac output, congestive heart failure, or arrhythmias may result. Since heart rate is a major determinant of oxygen requirements, angina or perhaps an increase in the size of an infarction may accompany persistent sinus tachycardia in patients with coronary artery disease.

Treatment. Therapy should be directed toward correcting the underlying disease state that caused the sinus tachycardia. Elimination of tobacco, alcohol, coffee, tea, or other stimulants (for example, sympathomimetic vasoconstrictors in nose drops) may be helpful. If sinus tachycardia is not secondary to a correctable physiologic stress, treatment with sedatives, reserpine, or clonidine is occasionally useful. The only currently available medication that consistently slows a sinus tachycardia directly is propranolol, administered orally, 10 to 60 mg, four times daily. Drugs that block the slow inward current (see Chapter 10), such as verapamil, may also slow the rate of sinus node discharge.

SINUS BRADYCARDIA
(Figs. 8-9 and 8-10)

In sinus bradycardia, impulses travel down the same pathway as in sinus rhythm, but the sinus node discharges at a rate less than 60 beats/minute. P waves have a normal contour and occur before each QRS complex with a constant PR interval exceeding 0.12 second. Sinus arrhythmia is frequently present.

Significance. Sinus bradycardia results from excessive vagal or decreased sympathetic tone or both. Eye surgery, meningitis, intracranial tumors, cervical and mediastinal tumors, and certain disease states such as myocardial infarction, myxedema, obstructive jaundice, and cardiac fibrosis may produce sinus bradycardia. In most instances, sinus bradycardia is a benign arrhythmia and may actually be beneficial by producing a longer period of diastole and increased ventricular filling. It occurs commonly in well-trained athletes, during sleep, vomiting, or vasovagal syncope and may be produced by carotid sinus stimulation or by the administration of parasympathomimetic drugs. Sinus bradycardia occurring in patients who have myocardial infarction, more commonly diaphragmatic or posterior, may compromise optimal myocardial function and predispose to premature systoles and sustained tachyarrhythmias. More recent data suggest sinus bradycardia actually is beneficial in some patients who have acute myocardial infarction because it reduces oxygen demands, may help to minimize the size of the infarction, and may lessen the frequency of some arrhythmias. Patients with acute myocardial infarction who have sinus bradycardia generally

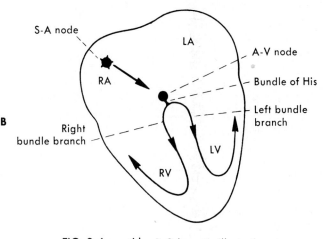

FIG. 8-6, cont'd.   B, Schematic illustration.

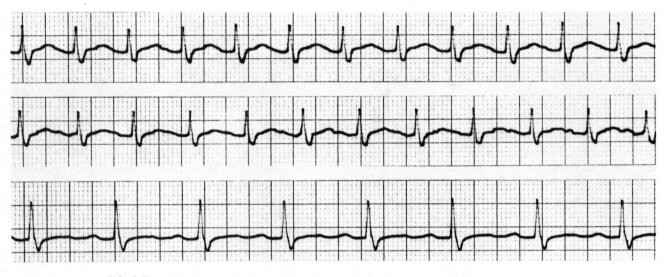

FIG. 8-7. Sinus tachycardia. Sinus tachycardia gradually slows to reveal clearer P waves in the bottom tracing, which is a sinus rhythm with a first degree AV block. Monitor lead.

Rate: Top, 125 beats/minute; middle, 122 beats/minute; bottom, 82 beats/minute.
Rhythm: Regular.
P waves: Difficult to see in top strip. Precede each QRS complex at a regular interval with unchanging contour in middle and bottom strip.
PR interval: Top, cannot measure; middle, 0.20 second; bottom, 0.24 second.
QRS: 0.09 second.

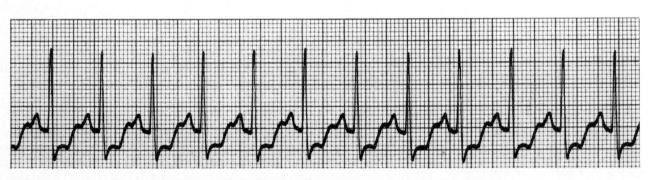

FIG. 8-8. Sinus tachycardia. Patient complained of chest pain and was noted to have sinus tachycardia with ST segment depression, consistent with anginal episode. Lead II.

Rate: 125 beats/minute.
Rhythm: Regular.
P waves: Normal; precede each QRS complex with regular contour at fixed interval.
PR interval: 0.16 second.
QRS: Normal, 0.08 second. ST segments are depressed.

have lower mortality than patients who have sinus tachycardia.

Treatment. Treatment of sinus bradycardia per se usually is not needed. If the patient with an acute myocardial infarction is asymptomatic, it is probably best not to try to speed the sinus rate. If the cardiac output is inadequate, or if arrhythmias are associated with the slow rate, atropine (0.5 mg IV as an initial dose, repeated if necessary) or isoproterenol (1 or 2 μg/minute IV) is usually effective.

These drugs should be used cautiously, with care taken not to produce too rapid a rate. In patients who have symptoms as a result of chronic sinus bradycardia, electrical pacing may be needed, since few, if any, drugs successfully speed sinus node discharge chronically without producing side effects. Theophylline drugs or dermally applied scopolamine may be tried, although they are not approved for those indications.

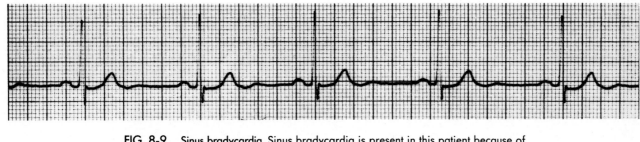

FIG. 8-9. Sinus bradycardia. Sinus bradycardia is present in this patient because of administration of propranolol. Lead II.

Rate: 46 beats/minute.
Rhythm: Regular.
P waves: Precede each QRS with a normal contour.
PR interval: 0.19 second.
QRS: 0.09 second.

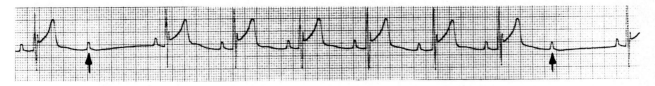

FIG. 8-10. Sinus bradycardia in a young patient. Type I (Wenckebach) AV block is also present and probably represents excessive vagal tone that may be normal in young individuals. Monitor lead. ST elevation is early repolarization.

Rate: Atrial, 55 beats/minute.
Rhythm: Atrial, regular; ventricular, irregular because of nonconducted P waves (arrows).
PR interval: Increasing slightly from 0.18 second to 2.2 seconds.
QRS: 0.09 second.

SINUS ARRHYTHMIA (Figs. 8-11 to 8-13)

Sinus arrhythmia is characterized by a phasic variation in cycle length exceeding 0.16 second during sinus rhythm. It is the most frequent form of arrhythmia and occurs as a normal phenomenon. The P waves do not vary in morphology, and the PR interval exceeds 0.12 second and remains unchanged, since the focus of discharge is fixed within the sinus node. Occasionally the pacemaker focus may wander within the sinus node, producing P waves of slightly different contour (but not retrograde) and a changing PR interval (but not less than 0.12 second). Sinus arrhythmia commonly occurs in the young or aged, especially with slower heart rates or following enhanced vagal tone from digitalis or morphine administration. Sinus arrhythmia appears in two basic forms. In the respiratory form the PP interval cyclically shortens during inspiration as a result of reflex inhibition of vagal tone or enhancement of sympathetic tone or both. Breath-holding eliminates the cycle length variation. Nonrespiratory sinus arrhythmia is characterized by a phasic variation unrelated to the respiratory cycle. In both forms, impulses are generated in the sinus node and travel over the normal pathway to the AV node.

Significance. Sinus arrhythmia commonly occurs in the young or aged especially with slower heart rates or from enhanced vagal tone after morphine or digitalis administration. Symptoms produced by sinus arrhythmias are rare, but on occasion, if the pauses between beats are excessively long, palpitations or dizziness may be experienced. Marked sinus arrhythmia can produce a sinus pause sufficiently prolonged to induce syncope if not accompanied by an escape rhythm.

Treatment. Treatment is usually not necessary. Increasing the heart rate by exercise or drugs will abolish sinus arrhythmia. Symptomatic individuals may experience relief from feelings of palpitations through the use of sedatives, tranquilizers, atropine, ephedrine, or isoproterenol administration, as in the treatment of sinus bradycardia.

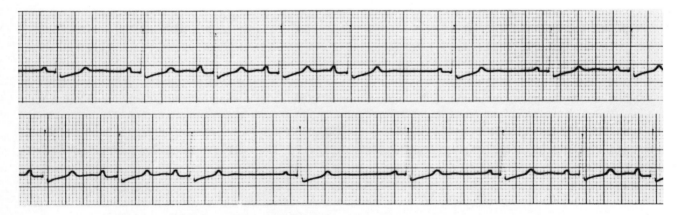

FIG. 8-11. Respiratory sinus arrhythmia. The phasic variation in heart rate corresponds to a respiratory rate of approximately 12 beats/minute. Monitor lead.

Rate: Sinus rate increases with inspiration and decreases with expiration at a rate of 53 to 80 beats/minute.
Rhythm: Irregular with repetitive phase variation in cycle length according to respiratory cycles. Cycle lengths vary by more than 0.16 second. Breath-holding eliminates the rate variations (not shown).
P waves: Precede each QRS complex with a normal, fairly constant contour.
PR interval: Normal, constant, 0.18 second.
QRS: Normal, 0.08 second.

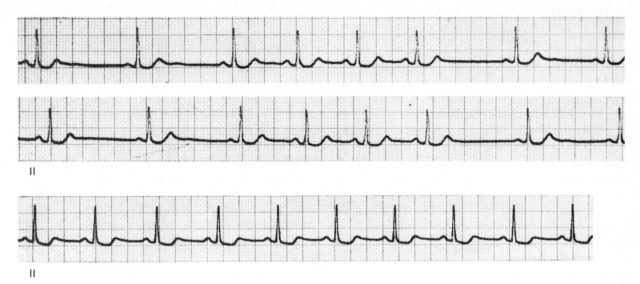

FIG. 8-12. Nonrespiratory sinus arrhythmia. In this instance it was caused by digitalis toxicity (A). One week following discontinuation of digitalis the nonrespiratory sinus arrhythmia disappeared (B).

Rate:	Rate increases and decreases independently of respiration in A (47 to 80 beats/minute). Rate constant (78 beats/minute) in B.
Rhythm:	A, Irregular with a repetitive phasic variation in cycle length which continues during breath-holding. B, Regular.
P waves:	Precede each QRS with a normal, fairly constant contour.
PR interval:	0.12 second.
QRS:	Normal, 0.06 second.

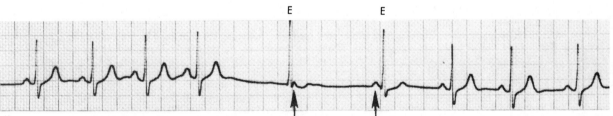

FIG. 8-13. Respiratory sinus arrhythmia. The first four P waves are fairly regular; the PR interval is 0.16 second and constant. Then the sinus node slows and the next two P waves occur much later *(arrows)*. The marked sinus slowing allows a latent pacemaker—possibly located in the His bundle or high in the fascicles—to escape sinus domination, depolarize automatically, and discharge the ventricles *(E, junctional escapes)*. A slight change in QRS contour is apparent in these beats. The sinus node then speeds up to resume control. This slightly complex arrhythmia is completely normal in an otherwise healthy person.

Rate:	Rate increases with inspiration and decreases with expiration (55 to 80 beats/minute).
Rhythm:	Irregular with a repetitive phasic variation in cycle length.
P waves:	Normal, fairly constant contour
PR interval:	0.16 second during sinus-conducted beats.
QRS:	Normal, 0.08 second during sinus-conducted beats.

SINUS ARREST (Figs. 8-14 and 8-15)

Failure of sinus node discharge results in absence of atrial depolarization and periods of ventricular asystole if escape beats produced by latent pacemakers do not discharge. Sinus arrest may be produced by involvement of the sinus node or the sinus node artery by acute myocardial infarction, digitalis toxicity, excessive vagal tone, or degenerative forms of fibrosis. It may occur as a side effect of therapy with certain drugs such as amiodarone.

Significance. Transient sinus arrest may have no clinical significance by itself if latent pacemakers promptly escape to prevent ventricular asystole (Fig. 8-14). Prolonged ventricular asystole results should the latent pacemakers fail to escape. Other arrhythmias may be precipitated by the slow rates (Fig. 8-15).

Treatment. Atropine (0.5 mg IV initially, repeated if necessary) or isoproterenol (1 or 2 μg/minute IV) may be tried as the first therapeutic approach. If these drugs are unsuccessful, atrial or ventricular pacing may be required. In patients who have a chronic form of sinus node disease characterized by marked sinus bradycardia or sinus arrest (sick sinus syndrome), permanent pacing is often necessary. Some of these patients experience sinus bradycardia alternating with periods of supraventricular tachycardia (bradycardia-tachycardia syndrome). These patients are best treated by a combination of drugs (to slow the ventricular rate during the supraventricular tachycardia) and implantation of a permanent demand pacemaker (to prevent the slow rate when the tachycardia terminates).

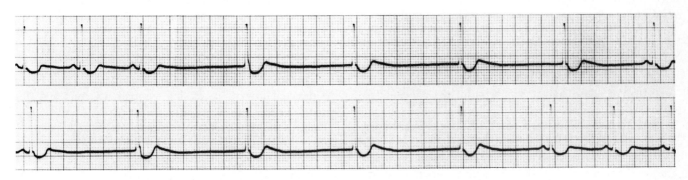

FIG. 8-14. Sinus arrest. After three sinus beats in the top strip, sinus arrest occurs followed by junctional escape beats. The sinus rhythm returns at the end of the strip and once again restores sinus rhythm. A similar event happens in the lower recording. Monitor lead.

Rate: Varying: junctional escape rate, 38 beats/minute; sinus rate, 70 beats/minute.
Rhythm: Irregular.
P waves: Normal contour, intermittently precedes QRS complexes.
PR interval: Constant when P waves precede QRS contours. 0.18 second.
QRS: Normal, 0.09 second.

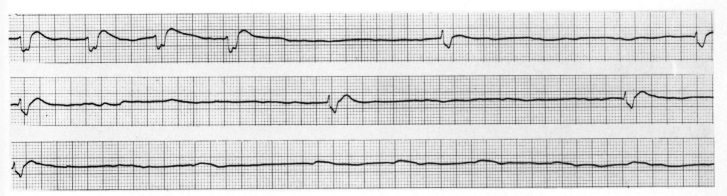

FIG. 8-15. Sinus arrest with asystole. These monitor lead tracings were recorded during a resuscitation procedure in a patient with recurrent syncope. No atrial activity is apparent, and the slight undulations in the baseline represent chest compression during resuscitation. The patient has intermittent junctional or most probably ventricular escapes and then develops complete atrial and ventricular asystole.

Rate: Varying.
Rhythm: Irregular.
P waves: Not seen.
PR interval: Not measurable.
QRS: 0.16 second.

SINUS EXIT BLOCK (Figs. 8-16 and 8-17)

Sinus exit block is a conduction disturbance during which an impulse formed within the sinus node is blocked from depolarizing the atria. Sinus exit block is indicated on the ECG by the absence of the normally expected P wave(s). The length of the pause between P waves is a multiple of the basic PP interval, approximately two, less commonly three or four times the normal PP interval (type II exit block). Type I (Wenckebach) sinus exit block may also occur, in which case the PP interval progressively shortens prior to the pause, and the duration of the pause is less than two PP cycles.

Significance. Sinus exit block may be caused by excessive vagal stimulation, by acute infections such as diphtheria or rheumatic carditis, by atherosclerosis involving the sinus nodal artery, or by fibrosis involving the atrium. Occlusion of the sinus nodal artery owing to acute myo-cardial infarction may result in an atrial infarction and produce sinus exit block. Medications such as quinidine, procainamide, amiodarone, and digitalis may lead to sinus exit block. Sinus exit block is usually transient and often of no clinical importance except to prompt a search for the underlying cause. Syncope may result if the sinus exit block is prolonged and unaccompanied by an AV junctional or ventricular escape rhythm. Digitalis produces type II sinus exit block (but not type I AV block).

Treatment. Therapy for symptomatic sinus exit block is directed toward increasing sympathetic tone and decreasing parasympathetic tone. Thus atropine and isoproterenol are useful, as described under sinus bradycardia. If the clinical situation demands therapy and pharmacologic measures are not effective, atrial or ventricular pacing may be indicated.

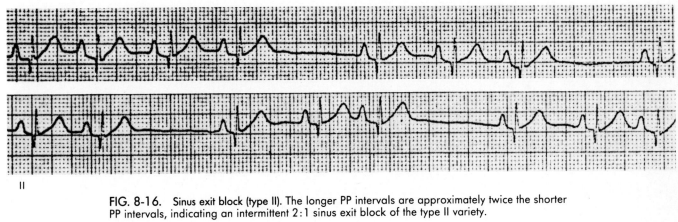

II

FIG. 8-16. Sinus exit block (type II). The longer PP intervals are approximately twice the shorter PP intervals, indicating an intermittent 2:1 sinus exit block of the type II variety.

Rate: Varying, slow (43 to 68 beats/minute).
Rhythm: Irregular; pauses are twice as long as the shorter intervals.
P waves: Contour normal, precede each QRS complex; intermittent loss of P wave.
PR interval: 0.16 second.
QRS: Normal, 0.08 second.

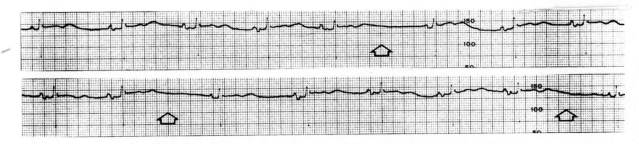

FIG. 8-17. Sinus exit block, type I (Wenckebach block). The following characteristics of this tracing suggest the diagnosis of a Wenckebach exit block from a sinus node. *1,* The PP intervals progressively shorten until *(2)* a pause in atrial activity occurs as depicted by the arrows. *3,* The duration of the pause is less than twice the shortest PP interval. *4,* The PP interval after the pause exceeds the PP interval preceding the pause, which is the shortest PP interval. Monitor lead.

Rate: Varying from 33 to 50 beats/minute.
Rhythm: The four features mentioned above.
P waves: Biphasic, but fairly constant contour; intermittent loss of P wave, producing a pause
             (arrows).
PR interval: 0.24 second.
QRS: 0.07 second.

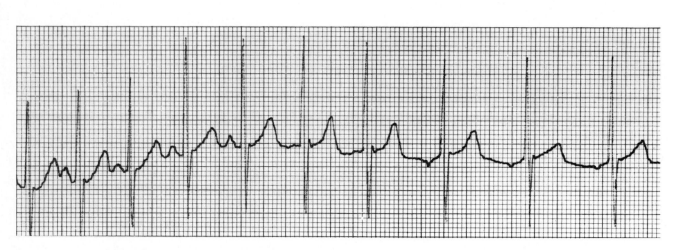

FIG. 8-18.   Wandering atrial pacemaker. When the heart rate is fast, the P wave is upright and gradually becomes inverted as the heart rate slows and the site of impulse formation shifts. Monitor lead.

Rate: Varying, 80 to 135 beats/minute.
Rhythm: Irregular with a repetitive phasic variation in cycle length, as in sinus arrhythmia.
P waves: Varying contour, indicating shift in pacemaker site or change in activation
              sequence.
PR interval: Constant, 0.13 second.
QRS: 0.10 second.

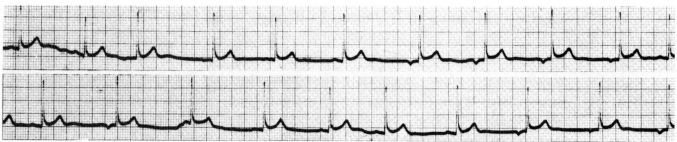

II-continuous

FIG. 8-19.   Wandering atrial pacemaker. As the heart rate slows, the P waves become inverted and then gradually revert toward normal as the heart rate speeds. The PR interval shortens to 0.14 second with the inverted P wave and is 0.16 second with the upright P wave.

Rate: Varying, slow (52 to 72 beats/minute).
Rhythm: Irregular with a repetitive phasic variation in cycle length as in sinus arrhythmia.
P waves: Varying contour, indicating shift in pacemaker site. Become negative in lead II.
PR interval: Varies, 0.14, 0.16 second.
QRS: Normal, 0.08 second.

WANDERING PACEMAKER
(Figs. 8-18 and 8-19)

Wandering pacemaker, a variant of sinus arrhythmia, involves the passive transfer of the dominant pacemaker focus from the sinus node to latent pacemakers with the next highest degree of automaticity, in other atrial sites or in the AV junctional tissue. Thus only one pacemaker is operative at a time. As with other forms of sinus arrhythmia, the change occurs in a gradual fashion over the duration of several beats. The ECG displays a cyclic increase of the RR interval, a PR interval that gradually shortens and may become less than 0.12 second, and a change in P wave configuration until it becomes negative in lead I or II or becomes buried in the QRS complex. A slight change in

QRS configuration may occur owing to aberrant conduction. Generally these changes occur in reverse as the pacemaker shifts back to the sinus node. Rarely a wandering pacemaker may appear without changes in rate.

Significance. Wandering pacemaker is a normal phenomenon that is often seen in the very young or in the aged, and particularly in athletes. Persistence of an AV junctional rhythm for long periods of time, however, usually indicates underlying heart disease.

Treatment. Treatment of a wandering pacemaker usually is not indicated. Sympathomimetic agents such as ephedrine or isoproterenol or parasympatholytic agents such as atropine can be used if necessary (see discussion of sinus bradycardia).

PREMATURE ATRIAL COMPLEXES
(Figs. 8-20 to 8-24)

Premature complexes are the most common cause of an intermittent pulse. They may originate in any area of the heart, most frequently in the ventricles, less often in the atria and the AV junctional region, and rarely in the sinus node. Although premature complexes arise in normal hearts, they are more often associated with organic disease, particularly in older patients.

The diagnosis of premature atrial complexes is indicated by a premature P wave and a PR interval greater than 0.12 second. Although the contour of the premature P wave may resemble the normal sinus P wave, it generally is different. Variations in the basic sinus rate at times may make the diagnosis of prematurity difficult, but differences in the contour of the P wave are usually quite apparent and indicate a different focus of origin. When a premature atrial complex occurs early in diastole, conduction may not be completely normal. The AV junction may still be refractory from the preceding beat and will prevent propagation of the impulse (blocked premature atrial complex) or cause conduction to be slowed in the AV junction (prolonged PR interval) or ventricle (functional bundle branch block). As a general rule, a short RP interval produced by an early premature atrial complex close to the preceding QRS complex is followed by a long PR interval. On occasion, when the AV junction has sufficiently repolarized to conduct normally, the supraventricular QRS complex may be aberrant in configuration because the ventricle has not completely repolarized (see discussion of supraventricular arrhythmias with abnormal QRS complexes, Figs. 8-23 and 8-24).

The length of the pause following any premature beat or series of premature beats is determined by the interaction of several factors. If the premature atrial complex occurs when the sinus node is not refractory, the impulse

may conduct to the sinus node, discharge it prematurely, and cause the next sinus cycle to begin from that point. The interval between the two normal beats flanking a premature atrial complex that has reset the timing of the basic sinus rhythm is less than twice the normal cycle, and the pause after the premature atrial complex is said to be "noncompensatory." The interval following the premature atrial complex is generally slightly longer than one sinus cycle, however. Less commonly the premature atrial complex may find the sinus node refractory, in which case the timing of the basic sinus rhythm is not altered, and the interval between the two normal beats flanking the premature atrial complex is twice the normal PP cycle. The interval following this premature atrial discharge is therefore said to be a "full compensatory pause." A *compensatory pause* is one of sufficient duration to make the interval between the two normal beats on each side of the premature beat equal to twice the basic cycle length. However, sinus arrhythmia may lengthen or shorten this pause.

Significance. Premature atrial complexes may occur in a variety of situations: for example, during infection, inflammation, or myocardial ischemia, or they may be provoked by a variety of medications, by tension states, or by tobacco and caffeine. Premature atrial complexes may precipitate or presage the occurrence of a sustained supraventricular tachycardia.

Treatment. In the absence of organic heart disease, treatment may not be necessary, unless the patient complains of symptoms such as palpitations or has recurrent tachycardias or an excessive number of premature atrial complexes. If treatment is indicated, for example, in a patient with acute myocardial infarction, initial therapy should probably be with digitalis, combined with quinidine or procainamide if digitalis alone is not successful. Sedation and/or omission of alcohol, caffeine, or smoking may be helpful in some patients.

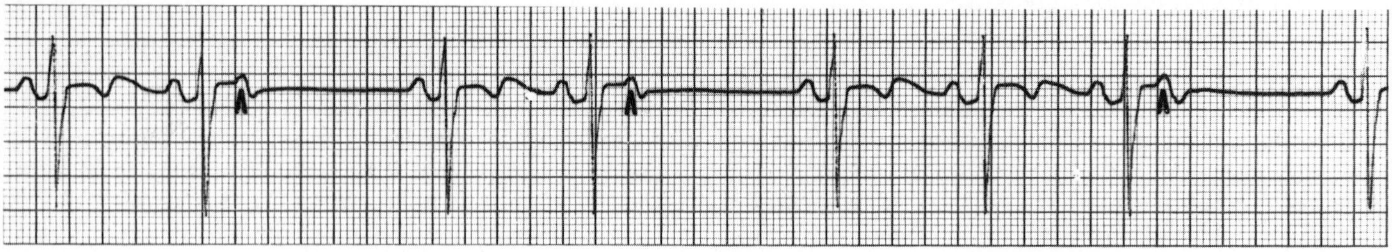

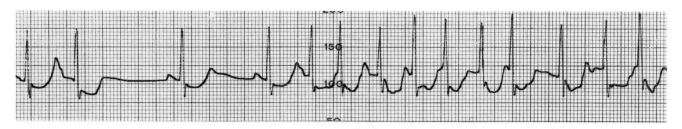

FIG. 8-20.   Premature atrial complexes, blocked and hidden in the T wave. The deformed T waves *(arrows)* indicate a nonconducted premature atrial complex that blocks within the AV node or His bundle. The premature atrial complex discharges the sinus node and delays its return so that the PP interval from the premature atrial complex to the next sinus P wave exceeds the normal sinus PP interval A noncompensatory pulse follows the blocked PACs. Monitor lead.

Rate: 67 beats/minute during sinus rhythm.
Rhythm: Varying because of premature atrial complexes.
P waves: Premature atrial complexes are hidden within and deform the T waves.
PR interval: Of normal sinus beats, 0.18 second.
QRS: 0.10 second.

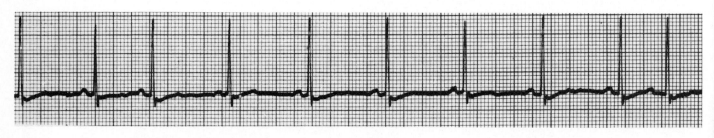

FIG. 8-21.   Premature atrial complex precipitating atrial flutter-fibrillation. A premature atrial complex is hidden within the T wave of the first QRS complex and occurs again in the T wave of the fourth QRS complex. This premature atrial complex precipitates atrial flutter fibrillation. Monitor lead.

Rate: Varying.
Rhythm: Varying due to premature atrial complexes and atrial flutter-fibrillation.
P waves: Premature atrial complexes hidden in the T waves.
PR interval: Of normally conducted beats, 0.14 second.
QRS: 0.08 second.

FIG. 8-22.   Premature atrial complexes. Third and tenth complexes represent premature atrial complexes. Monitor lead.

Rate: 68 beats/minute during sinus rhythm.
Rhythm: Varying due to premature atrial complexes.
P waves: Precede each QRS complex.
QRS interval: 0.06 second.

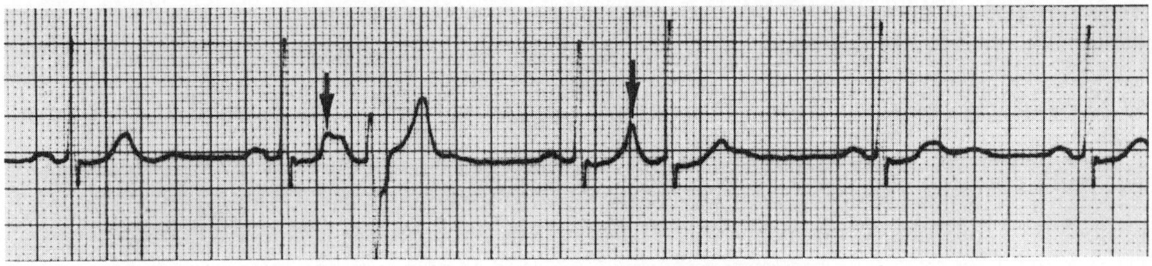

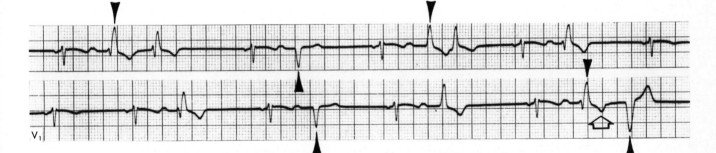

FIG. 8-23. Premature atrial complexes with and without aberrancy. The first premature atrial complex *(arrow)* occurs at a shorter RP interval than does the second premature atrial complex *(arrows)* and conducts with a bundle branch block contour (probably right bundle branch block in this monitor lead). The first premature atrial complex conducts with aberrancy while the second does not because the first reaches the bundle branch system before complete recovery of repolarization.

Rate: 50 beats/minute during the normally conducted complexes.
Rhythm: Irregular because of the premature atrial complexes.
P waves: Normal for the normally conducted sinus beats. Premature atrial complexes deform the T waves.
PR interval: Of premature atrial complexes, prolonged because the AV node and/or His bundle has incompletely recovered. PR interval of first premature atrial complex is approximately 0.26 second and that of the second premature atrial complex approximately 0.22 second. The PR interval of normally conducted sinus beats is 0.19 second.
QRS: Of normally conducted beats, 0.07 second; of aberrantly conducted QRS complex, 0.12 second.

FIG. 8-24. Premature atrial complexes that produce functional right and functional left bundle branch block. Upright arrowheads point to QRS complexes that conduct with complete or incomplete functional left bundle branch block while inverted arrowheads point to some of the QRS complexes that conduct with functional right bundle branch block. Note that the latter have both a monophasic and triphasic contour. The deformed T waves *(open arrow* at the end of the last strip) indicate a premature atrial complex. They occur singly and in pairs.

Rate: Varying because of premature atrial complexes.
Rhythm: Irregular because of premature atrial complexes.
P waves: During sinus rhythm, normal; P waves of premature atrial complexes are hard to discern because they occur in the preceding T wave.
PR interval: Of normal sinus beats, 0.12 second; of premature atrial complexes, prolonged and of differing durations because of differences in RP intervals.

AV NODAL REENTRY (Figs. 8-25 to 8-28)

The tachycardias formerly called paroxysmal atrial (PAT) and junctional (PJT) tachycardias are caused most commonly by AV nodal reentry or reentry over an accessory pathway. They are often called, nonspecifically, paroxysmal supraventricular tachycardia (PSVT) when the mechanism responsible for the tachycardia cannot be determined with certainty (Figs. 8-25 to 8-28). In this section AV nodal reentry is examined. Reentry over an accessory pathway is dealt with in the section on Wolff-Parkinson-White syndrome.

AV nodal reentry is characterized by a rapid, regular tachycardia of sudden onset and termination, occurring at rates generally between 150 and 250 beats/minute. Uncommonly the rate may exceed 250 beats/minute. Unless aberrant ventricular conduction exists, the QRS complex is normal in contour and duration. The retrograde P wave is usually lost within the QRS complex. AV nodal reentry is most commonly caused by reentry within the AV node, anterogradely over a slowly conducting pathway and retrogradely over a more rapidly conducting pathway (Fig. 8-28).

AV nodal reentry recorded at the onset begins abruptly, usually following a premature atrial complex that conducts with a prolonged PR interval; the abrupt termination is sometimes followed by a brief period of asystole, which results in part from tachycardia-induced depression of sinus nodal automaticity. The RR interval may shorten during the course of the first few beats at the onset or lengthen during the course of the last few beats preceding termination of the tachycardia. Variation in cycle length is usually caused by variation in AV nodal conduction time. The mechanism of the tachycardia is reentry within the AV node (see Fig. 8-91).

Significance. AV nodal reentry may occur at any age and is often unassociated with underlying heart disease. The arrhythmia may be related to specific inciting causes such as overexertion, emotional stimuli, and coffee and smoking, although this is often difficult to prove; it may follow a specific pattern, or its onset may be unrelated to any particular event.

Symptoms frequently accompany the attack and range from feelings of palpitations, nervousness, or anxiety to angina, frank heart failure, or shock, depending on the duration and rate of the AV nodal reentry and the presence of organic heart disease. The AV nodal reentry may cause syncope because of the rapid ventricular rate, reduced cardiac output, and cerebral circulation or because of asystole when the AV nodal reentry terminates. The prognosis for patients without heart disease is usually quite good.

Treatment. Treatment of the acute attack depends on the clinical situation, how well the AV nodal reentry is tolerated, the natural history of the attacks in the individual patient, and the presence of associated disease. For some patients, rest, reassurance, and sedation may be all that are required to abort an attack.

1. Simple vagal maneuvers, including carotid sinus massage, Valsalva, and gagging, serve as the first line

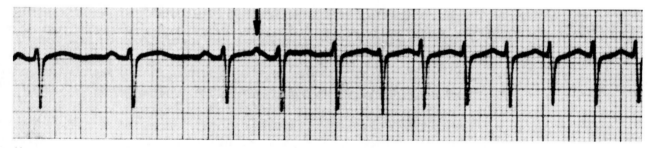

V₁

FIG. 8-25. Paroxysmal supraventricular tachycardia. Three sinus beats are interrupted by a premature atrial complex *(arrow)*, which conducts with PR prolongation and initiates the supraventricular tachycardia.

Rate:	Sinus rhythm, 83 beats/minute; paroxysmal supraventricular tachycardia, 190 beats/minute.
Rhythm:	Regular during sinus rhythm and during paroxysmal supraventricular tachycardia.
P waves:	Seen in first four beats but not afterward.
PR inverval:	Normal during sinus beats, 0.16 second; slightly prolonged (0.20 second) during premature atrial complex.
QRS:	Normal, 0.08 second.
Arrhythmia:	Sudden initiation of paroxysmal supraventricular tachycardia by a premature atrial complex that conducts with PR prolongation. In the absence of a recognizable P wave (probably buried in the QRS complex). The tachycardia is most likely AV nodal reentry.

of therapy and either terminate AV nodal reentry by prolonging AV nodal refractoriness or leave it unaffected (actually, slight slowing may occur during vagal stimulation). These maneuvers should be retried after *each* pharmacologic approach.

2. Verapamil, a calcium antagonist, at a dose of 5 to 10 mg IV, terminates AV nodal reentry successfully in about 2 minutes in over 90% of instances. A second injection may be administered in 30 minutes if necessary. It has become the preferred treatment if the simple vagal maneuvers fail.[13,14]

3. Cholinergic drugs, particularly edrophonium chloride (Tensilon), a shortacting cholinesterase inhibitor, may terminate AV nodal reentry when administered initially at a dose of 3 to 5 mg IV and, if unsuccessful, repeated at a dose of 10 mg IV. Its action is rapid in onset and short in duration, with minimal side effects. Edrophonium chloride should be used cautiously or not at all in patients who are hypotensive or who have lung disease, especially asthmatics.

4. Pressor drugs may terminate AV nodal reentry by inducing reflex vagal stimulation mediated via baroreceptors in the carotid sinus and aorta when the systolic blood pressure is acutely elevated to levels of about 180 mm Hg. One of the following drugs,

diluted in 5 to 10 ml of 5% dextrose and water, may be given over a period of 1 to 3 minutes; phenylephrine hydrochloride (Neo-Synephrine), 0.5 to 1.0 mg; methoxamine hydrochloride (Vasoxyl), 3 to 5 mg; or metaraminol (Aramine), 0.5 to 2.0 mg. Pressor drugs should be used cautiously or not at all in the elderly or in patients with organic heart disease, significant hypertension, hyperthyroidism, or acute myocardial infarction. This potentially dangerous and almost always uncomfortable procedure is rarely needed any longer, unless the patient is also hypotensive. Other, safer procedures are preferred.

5. If these approaches are unsuccessful, IV digitalis administration may be attempted next, using one of the following short-acting digitalis preparations: ouabain, 0.25 to 0.50 mg IV, followed by 0.1 mg every 30 to 60 minutes if needed, keeping the total dose less than 1.0 mg within a 24-hour period; digoxin (Lanoxin), 0.5 to 1.0 mg IV, followed by 0.25 mg every 2 to 4 hours, with a total dose less than 1.5 mg within a 24-hour period; or deslanoside (Cedilanid-D), 0.8 mg IV, followed by 0.4 mg every 2 to 4 hours, restricting the total dose to less than 2.0 mg within a 24-hour period. Oral digitalis administration to terminate an acute attack is generally not indicated. Vagal maneuvers, previously ineffec-

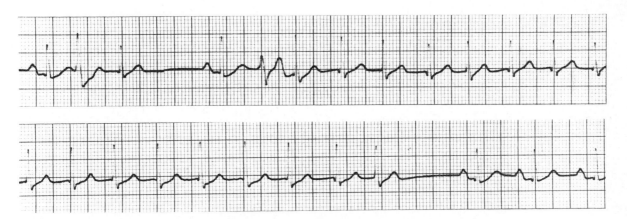

FIG. 8-26.   Initiation of paroxysmal supraventricular tachycardia (PSVT) following a premature ventricular complex and spontaneous termination of PSVT. In the top panel, PSVT begins following the fifth QRS complex, which is a premature ventricular complex (PVC). Two interpretations are possible. The first possibility is that the normally conducted sinus complex occurs in the T wave of the PVC and conducts with a prolonged PR interval (i.e., the PVC is interpolated) and initiates PSVT. The second possibility is that the PVC conducts retrogradely to the atrium and initiates the PSVT in that manner. In the bottom strip, the PSVT terminates spontaneously with a slight pause. Monitor lead.

Rate: During PSVT, 120 beats/minute.
Rhythm: Fairly regular during PSVT.
P waves: Cannot be seen during PSVT.
PR interval: Cannot determine during PSVT.
QRS: Normal, 0.07 second.
Arrhythmia: Probably AV nodal reentry.

tive, may terminate AV nodal reentry following digitalis administration and therefore should be repeated.

6. Propranolol (Inderal) given IV at a rate of 0.5 to 1 mg/minute for a total dose of 1 to 3 mg may be tried if digitalis administration is unsuccessful. Propranolol must be used cautiously, if at all, in patients who have heart failure or chronic lung disease because its adrenergic beta-receptor blocking action depresses myocardial contractility and may produce bronchospasm.

Prior to administering digitalis or propranolol, it is advisable to reassess the clinical status of the patient and consider whether DC cardioversion may be advisable at this stage. DC shock, administered to patients who have received excessive amounts of digitalis, may be dangerous and result in serious postshock ventricular arrhythmias (see Chapter 12 for discussion).

7. Particularly if signs or symptoms of cardiac decompensation occur, DC electrical shock should be attempted next. DC shock, synchronized to the QRS complex to avoid precipitating ventricular fibrillation, successfully terminates AV nodal reentry with energies in the range of 10 to 50 watt-seconds; higher energies may be required in some instances. Short-acting barbiturates like sodium methohexital (Brevital), 50 to 120 mg given IV at a rate of 50 mg/30 seconds, may be used to provide anesthesia, or diazepam (Valium), 5 to 15 mg given IV at a rate of 5 mg/minute, may be used to provide sedation and amnesia. Doses must be individualized and in general should be reduced for patients who have heart failure, hypotension, or liver disease. During DC cardioversion a physician skilled in airway management should be in attendance, an IV route established, and all equipment and drugs necessary for emergency resuscitation immediately accessible. One hundred percent oxygen is administered throughout the procedure, employing manually assisted ventilation if necessary.

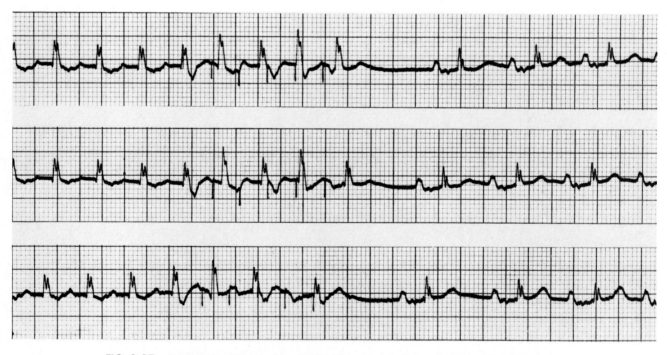

FIG. 8-27. Pacing-induced termination of PSVT. The patient had recurrent episodes of PSVT that were easily terminated by rapid atrial pacing. Pacing stimuli can be seen before the onset of sinus rhythm in the midportion of each monitor lead tracing.

Rate: During PSVT, 150 beats/minute.
Rhythm: During PSVT, regular.
P waves: Not seen during PSVT. P waves during sinus rhythm are abnormal with a low-amplitude biphasic component following an initial positive component.
PR interval: During sinus rhythm, 0.24 second; during PSVT, cannot be discerned.
QRS: 0.08 second.
Arrhythmia: AV nodal reentry (documented by invasive electrophysiologic study).

If DC shock becomes necessary in patients who have received large amounts of digitalis, one should begin with 1 to 5 watt-seconds and gradually increase the energy level in increments of approximately 25 to 50 watt-seconds as long as premature ventricular systoles do not result. If premature ventricular systoles occur but can be suppressed with lidocaine or phenytoin, the next higher energy level may be tried.

8. In the event that digitalis has been given in large doses and DC shock is contraindicated, right atrial pacing may restore sinus rhythm, presumably by prematurely depolarizing one of the pathways required for continued reentry (Fig. 8-27). In some patients, right atrial pacing may precipitate atrial fibrillation; however, because the latter is generally accompanied by a slower ventricular rate, the patient's clinical status improves.

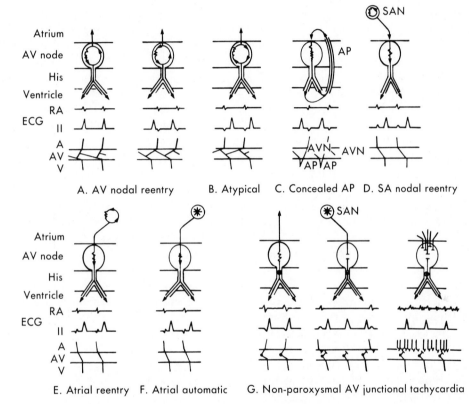

FIG. 8-28. Diagrammatic representation of various tachycardias. In the top portion of each example is a schematic representation of the presumed anatomic pathways. In the lower portion the ECG presentation in the explanatory ladder diagram is depicted. A, AV nodal reentry. *Left,* reentrant excitation is confined to the AV node with retrograde atrial activity occurring simultaneously with ventricular activity, owing to anterograde conduction over the slow AV nodal pathway and retrograde conduction over the fast AV nodal pathway. *Right,* atrial activity occurs slightly later than ventricular activity, owing to retrograde conduction delay. B, Atypical AV nodal reentry as a result of anterograde conduction over a fast AV nodal pathway and retrograde conduction over a slow AV nodal pathway. C, Concealed accessory pathway (AP). Reciprocating tachycardia is caused by anterograde conduction over the AV node and retrograde conduction over the accessory pathway. Retrograde P waves occur after the QRS complex. D, Sinus nodal reentry. The tachycardia occurs as a result of reentry within the sinus node, which then conducts to the rest of the heart. E, Atrial reentry. Tachycardia is caused by reentry within the atrium, which then conducts to the rest of the heart. F, Automatic atrial tachycardia. Tachycardia is result of automatic discharge in the atrium, which then conducts to the rest of the heart. It is difficult to distinguish this tachycardia from tachycardia caused by atrial reentry. G, Nonparoxysmal AV junctional tachycardia. Various presentations of this tachycardia are depicted with retrograde atrial capture, AV dissociation with the sinus node in control of the atria, and AV dissociation with atrial fibrillation. (From Zipes, D.P.: Specific arrhythmias: diagnosis and treatment. In Braunwald, E., editor: Heart disease: textbook of cardiovascular medicine, Philadelphia, 1984, W.B. Saunders Company.)

9. Procainamide (Pronestyl), quinidine, or disopyramide (Norpace) may be required to terminate AV nodal reentry in some patients. Unless contraindicated, DC cardioversion should be employed prior to using these agents, which are more often administered to prevent recurrences.

Prevention of recurrences is often more difficult than terminating the acute episode. Smoking, alcohol, or excessive fatigue, if identified as precipitating factors, should be avoided. Initially, one must decide whether the frequency and severity of the attacks warrant drug prophylaxis. For example, an attempt should probably not be made to suppress AV nodal reentry occurring twice yearly in an otherwise healthy patient.

1. If drug prophylaxis is indicated, digitalis is the initial drug of choice. The speed at which digitalization is achieved is determined by the clinical situation. Using digoxin, rapid oral digitalization can be accomplished in 24 to 36 hours with an initial dose of 1.0 to 1.5 mg, followed by 0.25 to 0.5 mg every 6 hours for a total dose of 2.0 to 3.0 mg. A less rapid oral regimen digitalizes in 2 to 3 days with an initial dose of 0.75 to 1.0 mg, followed by 0.25 to 0.5 mg every 12 hours for a total dose of 2.0 to 3.0 mg. Alternatively, digoxin administered as a maintenance dose of 0.125 to 0.5 mg achieves digitalization in about 1 week. Because of its shorter half-life, digoxin may provide more effective control when administered twice daily. Digitoxin, which has a longer duration of action, may be used instead of digoxin. Oral digitalization with digitoxin may be accomplished in 24 to 36 hours with an initial dose of 0.5 to 0.8 mg, followed by 0.2 mg every 6 to 8 hours until reaching a total dose of 1.2 mg. A slower approach involves administering 0.2 mg three times daily for 2 to 3 days. Complete digitalization can also be accomplished in about 1 month by simply giving a maintenance dose of 0.05 to 0.2 mg daily.

2. If digitalis alone is unsuccessful, one can then add quinidine, 200 to 400 mg every 6 hours, or propranolol (Inderal), 10 to 40 mg every 6 hours. Verapamil (80 to 120 mg every 6 to 8 hours) combined with digitalis may be very effective treatment.

3. If a combination of digitalis and quinidine or digitalis and propranolol is unsuccessful, concomitant administration of all three drugs, that is, digitalis, quinidine, and propranolol, may be tried. If this regimen also fails, empiric trials with other antiarrhythmic agents such as procainamide or disopyramide may be warranted. Flecainide or amiodarone often is effective in patients with supraventricular tachycardia but is investigational for that purpose.

4. For many patients, pacemaker implantation is an acceptable treatment. Rapid atrial pacing promptly terminates AV nodal reentry, restoring sinus rhythm immediately or sometimes after a transient episode of atrial fibrillation. Some pacemaker units need to be activated by the patient when AV nodal reentry occurs; other units discharge automatically when they detect the onset of AV nodal reentry. Such pacing devices can be combined with drug therapy (see Chapter 11).

5. Ablation of the AV node–His bundle area by catheter or surgical techniques may be indicated on occasion to eliminate episodes of the tachycardia. Such an approach may make the patient pacemaker-dependent if complete AV heart block results.

PREEXCITATION (WOLFF-PARKINSON-WHITE) SYNDROME (Figs. 8-29 to 8-38)

Ventricular preexcitation[1,8,15] exists when the atrial impulse activates the whole or some part of ventricular muscle earlier than would be expected if the atrial impulse reached the ventricles by way of the normal specialized conduction system only. Four basic features typify the usual ECG of a patient with the preexcitation (Wolff-Parkinson-White) syndrome: (1) PR interval less than 0.12 second during sinus rhythm, (2) QRS complex duration greater than 0.12 second with a slurred, slow-rising onset of the R wave upstroke in some leads (delta wave) and usually normal terminal QRS portion, (3) secondary ST-T wave changes that are usually directed opposite the major delta and QRS vectors, and (4) paroxysmal tachyarrhythmias in many patients (the exact percentage varies widely, from 4% to 80%, and depends on the patient population studied). The ex-

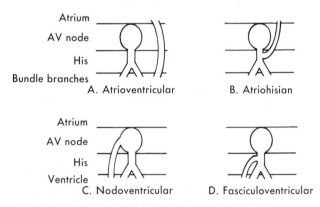

FIG. 8-29.   Schematic representation of accessory pathways. A, The usual atrioventricular connection often called a Kent bundle. B, Atriohisian bypass tract in which the connection is from the atrium to the His bundle, thus bypassing the AV node. C, Nodoventricular connection from the AV node to the ventricle. D, Fasciculoventricular connection from the His bundle or bundle branches to the ventricle. (From Zipes, D.P.: Specific arrhythmias: Diagnosis and treatment. In Braunwald, E., editor: Heart disease: a textbook of cardiovascular medicine, Philadelphia, 1984, W.B. Saunders Company.)

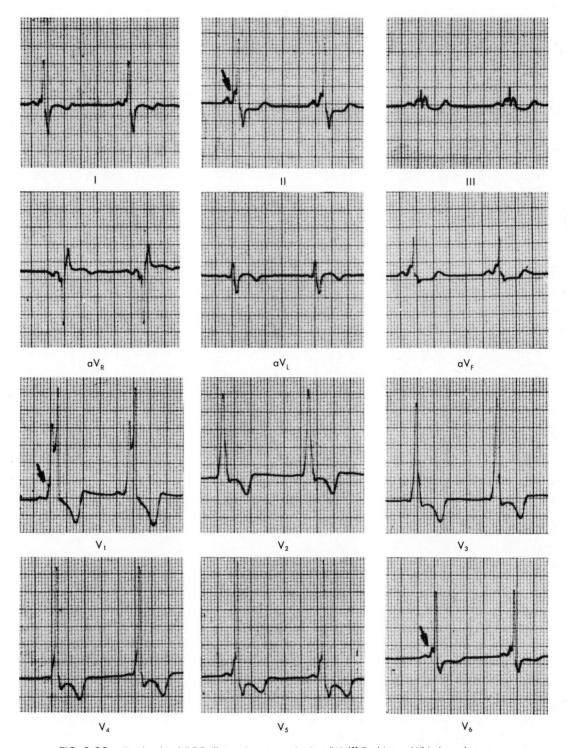

I   II   III

aV_R   aV_L   aV_F

V_1   V_2   V_3

V_4   V_5   V_6

FIG. 8-30.   Twelve-lead ECG illustrating preexcitation (Wolff-Parkinson-White) syndrome. Arrows indicate delta waves. The short PR interval is apparent. The vector of the delta wave suggests that the accessory pathway is in a left anterior (position 9) or left anterior paraseptal (position 10) position. See Fig 8-34 for position.

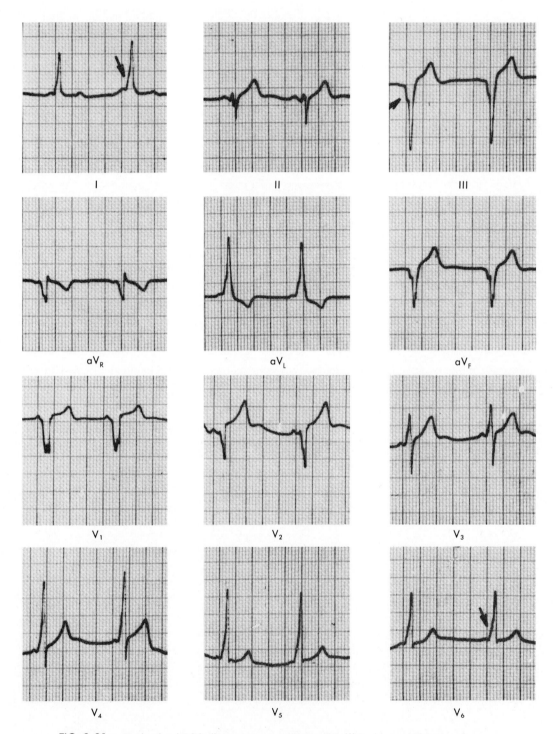

FIG. 8-31. Twelve-lead ECG illustrating preexcitation (Wolff-Parkinson-White) syndrome. Arrows indicate delta waves. The short PR interval is apparent. The vector of the delta wave suggests accessory pathway is located in a right lateral (area 3) position (see Fig. 8-34).

planation for those ECG findings is the presence of a rapidly-conducting muscular accessory pathway connection that bypasses the AV node by communicating directly from atrium to ventricle. Other patients may possess variants of the preexcitation syndrome that are explained by the presence of bypass tracts between the AV node and ventricle (nodoventricular) or between the fascicles and ventricle (fasciculoventricular). The group of patients who have a short PR interval (less than 0.12 second) and a normal QRS complex with supraventricular tachycardias most often do not have a bypass tract from atrium to His bundle (so-called Lown-Ganong-Levine syndrome). These patients may simply possess an AV node that conducts rapidly and also have episodes of supraventricular tachycardia (Fig. 8-29).

The site of the accessory pathway can be determined by a careful analysis of the spatial direction of the delta wave in maximally preexcited QRS complexes (Fig. 8-34), as well as from electrical recordings made directly on the heart using catheters during an electrophysiologic study or at the time of open heart surgery. Once identified, the accessory pathway can be interrupted surgically or by other ablation techniques.

Because of the accessory pathway, two parallel routes of AV conduction are possible, one subject to physiologic delay over the AV node and the other passing directly without delay over the accessory pathway from atrium to ventricle. This produces the typical QRS complex that is a fusion beat caused by depolarization of the ventricle in part by the wavefront traveling over the accessory pathway and in part by the wavefront traveling over the normal AV node–His bundle route. The delta wave represents ventricular activation from input over the accessory pathway. The extent of contribution to ventricular depolarization by the wavefront over each route depends upon the relative activation time of each wavefront.

The usual tachycardia is characterized by anterograde conduction over the normal pathway and retrograde conduction over the accessory pathway, which results in a normal QRS complex at rates of 150 to 250/minute. Because the reentrant loop involves atria and ventricles, the tachycardia is called an atrioventricular reciprocating tachycardia (AVRT). In contrast to most patients who have AV nodal reentry, the retrograde P wave during AVRT occurs in the ST segment.

The rhythm of AVRT may change spontaneously into atrial flutter or atrial fibrillation, and patients with Wolff-Parkinson-White syndrome may have other types of tachycardia as well. Patients who have atrial fibrillation almost always have AVRT that can be induced during electrophysiologic study. Atrial fibrillation presents a potentially serious risk because of the possibility for rapid conduction over the accessory pathway and rapid ventricular rates. On occasion, ventricular fibrillation may result.

Significance. The reported incidence of the preexcitation syndrome averages about 1.5 in 1000 persons, although the actual incidence is unknown. It occurs in all age groups and more often (60% to 70%) in males. Two thirds of patients with the short PR interval and normal QRS complex are female. Patients may seek help because of recurrent supraventricular tachycardia, atrial fibrillation with a rapid ventricular response, heart failure, syncope, or symptoms related to associated cardiac anomalies; or the symptoms may be discovered during examination for

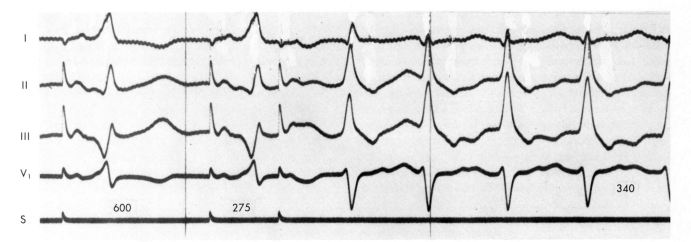

FIG. 8-32.   Onset of reciprocating tachycardia in a patient with preexcitation (WPW) syndrome. The first two beats are paced from the right atrium (cycle length 600 msec) and conduct over the accessory pathway. The third beat is premature (275 msec) and conducts over the normal AV node–His bundle (note loss of delta wave). Following this a reciprocating tachycardia in a patient with Wolff-Parkinson-White syndrome. S, Stimulus.

noncardiac-related reasons. Of adults with preexcitation syndrome, 60% to 70% have normal hearts; a higher proportion of children have heart disease. A variety of acquired and congenital cardiac defects have been reported in patients with the preexcitation syndrome, including Ebstein's anomaly, cardiomyopathies, and mitral valve prolapse.

Of patients with the preexcitation syndrome who have recurrent tachyarrhythmias, 80% have AVRT, 15% to 30% have atrial fibrillation, and 5% have atrial flutter. Ventricular tachycardia rarely occurs, and most reports have misdiagnosed as ventricular tachycardia the aberrant QRS complexes caused by anomalous conduction. Recognition of the preexcitation syndrome is clinically important, since the tachyarrhythmias at times do not respond to conventional therapy and may be associated with very rapid ventricular rates. For example, digitalis may accelerate the ventricular rate in some patients who have atrial fibrillation and the WPW syndrome. The anomalous complexes may mask or mimic myocardial infarction, bundle branch block, or ventricular hypertrophy, and the presence of the preexcitation syndrome may call attention to an associated cardiac defect.

The prognosis is excellent in patients without tachycardia or associated cardiac anomaly. In most patients with recurrent tachycardia the prognosis is good, but sudden unexpected death can occur, especially when the ventricular rate during atrial fibrillation is rapid or associated congenital defects are present. Ventricular fibrillation has been

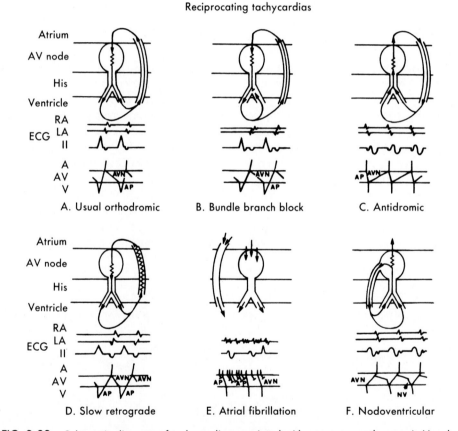

Reciprocating tachycardias

A. Usual orthodromic B. Bundle branch block C. Antidromic

D. Slow retrograde E. Atrial fibrillation F. Nodoventricular

FIG. 8-33. Schematic diagram of tachycardia associated with accessory pathways. A, Usual (orthodromic) form of tachycardia with anterograde conduction over the AV node–His bundle route and retrograde conduction over the accessory pathway (left-sided as depicted here by left atrial activation preceding right atrial activation). B, Usual (orthodromic) form of tachycardia and functional bundle branch block on the same side as the accessory pathway. C, Unusual (antidromic) form of tachycardia with anterograde conduction over the accessory pathway and retrograde conduction over the AV node–His bundle route. D, Orthodromic tachycardia with a slowly conducting accessory pathway. E, Atrial fibrillation conducting over the accessory pathway and the AV node. F, Nodoventricular tachycardia with anterograde conduction over a portion of the AV node and a nodoventricular pathway and retrograde conduction over the AV node. (From Zipes, D.P.: Specific arrhythmias: Diagnosis and treatment. In Braunwald, E., editor: Heart disease: a textbook of cardiovascular medicine, Philadelphia, 1984, W.B. Saunders Company.)

documented in humans and in dogs with WPW syndrome and is probably caused by extremely rapid ventricular rates, permitted by the bypass during atrial flutter or fibrillation that exceed the ability of the ventricle to follow in an organized fashion. Consequently, fragmented, disorganized ventricular activation results and leads to ventricular fibrillation. Alternatively, supraventricular discharge, bypassing the AV nodal delay, may activate the ventricle during the vulnerable period of the antecedent T wave and precipitate ventricular fibrillation.

Treatment.[7,9,15] Patients with ventricular preexcitation who have none or only occasional episodes of tachyarrhythmias unassociated with significant symptoms do not require electrophysiologic evaluation or therapy. However, if the patient has frequent episodes of tachyarrhythmias and/or the arrhythmias cause significant symptoms, therapy should be instituted.

Drugs that increase the refractory period, slow conduction, or cause block in one of the reentrant pathways may suppress reciprocating tachycardia. Verapamil, pro-

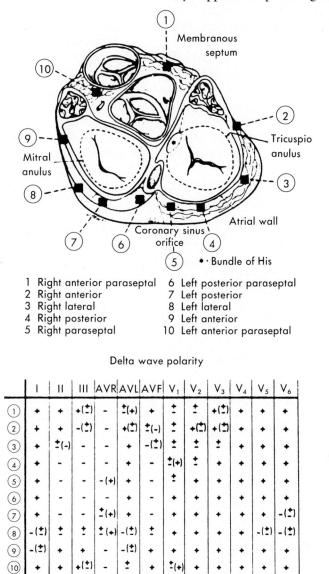

1 Right anterior paraseptal
2 Right anterior
3 Right lateral
4 Right posterior
5 Right paraseptal
6 Left posterior paraseptal
7 Left posterior
8 Left lateral
9 Left anterior
10 Left anterior paraseptal

Delta wave polarity

	I	II	III	AVR	AVL	AVF	V1	V2	V3	V4	V5	V6
1	+	+	+(±)	-	±(+)	+	±	±	+(±)	+	+	+
2	+	+	-(±)	-	+(±)	±(-)	±	+(±)	+(±)	+	+	+
3	+	±(-)	-	-	+	-(±)	±	±	±	+	+	+
4	+	-	-	-	+	-	±(+)	±	+	+	+	+
5	+	-	-	-(+)	+	-	±	+	+	+	+	+
6	+	-	-	-	+	-	+	+	+	+	+	+
7	+	-	-	±(+)	+	-	+	+	+	+	+	-(±)
8	-(±)	±	±	±(+)	-(±)	±	+	+	+	+	-(±)	-(±)
9	-(±)	+	+	-	-(±)	+	+	+	+	+	+	+
10	+	+	+(±)	-	±	+	±(+)	+	+	+	+	+

± · Initial 40 msec delta isoelectric
+ · Initial 40 msec delta positive
- · Initial 40 msec delta negative

FIG. 8-34. In this schematic representation *(top)*, sites of the potential position of the accessory pathways are indicated by filled boxes numbered 1 through 10. Delta wave polarity in the 12-lead ECG for each of the 10 sites is depicted in the table at the bottom. (From Gallagher, J.J., et al.: The preexcitation syndromes, Prog. Cardiovasc. Dis. 20:285, 1978.)

pranolol, and digitalis prolong conduction time and refractoriness in the AV node. Verapamil and propranolol do not directly affect conduction in the accessory pathway, whereas digitalis has variable effects. However, because digitalis has been reported to shorten refractoriness in the accessory pathway and speed the ventricular response in some patients with atrial fibrillation, it is advisable not to use digitalis as a single drug in patients with the WPW syndrome who have or may develop atrial flutter or atrial fibrillation. Since many patients may develop atrial flutter or fibrillation during the reciprocating tachycardia, the caveat about digitalis probably applies to all patients who have tachycardia and the WPW syndrome.

Drugs, such as quinidine (see table), that prolong the refractory period in the accessory pathway should be used to treat patients with atrial flutter or fibrillation. Lidocaine does not prolong refractoriness of the accessory pathway in patients whose effective refractory period is less than 300 msec. Verapamil and lidocaine given intravenously may increase the ventricular rate during atrial fibrillation in patients with the WPW syndrome.

DRUG THERAPY IN WPW SYNDROME		
Affects AV node	Affects accessory pathway	Affects both
Digitalis	Quinidine	Flecainide
Propranolol	Procainamide	Encainide
Verapamil	Disopyramide	Amiodarone
Vagal stimulation		

Termination of the acute episode of AVRT, suspected electrocardiographically by a normal QRS complex, regular RR intervals at rate of about 200 beats/minute, and a P wave in the ST segment, should be approached as for AV nodal reentry. For atrial flutter or fibrillation, drugs that prolong refractoriness in the accessory pathway—often coupled with drugs that prolong AV nodal refractoriness (for example, quinidine and propranolol) or a drug that affects both pathways (for example, encainide or amio-

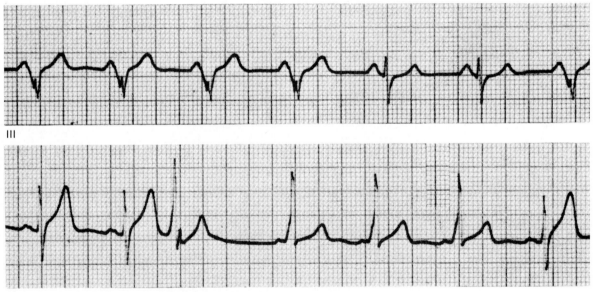

III

V₃

FIG. 8-35.   Preexcitation (Wolff-Parkinson-White) syndrome. Spontaneous onset and termination of preexcitation conduction account for the variable QRS conduction in lead III and V₃. The fifth and sixth QRS complexes in III and the first, second, and last QRS complexes in V₃ are normally conducted. In lead V₃ the onset of anomalous conduction follows a premature atrial complex (third QRS) with a Wolff-Parkinson-White pattern. This patient was erroneously admitted to the coronary care unit because of the Q waves in lead III, which were misinterpreted as indicating an inferior myocardial infarction.

Rate:	78 beats/minute.
Rhythm:	Regular.
P waves:	Normal.
PR interval:	Varies between 0.10 and 0.13 second.
QRS:	Normal (0.08 second) during conduction over the AV node with a normal PR interval; abnormal (0.12 second) during conduction over the bypass tract with a short PR interval.

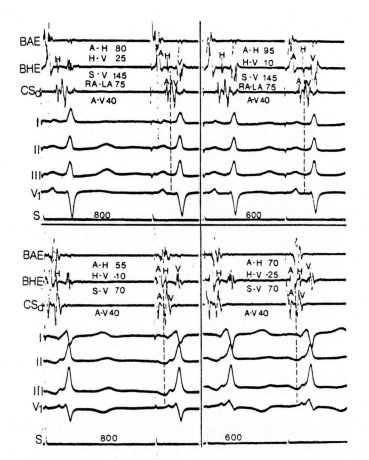

FIG. 8-36. Influence of pacing site and cycle length on the degree of preexcitation. In this patient with a left anterolateral accessory pathway (site 9 in FIG. 8-34), pacing the high right atrium at a cycle length of 800 msec *(top left panel)* produced an A-H interval of 80 msec and an H-V interval of 25 msec. The interval from the stimulus to the onset of ventricular activity *(S-V)* was 145 msec and the right-to-left atrial activation time was 75 msec. The interrupted line indicates the onset of the delta wave. Little preexcitation is seen in the ECG because the fairly rapid AV conduction time over the normal pathway allows much of the ventricle to be activated normally before the impulse traveling from right to left atrium and then over the accessory pathway can depolarize the ventricles. Shortening the pacing cycle length to 600 msec *(top right panel)* without changing the pacing site lengthened the A-H interval by 15 msec and shortened the H-V interval by 10 msec. The other intervals remained the same and the QRS complex changed very slightly. The coronary sinus is paced at a cycle length of 800 msec *(bottom left panel)*. Even though the A-H interval shortens to 55 msec because of coronary sinus pacing, the S-V shortens to 70 msec, His bundle activation follows the onset of ventricular depolarization by 10 msec, and the QRS complex becomes more aberrant. By pacing at a site near the atrial insertion of the accessory pathway, conduction rapidly reaches the ventricle over the accessory pathway to activate more of the ventricle than when pacing the right atrium at the same cycle length. Shortening the pacing cycle length to 600 msec *(bottom right panel)* lengthens the A-H interval 15 msec, and His bundle activation begins 25 msec after the onset of QRS complex. S-V and A-V intervals remain unchanged and the QRS complex becomes even more aberrant. (From Zipes, D.P.: Specific arrhythmias: diagnosis and treatment. In Braunwald, E., editor: Heart disease: a textbook of cardiovascular medicine, Philadelphia, 1984, W.B. Saunders Company.)

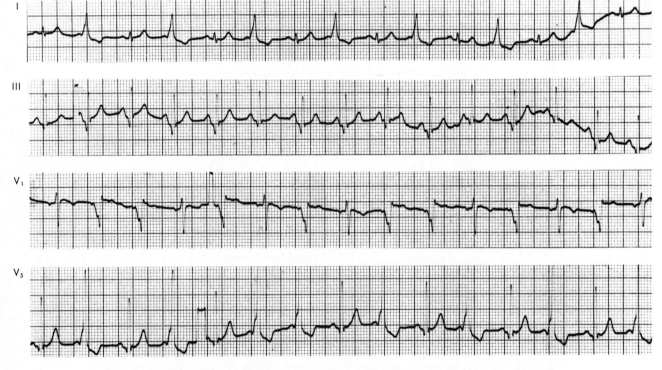

FIG. 8-37. Alternating conduction over the accessory pathway in preexcitation (Wolff-Parkinson-White) syndrome during normal sinus rhythm. Almost throughout the recording, the QRS complexes alternate between conduction over the accessory pathway and conduction over the normal pathway. Occasionally two consecutive beats conduct over the accessory pathway. Conduction over the accessory pathway is characterized by a short PR interval, delta wave, prolonged QRS duration, and secondary T wave changes. Such intermittent conduction over an accessory pathway suggests that its refractory period is prolonged and implies that extremely rapid rates during atrial flutter or atrial fibrillation, as seen in Fig. 8-38, would not occur.

Rate:	105 beats/minute.
Rhythm:	Regular.
P waves:	Normal.
PR interval:	Alternating between 0.08 and 0.12 second.
QRS:	Normal, 0.06 second during conduction over the AV node and abnormal, 0.12 second, during conduction over the accessory pathway.

darone)—must be used. In some patients, particularly those with a very rapid ventricular response during atrial fibrillation, electrical cardioversion should be the initial treatment of choice.

For long-term therapy to prevent a recurrence, drugs are selected on the basis of their effects on the AV node or accessory pathway. Invasive electrophysiologic studies are often necessary.

Some patients may require surgical ablation of the accessory pathway, particularly when symptomatic tachyarrhythmias are recurrent or incompletely controlled by drugs or are associated with rapid ventricular rates. Improved surgical techniques now permit surgery as a logical therapy for a young person who would otherwise face many years of drug management.

For patients who are symptomatic because of drug-refractory, recurrent tachycardia, surgery to interrupt the accessory pathway has been extremely useful.[7]

It is now known that some patients who have supraventricular tachycardia without any overt evidence of WPW may have an accessory pathway that only conducts retrogradely (concealed WPW).[15] The surface ECG during AVRT may provide some clues about the presence of a concealed accessory pathway by demonstrating the retrograde P wave to be in the ST segment (rather than simultaneous with the QRS, as in AV nodal reentry) and, if the accessory pathway is left-sided, a negative P wave in lead I. Naturally, the short PR interval, delta wave, and prolonged QRS duration during sinus rhythm are not present.

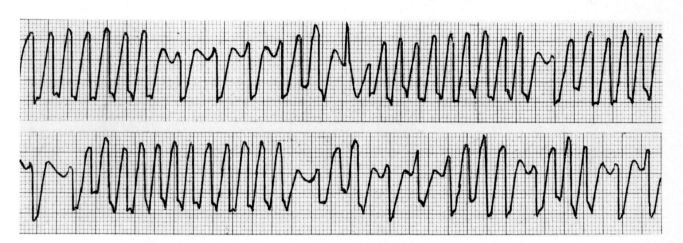

FIG. 8-38.   Atrial fibrillation with an extremely rapid ventricular response in a patient who has preexcitation (Wolff-Parkinson-White) syndrome. In this monitor lead the extremely rapid ventricular rates and gross irregularity of the RR intervals (remember, ventricular tachycardia can be irregular also; see Fig. 8-57) suggest the diagnosis of atrial fibrillation in a patient who has Wolff-Parkinson-White syndrome. The atrial fibrillatory impulses conduct to the ventricle over the accessory pathway, bypassing the AV node.

Rate: Atrial, indeterminant; ventricular, 150 to 350 beats/minute.
Rhythm: Irregular.
P waves: Cannot be seen.
PR interval: Cannot be determined.
QRS: Difficult to determine, but approximately 0.12 to 0.14 second.

ATRIAL FLUTTER (Figs. 8-39 to 8-42)

Atrial flutter is an atrial tachyarrhythmia characterized electrocardiographically by identically recurring, regular, sawtooth-shaped flutter waves and evidence of continual electrical activity (lack of an isoelectric interval between flutter waves), often best visualized in leads II, III, aV_F, or V_1. Commonly the flutter waves appear inverted in these leads. Less commonly the flutter waves are upright (positive) in these leads. In most instances, reentry in the atria causes atrial flutter. If the AV conduction ratio remains constant, the ventricular rhythm will be regular; if the ratio of conducted beats varies (usually the result of a Wenckebach AV block), the ventricular rhythm will be irregular. Impure flutter (flutter-fibrillation), occurring at a faster rate than pure flutter, shows variability in the contour and spacing of the flutter waves and may represent dissimilar atrial rhythms, that is, fibrillation in one atrium or part of the atrium and a slower, more regular rhythm in the opposite atrium.

The atrial rate during atrial flutter is usually 250 to 350 beats/minute; antiarrhythmic drugs such as quinidine or procainamide may reduce the rate to 200 beats/minute. In patients who have untreated atrial flutter the ventricular rate is usually half the atrial rate, that is, 150 beats/minute. A significantly slower ventricular rate (in the absence of drugs) suggests abnormal AV conduction. Atrial flutter in children, in patients who have the preexcitation syndrome or hyperthyroidism, and occasionally in otherwise normal adults may conduct to the ventricle in a 1:1 fashion, producing a ventricular rate of 300 beats/minute. In patients whose atrial flutter rate has been slowed by drugs, 1:1 conduction to the ventricle may also occur.

Significance. Atrial flutter is a less common tachyarrhythmia than is atrial fibrillation. Although paroxysmal atrial flutter usually indicates the presence of cardiac disease, it may occur in normal hearts. Chronic (persistent) atrial flutter rarely occurs in the absence of underlying heart disease. Atrial flutter usually responds to carotid sinus massage with a decrease in ventricular rate in stepwise multiples, reversing to the former ventricular rate at the termination of carotid massage. The ratio of conducted atrial impulses to ventricular responses is most often of an even number, for example, 2:1 or 4:1. Very rarely will sinus rhythm follow carotid sinus massage. Exercise, by enhancing sympathetic tone, lessening parasympathetic tone, or both, may reduce the AV conduction delay and produce an increase in the ventricular rate.

Treatment. Treatment for atrial flutter, aimed at slowing the ventricular rate, is as follows:

1. Synchronous DC cardioversion is commonly the preferred initial treatment for atrial flutter, since it promptly and effectively restores sinus rhythm with energies less than 50 watt-seconds. If DC shock results in atrial fibrillation, a second shock with a higher energy level may be used to restore sinus rhythm, or, depending on the clinical circumstance, the atrial fibrillation may be left untreated. The untreated fibrillation will usually revert to atrial flutter or sinus rhythm.

2. If the patient cannot be cardioverted or the DC cardioversion is contraindicated (for example, after administering large amounts of digitalis), rapid atrial pacing can effectively terminate atrial flutter in many patients.

3. If the patient cannot be cardioverted or if the atrial flutter recurs at frequent intervals, therapy with a short-acting digitalis preparation, such as digoxin should be prescribed. The dose of digitalis necessary to slow the ventricular response varies and at times may result in toxic levels because it is often difficult to slow the ventricular rate during atrial flutter. Frequently, atrial fibrillation develops after digitalization and may revert to normal sinus rhythm on withdrawal of digitalis; occasionally, normal sinus rhythm may occur without intervening atrial fibrillation.

4. Verapamil, in an initial bolus of 5 to 10 mg IV followed by a constant infusion at a rate of 0.005 mg/kg/minute, may be used to slow the ventricular response. Verapamil less commonly restores sinus rhythm in patients who have atrial flutter.

5. If the atrial flutter persists after digitalization, quinidine, 200 to 400 mg orally every 6 hours, is used to restore sinus rhythm. Large doses of quinidine, formerly used to terminate atrial flutter prior to the development of DC cardioversion, are no longer warranted. If atrial flutter persists after digitalis and quinidine administration, termination may be attempted with DC cardioversion and the patient maintained on both digitalis and quinidine following reversion to sinus rhythm. Sometimes, treatment of the specific, underlying disorder, for example, thyrotoxicosis, is necessary to effect conversion to sinus rhythm.

6. In certain instances atrial flutter may continue, and if the ventricular rate can be controlled with digitalis, conversion may not be indicated. Quinidine maintenance therapy should be discontinued if flutter remains. It is important to remember that quinidine and procainamide should *not* be used unless the patient is fully digitalized. Both drugs have a vagolytic action and also directly slow the atrial rate. These two effects may facilitate AV conduction sufficiently to result in a 1:1 ventricular response to the atrial flutter, unless digitalis has been administered previously.

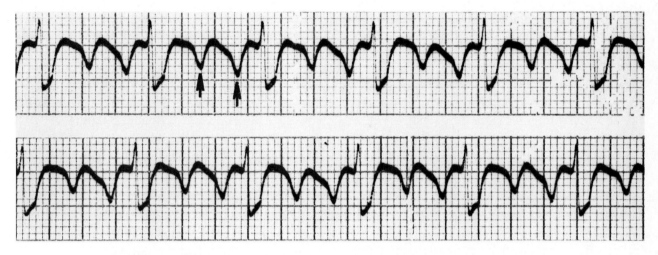

FIG. 8-39.   Atrial flutter. Flutter waves indicated by arrows. The conduction ratio is 3:1, that is, three flutter waves to one QRS complex and is a less common conduction ratio than is 2:1 or 4:1. Monitor lead.

Rate: Atrial, 270 beats/minute; ventricular, 90 beats/minute
Rhythm: Atrial, regular; ventricular, regular.
P waves: Flutter waves with regular oscillations resembling a sawtooth pattern are apparent.
PR interval: Flutter-R interval is constant. Assuming that the flutter wave immediately preceding the QRS complex conducts to the ventricle, the flutter-R interval is approximately 0.18 second.
QRS: 0.12 second.

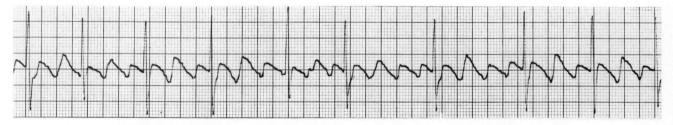

FIG. 8-40.   Atrial flutter rate slowed by an antiarrhythmic agent. The atrial flutter in this patient had a rate of 300 beats/minute before therapy but was slowed by an experimental antiarrhythmic agent, amiodarone. Monitor lead.

Rate: Atrial, 220 beats/minute; ventricular, 52 to 86 beats/minute.
Rhythm: Atrial, regular; ventricular, irregular.
P waves: Flutter waves are apparent.
PR interval: The flutter-R interval varies as the conduction ratio varies.
QRS: Normal, 0.08 second.

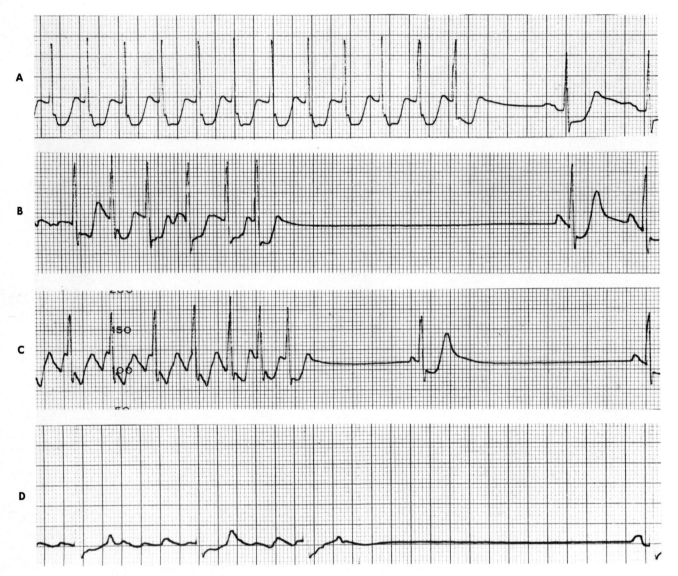

FIG. 8-41. Termination of multiple supraventricular tachycardias. In panel A, paroxysmal supraventricular tachycardia abruptly terminates with only a short pause before restoration of sinus rhythm. In panels B and C, atrial flutter-fibrillation and pure atrial flutter, respectively, terminate on separate occasions in the same patient. In panel B, a fairly long period of asystole results before restoration of the first sinus beat while the lengthy pause is interrupted by an escape beat in panel C. In panel D, termination of atrial flutter-fibrillation in another patient results in a long period of asystole before the first sinus beat occurs. The long pauses in B, C, and D are consistent with sick sinus syndrome and episodes of bradycardia-tachycardia. Monitor leads.

Rate:	158 beats/minute in panel A; varying ventricular rate, approximately 150 beats/minute in panel B; 136 beats/minute in panel C; 48 beats/minute in panel D.
Rhythm:	Atrial and ventricular rhythm regular in panel A; atrial and ventricular rhythm irregular in panel B; atrial rhythm regular and ventricular rhythm irregular in panel C; atrial rhythm and ventricular rhythm irregular in panel D.
PR interval:	Not measurable.
QRS:	Normal in all panels.

7. Propranolol effectively diminishes the ventricular response to atrial flutter and may be used together with digitalis in patients in whom the ventricular rate is not decreased after digitalization. Propranolol does not appear to affect the atrial rate during atrial flutter.

8. Uncommonly, atrial flutter may be resistant to cardioversion as well as to the AV blocking effects of digitalis. Rapid atrial pacing, on a temporary or permanent basis, may be used to convert flutter to fibrillation with a decrease in the ventricular rate.

9. Rarely, neostigmine (Prostigmin), 0.25 to 0.5 mg subcutaneously, or edrophonium (Tensilon), 0.25 to 2.0 mg/minute in an IV solution, may be administered over a few days to control the ventricular rate.

Prevention of recurrent atrial flutter is often difficult to achieve but should be approached as outlined for the prevention of PSVT caused by AV nodal reentry. If recurrences cannot be prevented, the aim of therapy is directed toward a controlled ventricular rate when the flutter does recur, with digitalis alone or combined with propranolol, or with oral verapamil.

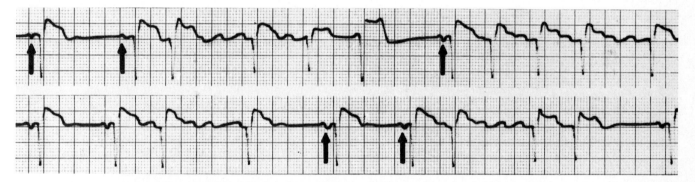

FIG. 8-42.   Intermittent atrial flutter. Atrial flutter starts and stops intermittently throughout this continuous recording. Monitor lead.

Rate and rhythm:	Both atrial and ventricular rate and rhythm vary.
P waves:	Precede some QRS complexes. Atrial flutter waves precede other QRS complexes. Several P waves indicated by arrows.
PR interval:	0.14 second when it can be measured.
QRS:	0.08 second.

ATRIAL FIBRILLATION
(Figs. 8-43 and 8-44)

Atrial fibrillation is characterized by a total disorganization of atrial activity without effective atrial contraction. The ECG reveals small deflections appearing for the most part as irregular base-line undulations of variable amplitude and contour at a rate of 305 to 600/minute. The ventricular response is totally irregular, and if the patient is untreated, the rate is usually between 100 and 160 beats/minute. Carotid sinus massage slows the ventricular rate, but the ventricular rhythm remains completely irregular. The conversion of atrial flutter to atrial fibrillation is usually accompanied by a *slowing* of the ventricular rate because more atrial impulses become blocked at the AV node. As a result, it is generally easier to slow the ventricular rate with digitalis during atrial fibrillation than during atrial flutter. When the ventricular rhythm becomes regular in patients with atrial fibrillation, four explanations are possible: conversion to sinus rhythm, conversion to atrial flutter, development of atrial tachycardia, or development of an independent junctional or ventricular rhythm (or tachycardia) controlling the ventricles and giving rise to AV dissociation. In the last two instances, digitalis intoxication must be suspected. If after a period of regularization the ventricular rhythm becomes irregular again in a patient who has been given an excessive amount of digitalis, it may be due to an exit block, generally of the Wenckebach type (see p. 202), from the junctional or ventricular focus.

Because irregular ventricular cycle lengths cause changes in ventricular refractoriness (long cycles lengthening refractoriness and short cycles shortening refractoriness), when a short ventricular cycle follows a long ventricular cycle, aberrant ventricular conduction may occur, generally of right bundle branch block configuration. This is called the Ashman phenomenon (see Figs. 8-103 and 8-109).

Significance. Similar to other tachyarrhythmias, atrial fibrillation may be chronic or intermittent; the former is almost always associated with underlying heart disease, whereas the latter may occur in clinically normal patients. Underlying heart disease is more frequent in patients who have atrial fibrillation than in patients who have atrial flutter. The arrhythmia is commonly seen in patients who have rheumatic mitral stenosis, thyrotoxicosis, cardiomyopathy, hypertensive heart disease, pericarditis, and coronary heart disease.

Approximately 30% of all patients who have atrial fibrillation have systemic or pulmonary emboli. Such a catastrophe is most common in patients who have rheumatic mitral valvular disease. Of the emboli that occur in patients with mitral stenosis, 90% occur in patients who have atrial fibrillation.

Treatment. It is of paramount importance in treating the patient who has atrial fibrillation for the first time to search for a precipitating cause. Thyrotoxicosis, mitral stenosis, acute myocardial infarction, pericarditis, and other known associated causes should be considered.

1. Initial therapy is determined by the patient's clinical status. The primary therapeutic objective is to slow the ventricular rate and, secondarily, to restore atrial systole. DC cardioversion may accomplish both of these objectives. If the sudden onset of atrial fibrillation with a rapid ventricular rate results in acute cardiovascular decompensation, DC cardioversion is the preferred treatment, beginning with 50 to 100 watt-seconds.

2. In the absence of hemodynamic decompensation the patient may be given digitalis to maintain a resting apical rate of 60 to 80 beats/minute, which does not exceed 100 beats/minute after slight exercise. The speed, route, dosage, and type of digitalis preparation administered are determined by the degree of cardiovascular compensation (see the discussion of the treatment of AV nodal reentry). The ventricular rate cannot be slowed sufficiently by digitalis administration in some patients, and digitalis toxicity may result before slowing the ventricular rate. In such cases, complicating factors such as pulmonary emboli, atelectasis, myocarditis, infection, congestive heart failure, and hyperthyroidism should be excluded and treated if found. In some instances[11] verapamil may be useful (see atrial flutter).

3. The combined use of digitalis and propranolol or digitalis and verapamil may be used to slow the ventricular rate when digitalis alone fails. Occasionally, conversion of atrial fibrillation to normal sinus rhythm may result from this combination or following the administration of digitalis alone.

4. Most often the use of quinidine to maintain a controlled ventricular rate, together with digitalis administration[1] is necessary to convert the atrial fibrillation to sinus rhythm medically. Because of the availability and safety of the electrical cardioverter, it is preferable not to administer the large doses of quinidine that were used formerly to produce drug reversion to normal sinus rhythm. Rather, maintenance doses in the range of 1.2 to 2.4 g/day should be administered for a few days prior to the planned DC cardioversion. During this time, 10% to 15% of patients establish a normal sinus rhythm. If sinus rhythm does not occur, DC cardioversion is carried out. Recent experience suggests that digitalis may not have to be discontinued prior to cardioversion if the patient has not received an excessive amount of digitalis. Pretreatment with quinidine establishes an effective tissue concentration, determines whether the drug will be tolerated, improves chances of main-

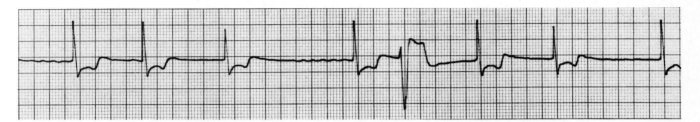

FIG. 8-43. Atrial fibrillation. Atrial activity is present as the undulating wavy baseline seen in the midportion of the ECG strip. Note that the premature ventricular complex follows the longest RR cycle. This conforms to a phenomenon known as the *rule of bigeminy,* that is, ventricular ectopy during atrial fibrillation more commonly follows the long RR cycles. The premature ventricular complex would have to be differentiated from aberrant supraventricular conduction. Monitor lead.

Rate: Atrial, cannot be determined accurately; ventricular, 36 to 105 beats/minute.
Rhythm: Atrial and ventricular are both irregularly irregular.
P waves: Only the fibrillatory *(F)* waves of atrial fibrillation can be seen.
PR interval: Not measurable.
QRS: 0.08 second.

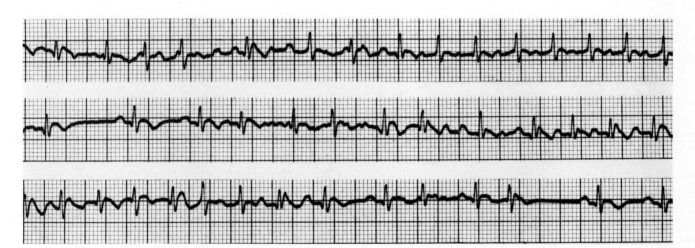

FIG. 8-44. Intermittent, "coarse" atrial flutter-fibrillation. Throughout this recording sinus beats are interrupted by premature atrial complexes that initiate episodes of atrial flutter-fibrillation. The fibrillatory waves appear more coarse than usual, and the flutter waves are irregularly spaced and of varying amplitude. Such atrial rhythms are often called *coarse atrial flutter* and are probably caused by portions of the atria that are fibrillating and other portions that are fluttering. A more appropriate term might be *flitter.* Monitor lead.

Rate: Atrial, varying; ventricular, 69 to 150 beats/minute.
P waves: Appear before the sinus beats; otherwise the undulating base line indicates flutter-fibrillation.
PR interval: 0.16 second for the sinus beats.
QRS: 0.08 second.

taining normal sinus rhythm after cardioversion, and reduces the number of shocks and level of energy required to restore normal sinus rhythm. Successful establishment of normal sinus rhythm by electrical DC cardioversion occurs in over 90% of patients; with maintenance quinidine therapy approximately 30% to 50% continue to have normal sinus rhythm for 12 months. In patients who do not tolerate quinidine, disopyramide or procainamide may be tried. Amiodarone is very effective in maintaining sinus rhythm but is investigational for that purpose.

Certain patients should *not* be considered for cardioversion. These include patients who have (1) known sensitivity or intolerance to quinidine or other antiarrhythmic agents (according to some studies, the recurrence rate of atrial fibrillation is higher in the absence of prophylactic quinidine administration), (2) repetitive paroxysmal atrial fibrillation that cannot be prevented by drugs, (3) digitalis intoxication, (4) numerous conversion procedures without clinical improvement or preservation of sinus rhythm, (5) difficult-to-control atrial tachyarrhythmias that finally eventuate into atrial fibrillation with clinical improvement and stability of arrhythmia, (6) cardiac surgery planned in the near future, (7) a high degree of partial or complete AV block and thus a slow ventricular response, and (8) sick sinus syndrome (Fig. 8-41).

Many elderly patients in the last two groups tolerate the atrial fibrillation well because the ventricular rate is slow, and they often do not require treatment with digitalis, unless the ventricular rate increases or congestive heart failure develops. These patients may demonstrate serious supraventricular and ventricular arrhythmias after cardioversion because concomitant sinus node disease becomes manifest. A related group of patients may have supraventricular tachycardias that alternate with bradycardias; these patients represent a subgroup of the sick sinus syndrome called "bradycardia-tachycardia syndrome."[16] Usually, these patients are best treated with a ventricular pacemaker (to correct the slow rates) and digitalis (to control the ventricular rates during the supraventricular tachycardia).

In general, all other patients in whom improved circulatory hemodynamics are desirable may be considered candidates for electrical cardioversion. Failure to maintain normal sinus rhythm after electrical reversion is related to the duration of atrial fibrillation, the functional classification of the patient, and the cause of the underlying heart disease. The likelihood of establishing and maintaining sinus rhythm should be weighed against the risks of cardioversion or other forms of therapy. The presence of multiple factors that adversely affect maintenance of sinus rhythm militates against cardioversion attempts.

Anticoagulation before cardioversion is indicated in patients with a high risk of emboli, that is, those who have mitral stenosis, recent onset of atrial fibrillation, recent or recurrent emboli, or enlarged heart.[17] The incidence of embolization during conversion to normal sinus rhythm is 1% to 3%. Some experts suggest anticoagulation for patients for 2 weeks before elective cardioversion of atrial fibrillation present for more than 1 to 2 weeks, if no contraindications to anticoagulation exist, and continuing anticoagulation for 2 additional weeks. However, few controlled studies exist to establish that approach definitively.

ATRIAL TACHYCARDIA WITH AND WITHOUT AV BLOCK (Figs. 8-45 and 8-46)

The atrial rate is usually between 150 and 200 beats/minute, with a range similar to AV nodal reentry, 150 to 250 beats/minute. When caused by digitalis excess, the atrial rate is generally less than 200 beats/minute and may be noted to increase gradually as the digitalis is continued. The PR interval also may gradually lengthen until Wenckebach second-degree AV block develops. On occasion the degree of AV block may be more advanced. Frequently other manifestations of digitalis excess, such as premature ventricular complexes coexist. In nearly 50% of cases of atrial tachycardia with block the atrial rate is irregular, whereas in AV nodal reentry the atrial rate is generally exceedingly regular. Characteristic isoelectric intervals between P waves, in contrast to atrial flutter, are usually present in all leads. However, at rapid atrial rates the distinction between atrial tachycardia with block and atrial flutter may be quite difficult. As in atrial flutter, carotid sinus massage slows the ventricular rate by increasing the degree of AV block but does not terminate the tachycardia.

Significance. Atrial tachycardia with block occurs most commonly in patients who have significant organic heart disease such as coronary artery disease or cor pulmonale. It is associated with digitalis excess in 50% to 75% of such patients.

A different type of atrial tachycardia, multifocal atrial tachycardia, is characterized by atrial rates of 100 to 250 beats/minute and marked variation in P wave morphology and in the PP interval, is associated with a high mortality, and is rarely produced by digitalis. Verapamil may be effective therapy.

Treatment. If the ventricular rate is within a normal range and the patient is asymptomatic, often no therapy at all may be necessary.

1. Very slow ventricular rates may respond to atropine (0.5-mg increments IV) or, rarely, require ventricular pacing.
2. Atrial tachycardia with block in a patient who is not taking digitalis may be treated with digitalis to slow the ventricular rate.

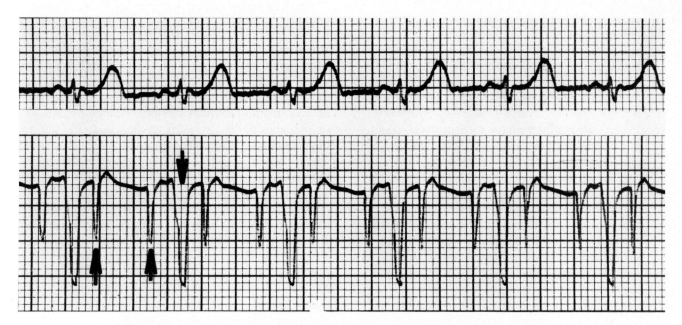

FIG. 8-45. Atrial tachycardia with 2:1 block. In the top tracing (lead II) alternate P waves cannot be seen because they are lost within the ST segment and the ECG appears to be sinus rhythm at a rate of 95 beats/minute. The extra deflection in the terminal portion of the T wave suggests the presence of a second P wave, which is revealed in the esophageal recording *(bottom tracing)*. The atrial rate actually is 190 beats/minute with 2:1 conduction to the ventricle. Upright arrows indicate P waves, inverted arrow indicates QRS complex. Monitor lead.

Rate:	Atrial, 190 beats/minute; ventricular, 95 beats/minute.
Rhythm:	Atrial and ventricular, regular.
P waves:	Seen with clarity in the esophageal recording.
PR interval:	0.14 second for the conducted beats.
QRS:	0.07 second.

↑ CSM

FIG. 8-46. Atrial tachycardia with 1:1 conduction becoming 2:1 conduction during carotid sinus massage. At the left portion of the ECG, P waves can be seen to conduct to each QRS complex. Carotid sinus massage (CSM) performed at the large arrow, precipitates 2:1 conduction. Clear atrial activity can be seen *(arrows)* as 2:1 conduction occurs. Monitor lead.

Rate:	Atrial, 150 beats/minute; ventricular, 150 beats/minute in left portion and 75 beats/minute in right portion.
Rhythm:	Atrial, regular; ventricular, regular.
P waves:	Can be seen in the ST segment in the left portion of the tracing and are quite clear in the right portion of the tracing.
PR interval:	Difficult to measure in the left portion of the tracing, but P waves conduct with a PR interval of 0.25 second in the right portion of the tracing.
QRS:	0.09 second.

3. If atrial tachycardia with block remains after digitalization, oral quinidine, disopyramide, or procainamide may be added. Amiodarone or flecainide may be tried, but they are investigational for this purpose.

4. The rhythm in some patients may resist termination by pharmacologic means, and, if digitalis excess is not the cause, DC cardioversion may be tried.

5. If atrial tachycardia with (or without) block appears in a patient receiving digitalis, it should be assumed initially that the digitalis is responsible for the arrhythmia, especially if the patient recently has received diuretics, the serum potassium level is low, the digitalis dose has been increased, quinidine has been added to the therapeutic regimen, or multiple premature ventricular complexes are also present. In such patients, initial therapy includes omission of digitalis and potassium-depleting diuretics (discontinuation of quinidine if it has been started recently) and the administration of potassium chloride, orally (30 to 45 mEq initially, repeated if necessary in 1 hour) or intravenously (0.5 mEq/minute in 5% dextrose and water during constant electrocardiographic monitoring, for a total of 30 to 60 mEq initially). A gradual slowing of the atrial rate with a decrease in AV block usually occurs if the arrhythmia is caused by digitalis. In the presence of advanced AV block, potassium, as well as other antiarrhythmic agents, must be given with great caution and under constant electrocardiographic monitoring. It should be remembered that renal dysfunction, acidosis, and excess digitalis predispose to the development of hyperkalemia, and therefore potassium must be administered cautiously, along with frequent ECG, serum potassium, and blood urea nitrogen (BUN) checks.

6. Propranolol, 0.5 to 1 mg/min IV for a total dose of 0.5 to 3 mg, or phenytoin, 50 to 100 mg IV every 5 minutes until the tachycardia terminates, the patient develops signs of toxicity such as nystagmus, vertigo, or nausea, or a total dose of 1 g is given, may be quite useful for digitalis-induced arrhythmias, including atrial tachycardia with block. The latter agent, since it does not appear to slow AV conduction, may be particularly useful.

7. If these agents are not effective, further short-acting digitalis preparations may be given cautiously, assuming that the development of atrial tachycardia with block was not caused by digitalis.

PREMATURE AV JUNCTIONAL COMPLEXES (Fig. 8-47)

Rhythms formerly called nodal, coronary nodal, and coronary sinus are now termed AV *junctional*. This term, which includes the AV nodal–His bundle area, is preferred to terms that imply a more exact site of impulse origin because the exact location at which the impulse originates often cannot be determined from the surface ECG. A premature AV junctional complex arises in the AV junction and spreads in an anterograde and retrograde fashion. If unimpeded in its course, the impulse discharges the atrium to produce a premature retrograde P wave and a QRS complex with a supraventricular contour. Retrograde atrial activation generally results in a negative P wave in leads II, III, aV_F, and V_6, with positive P waves in leads I, aV_L, aV_R, and V_1. The retrograde P wave may occur before, be buried in, or (less commonly) follow the QRS complex. The site at which the impulse originates, as well as the relative speeds of anterograde and retrograde conduction, determines the relationship of the P wave to the QRS complex. A compensatory pause commonly follows a premature AV junctional complex, but if the atrium and sinus node are discharged retrogradely, a noncompensatory pause results.

Significance and Treatment. The significance and treatment of premature AV junctional complexes is discussed under premature ventricular complexes.

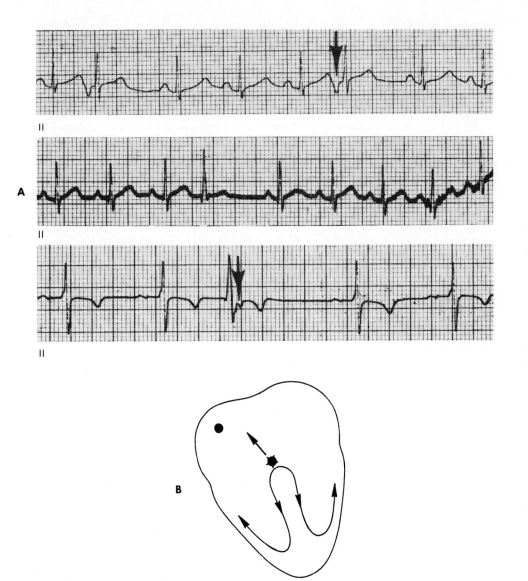

II

A

II

II

B

FIG 8-47. A, Premature AV junctional complexes. Premature junctional complexes seen in the top, middle, and bottom tracings were formerly called upper, middle, and lower nodal premature complexes, respectively, because the regrograde P wave was inscribed before, during, and after the QRS complex. Since not only the site of origin, but also the relative speeds of anterograde and retrograde conduction determine the P-QRS complex relationships during a premature AV junctional complex, it is best to use the nonspecific term *premature AV junctional complex* for all three types. Note that the QRS complex maintains an almost identical contour to the normally conducted beats. Slight QRS aberration occurs in the middle recording. Monitor lead from three different patients; arrows indicate P waves. In B, schematic illustration is presented.

Rate: Determined by basic rate and number of premature complexes.

Rhythm: Irregular because of premature complexes; may be a regular irregularity, as in bigeminy or trigeminy.

P waves: Atria discharged in a retrograde direction, producing negative (inverted) P waves in lead II. P waves occur before *(top tracing),* during *(middle tracing),* and after *(bottom tracing)* the QRS complex, depending on the site of origin of the premature complex and the status of anterograde and retrograde conduction.

PR interval: Less than 0.12 second.

RP interval: If P wave follows QRS, less than 0.20 second.

QRS: Normal, 0.08 second, reflecting normal anterograde conduction to the ventricles. Contour may differ slightly from normal.

AV JUNCTIONAL RHYTHMS
(Figs. 8-48 to 8-50)

An AV junctional escape beat occurs when the rate of impulse formation of the primary pacemaker (usually sinus node) becomes less than that of the AV junctional pace-ecmaker, or when impulses from the primary pacemaker do not penetrate to the region of the escape focus (AV block). The interval from the last normally conducted beat to the escape beat therefore exceeds the normal RR interval and is a measure of the initial rate of discharge of the AV junctional focus. The inherent discharge rate of the AV junctional escape focus (usually 40 to 60 per minute) determines when the junctional escape beat occurs. A continued series of AV junctional escape beats is called an AV junctional rhythm. An AV junctional escape rhythm is usually fairly regular. Intervals between subsequent escape beats after the initial escape beat may gradually shorten as the rate of discharge of the escape focus increases (rhythm of development). The configuration of the QRS complex may differ from the normal sinus-initiated QRS complex; usually, it maintains the same contour as the normally conducted QRS.

The atria may be under retrograde control of the AV junctional pacemaker, or the atria may discharge independently (see discussion of AV dissociation).

Significance. An AV junctional escape beat(s) or rhythm may be a normal phenomenon owing to the effects of vagal tone on higher pacemakers, or it may occur during pathologic slow sinus discharge and heart block. The escape beat or rhythm serves as a safety mechanism that assumes control of the cardiac rhythm owing to *default* of the primary pacemaker, so as to prevent the occurrence of complete ventricular asystole.

Treatment. Treatment, if indicated, lies in increasing the discharge rate of higher pacemakers or improving conduction with atropine or isoproterenol. Rarely, pacing may be needed.

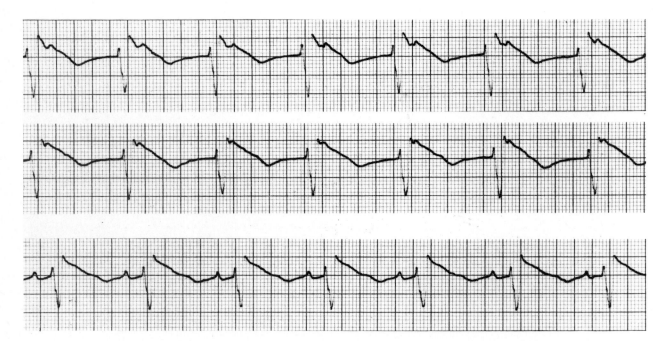

FIG. 8-48. AV junctional rhythm. The top tracings are a continuous recording, whereas the bottom tracing is recorded some time later. In the top two tracings, isorhythmic AV dissociation is present. P waves are in the ST segment and gradually move into the QRS complex (compare the QRS-P relationship in the first complex in the top strip with the last complex in the second strip). In the top strip, sinus slowing initially allowed the escape of the junctional rhythm (not shown). Monitor lead.

Rate:	Top two strips, atrial is 60 beats/minute and ventricular is 58 beats/minute; bottom strip, atrial and ventricular rate 57 beats/minute.
Rhythm:	Atrial, regular; ventricular, regular.
P waves:	Normal.
PR interval:	Varying in the top two strips; regular (0.22 second) in the bottom strip.
QRS:	0.10 second (appears prolonged in this monitor lead but was normal by 12-lead ECG).

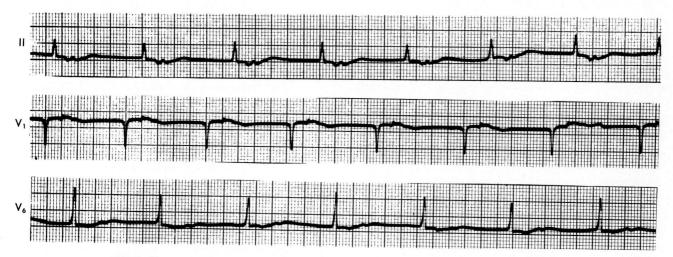

FIG. 8-49.   AV junctional rhythm. The patient has an AV junctional rhythm with 1:1 retrograde capture. Thus AV dissociation is not present.

Rate: Atrial and ventricular, 55 beats/minute.
Rhythm: Regular.
P waves: Retrograde.
RP interval: 0.18 second.
QRS: 0.06 second.

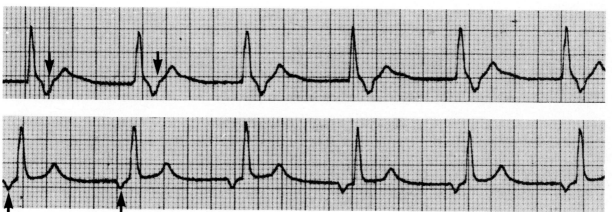

FIG. 8-50.   AV junctional rhythm with a changing P-QRS relationship. In the top tracing, retrograde atrial activity (↓) follows the QRS complex. In the bottom tracing, retrograde atrial activity (↑) precedes the QRS complex. Thus, with the same AV junctional rhythm in the same patient, atrial activity first followed and then preceded the QRS complex.

Rate: Atrial, 65 beats/minute; ventricular, 65 beats/minute.
Rhythm: Regular.
P waves: Inverted; follow QRS in top tracing; precede QRS in bottom tracing.
PR interval: 0.12 second, bottom.
RP interval: 0.12 second, top.
QRS: Generally normal, 0.08 second.

NONPAROXYSMAL AV JUNCTIONAL TACHYCARDIA (Figs. 8-51 and 8-52)

Accepted terminology confers the label of tachycardia to rhythms that exceed 100 beats/minute. However, since rates greater than 60 to 70 beats/minute represent, in effect, a tachycardia for the AV junctional tissue, the term *nonparoxysmal AV junctional tachycardia* (NPJT), although not entirely correct, has been generally accepted when the rate of junctional discharge exceeds 60 to 70 beats/minute.[16] NPJT usually has a more gradual onset and termination than does AV nodal reentry, with a ventricular rate commonly between 70 and 130 beats/minute. The rate sometimes may be slowed by vagal maneuvers, as in sinus tachycardia, and the rhythm may not always be entirely regular. Although retrograde atrial activation may occur, more commonly the atria are controlled by an independent sinus or atrial focus resulting in AV dissociation.

Significance. The distinction between NPJT and AV nodal reentry is etiologically and therapeutically quite important. NPJT occurs most commonly in patients who have underlying heart disease, such as inferior wall infarction and acute rheumatic myocarditis, and following open-heart surgery. Probably the most important cause is excessive digitalis, which only rarely produces AV nodal reentry. It is especially important to recognize slowing and regularization of the ventricular rhythm caused by NPJT as an early sign of digitalis intoxication in a patient who has atrial fibrillation.

Treatment. The treatment for NPJT is as follows:

1. If the ventricular rate is rapid, the cardiovascular status compromised, and the patient is not taking digitalis, digitalization should be the first measure.
2. Uncommonly in an emergency situation or if the arrhythmia does not respond to digitalization and is *clearly not induced by digitalis,* electrical DC cardioversion may be employed.
3. However, if the patient tolerates the arrhythmia well, careful monitoring and attention to the underlying heart disease is usually all that is needed. The arrhythmia will usually abate spontaneously.
4. If digitalis toxicity is the causative factor, the drug must be immediately stopped. Potassium may be given (see discussion of treatment of atrial tachycardia with block). The ECG should be monitored, since the blocking effects of potassium administration and digitalis are additive in the AV junctional tissue, and advanced AV heart block may result. The rate of potassium administration is important, since a rapid infusion of the potassium, especially in a potassium-depleted patient, may result in transient cardiac arrest or depression of AV conduction.
5. Lidocaine, propranolol, phenytoin, or verapamil also may be tried.

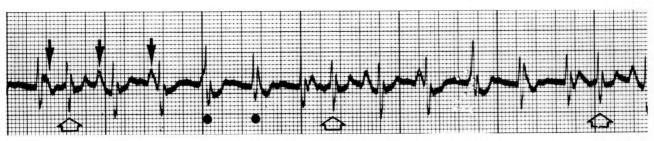

Lead II

FIG. 8-51.   Nonparoxysmal AV junctional tachycardia. Atrial activity *(inverted dark arrows)* intermittently capture the ventricles *(upright arrow outlines)* to produce incomplete AV dissociation. The junctional tachycardia fails to capture the atria retrogradely, but the sinus tachycardia intermittently captures the ventricles. Unidirectional block (i.e., retrograde) is present. Incomplete AV dissociation occurs because of the accelerated AV junctional discharge. Two uninterrupted junctional cycles indicated by filled circles.

Rate: Atrial, 111 beats/minute; ventricular, 125 beats/minute.
Rhythm: Atrial, regular; ventricular, fairly regular with intermittent speeding due to sinus
               captures.
P waves: Normal and can be "marched out." P waves are not influenced by ventricular
               activity.
PR interval: Difficult to measure but prolonged before the captures.
QRS: 0.06 second.

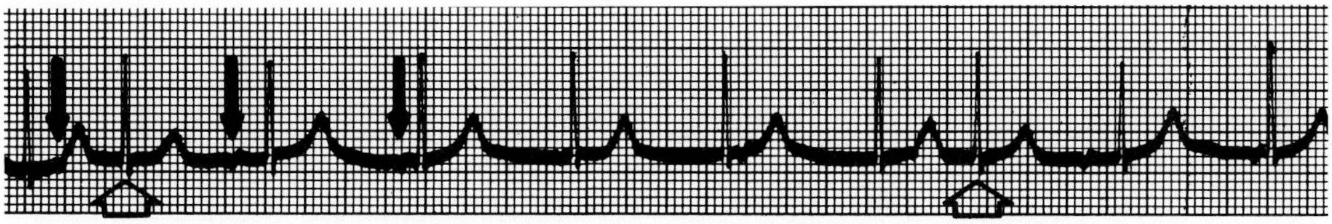

Lead I

FIG. 8-52.   Nonparoxysmal AV junctional tachycardia. Atrial activity *(inverted dark arrows)* can be seen as small inverted P waves that occur regularly throughout the QRS complex, uninfluenced by ventricular activity. The ventricular rhythm is regular except for intermittent atrial captures indicated by the unfilled upright arrows. The rhythm is explained as in Fig. 8-51 except that an ectopic pacemaker, rather than a sinus pacemaker, controls the atria. This ectopic pacemaker could be an atrial focus or an upper junctional focus. Incomplete AV dissociation is present with unidirectional conduction from atria to ventricles but retrograde block (the ventricular rhythm does not capture the atria retrogradely).

Rate: Atrial, 72 beats/minute; ventricular, 79 beats/minute.
Rhythm: Atrial, regular; ventricular, irregular due to intermittent atrial captures.
P waves: Abnormal.
PR interval: Prolonged during ventricular captures.
QRS: 0.06 second.

VENTRICULAR ESCAPE BEATS (Fig. 8-53)

A ventricular escape beat results when the rate of impulse formation of supraventricular pacemakers (sinus node and AV junctional) becomes less than that of potential ventricular pacemakers or when supraventricular impulses do not penetrate to the region of the escape focus because of SA or AV block. The inherent rate of discharge of ventricular escape pacemakers is usually 20 to 40 per minute. A continued series of ventricular escape beats is called a ventricular escape rhythm. The ventricular rhythm is usually fairly regular, although the rhythm may accelerate for a few complexes shortly after its onset (rhythm of development). The duration of the QRS complexes is prolonged to greater than 0.12 second because the origin of ventricular discharge is located in the ventricles. Sometimes the escape focus may shift from one to another portion of ventricle and may generate QRS complexes with a different contour and rate.

Significance. The presence of ventricular escape beats indicates significant slowing of supraventricular pacemakers or a fairly high degree of SA or AV block and would therefore generally be considered abnormal.

Treatment. Depending on the cause, atropine, isoproterenol, or pacing generally would represent the therapeutic approach.

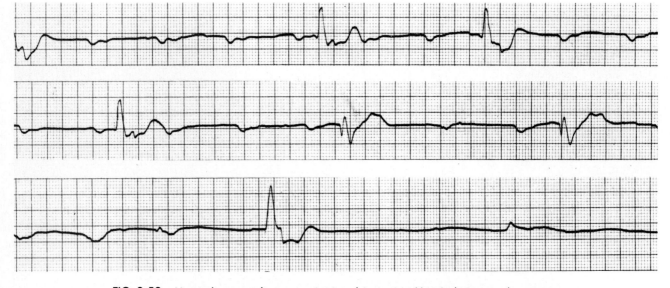

FIG. 8-53. Ventricular escape beats occurring in a dying patient. Ventricular escape beats occur with changing contour and at irregular intervals in this ECG from a dying patient. AV block is also present, since the P waves do not appear to conduct to the ventricles. The changing QRS contour may be caused by shifting pacemakers or changing activation sequence.

Rate:	Varying.
Rhythm:	Atrial and ventricular rhythms are varying.
P waves:	Can be seen in the top strip and then more intermittently in the second and third strips.
PR interval:	Varying.
QRS:	Varying but approximately 0.16 second.

PREMATURE VENTRICULAR COMPLEXES
(Figs. 8-54 to 8-56)

A premature ventricular complex is characterized by the premature occurrence of a QRS complex, initiated in the ventricle, that has a contour different from the normal supraventricular complex and a duration usually greater than 0.12 second. The T wave is generally large and opposite in direction to the major deflection of the QRS. The QRS complex generally is not preceded by a premature P wave but may be preceded by a sinus P wave occurring at its expected time. However, these criteria may be met by a supraventricular complex or rhythm that conducts aberrantly through the ventricle; in fact, aberrant supraventricular conduction may mimic all the manifestations of ventricular arrhythmia except ventricular fibrillation (see p. 198).

Retrograde transmission to the atria from premature ventricular complex occurs more frequently than has often been affirmed but still probably does not occur commonly. The retrograde P wave produced in this fashion is often obscured by the distorted QRS complex. Usually a fully compensatory pause follows a premature ventricular complex. If the retrograde impulse discharges the sinus node prematurely and resets the basic timing, it may produce a pause that is not fully compensatory. A compensatory pause results when the premature complex does not alter the discharge rate or rhythm of the sinus node, so that a P wave occurs at its normal time. The P wave does not reach the ventricle, since the AV node is refractory because of (concealed) retrograde penetration into the AV node by the premature junctional or ventricular complex. Therefore the RR interval produced by the two QRS complexes on either side of the premature complex equals twice the normally conducted RR interval. A compensatory pause occurs more commonly with ventricular and AV junctional premature complex, but the presence of a compensatory pause is not invariably diagnostic of the site of origin of the premature complex.

The normal sinus P wave following a premature ventricular complex may conduct to the ventricles with a long PR interval, in which case a pause does not follow the premature ventricular complex, and the premature complex is said to be *interpolated*. A *ventricular fusion beat* (the simultaneous activation of one chamber by two foci) represents a blend of the characteristics of the normally conducted beat and the beat originating in the ventricles, indicating that the ventricle has been depolarized from both atrial and ventricular directions. *Atrial fusion beats* may occur during ectopic atrial discharge and represent a blend of the characteristics of the sinus-initiated and ectopic atrial P waves. Whether a compensatory or noncompensatory pause, a retrograde atrial excitation, an interpolated complex, a fusion complex, or an echo beat (see Fig. 8-54)

occurs is merely a function of how well the AV junction conducts and the timing of the events taking place.

The term *bigeminy* refers to pairs of beats or two complexes and may be used to indicate couplets of normal and ectopic ventricular complex. Premature ventricular complexes may have differing contours and often are called multifocal. More properly they should be called multiform, since it is not known from a surface ECG recording that there are multiple foci discharging.

Significance. The frequency of premature ventricular complexes increases with age. The presence of premature complexes may be manifested by symptoms of palpitations or discomfort in the chest or neck; this is caused by the greater than normal contractile force of the postectopic beats or the feeling that the heart has stopped during the long pause after the premature complexes. Long runs of premature complexes in patients who have heart disease may produce angina or hypotension. Frequent interpolated premature complexes actually represent a doubling of the heart rate and may compromise the patient's hemodynamic status. In the absence of underlying heart disease the presence of premature complexes may have no significance and not require suppression. Premature ventricular complexes and complex ventricular arrhythmias occurring in asymptomatic healthy subjects portends no increased risk of death and their long term prognosis is similar to that of the healthy U.S. population. Ventricular ectopy recorded after myocardial infarction represents an indendent risk factor for subsequent death. However, it has not been demonstrated that the premature ventricular complexes or complex ventricular arrhythmias play a *precipitating* role in the genesis of sudden death; they may be simply a marker of heart disease. Nor has it been shown unequivocally that antiarrhythmic therapy given to suppress the premature ventricular complexes or complex ventricular arrhythmias reduces the incidence of sudden death in these patients.

Most of the drugs used to suppress premature complexes also may produce them on certain occasions. This is especially true of the digitalis preparations. On the other hand, digitalis may be effective in controlling premature atrial and ventricular complexes, especially those related to the presence of congestive heart failure. In patients suffering from acute myocardial infarction, it has been commonly held that so-called warning arrhythmias (premature ventricular complexes occurring close to the preceding T wave, greater than five or six per minute, bigeminal, multiform, or occurring in salvos of two, three, or more) may presage or precipitate ventricular tachycardia or fibrillation. However, it has been demonstrated that about half of the patients who develop ventricular fibrillation have no warning arrhythmias, and half of those who do have warning arrhythmias do not develop ventricular fibrillation.

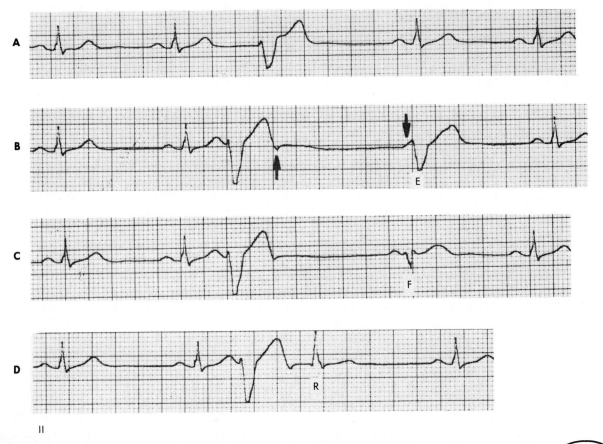

II

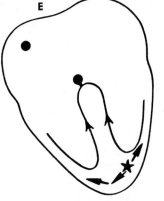

FIG. 8-54. Premature ventricular complexes. All four tracings were recorded from the same patient. In A a relatively late premature ventricular complex is followed by a full compensatory pause. Sinus slowing makes the pause after the ventricular complex minimumly greater than compensatory, but its characteristics are essentially the same, that is, the interval between the two normal QRS complexes flanking the premature ventricle complex is twice the basic RR interval. In B an earlier premature ventricular complex in the same patient retrogradely discharges the atria (↑). This resets the sinus node and a ventricular escape beat (E) escapes before the next P wave (↓) can conduct to the ventricles. In strip C the sequence is the same as in B, except that the atrial rate is faster. This permits the P wave, following the premature ventricular complex and retrograde P wave, to partially depolarize the ventricles at the same time the ventricular escape beat occurs, resulting in a fusion beat (F). In D, the sequence is the same as in C, except that after the impulse from the ventricle retrogradely discharges the atria, it returns to the ventricles to produce a ventricular echo, or reciprocal beat (R). In E, a schematic illustration is presented.

Rate:	Determined by basic rate and number of ventricular complexes.
Rhythm:	Irregular because of premature complexes.
P waves:	Generally normal; may be captured retrogradely; often lost in QRS or T wave of premature ventricular complex.
PR interval:	Determined by whether P wave is blocked, conducted with a prolonged PR interval, or retrogradely activated.
QRS:	0.14 second.

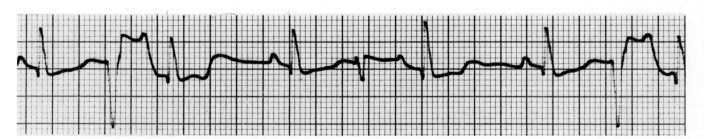

FIG. 8-55.   Interpolated premature ventricular complexes. The second, fifth, and eighth QRS complexes are premature ventricular complexes. The sinus P wave that follows those premature ventricular complexes conducts to the ventricle with a long PR interval. Thus the normally expected compensatory pause is not present. The premature ventricular complex does not replace a normally conducted complex (see Fig. 8-54,A) but occurs in addition to the normally conducted complex. The PR interval following the premature ventricular complex is prolonged due to incomplete recovery of the AV node because of partial retrograde penetration by the interpolated premature ventricular complex. Monitor lead.

Rate and rhythm: Varying because of the premature ventricular complexes.
P waves: Normal.
PR interval: 0.16 second for the normally conducted beats and 0.20 to 0.25 second after the interpolated premature ventricular complexes.
QRS: 0.09 second for the normal beats and 0.12 second for the premature ventricular complexes.

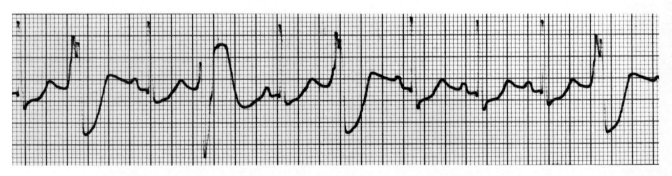

FIG. 8-56.   Multiform premature ventricular complexes. Each sinus beat is followed by premature ventricular complexes that have two contours, one predominantly upright and the other predominantly negative. These premature ventricular complexes of different contours are more properly called multiform rather than multifocal, since one cannot be certain if more than one focus is active or if different activation sequences are emerging from the same focus. Monitor lead.

Rate: 100 beats/minute but varying.
Rhythm: Varying due to premature ventricular complexes.
P waves: Normal preceding the normally conducted beats.
PR interval: 0.14 second preceding the normally conducted beats.
QRS: 0.09 second for the normally conducted beats and 0.16 second for the premature ventricular complexes.

Treatment. In the hospitalized patient with or without an acute myocardial infarction, lidocaine IV is the initial drug of choice when suppression of premature ventricular complexes is deemed necessary.

IMMEDIATE SUPPRESSION

1. Lidocaine, 1 to 2 mg/kg (50 to 100 mg) given as an IV bolus (at a rate of 20 to 50 mg/min) followed by an IV drip in a dosage of 1 to 4 mg/minute, is administered initially. A second or third IV injection using half the initial dose may be given at approximately 20- to 60-minute intervals after the first dose if necessary, but care should be taken not to exceed 400 to 500 mg/hour. A loading dose may also be given by rapid infusion, with an effective serum concentration maintained by constant infusion. In some instances, lidocaine may be given intramuscularly in a dose of 250 to 300 mg. The onset of action of lidocaine given IV is 45 to 90 seconds and the duration of action is 10 to 20 minutes. Lidocaine produces less hypotension and negative inotropic effects than procainamide or quinidine in doses having equivalent antiarrhythmic effects. It is ideal for use in patients who have renal disease, since less than 10% is excreted unaltered in the kidney and the rest is metabolized by the liver. In patients exhibiting allergic reactions to quinidine or procainamide, lidocaine is useful, since there appears to be no cross-sensitivity.

2. If maximum doses of lidocaine are unsuccessful, then procainamide, administered IV (0.14 mg/kg, maximum 1200 mg at 50 mg/minute if no hypotension occurs, or until suppression of the premature ventricular complexes occurs, toxic effects such as QRS widening or hypotension result, or 750 to 1000 mg is administered) may be tried. If successful, procainamide may then be given as a continuous IV infusion (2 to 6 mg/min). Quinidine given IV may produce significant hypotension and is used uncommonly by that route.

LONG-TERM SUPPRESSION

1. Oral maintenance therapy can be achieved with procainamide, 375 to 500 mg every 3 to 4 hours to produce therapeutic blood levels of 4 to 8 mg/L, or with quinidine sulfate, 200 to 400 mg every 6 hours to produce serum levels of 3 to 6 mg/L. A long-acting procainamide preparation can be given at a dose of 750 to 1000 mg every 6 hours.

2. Disopyramide (Norpace), 100 to 250 mg every 6 hours, may be useful at serum concentrations of 2 to 5 µg/ml.

3. Tocainide (Tonocard) 400 to 600 mg every 8 to 12 hours achieving serum concentrations of 4 to 10 µg/ml may be effective, particularly if lidocaine has successfully suppressed the arrhythmia.

4. Flecainide (Tambocor), recently approved by the Food and Drug Administration, is given in doses of 100 to 200 mg every 12 hours to produce serum concentrations in the range of 0.6 µg/ml, and may be useful.

5. Amiodarone (Cordarone), also approved by the FDA recently, is generally given in a loading dose of 800 to 1600 mg/day for 1 to 2 weeks and then at maintenance doses of 400 to 800 mg/day (or less), titrating the dose to the lowest effective amount. Therapeutic serum concentrations range between 1 and 3.5 µg/ml.

6. Mexiletine (Mexitel), just approved by the FDA, may be tried in doses of 250 to 400 mg every 8 hours to achieve plasma concentrations of 1 to 2 µg/ml.

7. Propranolol or phenytoin may be tried if the above drugs fail (see discussion of treatment of ventricular tachycardia).

VENTRICULAR TACHYCARDIA
(Figs. 8-57 to 8-59)

Ventricular tachycardia is usually an ominous finding, indicating the presence of significant underlying cardiac disease. In many instances the responsible electrophysiologic mechanism is probably reentry.[1] Although ventricular tachycardia occurs most commonly in patients who have acute myocardial infarction and coronary artery disease, this arrhythmia also occurs in patients who have a variety of cardiac diseases, including cardiomyopathy, mitral valve prolapse, prolonged QT syndrome, and other problems. It has been reported in patients who have no evidence of structural heart disease.

The electrocardiographic diagnosis of ventricular tachycardia is suggested when a series of three or more bizarre, premature ventricular complexes occur that have a duration exceeding 0.12 second, with the ST-T vector pointing opposite to the major QRS deflection. The ventricular rate is between 110 and 250 beats/minute, and the RR interval may be exceedingly regular, or it may vary. Atrial activity may be independent of ventricular activity (AV dissociation) or the atria may be depolarized by the ventricles in a retrograde fashion (in which case AV dissociation is *not*

present). Ventricular tachycardia may be sustained (defined in the electrophysiology laboratory as lasting longer than 30 seconds or requiring termination because of hemodynamic deterioration) or nonsustained (lasting less than 30 seconds), and the patient's prognosis as well as the electrophysiologic mechanism may differ for the two forms. One type of nonsustained ventricular tachycardia is characterized by repetitive bursts of premature ventricular complexes separated by a series of sinus beats. Another type of ventricular tachycardia that may be sustained or nonsustained is called *torsades de pointes* and is characterized by a QRS contour that gradually changes its polarity from negative to positive or vice versa over a series of beats. It often occurs in a setting of QT prolongation.[8]

The distinction between supraventricular and ventricular tachycardia may be difficult at times because the features of both arrhythmias frequently overlap, and under certain circumstances a supraventricular tachycardia can mimic the criteria established for ventricular tachycardia. Ventricular complexes with abnormal configurations indicate only that conduction through the ventricle is not normal; they do not necessarily indicate the origin of impulse formation or the reason for the abnormal conduction

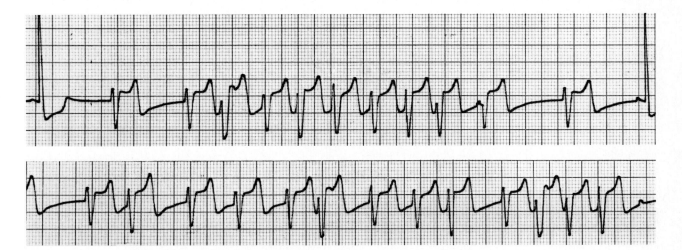

FIG. 8-57. Ventricular tachycardia. Ventricular tachycardia may be irregular at times, as exemplified in this ECG. The origin of the ventricular tachycardia was documented by electrophysiologic study. The interectopic intervals do not conveniently fit a diagnosis of exit block. Monitor lead.

Rate:	Atrial, cannot be determined; ventricular, varying.
Rhythm:	Atrial, cannot be determined; ventricular, irregular.
P waves:	Can be seen occasionally and precede the first and next to last QRS complexes in the top strip, which are the only normally conducted QRS complexes. The nonconducted P wave at the terminal portion of the bottom strip is probably due to incomplete AV nodal recovery of refractoriness caused by retrograde penetration from the last beat in the ventricular tachycardia.
PR interval:	0.12 second for the normally conducuted beats.
QRS:	0.08 second for the normally conducted beat and 0.11 second for the ventricular tachycardia.

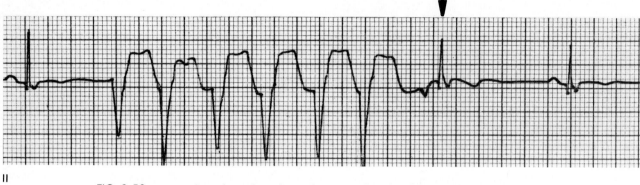

II

FIG. 8-58.   Ventricular tachycardia ending with a ventricular echo. Six beats of ventricular tachycardia occur following the first sinus beat. The last ventricular tachycardia beat conducts retrogradely to the atrium (note the small negative P wave in lead II), which then returns to reexcite the ventricle (ventricular echo, *arrow*).

Rate: Atrial, 55 to 75 beats/minute; ventricular, approximately 150 beats/minute.
Rhythm: Atrial, cannot be determined during ventricular tachycardia; regular during sinus rhythm. Ventricular, slightly irregular during ventricular tachycardia.
P waves: Normal during sinus-conducted beats; retrograde P wave following the last ventricular tachycardia beat.
PR interval: 0.16 second during sinus rhythm. RP interval following the last ventricular tachycardia beat, 0.52 second.
QRS: 0.08 second during sinus rhythm and 0.10 second during ventricular tachycardia.

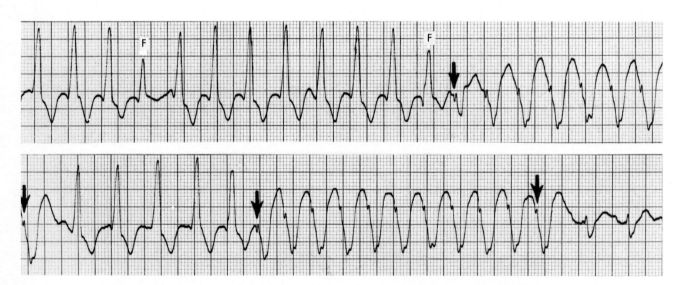

FIG. 8-59.   Termination of ventricular tachycardia by rapid ventricular pacing. Intermittent fusion beats *(F)* in the top strip support the diagnosis of ventricular tachycardia. Between the first and second arrows, competitive ventricular pacing is performed at a rate of 166 beats/minute, but the ventricular tachycardia continues. Between the third and fourth arrows, competitive ventricular pacing is performed at a rate of 176 beats/minute, and following cessation of pacing, sinus rhythm occurs. Monitor lead.

Rate: Atrial, cannot be determined; ventricular 136 beats/minute.
Rhythm: Atrial, cannot be determined; ventricular, fairly regular.
P waves: Cannot be seen.
PR interval: Cannot be determined.
QRS: 0.13 second.

(see discussion of supraventricular arrhythmia with abnormal QRS complex, p. 216).

The presence of *fusion* and *capture* beats provides evidence in favor of ventricular tachycardia. Fusion beats indicate simultaneous activation of the ventricles by two separate impulses (suggesting that one of the impulses arose in the ventricles), whereas the capture beats signal supraventricular control of the ventricles, generally at a rate faster than the ventricular tachycardia. This proves that normal ventricular conduction can occur at cycle lengths equal to or shorter than the tachycardia in question, again implying that the origin of the wide QRS complexes lies in the ventricles rather than in aberrant supraventricular conduction.

Significance. Symptoms occurring during ventricular tachycardia depend on the ventricular rate, the duration of the tachyarrhythmia; and the severity of the underlying heart disease. The location of impulse formation and therefore the way in which the depolarization wave spreads across the myocardium also may be important because it influences the ventricle's contraction. The immediate significance of ventricular tachycardia to the patient relates to the hemodynamic dysfunction it produces and the possible development of ventricular fibrillation.

A premature ventricular (rarely, atrial) complex can initiate ventricular tachycardia or ventricular fibrillation when the premature complex occurs during the vulnerable period of the antecedent T wave. The vulnerable period represents an interval of 20 to 40 msec located near the apex of the T wave during which the heart, when stimulated, is prone to develop ventricular tachycardia or fibrillation (see discussion of ventricular fibrillation). The stimulus may be from an intrinsic source such as a spontaneous premature complex or from an extrinsic source such as a pacemaker or DC shock. During the interval of the vulnerable period, maximal electrical nonuniformity in the ventricular muscle is present; that is, ventricular muscle fibers are at varying stages of recovery of excitability. Some fibers may have completely repolarized, others may have only partially repolarized, and still others may be completely refractory. Therefore stimulation during this period establishes nonuniform conduction with some areas of slowed conduction or actual block and sets the stage for repetitive ventricular discharge possibly caused by reentrant excitation. Equally important, however, is that ventricular tachycardia or fibrillation may begin without preexisting or precipitating premature ventricular complexes or may be ushered in by a *late* premature ventricular complex. In fact, the majority of recorded episodes of ventricular tachycardia begin with a late premature ventricular complex that occurs after the vulnerable period has ended.

Treatment. The treatment for ventricular tachycardia is as follows:

1. Striking the patient's chest, sometimes called *"thumpversion,"* may terminate ventricular tachycardia by mechanically inducing a premature ventricular complex that presumably interrupts the reentrant pathway necessary to support the ventricular tachycardia. It is a simple treatment to try initially. Stimulation at the time of the vulnerable period during ventricular tachycardia may provoke ventricular fibrillation.

2. Acute termination of ventricular tachycardia that does not cause any hemodynamic decompensation may be achieved medically, by administering lidocaine IV in an initial bolus of 1 to 2 mg/kg body weight. A second or third IV injection of one half the initial dose may be given at approximately 20- to 40-minute intervals if necessary, but care should be taken not to exceed 400 to 500 mg/hr. The dosage should be reduced in patients who have liver disease, heart failure, or shock. If lidocaine abolishes the ventricular tachycardia, then a continuous IV infusion of about 40 mg/kg/minute or 1 to 4 mg/minute can be given to the patient. Other infusion schedules also are effective.[7]

3. If maximum doses of lidocaine are unsuccessful, procainamide administered IV (up to 100 mg/1 minute until termination of the tachycardia occurs, toxic effects such as QRS widening or significant hypotension result, or 750 to 1000 mg is administered) may be tried. If successful, procainamide may then be given as a continuous IV infusion (2 to 6 mg/minute).

4. When first-line antiarrhythmic agents such as lidocaine or procainamide have failed, IV bretylium at a dose of 5 mg/kg is given over several minutes and may be increased to 10 mg/kg 15 to 30 minutes later. Doses may be repeated at 15- to 30-minute intervals, not to exceed a total of 40 mg/kg. A continuous infusion at 1 to 2 mg/min can be initiated.

5. If the arrhythmia does not respond to medical therapy, electrical DC cardioversion may be used. Ventricular tachycardia that precipitates hypotension, shock, angina, or congestive heart failure should be treated *promptly* with DC cardioversion. Very low energies (10 to 50 watt-seconds) may terminate ventricular tachycardia (see discussion of treatment of ventricular fibrillation). Digitalis-induced ventricular tachycardia is best treated medically. After reversion of the arrhythmia to a normal rhythm, it is essential to institute measures to prevent a recurrence (see Chapter 8 for discussion of cardioversion).

6. In patients who have recurrent ventricular tachycardia a pacing catheter can be inserted into the right ventricle, and single, double, or multiple stimuli can

be introduced competitively to terminate the ventricular tachycardia (Fig. 8-59). This procedure incurs the risk of accelerating the ventricular tachycardia to ventricular flutter or ventricular fibrillation. A new catheter electrode has been recently developed through which synchronized cardioversion can be performed. In the awake, conscious patient shocks of 0.25 watt-seconds that successfully terminate ventricular tachycardia can be delivered through this catheter electrode.[18]

7. A search for reversible conditions contributing to the initiation and maintenance of ventricular tachyarrhythmias should be made and the conditions corrected if possible. For example, ventricular arrhythmia related to hypotension or hypokalemia at times may be terminated by vasopressors or potassium, respectively. Slow ventricular rates that are caused by sinus bradycardia or AV block may permit the occurrence of premature ventricular complexes and ventricular tachyarrhythmias that can be corrected by administering atropine, 0.5 to 2.0 mg IV, temporary isoproterenol administration (1 to 2 μg/minute in an IV drip), or temporary transvenous pacing.

8. Intermittent ventricular tachycardia, interrupted by one or more supraventricular beats, generally is best treated medically. Lidocaine or procainamide should be tried. If they prove unsuccessful, then quinidine, disopyramide (IV administration is approved for investigational use only), propranolol, or recently approved drugs such as flecainide and amiodarone (IV administration investigational) may be tried.

Prevention of recurrences may be difficult at times.[19]

1. Initial preventive drug therapy for recurrent ventricular arrhythmias in the ambulatory patient should be with quinidine, procainamide, disopyramide, flecainide, or tocainide. Amiodarone is reserved for the patient in whom these other drugs fail to work or who cannot tolerate them. Procainamide is given as a loading dose of 0.5 to 1 g orally, followed by 375 to 500 mg three to six times daily. Because procainamide has a shorter duration of action than quinidine, the long-acting preparation must be used when giving procainamide at 6-hour intervals to provide therapeutic blood levels (4 to 8 mg/L) for the entire 6-hour period. Hard-to-control arrhythmias may reflect poor absorption of the drug or nontherapeutic blood levels between two widely spaced doses.

2. Alternatively, quinidine may be used, administered at a dose of 200 to 400 mg four times daily, to achieve therapeutic blood levels of 3 to 6 mg/L.

3. If quinidine is unsuccessful, disopyramide, 100 to 250 mg every 6 hours, flecainide, 50 to 300 mg every 12 hours, or tocainide, 400 to 600 mg every 8 to 12 hours, may be tried. Amiodarone, after a loading dose of 800 to 1600 mg/day for 1 to 2 weeks, is given at a maintenance dose of 400 to 800 mg/day working down to the lowest effective dose daily.

4. Following an initial approach with the above drugs, phenytoin or propranolol may be tried; these two drugs are often not very effective in preventing recurrences of ventricular tachyarrhythmias.

5. Combinations of drugs with different mechanisms of action may be successful and allow one to use low doses of both agents rather than high or toxic doses of one drug. For example, propranolol, 40 mg daily, combined with average doses of quinidine or procainamide may be efficacious. Similarly, procainamide or quinidine might be effectively combined with amiodarone.

6. Administration of potassium to maintain serum potassium levels in the 5+ range, in addition to antiarrhythmic agents, may be helpful on occasion.

7. A trial of ventricular or atrial pacing, combined with antiarrhythmic agents if necessary, may be tried empirically; if successful, permanent pacing may be instituted. Generally, unless the initiation of the ventricular tachycardia is related to significant bradycardia, such as ventricular rates in the 30s caused by complete AV block, attempts at rapid "overdrive" pacing are often ineffective long term.

8. Surgery[20] may be used in selected patients to treat ventricular tachycardia. Multiple surgical techniques are available and include a single ventriculotomy in some patients, cryosurgery, and encircling endocardial ventriculotomy to isolate the arrhythmogenic area or endocardial resection to remove the arrhythmogenic area (preferably directed by electrophysiologic mapping techniques) in patients who have ventricular tachycardia related to coronary artery disease (Fig. 8-60). If the surgery alone fails to eliminate recurrences of the arrhythmias, it may make previously ineffective drug regimens efficacious. Coronary bypass surgery alone, without electrophysiologic mapping and myocardial resection, in patients who do not have ventricular tachycardia definitely associated with ischemia, for example, ventricular tachycardia induced by stress testing, has not been very successful.

9. A number of new antiarrhythmic agents (see Chapter 10) offer promise to control recurrent, life-threatening ventricular tachyarrhythmias.[21]

10. Implantable electrical devices that competitively pace, synchronously cardiovert or defibrillate may be very effective in some patients (see Chapter 11).

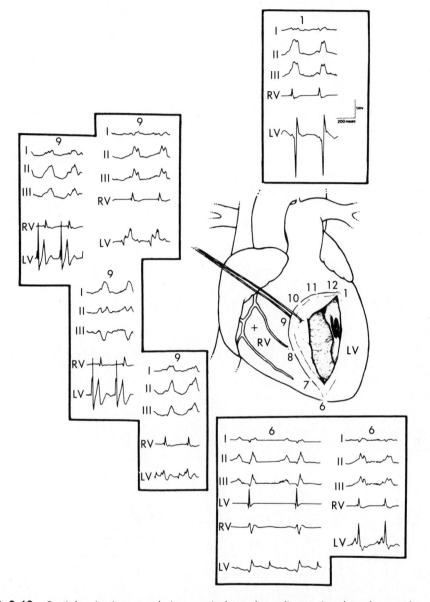

FIG. 8-60.   Partial activation map during ventricular tachycardia; tracings have been redrawn for clarity. Left ventricular aneurysm is opened and numbered in a clockwise fashion. Left ventricular endocardial recordings *(LV)* from a handheld exploring electrode are shown in the inserts for sites 1, 6, and 9. A stationary right ventricular epicardial electrode *(RV)* was sewn in place (+ on right ventricle). Ventricular tachycardia with four different contours (see surface leads, insert 9) was initiated. Left ventricular endocardial recordings at site 9 showed earliest activation during each ventricular tachycardia *(arrows)*. Left ventricular recordings at site 6 (right portion of insert 6) show activation starting later than the left ventricular recordings at site 9 but before the left ventricular recording at site 1, which is relatively normal and late in the QRS complex. However, during sinus rhythm (left portion of insert 6), recording at site 6 shows a split, late potential *(arrow)*. Endocardial resection was carried out between sites 6 and 9 with elimination of ventricular tachycardia.(From Braunwald, E., editor: Heart disease: a textbook of cardiovascular medicine, Philadelphia, 1984, W.B. Saunders Company.)

Evaluation of Therapy. Evaluating the adequacy of drug therapy in patients who have widely spaced episodes of ventricular tachycardia is a difficult problem because there exists no adequate end point to judge therapy until the patient has another spontaneous recurrence. Because of this, many groups have taken a more aggressive approach. The patient undergoes a control electrophysiologic study, during which the ventricular tachycardia is initiated and a variety of electrophysiologic and hemodynamic parameters are assessed. Then the patient is treated with a drug and the electrophysiologic study is repeated. If the drug prevents reinduction of the ventricular tachycardia, there is a high likelihood that the drug will also prevent spontaneous recurrences. If the drug fails to prevent reinitiation of the tachycardia, in many instances the drug may still be successful clinically by slowing the rate of the ventricular tachycardia, converting a sustained form to a non-

sustained episode, or preventing a recurrence.[22] See Chapter 10 for a more detailed discussion.

Torsades de Pointes

The term *torsades de pointes* refers to a ventricular tachycardia characterized by QRS complexes of changing amplitude and morphology that appear to twist around the isoelectric line and occur at rates of 200 to 250 beats/min (Fig. 8-61). The peaks of the QRS complexes appear successively on one side and then the other of the isoelectric baseline, giving the typical twisting appearance with continuous and progressive changes in QRS contour and amplitude. Torsades de pointes connotes a *syndrome* characterized by prolonged ventricular repolarization with corrected QT intervals generally exceeding 500 msec. The U wave also may be prominent but its role in this syndrome and in the long QT syndrome is not clear. Patients expe-

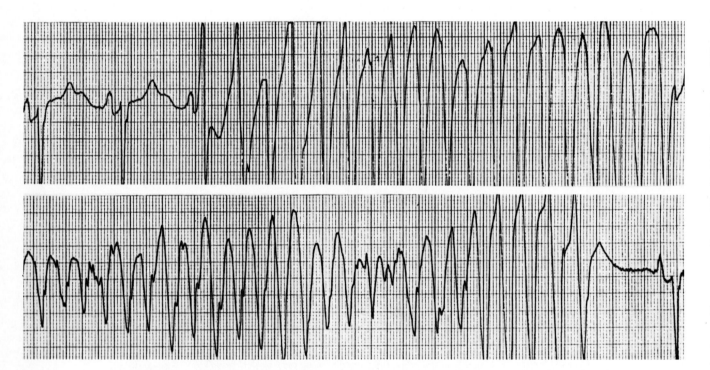

FIG. 8-61.   Long QT interval and torsades de pointes. Congenital long QTU interval (approximately 680 msec, uncorrected) in a 16-year-old with recurrent syncope. Characteristic contour of torsades de pointes is present in the lower recording just before termination of the ventricular tachycardia.

Monitor lead:	Continuous recording.
Rate:	Atrial 60 beats/minute. Ventricular irregular.
Rhythm:	Atrial regular. Ventricular irregular.
P waves:	Normal when visible.
PR interval:	0.18 second during sinus rhythm.
QRS:	Normal during sinus rhythm. QT interval prolonged.
Arrhythmia:	Torsades de pointes.

rience recurrent episodes of ventricular tachycardia often precipitated by a late premature complex. Tachycardia may terminate with progressive prolongation of cycle lengths and larger and more distinctly formed QRS complexes. Rarely ventricular fibrillation supervenes. Of interest is the fact that cycle length changes that occur immediately before the onset of torsades de pointes often show a long-short RR cycle sequence: a pause in the supraventricular rhythm, caused by sinus bradycardia or the compensatory pause following a premature ventricular complex, is followed by the next sinus beat that has a premature ventricular complex in its T wave. The premature ventricular complex appears to initiate torsades de pointes.

Significance. Severe bradycardia, potassium depletion, or drugs such as quinidine, disopyramide, procainamide or some antidepressant drugs may cause torsades de pointes. Patients with the long QT syndrome (see below) may also experience torsades de pointes.

Treatment. Treatment of ventricular tachycardia that has a polymorphic pattern depends on whether or not the QT interval is prolonged. Thus it is important to restrict the definition of torsades de pointes to the typical electrocardiographic morphology described above that occurs in the setting of a long QT and/or long Q-T U wave. In patients with torsades de pointes, administration of antiarrhythmic agents such as quinidine, disopyramide and procainamide tends to increase the abnormal QT interval and worsen the arrhythmia.

1. Temporary ventricular or atrial pacing should be instituted. Pacing at rapid rates suppresses the ventricular tachycardia, which often does not recur after cessation of pacing. Isoproterenol can be tried until pacing is instituted.
2. Magnesium sulfate given intravenously has been reported to suppress torsades de pointes in a small number of patients.
3. The cause of the long QT interval and torsades de pointes should be determined and corrected if possible.
4. Antiarrhythmic drugs that do not prolong the QT interval, such as lidocaine, mexiletine, or tocainide, may be tried.

Long QT Syndrome

Long QT syndrome exists when an abnormally prolonged QT interval is present that exceeds 0.44 seconds after correction for rate, or when the Q-T U pattern appears abnormal in configuration. The nature of the U wave and its relationship to the long QT syndrome are not clear. Notched, bifid and sinusoidal T waves may occur.

Significance. Repolarization abnormalities can be divided into two groups: 1) a primary or idiopathic group that includes a congenital, often familial disorder sometimes, but not always, associated with deafness, and 2) an acquired group caused by various drugs like quinidine, disopyramide and procainamide, phenothiazines and tricyclic antidepressants, metabolic abnormalities such as hypokalemia, central nervous system lesions, autonomic nervous system dysfunction, coronary artery disease with myocardial infarction, and other problems. Symptomatic patients with the long QT syndrome develop ventricular tachycardias that, in many instances, are caused by torsade de pointes. Since sudden death may occur in this group of patients, it is obvious that, in some, the ventricular arrhythmia becomes sustained and probably results in ventricular fibrillation. Patients with congenital long QT syndrome who are at increased risks for developing sudden cardiac death include those who have family members who died suddenly at an early age and those who have experienced syncope.

Treatment. 1) For patients who do not have syncope, complex ventricular arrhythmias or a family history of sudden cardiac death, no therapy is recommended; 2) in asymptomatic patients with complex ventricular arrhythmias or a family history of premature sudden cardiac death, beta blockers at maximally tolerated doses are recommended; 3) in patients with syncope, beta blockers at maximally tolerated doses, at times combined with phenytoin and phenobarbital, are suggested; 4) patients who continue to have syncope despite triple drug therapy, left-sided cervicothoracic sympathetic ganglionectomy that interrupts the stellate ganglion and the first three or four thoracic ganglia has been proposed; 5) finally, implantable automatic defibrillators may be needed in the symptomatic patient who has not responded to other therapy.

ACCELERATED IDIOVENTRICULAR RHYTHM (Figs. 8-62 and 8-63)

The ventricular rate, commonly between 50 and 110 beats/minute, usually hovers within 10 beats of the sinus rate so that control of the cardiac rhythm may be passed back and forth between these two competing pacemaker sites. Consequently, long runs of fusion beats often appear at the onset and termination of the arrhythmia as the pacemakers vie for control of ventricular discharge. Because of the slow rates, capture beats are common. The onset of this arrhythmia is generally gradual (nonparoxysmal) and occurs when the rate of ectopic ventricular discharge exceeds the sinus rate because of sinus slowing, or SA or AV block. The ectopic mechanism may also begin following a premature ventricular complex or the ectopic ventricular rate may simply accelerate sufficiently to overtake the sinus focus. The slow rate and nonparoxysmal onset usually avoid the problems initiated by excitation during the vulnerable period, and consequently, precipitation of more rapid ventricular arrhythmias is rarely seen. Termination of the rhythm generally occurs gradually as the dominant sinus rhythm accelerates or the ectopic ventricular rhythm decelerates. Occasionally, an accelerated idioventricular rhythm may be present in a patient who also has a more rapid ventricular tachycardia at other times.

Significance. The arrhythmia occurs as a rule in patients with heart disease such as in a setting of acute myocardial infarction or as an expression of digitalis toxicity. Generally it is transient and intermittent, with episodes lasting a few seconds to a minute, and does not appear to seriously affect the course or prognosis of the disease. Suppressive therapy is usually unnecessary because the ventricular rate is commonly less than 100 beats/minute. Basically, five conditions exist during which therapy may be considered: (1) when AV dissociation results in loss of sequential AV contraction and, with it, the hemodynamic benefits of atrial contraction; (2) when accelerated idioventricular rhythm occurs together with more rapid forms of ventricular tachycardia; (3) when accelerated idioventricular rhythm begins with a premature ventricular com-

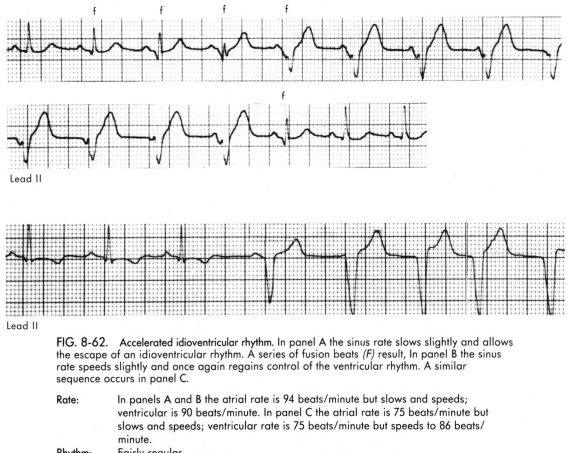

FIG. 8-62.   Accelerated idioventricular rhythm. In panel A the sinus rate slows slightly and allows the escape of an idioventricular rhythm. A series of fusion beats *(F)* result, In panel B the sinus rate speeds slightly and once again regains control of the ventricular rhythm. A similar sequence occurs in panel C.

Rate:	In panels A and B the atrial rate is 94 beats/minute but slows and speeds; ventricular is 90 beats/minute. In panel C the atrial rate is 75 beats/minute but slows and speeds; ventricular rate is 75 beats/minute but speeds to 86 beats/minute.
Rhythm:	Fairly regular.
P waves:	Normal P waves preceding each normally conducted QRS complex.
PR interval:	0.14 second for the normally conducted beats.
QRS:	0.06 second for the normally conducted beats and 0.14 second for the accelerated idioventricular beats.

plex that initiates more rapid ventricular tachycardia; (4) when the ventricular rate is too rapid and produces symptoms; and (5) if ventricular fibrillation develops. The latter appears only rarely.

Treatment. Treatment for accelerated idioventricular rhythm is as follows:

1. The best initial therapeutic approach would appear to be close observation, rhythm monitoring, and care for the underlying heart disease.

2. Digitalis administration should be discontinued if the drug is implicated in the genesis of the arrhythmia.

3. Atropine, 0.5 mg IV initially, repeated if necessary, may be used to speed the sinus rate and capture the ventricles. Rarely, pacing may be considered to speed the basic heart rate and suppress the accelerated idioventricular rhythm.

4. Lidocaine or other antiarrhythmic drugs may be given to suppress the ectopic ventricular focus.

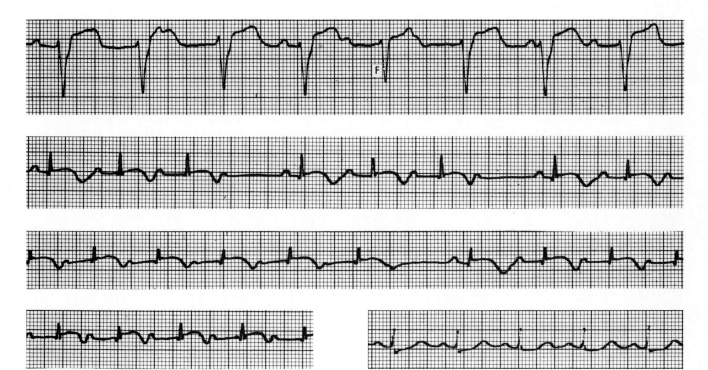

FIG. 8-63. Accelerated idioventricular rhythm and second-degree AV block. This series of tracings was recorded over a period of several days in a patient who had an acute inferior myocardial infarction. In panel A an acceelerated idioventricular rhythm occurs at a rate of 70 beats/minute. Note the fusion QRS complex (F) in the midportion of the strip preceded by a long PR interval. The long PR interval suggests the presence of an AV conduction disturbance, but its exact degree cannot be determined from this ECG. Thus incomplete AV dissociation is present, caused by a combination of accelerated idioventricular rhythm and AV block. In panel B the accelerated idioventricular rhythm has stopped, but Wenckenbach second-degree AV block is present with a conduction ratio of 4:3. In panel C the Wenckebach second-degree AV block is still present, but the conduction ratio has increased significantly. On the following day (D) the second-degree AV block has disappeared and is now replaced by first-degree AV block. Finally, after several days the first-degree AV block is barely present (E). A, Monitor lead. B-E, Lead II.

Rate:	Panel A: atrial, 88 beats/minute; ventricular, 70 beats/minute. Panel B: atrial, 87 beats/minute; ventricular, varying. Panel C: atrial, 86 beats/minute; ventricular, varying. Panel D; atrial and ventricular, 88 beats/minute. Panel E: atrial and ventricular, 88 beats/minute.
Rhythm:	Panel A: atrial and ventricular, regular. Panel B: atrial, regular; ventricular, irregular. Panel C: atrial, regular; ventricular, irregular. Panel D: atrial and ventricular, regular. Panel E: atrial and ventricular, regular.
P waves:	Normal in all traces.
PR interval:	Not measurable in panel A, progressively increasing in panels B and C, regular at 0.3 second in panel D, and regular at 0.20 second in panel E.
QRS:	0.12 second in panel A and 0.06 second in panels B to E.

VENTRICULAR FLUTTER AND VENTRICULAR FIBRILLATION
(Figs. 8-64 to 8-66)

Ventricular flutter and ventricular fibrillation represent severe derangements of the heartbeat that usually terminate fatally within 3 to 5 minutes unless they are promptly stopped. Ventricular flutter resembles a sine wave in appearance, with regular, large oscillations occurring at a rate between 150 and 300 beats/minute, usually exceeding 200 beats/minute. Ventricular fibrillation is recognized by the presence of irregular undulations of varying contour and amplitude. Distinct QRS complexes, ST segment, and T waves are absent. The difference between rapid ventricular tachycardia and ventricular flutter may be difficult to discern and is usually of academic interest only.

Significance. Ventricular fibrillation occurs in a variety of clinical situations but is most commonly associated with coronary heart disease, acute myocardial infarction, and cardiomyopathy. The arrhythmia occurs frequently as the terminal event in a variety of diseases. It also may be seen during cardiac pacing, cardiac catheterization, operation, anesthesia, drug toxicity (for example, antiarrhythmic drugs), and hypoxia. It may occur after electric shock administered during cardioversion or accidentally by improperly grounded equipment. Premature stimulation during the vulnerable period (R-on-T phenomenon; see discussion of ventricular tachycardia) may precipitate ventricular tachycardia, flutter, or fibrillation, particularly when the electrical stability of the heart has been altered by the ischemia of an acute myocardial infarction, for example. In many patients, sustained ventricular tachycardia may precede ventricular fibrillation.[22] However, ventricular fibrillation may occur without antecedent or precipitating ventricular tachycardia or premature ventricular complexes. Experimentally, it may occur when a previously occluded coronary artery undergoes sudden restoration of flow. Clinically, this condition may be replicated by streptokinase infusion or percutaneous transluminal angioplasty (PTCA) that restores flow to an occluded coronary artery, or possibly when coronary spasm relaxes. Conceivably, the latter event could result in ventricular fibrillation without myocardial infarction.

Ventricular flutter or fibrillation results in faintness followed by loss of consciousness, seizures, apnea, and, if the rhythm continues untreated, death. The blood pressure is unobtainable, and heart sounds are usually absent. The atria may continue to beat at an independent rhythm or be retrogradely captured for a time. Eventually, electrical activity of the heart is completely absent.

Many patients who suffer ventricular fibrillation out of hospital have been resuscitated. It is interesting that only 20 to 30% of them develop a myocardial infarction, and those that do have a myocardial infarction experience a 2% to 3% recurrence rate of ventricular fibrillation in the first year. However, those patients who are resuscitated from out-of-hospital ventricular fibrillation but do not develop a myocardial infarction have a 1-year recurrence rate of almost 25% (see Chapter 9).

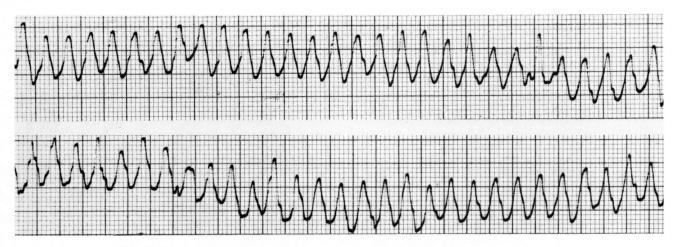

FIG. 8-64. Ventricular flutter. During ventricular flutter, ventricular depolarization and repolarization appear as a sine wave with regular oscillations. The QRS complex cannot be distinguished from the ST segment or T wave. Monitor lead is continuous recording.

Rate: Ventricular, 300 beats/minute.
Rhythm: P waves cannot be seen; ventricular, fairly regular.
PR interval: Not measurable.
QRS: 0.18 second.

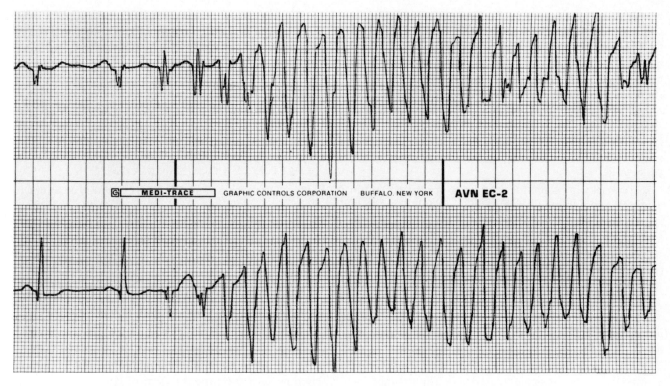

FIG. 8-65.   Ventricular tachycardia to fibrillation. During a 24-hour ambulatory ECG recording the patient experienced sudden death. The ECG demonstrated the development of a rapid ventricular tachycardia that progressed promptly to ventricular fibrillation. Ventricular fibrillation at its onset may appear fairly regular. Dual tracing records simultaneously.

Rate:	During sinus rhythm, 65 beats/minute; ventricular rate during the rapid ventricular tachycardia is approximately 300 beats/minute.
Rhythm:	During sinus rhythm, regular; during rapid ventricular tachycardia, grossly iregular.
P waves:	Normal during sinus rhythm. Cannot be seen during ventricular tachycardia-fibrillation.
PR interval:	0.16 second during sinus rhythm.
QRS:	0.08 second during sinus rhythm. Cannot be measured accurately during the ventricular tachycardia-fibrillation.

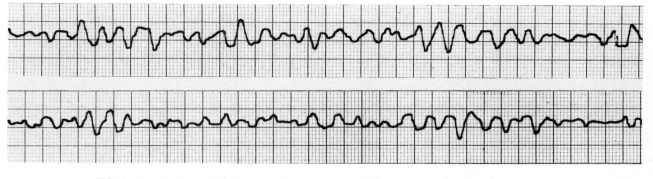

FIG. 8-66.   Ventricular fibrillation. In this monitor lead the irregular, undulating baseline without any electrical evidence of organized ventricular activity is characteristic of ventricular fibrillation. The rhythm in Fig. 8-65 proceeded to degenerate and resemble the rhythm in 8-66.

Rate:	Cannot be determined.
Rhythm:	Grossly irregular.
P waves:	Cannot be seen.
PR interval:	Cannot be determined.
QRS:	Cannot be measured.

Treatment. Ventricular flutter and ventricular fibrillation are totally unphysiologic life-threatening arrhythmias for which immediate electrical (nonsynchronized) DC cardioversion, using 200 to 400 watt-seconds, is the only reliable treatment. When ventricular tachycardia produces the same hemodynamic response as ventricular flutter or fibrillation, it also must be terminated immediately by DC shock. A sharp blow to the chest may terminate some forms of ventricular tachyarrhythmias ("thumpversion"), but time should not be wasted on this procedure if one or two sharp blows fail.

Termination of ventricular flutter or fibrillation within 30 to 60 seconds prevents the biochemical derangements accompanying ventricular fibrillation, eliminates the need for endotracheal intubation, and significantly increases the success rate of such procedures. If necessary, artificial ventilation by means of mouth-to-mouth resuscitation or a well-fitting rubber face mask and an Ambu bag is quite satisfactory and eliminates the delay attending intubation by inexperienced personnel. Chest compression to achieve cardiac massage may be instituted, but *there must be no delay in administering the DC shock.* If the patient is not monitored and it cannot be established whether asystole or ventricular fibrillation has caused the cardiovascular collapse, the electric shock should be administered *without* wasting precious seconds attempting to record the ECG. The DC shock may cause the asystolic heart to begin discharging, as well as terminate ventricular fibrillation if the latter is present. Following a successful cardioversion, measures must be taken to prevent a second episode of ventricular fibrillation, including monitoring of the cardiac rhythm, administration of lidocaine, procainamide, or bretylium, and so forth.

Ventricular fibrillation is quickly followed by severe metabolic acidosis, and sodium bicarbonate, 1 to 2 ampules containing 44 mEq of sodium bicarbonate per ampule, may be used initially depending on the pH, which in turn is related to the duration of the ventricular fibrillation. An additional ampule is given every 5 to 8 minutes until adequate cardiorespiratory function is achieved. Blood gases and pH should be obtained as soon as possible and further bicarbonate administration adjusted accordingly.

ATRIOVENTRICULAR BLOCK[23]

The conduction of an impulse may be slowed or completely blocked at sites along the conduction pathway. If the site of conduction impairment is in the AV node, His bundle or surrounding tissue, the resultant conduction abnormality is called an AV block. AV blocks are further described as first degree, second degree, (Type I and Type II), or third degree based on the following criteria.

FIRST-DEGREE AV BLOCK
(Figs. 8-67 and 8-68)

During first-degree heart block, every atrial impulse is conducted to the ventricles producing a regular ventricular rhythm. However, the duration of AV conduction is abnormally prolonged which is manifested by a PR interval exceeding 0.20 second in the adult. PR intervals as long as 1.0 second have been recorded. First-degree AV Block may be a precursor to more advanced degrees of block.

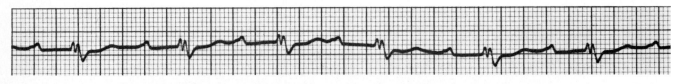

FIG. 8-67. First-degree heart block. In this monitor lead one cannot be certain of the type of intraventricular conduction delay. The prolonged AV conduction time may be caused by conduction delay within the AV node and/or His-Purkinje system (see His bundle section).

Rate: 60 to 70 beats/minute.
Rhythm: Regular.
P waves: Normal contour and precede each QRS complex.
PR interval: Prolonged 0.36 to 0.40 second.

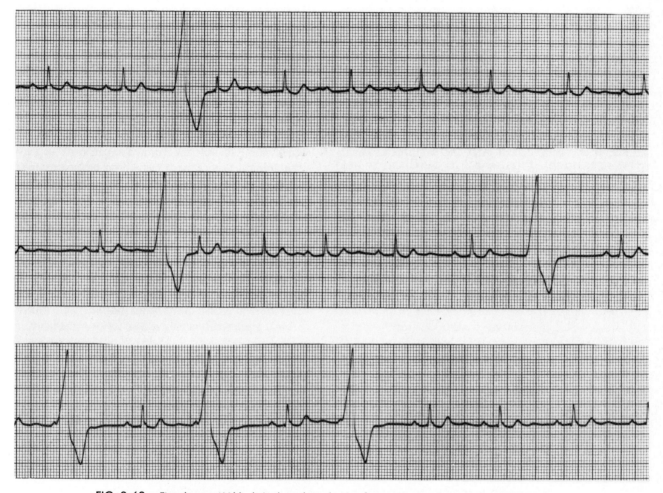

FIG. 8-68. First-degree AV block. In the selected strips from a continuous recording of lead 1, premature ventricular complexes occur and are either interpolated (PVC in the first strip and first PVC in the second strip) or result in a compensatory pause. The PR interval of the QRS complexes preceding the PVC is slightly prolonged. However, following the interpolated PVC the PR interval prolongs further and remains prolonged for a series of beats, finally returning to the resting PR interval duration. When the premature ventricular complex produces a compensatory pause, additional PR prolongation does not occur. Monitor lead.

Rate: 63 beats/minute.
Rhythm: Regular for the most part; irregularities caused by premature ventricular complexes.
P waves: Normal.
PR interval: 0.22 to 0.24 second prior to the interpolated premature ventricular complexes, lengthening to 0.4 second immediately following the interpolated premature ventricular complex.
QRS: 0.07 second for the normally conducted beats and 0.16 second for the PVC.

SECOND-DEGREE AV BLOCK
(Figs. 8-69 to 8-73)

Failure of some atrial impulses to conduct to the ventricles at a time when physiologic interference would not be expected constitutes second-degree AV block. The nonconducted P wave may be intermittent, frequent, or infrequent, occur at regular or irregular intervals, and may be preceded by fixed or lengthening PR intervals. A distinguishing feature is that conducted P waves relate to a QRS complex with recurring PR intervals, that is, the association of P with QRS is not random. The two types of second-degree AV block can be distinguished with an acceptable degree of accuracy by analysis of the PR intervals.

Second-Degree AV Block Type I (Wenckebach) (Figs. 8-69 to 8-70)

In a classic type I (Wenckebach) second-degree AV block a gradual lengthening of the PR interval occurs because of lengthening AV conduction time, until an atrial impulse is nonconducted. Then the sequence begins again. The ratio of atrial impulses to ventricular responses is frequently 5:4, 4:3, 3:2, or 3:1. The duration of the QRS complex may be normal or prolonged. Type I AV block occurs most commonly in the AV node but can occur in the His-Purkinje system as well. Because the increment in conduction time is greatest in the second beat of the Wenckebach group and then *decreases* progressively over succeeding cycles,

1) the interval between successive RR cycles prior to the nonconducted P wave progressively *decreases*,

2) the duration of the pause produced by the nonconducted P wave is less than twice the shortest cycle,

3) the duration of the RR cycle following the pause exceeds the RR cycle preceding the pause.

In atypical Wenckebach (which occurs commonly) the increment in AV conduction time may increase in the last beat so that the last RR cycle preceding the blocked P wave lengthens rather than shortens.

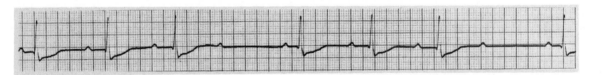

FIG. 8-69. Second-degree AV heart block (type I, Wenckebach). In this monitor lead classic AV Wenckebach heart block is characterized by four features in the surface electrodiogram: (1) progressive PR prolongation preceding the nonconducted P wave; (2) progressive shortening of the RR interval because the increment in PR interval decreases in succeeding cycles; (3) the duration of the pause (generated by the blocked P wave) is less than twice the duration of the shortest cycle, which is the cycle that precedes the nonconducted P wave; and (4) the duration of the RR cycle following the pause exceeds the duration of the RR cycle preceding the pause. The increment in PR interval is greatest in the second cycle following the pause. Wenckebach AV block often may be "atypical"; the increment in PR interval does not decrease but rather increases, so that the last RR interval preceding the nonconducted P wave lengthens rather than shortens. In the setting of a normal QRS complex, Wenckebach AV heart block almost always occurs at the level of the AV node.

Rate:	Atrial, 54 beats/minute; ventricular, varying.
Rhythm:	Atrial, regular; ventricular, varying.
P waves:	More numerous than QRS complexes but are related to ventricular beats in a consistent repetitive fashion.
PR interval:	Progressive PR prolongation preceding the nonconducted P wave. Finally, one P wave is blocked, and the cycle then repeats.
QRS:	Prolonged, 0.14 second. Therefore in this tracing one cannot be certain that the level of block is at the AV node but indeed could occur distal to the His bundle recording site (see His bundle section).

Second-Degree AV Block Type II
(Figs. 8-72 and 8-73)

In type II second-degree AV block a P wave is blocked without progressive antecedent PR prolongation and occurs almost always in a setting of bundle branch block. The PR interval of the conducted atrial impulses may be prolonged or normal but usually remains fairly constant.

The pause caused by the nonconducted P wave is equal to or may be slightly less than twice the normal RR interval. Sinus arrhythmia, premature beats, AV junctional escape beats, or changes in neurogenic influences may disturb the timing of the expected pauses. Type II AV block almost always occurs in the His-Purkinje system.

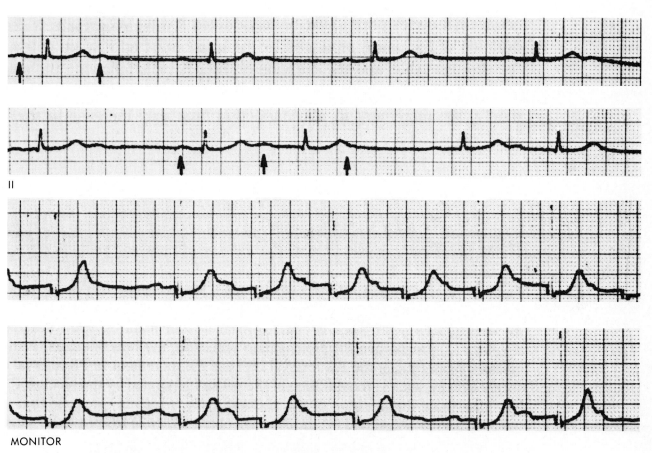

II

MONITOR

FIG. 8-70. Second-degree AV heart block (type I Wenckebach). In A, 2:1 conduction occurs (arrows indicate P waves). Since 2:1 conduction can occur with either type I or type II second-degree heart block, sometimes the two cannot be readily differentiated. However, the presence of a normal QRS complex is an indicator of type I second-degree AV heart block. In B the 2:1 AV heart block becomes 3:2 and PR prolongation for the second conducted P wave *(second arrow)* establishes the diagnosis of type I second-degree AV heart block. C (continuous recording) illustrates the response of Wenckebach AV block to intravenous atropine. Both the atrial rate and the conduction ratio increase.

Rate:	Atrial: in A and B, 72 beats/minute; in C, 79 beats/minute; ventricular: in A, 36 beats/minute; in B, varying; in C, varying but increased.
Rhythm:	Atrial, regular; ventricular, varying, depending on the degree of AV block.
P waves:	Normal.
PR interval:	Progressive increase in PR interval until one P wave fails to conduct.
QRS:	Normal, 0.07 second.

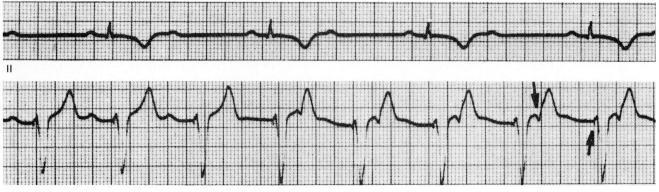

II

MONITOR lead

FIG. 8-71. 2:1 anterograde AV block 1:1 retrograde VA conduction. In the top tracing alternate P waves conduct to the ventricles. In the lower tracing (same patient) ventricular pacing (upright arrow indicates pacemaker artifact) establishes 1:1 retrograde atrial conduction beginning with the fourth paced QRS complex. Inverted arrow indicates retrograde atrial activation.

Rate:	Atrial: top tracing, 68 beats/minute; bottom tracing, 70 beats/minute; ventricular: top tracing, 34 beats/minute; bottom tracing, 70 beats/minute.
Rhythm:	Atrial, regular; ventricular, regular.
P waves:	Top tracing, normal; bottom tracing, normal and retrograde.
PR interval:	Top tracing, 0.20 second; conduction of alternate P waves.
RP interval:	Bottom tracing, 0.16 second.
QRS:	Top tracing. 0.08 second; bottom tracing, 0.14 second.

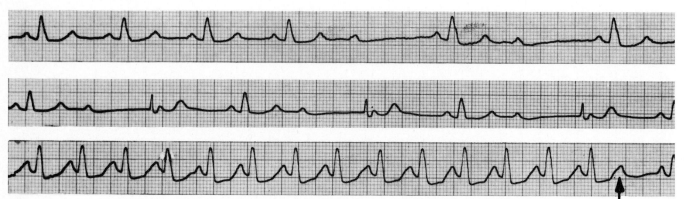

Isoproterenol

FIG. 8-72. Second-degree AV heart block, type II. Left bundle branch block is present in this recording of lead I. Sudden failure of AV conduction results without antecedent PR prolongation. In the second strip the escape beats interrupt the pause produced by the blocked P wave. In the bottom strip isoproterenol infusion has increased the atrial rate and also increased the conduction ratio significantly. Only one nonconducted P wave occurs *(arrow).*

Rate:	Atrial, 62 beats/minute in the top strip. 71 beats/minute in the middle strip, and 122 beats/minute in the bottom strip; ventricular, varying.
Rhythm:	Atrial, regular; ventricular, varying, depending on the degree of AV block.
P waves:	Normal.
PR interval:	Normal and constant at 0.19 second in the top and middle strips and difficult to measure in the bottom strip.
QRS:	Prolonged to 0.12 second with a left bundle branch block contour.

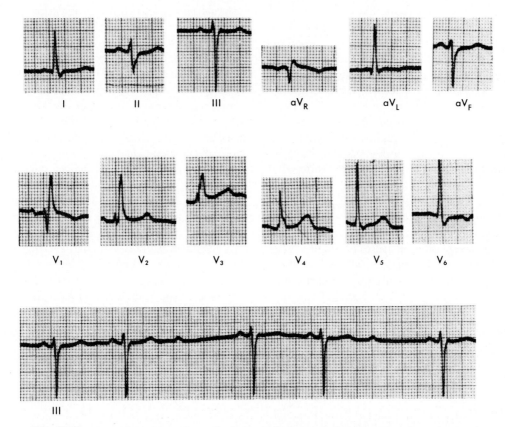

FIG. 8-73.   Second-degree AV heart block, type II. The 12-lead ECG indicates the presence of left anterior fascicular block and right bundle branch block. In the rhythm recording (lead III) sudden failure of AV conduction results without antecedent PR prolongation.

Rate: 62 beats/minute.
Rhythm: Atrial, regular; ventricular, varying, depending on the degree of AV block.
P waves: Normal.
PR interval: Normal, constant (0.14 second) or may be prolonged, constant; sudden failure of conduction.
QRS: Prolonged, 0.12 second.

COMPLETE AV BLOCK (Figs. 8-74 to 8-76)

Complete AV block occurs when no P waves are conducted to the ventricles. The atria and ventricles are controlled by independent pacemakers, and, as such, complete AV block constitutes one form of complete AV dissociation. The atrial pacemaker may be of sinus, ectopic atrial or (uncommonly) junctional origin (tachycardia, flutter, or fibrillation). The ventricular focus may be above or below the His bundle bifurcation, depending on the site of the block. In congenital complete AV block, the block is usually at the level of the AV node, proximal to the His bundle. The escape focus is supraventricular and, as such, is more stable and faster than that which occurs with distal His block. The rhythm, usually regular, may vary because of premature ventricular beats, a shift in pacemaker site, or an irregularly discharging pacemaker focus. The QRS is normal, and Adams-Stokes syncope occurs less often. In acquired complete AV block, the ventricular rate is 30 to 40 beats/minute because the site of block is distal to the His bundle and consequently the escape focus is in the bundle branch–Purkinje system (Fig. 8-62). Less commonly, block within the bundle of His may occur (Fig. 8-76).

Significance. In the adult, drug toxicity (predominantly digitalis, but other drugs as well) and degenerative heart disease are the most common causes of acquired AV heart block. The degenerative process produces partial or complete anatomic or electrical disruption within the AV nodal region, the His bundle, or both bundle branches. Multiple factors may contribute to this degenerative process. They include fibrosclerosis of the cardiac skeleton,

fibrosis of the conduction system, coronary artery disease, myocarditis, and cardiomyopathies. Cardiac surgery has become an infrequent but still important cause of heart block. Less commonly, electrolyte disturbances, endocarditis, myocarditis, tumors, Chagas' disease, syphilitic gummas, rheumatoid nodules, myxedema, infiltrative processes such as amyloidosis, sarcoidosis, or scleroderma, and other systemic illnesses may lead to AV heart block. Calcium deposition in the region of the aortic and mitral valves may extend to involve the conduction pathways. Digitalis excess produces type I, not type II, second-degree AV block.

AV heart block occurring during a myocardial infarction may be divided into two groups: that which occurs during an anterior or anteroseptal infarction and that which occurs during a diaphragmatic (inferior) infarction. When an anterior wall infarction produces AV block, it is usually the result of extensive necrosis of the summit of the interventricular septum, which spares the AV node and His bundle but inflicts severe damage to the bundle branches. Consequently, the block is apt to be distal to the His bundle (type II) and associated with right bundle branch block and a form of fascicular block. Complete AV block may develop, during which the ventricular rate is less than 40 beats/minute, asystole and syncope occur more commonly, and mortality is 75% or higher. Death results from pump failure or shock, owing to the large size of the infarction.

When AV block results from diaphragmatic infarction, the block, type I, usually occurs in the region of the AV node, owing to inflammation or edema that results from ischemia or infarction of neighboring myocardium. The

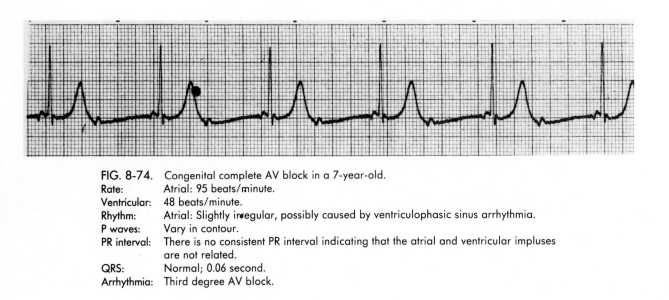

FIG. 8-74.   Congenital complete AV block in a 7-year-old.
Rate: Atrial: 95 beats/minute.
Ventricular: 48 beats/minute.
Rhythm: Atrial: Slightly irregular, possibly caused by ventriculophasic sinus arrhythmia.
P waves: Vary in contour.
PR interval: There is no consistent PR interval indicating that the atrial and ventricular impulses
               are not related.
QRS: Normal; 0.06 second.
Arrhythmia: Third degree AV block.

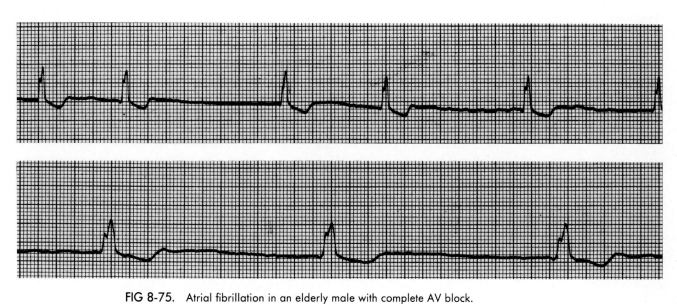

FIG 8-75. Atrial fibrillation in an elderly male with complete AV block.

Rate: 20 to 70 beats/minute.
Rhythm: Irregular.
P waves: Irregular baseline indicates atrial fibrillation.
PR interval: Not measurable.
QRS interval: 0.10 second in top strip to 0.14 second in bottom strip.
Arrhythmia: The underlying atrial rhythm is atrial fibrillation. In the bottom strip there is
               complete AV dissociation (as a result of complete AV block) manifested by
               ventricular escape beats while the atria continue to fibrillate.

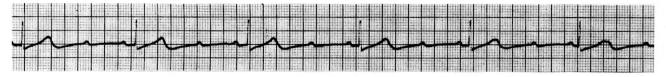

FIG. 8-76. Third-degree (complete) AV heart block. This tracing was recorded from an
80-year-old man who had recurrent syncope caused by an acquired complete AV block. The
ECG is uncommon, since the QRS complexes are normal in this monitor lead and suggest that
the site of block is AV nodal or, more likely, intrahisian. Congenital complete AV block has this
appearance, although with a faster ventricular rate. His bundle recording would be necessary to
establish site of block.

Rate: Atrial, 107 beats/minute; ventriclar, 36 beats/minute.
Rhythm: Atrial, regular; ventricular, regular.
P waves: Normal.
PR interval: Totally variable.
QRS: Normal, 0.6 second.

ventricular pacemaker is faster and more stable, located in the region of the AV node or His bundle, and the block is usually transient, without residua. Advanced block and syncope are uncommon, and the mortality in patients without associated heart failure does not appear to be increased. Some overlap occurs between these two divisions.

Atropine, isoproterenol, and exercise normally shorten the PR interval as the atrial rate increases; when the atrial rate is increased by atrial pacing, the PR interval lengthens. Steroids and thyroid hormones tend to improve AV conduction, which may lengthen during adrenal insufficiency or myxedema. In patients with type II AV block occurring in the His-Purkinje system, an increase in the atrial rate following atropine, isoproterenol or exercise may not concomitantly improve AV conduction and result in a greater number of blocked P waves.

Symptoms during second-degree AV block are infrequent unless periods of complete AV block occur. The slow ventricular rate during complete heart block may not maintain circulation effectively and may result in angina, congestive heart failure, or syncope. Ventricular asystole may occur or the slow rate may initiate premature ventricular systoles or tachyarrhythmias.

Treatment

FIRST-DEGREE AV BLOCK. Generally no therapy is required. If digitalis, quinidine, or procainamide is implicated, the offending drug must be stopped or its dosage reduced.

SECOND-DEGREE AV BLOCK

Type 1. Generally no therapy is required. Treatment may be necessary for patients who are symptomatic with very slow ventricular rates. This may be more common in elderly patients who develop type I AV block. Atropine, in 0.5-mg increments IV, or isoproterenol, 1 or 2 μg/minute, may be tried initially, with care taken not to produce a sinus tachycardia in patients who have an acute myocardial infarction. If there is no response or if the block remains for prolonged periods, pacemaker therapy may be used. Digitalis, if implicated, must be stopped.

Type II. If type II block develops in the setting of an acute myocardial infarction, temporary transvenous pacing is necessary because this form of block often presages the occurrence of sudden complete AV block with ventricular asystole and Adams-Stokes syncope. Prior to pacemaker insertion, isoproterenol may be used temporarily. Atropine, by increasing the atrial rate without decreasing the

AV block, may cause more P waves to block and reduce the ventricular rate. Symptomatic (for instance, with syncope, or presyncope) patients who do not have an acute myocardial infarction should receive a permanent pacemaker. For asymptomatic patients, many physicians recommend permanent pacemaker implantation prophylactically, since the natural history of type II AV block is to progress to complete AV block.

THIRD-DEGREE (COMPLETE) AV BLOCK. If third-degree (complete) AV block develops in a setting of an acute myocardial infarction, temporary transvenous pacing is necessary; isoproterenol may be used initially if required. Asymptomatic patients with chronic stable complete AV block may need no specific therapy, although many physicians recommend prophylactic pacemaker implantation for them, to prevent an Adams-Stokes attack. For those patients with symptoms of congestive heart failure or Adams-Stokes syncope, caused by ventricular asystole, severe ventricular bradycardia, or ventricular tachyarrhythmias occurring as a result of the AV block, long-term drug therapy is generally unreliable, and permanent pacemaker implantation is indicated. It has been suggested that patients who develop transient high-degree AV block during myocardial infarction and survive should receive prophylactic permanent pacemaker implantation even though the block resolves.[24] This conclusion needs to be supported by other studies.

BUNDLE BRANCH BLOCK
(Figs. 8-77 and 8-78)

Anatomic or functional discontinuity in one of the bundle branches may prevent or slow conduction so that the ventricle on the affected side becomes activated late, because this ventricle, normally supplied by the blocked bundle branch, must be activated by impulses traveling through the ventricular wall and interventricular septum from the unaffected side. Conduction along this circuitous route proceeds more slowly, and therefore the QRS complex becomes widened to 0.10 to 0.12 second (incomplete) or more than 0.12 second (complete right or left bundle branch block). Transient bundle branch block may occur as a result of tachycardia, bradycardia, pulmonary embolism, anemia, infection, myocardial ischemia or infarction, congestive heart failure, metabolic derangements, hypoxia, and other causes.

LEFT BUNDLE BRANCH BLOCK (Fig. 8-77)

In complete left bundle branch block (LBBB) the QRS complex becomes prolonged more than 0.12 second, with the major slowing occurring in the middle and terminal forces. The initial forces are deformed and prevent the development of the normal septal Q wave in I or V_6. Initial R waves in V_1 to V_3 are small or absent, followed by deep, large, slurred S waves, and large, prolonged R waves in V_5 and V_6. Significant mean axis deviation is usually absent. The ST segment and T wave shift are characteristically 180 degrees opposite the major QRS deflection.

Significance. LBBB is often associated with serious heart disease such as coronary artery disease, valvular heart disease, and hypertension. Although both RBBB and LBBB can occur in patients without apparent heart disease, LBBB correlates significantly with cardiomegaly and suggests a more serious prognosis. The conduction defect caused by LBBB alters the initial QRS vector, often obscuring the normal ECG signs of an acute myocardial infarction.

RIGHT BUNDLE BRANCH BLOCK (Fig. 8-78)

In uncomplicated complete right bundle branch block (RBBB) the QRS complex is 0.11 second or wider. The initial and middle forces of the vector loop are in a normal direction, and the terminal force is directed to the right and anteriorly. These changes produce large S waves in I, II, V_5, and V_6, often a terminal R wave in III, and R′ in V_1 and V_2. Incomplete RBBB is associated with the same electrocardiographic pattern, but the QRS complex is 0.10 second or less.

Significance. In a young individual, right ventricular hypertrophy may produce RBBB; in an older patient, coronary artery disease is a more likely cause. Early supraventricular complexes that are conducted aberrantly through the ventricle are more likely to develop RBBB than LBBB, presumably because the right bundle branch takes longer to repolarize than does the left bundle branch. The initial forces in RBBB are not altered, and therefore the ECG signs of myocardial infarction are not obscured.

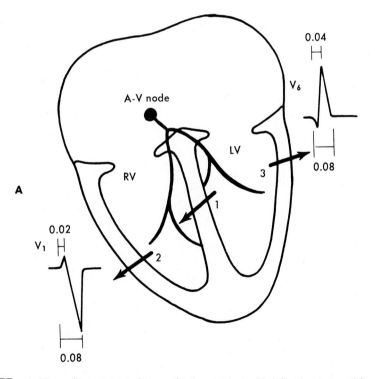

FIG. 8-77. A, Normal intraventricular conduction. Intrinsicoid deflection (interval from onset of QRS complex to peak of R wave, upper brackets) is usually about 0.02 second in right precordial leads and 0.03 to 0.04 second in left precordial leads. The intrinsicoid deflection prolongs during bundle branch block. *Continued.*

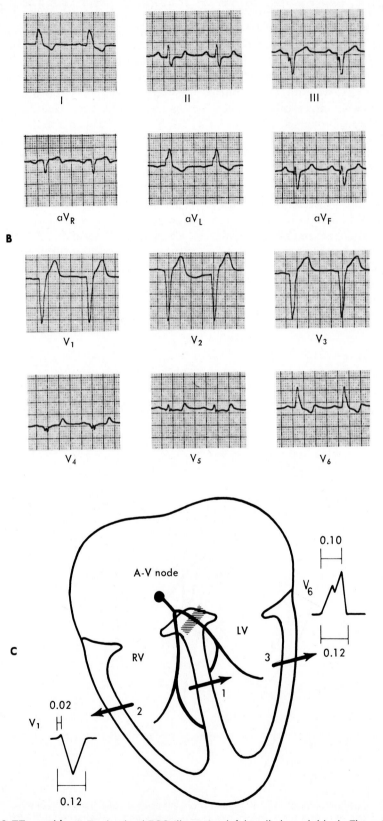

FIG. 8-77, cont'd. B, Twelve-lead ECG illustrating left bundle branch block. The axis is −30 degrees. C, Schematic illustration is presented.

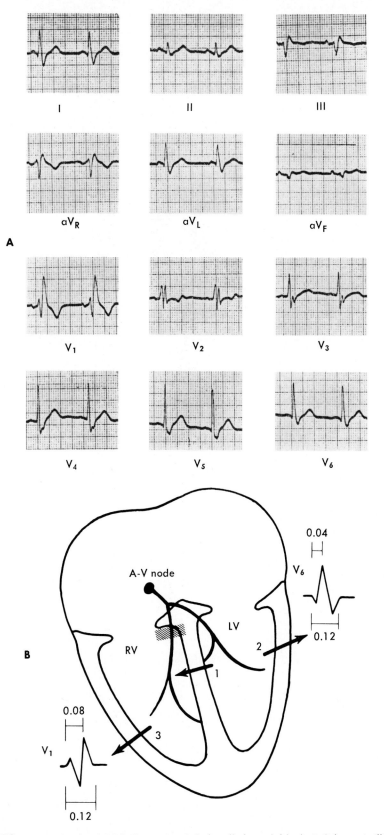

FIG. 8-78. A, Twelve-lead ECG illustrating right bundle branch block. B, Schematic illustration is presented.

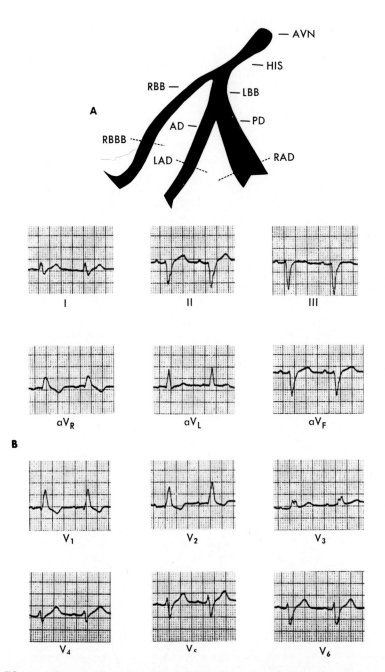

FIG. 8-79.   A, Schematic illustration of the trifascicular nature of ventricular conduction. *AVN,* Atrioventricular node; *HIS,* bundle of His; *RBB,* right bundle branch; *LBB,* main portion of left bundle branch; *AD,* anterior division (fascicle) of left bundle branch; *PD,* posterior division (fascicle) of left bundle branch. Interrupted lines indicate block or delay in conduction, with resultant right bundle branch block *(RBBB),* left axis deviation *(LAD),* right axis deviation *(RAD).* LAD and RAD, in this context, are called left anterior fascicular and left posterior fascicular block, respectively. B, Twelve-lead ECG illustrating right bundle branch block and left anterior fascicular block. See also Fig. 8-72.

FASCICULAR BLOCKS
(Figs. 8-79 and 8-80)

According to electrocardiographic concepts, the left bundle branch divides into anterior and posterior divisions or fascicles.[1] Block may occur in one or the other division (hemiblock) and give rise primarily to a shift in the frontal plane QRS axis without significant QRS prolongation. *Left anterior fascicular block* results in a QRS angle in the frontal plane of about −60 degrees, an initial Q wave in lead I, a terminal S wave in lead III, and a normal or slightly prolonged QRS duration. *Left posterior fascicular block* produces a QRS angle in the frontal plane of about +120 degrees, an initial Q wave in lead III, and a terminal S wave in lead I; forces of the first half of the QRS complex are also directed toward +120 degrees. Right ventricular hypertrophy and a vertical heart must be excluded. Fascicular blocks may combine with RBBB, thus representing examples of bilateral bundle branch block.

Significance. Fascicular blocks may result from coronary artery disease, particularly in the setting of an acute anteroseptal myocardial infarction that simultaneously involves the right bundle branch and one of the divisions of the left bundle branch. Two large groups of patients develop ventricular conduction disorders owing to a sclerodegenerative process limited to the conduction system (Lenegre's disease) or to fibrosclerosis of structures adjacent to the conduction system (Lev's disease). Patients with Lenegre's disease appear to be younger than those with Lev's disease and more prone to developing AV block.

If left anterior or left posterior fascicular block is present with RBBB, it must be remembered that the unblocked fascicle may constitute the only conduction pathway from the His bundle to the ventricle. The posterior division of the left bundle branch seems to be the least vulnerable segment of the specialized ventricular conduction system and, therefore, left posterior fascicular block, with or without RBBB, occurs least often. When lesions are sufficiently extensive to involve the posterior fascicle, they often involve the anterior fascicle and right bundle branch as well. Left posterior fascicular block carries a worse prognosis than does left anterior fascicular block, with increased likelihood to progress to more advanced stages of AV block.

Treatment. In the presence of an acute myocardial infarction, the development of RBBB with left anterior or posterior fascicular block generally requires prophylactic temporary transvenous pacemaker insertion because more advanced AV block may follow. Pacemaker implantation usually is not necessary for the asymptomatic patient without acute myocardial infarction who develops one of the chronic forms of unilateral or bilateral bundle branch block as a result of degenerative cardiac changes, since their rate of progression to forms of symptomatic AV block is fairly slow. Also, these patients do not require temporary prophylactic pacing prior to undergoing surgical procedures.

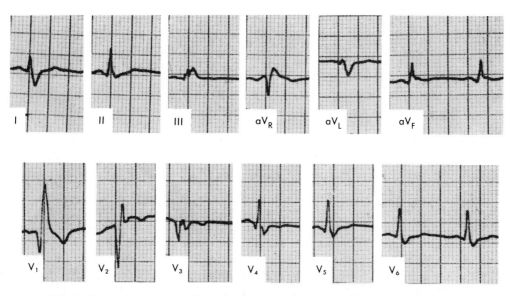

FIG. 8-80.   Twelve-lead ECG illustrating right bundle branch block and left posterior fascicular block. The abnormal Q waves in leads V₁ to V₄ indicate the presence of an anteroseptal myocardial infarction.

PARASYSTOLE (Fig. 8-81)

Premature complexes that lack a fixed relationship to the preceding complex (varying coupling intervals) may result from parasystole. As classically defined, a parasystolic focus is a protected pacemaker focus that discharges at a fixed rate. Parasystolic discharge becomes manifest when the area in which the parasystolic focus originates has recovered excitability. The parasystolic focus then may depolarize the atrium or ventricle to produce a premature complex. The resulting P wave or QRS complex has a configuration different from that of the dominant rhythm, depending on the site of origin. Although the dominant rhythm may be discharged by the parasystolic focus, the dominant rhythm does not depolarize the parasystolic focus because the latter is protected by unidirectional entrance block; that is, impulses may exit from the parasystolic focus to discharge the surrounding myocardium, but no impulse may enter the parasystolic focus and discharge it. For learning purposes, it can be thought of as a fixed-rate pacemaker that does not sense spontaneous complexes, is not reset by them but does cause depolarization of the rest of the heart. The manifest parasystolic rate may be much less than the actual rate because of exit block from the parasystolic focus. That is, the parasystolic focus may discharge at more rapid rates

than are apparent in the ECG because many of the discharges fail to exit and depolarize the surrounding myocardium. Exit block from the parasystolic focus may produce irregular spacing of the interectopic intervals. However, since the rate of discharge of the parasystolic focus is constant, the interectopic intervals between parasystolic impulses reduce to a common denominator. Premature complexes that are caused by a parasystolic focus ordinarily have no fixed relationship to the basic rhythm and often result in the production of fusion beats.

Recent experimental and clinical data suggest that these comments about parasystole are too restrictive, and that the dominant cardiac rhythm can and does modulate the discharge rate and rhythm of the parasystolic focus.[2] Further discussion of this concept is beyond the scope of this chapter, however.

Significance. Atrial and junctional parasystole may occur in patients without clinical evidence of heart disease. Ventricular parasystole generally manifests in patients with heart disease; it is rarely, if ever, caused by digitalis excess.

Treatment. The therapeutic approach is basically the same as that discussed for premature atrial, junctional, and ventricular complexes.

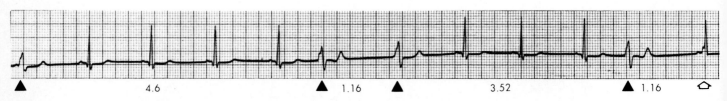

FIG. 8-81.   Ventricular parasystole. The parasystolic ventricular beats are indicated by the solid triangles and the open arrow. The interval between parasystolic ventricular complexes is 1.16 seconds. The intervals of 4.6 and 3.52 seconds are four times and three times, respectively, the interectopic interval of 1.16 seconds. Note that the coupling interval varies and that a fusion beat (next to last QRS complex, indicated by open arrow) is also present. Ventricular refractoriness prevents emergence of the parasystolic ventricular rhythm during the long intervals in which it is absent. This tracing was recorded from an otherwise healthy 15-year-old boy.

Rate:	65 beats/minute, with some variation; parasystolic rate, 63 beats/minute.
Rhythm:	Atrial and ventricular rhythms during normally conducted beats, regular; parasystolic ventricular interval, regular.
P waves:	Normal.
PR interval:	0.11 second during the normally conducted beats.
QRS:	Of normally conducted beats, 0.09 second; or parasystolic ventricular beats, 0.12 second.

AV DISSOCIATION

As the words imply, AV dissociation means that atria and ventricles are dissociated; they are controlled by separate pacemakers for one or more beats. The term used generically tells nothing about the nature of atrial or ventricular activity, except that these chambers are beating independently for a period of time. It is as if the term described a "symptom" without indicating what caused it. The atria may be fibrillating, fluttering, or responding to an ectopic tachycardia or sinus impulses; the ventricles may be controlled by AV junctional or ectopic ventricular beating. The only fact conveyed is that whatever controls one chamber does not also control the other during the period of AV dissociation.

AV dissociation is *never* a primary disturbance of rhythm but rather a consequence of a more basic disorder; for the term to be used properly, the cause(s) producing AV dissociation must also be described. Examples can be found throughout this chapter; some of them are as follows:

1. Slowing of the primary pacemaker to allow the escape of a subsidiary (latent) focus. In Fig. 8-13, sinus slowing allows two ventricular beats to escape under the control of a separate focus while the sinus node still controls the atria. During these two beats, AV dissociation exists.
2. Accelerated discharge of subsidiary focus. In Fig. 8-51, accelerated AV junctional discharge results in a nonparoxysmal AV junctional tachycardia without retrograde atrial capture. Since the atria remain under sinus domination, separate pacemakers control atria and ventricles, resulting in AV dissociation. Fig. 8-135 presents a similar example, called "isorhythmic" AV dissociation because atria and ventricles maintain similar rates and rhythms. AV dissociation may also occur during ventricular tachycardia if retrograde atrial capture does not ensue (see Figs. 8-57 to 8-62).
3. AV block. In Fig. 8-73, AV block reduces the number of effective (conducted) atrial impulses; this allows the escape of a subsidiary focus to produce AV dissociation. When AV block results in AV dissociation, the atrial rate generally exceeds the ventricular rate (see Fig. 8-162).
4. Combinations of 1, 2, or 3 may initiate AV dissociation, as, for example, when digitalis causes both first-degree (or Wenckebach) AV block and NPJT, or when acute myocardial infarction produces AV block and an accelerated idioventricular rhythm (Fig. 8-63).

In all these examples, but for diverse reasons, the ventricular rate either exceeds or becomes equal or nearly equal to the effective (conducted) atrial rate. It is this fact that allows AV dissociation to occur.

The preceding discussion makes it apparent that the presence or absence of AV dissociation depends on the rate and temporal relationships of the two pacemakers and the intactness of AV and VA conduction. Should the atrial pacemaker capture control of the ventricle, or vice versa, AV dissociation would be terminated during that period of capture (incomplete AV dissociation).

SUPRAVENTRICULAR ARRHYTHMIA WITH ABNORMAL QRS COMPLEXES[25]
(Figs. 8-82 to 8-85)

Wide, bizarre QRS complexes may occur during isolated supraventricular beats or sustained supraventricular rhythms. The term *aberrant ventricular conduction* is commonly applied to such complexes. Thus QRS contours that display prolonged abnormal configuration indicate that conduction through the ventricle is abnormal; they do not necessarily mean that the impulse *originated* in the ventricles.[26] The presence of fusion and capture complexes strongly supports the diagnosis of ventricular tachycardia

or accelerated ventricular rhythm. However, the electrocardiographic manifestations of ventricular tachycardia, including the presence or absence of AV dissociation, and complexes that appear to represent capture or fusion beats, may be mimicked, under certain circumstances, by supraventricular arrhythmias.

Intraventricular conduction defects, bundle branch blocks, and anomalous pathway conduction all may initiate abnormal ventricular depolarization with widened QRS complexes. Also, premature supraventricular stimulation may conduct to the ventricles before ventricular repolarization has been completed, causing the impulse to conduct aberrantly. The resulting widened QRS complex may dis-

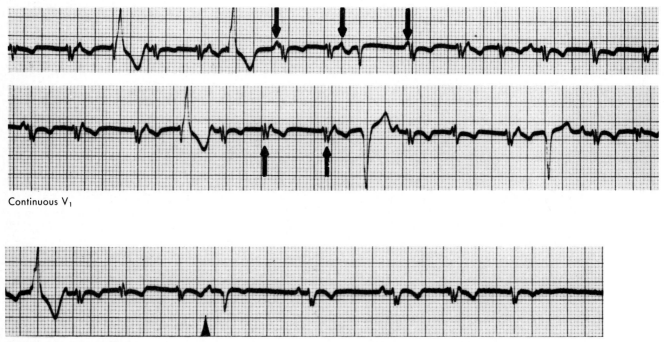

Continuous V₁

Carotid sinus massage V₁

FIG. 8-82. Nonparoxysmal AV junctional tachycardia with intermittent atrial captures producing functional right and functional left bundle branch block. The nonparoxysmal AV junctional tachycardia discharges at a slightly irregular rate and accounts for the W-shaped QRS complexes *(upright arrows)*. Intermittent sinus captures (P waves indicated by inverted arrows) shorten the cardiac cycle and result in either a normal, W-shaped QRS complex, functional right bundle branch block, or functional left bundle branch block. Carotid sinus massage (in the bottom tracing at the arrowhead) slows both the sinus and junctional discharge rates. This tracing was recorded from a 13-year-old boy with no heart disease other than the cardiac arrhythmia. Therapy with digitalis slowed the junctional rate sufficiently so that the patient remained asymptomatic and had resting rates of 70 to 80 beats/minute with a normal response to exercise.

Rate:	Atrial, approximately 88 beats/minute but varying; ventricular, approximately 88 beats/minute but varying.
Rhythm:	Irregular; incomplete AV dissociation.
P waves:	Normal.
PR interval:	0.14 second when premature capture does not occur.
QRS:	Normal, functional right and functional left bundle branch block with a duration of 0.12 second.

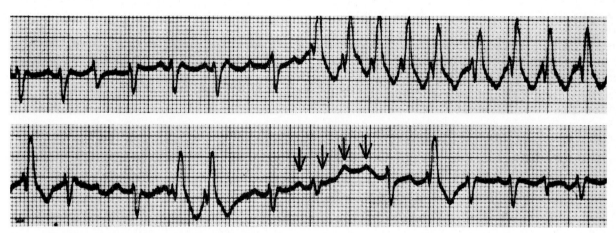

V₁—continuous

FIG. 8-83. Functional right bundle branch block. At first glance the tracing appears to be sinus rhythm interrupted by a burst of ventricular tachycardia and intermittent premature ventricular systoles. Closer inspection reveals flutter waves *(arrows)* when the ventricular rate slows slightly and suggests that the widened QRS complexes may be aberrantly conducted supraventricular beats. These beats conform in all respects to criteria established to differentiate supraventricular aberration from ventricular tachycardia. (See text.) The patient requires digitalis to slow the ventricular rate rather than lidocaine to suppress ectopic ventricular discharge.

Rate:	Atrial, 280 beats/minute; ventricular, 90 to 200 beats/minute.
Rhythm:	Atrial, regular; ventricular, irregularly irregular.
P waves:	Flutter waves *(arrows)* can be seen when the ventricular rate slows and can be marched out with regularity.
PR interval:	Flutter-R interval varies.
QRS:	Varying contour between normal and functional right bundle branch block.

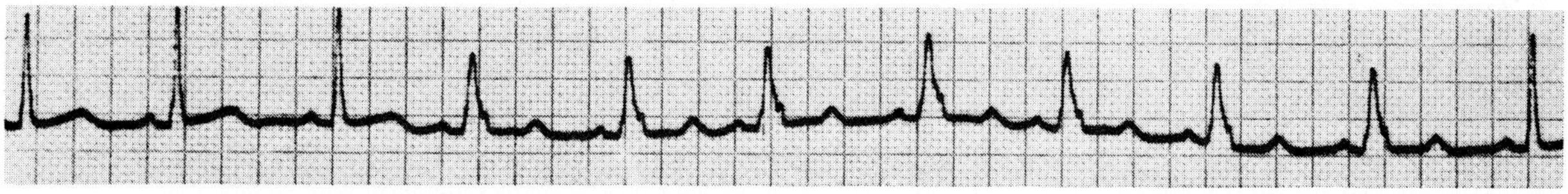

FIG. 8-84. Rate-dependent aberrancy of the left bundle branch block type. Gradual acceleration of the sinus rate results in a functional left bundle branch block that remains until the sinus rate slows sufficiently at the end of the tracing. This type of aberrancy is much more commonly of the left bundle rather than the right bundle branch block type and is more apt to be associated with cardiac disease than is functional right bundle branch block.

Rate:	60 to 78 beats/minute.
Rhythm:	Slightly irregular.
P waves:	Normal.
PR interval:	Normal and constant, 0.14 second.
QRS:	Varies between normal and functional left bundle branch block.

play characteristic features that distinguish it from those beats arising in the ventricles during a true ventricular tachycardia. The following analysis may be helpful in distinguishing aberrant ventricular conduction initiated by a supraventricular impulse from ventricular tachycardia.

Identification of Atrial Activity. During sinus rhythm or an ectopic supraventricular rhythm, identification of distinct atrial activity initiating ventricular depolarization, regardless of how deformed the QRS complex may appear, establishes the diagnosis of supraventricular rhythm with QRS aberration. A casual relationship between the P and QRS complexes may be demonstrated in one or more of the following ways, depending on the nature of the supraventricular rhythms:

1. P waves with a normal contour precede and maintain a constant relationship to each QRS complex during sinus rhythm.
2. Interventions that alter the sinus rate, such as carotid sinus massage or exercise, secondarily alter the ventricular rate in exactly the same manner and maintain the same, or nearly the same, PR interval. This indicates that ventricular activation follows as a consequence of atrial discharge. Atrial pacing can be employed to alter the atrial rate during a tachycardia characterized by wide QRS complexes, and a diagnosis of ventricular tachycardia is considered likely when fusion and capture complexes result.
3. When atrial flutter, atrial fibrillation, or atrial tachy-

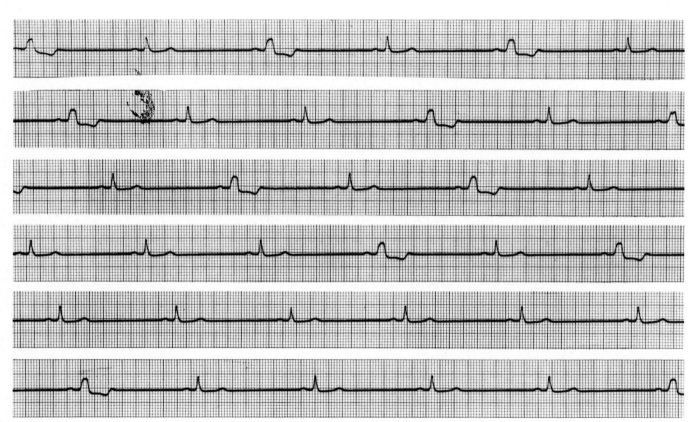

Continuous lead I

FIG. 8-85. Bradycardia-dependent left bundle branch block. In this unusual tracing the patient has a sinus bradycardia. When the sinus cycle increases, the P wave conducts with a left bundle branch block. Shorter sinus cycles are ended with a normally conducted QRS complex. Very small changes in the sinus rate account for these differences.

Rate:	34 to 38 beats/minute.
Rhythm:	Fairly regular.
P waves:	Normal and precede each QRS complex.
PR interval:	0.19 second.
QRS:	Normal and left bundle branch block, 0.14 second.

cardia exists, carotid sinus massage, digitalis, verapamil, or edrophonium chloride (Tensilon) administration produces characteristic slowing of the ventricular response (at times also normalizing the QRS complex); during AV nodal reentry or AVRT the rhythm may remain unchanged or terminate and allow sinus rhythm to resume.

4. Atrial and ventricular rhythms may be so related as to suggest dependency of the latter on the former, during typical AV Wenckebach cycles, for example.

5. When atria and ventricles are dissociated, finding ventricular captures that have the same contour as the QRS of the tachyarrhythmia in question indicates a supraventricular rhythm.

6. Bursts of an intermittent tachycardia that are always initiated by a premature atrial complex provide indirect evidence supporting a supraventricular diagnosis. However, it is important to remember that, under certain circumstances, a premature atrial complex can initiate a ventricular tachycardia.

7. During retrograde atrial capture the RP interval is of too short a duration to be explained by retrograde conduction from a ventricular focus (about 0.10 second or less).

8. If the rate and rhythm of abnormal QRS complexes are the same as the rate and rhythm of a known supraventricular tachycardia, this provides some support in favor of aberration.

9. The presence of AV dissociation during a wide QRS tachycardia is much more consistent with ventricular than supraventricular tachycardias.

Analysis of QRS Contours and Intervals. The following clues suggest aberrant ventricular conduction initiated by a supraventricular impulse:

1. The contour of the QRS is a triphasic rsR' in V_1. RBBB patterns occur more frequently than LBBB patterns because, at a slower heart rate, the right bundle branch appears to require more time to repolarize than the left. Therefore premature discharge is more likely to encounter a refractory right bundle branch and produce RBBB.

2. Monophasic or diphasic complexes in V_1 or an LBBB pattern favor the diagnosis of ventricular tachycardia, as does a frontal QRS axis that is directed superiorly and to the right.

3. Faster rates speed repolarization, whereas slower rates retard it; the refractory period is proportional to the preceding cycle length. Therefore the heart takes longer to repolarize following a long cycle than it does after a short cycle. Because of this, when an early beat succeeds a long cycle, the early beat may encounter refractory tissue and conduct aberrantly. A comparison of such long-short cycle sequences aids in determining aberrant conduction.

4. During atrial flutter or fibrillation or a series of premature atrial complexes, aberrantly conducted beats persist in runs rather than maintain a bigeminal pattern and then lack a compensatory pause after their termination.

5. The initial vectors of aberrant and normal beats are similar during functional RBBB, since RBBB preserves the normal initial forces.

6. Aberrantly conducted supraventricular QRS complexes are not wildly bizarre or lengthened; most of the QRS prolongation occurs in the latter portion of the beat. QRS complexes with a duration exceeding 0.14 second are more likely to indicate ventricular tachycardia.

7. A fixed coupling interval between the normal and aberrant beats is absent during atrial flutter or atrial fibrillation. Conversely, fixed coupling during atrial flutter or fibrillation favors ventricular ectopy.

8. The aberrant beats are not excessively premature.

9. During a narrow QRS supraventricular tachycardia (excluding atrial flutter and atrial fibrillation, the presence of alternation of QRS morphology favors the presence of a retrograde accessory pathway in the tachycardia circuit [i.e., AVRT associated with the WPW syndrome; see p. 160]).[27]

10. The QRS configuration appears the same as that resulting from known supraventricular conduction at similar rates. Conversely, if the QRS contour is the same as that resulting from known ventricular conduction, the tachycardia is probably ventricular in origin.

11. Vagal maneuvers remain a most important differentiating point, since vagal discharge does not usually affect ventricular tachycardia, whereas it slows the ventricular rate in most supraventricular mechanisms. However, ventricular tachycardia terminated by vagal discharge has been reported.

12. The presence of fusion and capture beats (see p. 185), as stated earlier, provides the most important evidence in favor of ventricular tachycardia.

None of the aforementioned features can be used to establish unequivocally the diagnosis of ventricular tachycardia, and in many instances invasive electrophysiologic studies must be performed.

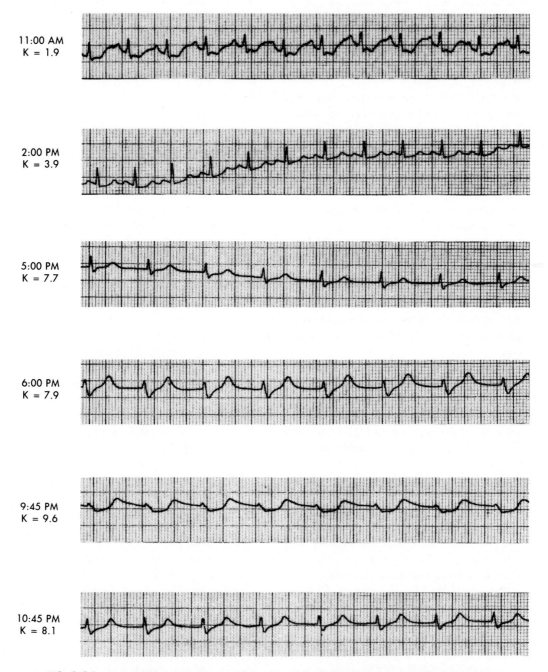

FIG. 8-86. Serial ECG tracings in a patient with marked changes in serum potassium level. In the 11:00 AM tracing the depressed ST segment and low amplitude T wave blending into a probable U wave (this cannot be seen with clarity because of the superimposed P waves) indicate the presence of hypokalemia. Following the administration of potassium the 2:00 PM tracing becomes relatively normal. Continued potassium administration results in hyperkalemia with the disappearance of atrial activity on the ECG and some prolongation of the QRS complex. By 7:00 PM the QRS complex is more prolonged, and by 9:45 PM the QRS complex is greatly prolonged. Secondary ST-T wave changes are present. Improvement follows the administration of bicarbonate, glucose, and insulin at 10:45 PM with reduction in serum potassium level; improvement in the ECG results.

ELECTROLYTE DISTURBANCES[28]
Potassium (Figs. 8-86 and 8-87)

During induced hyperkalemia in animals, the ECG correlates closely with the potassium blood level. The T wave peaks when potassium concentration reaches about 5.5 mEq/L; the corrected QT interval is normal or shortens initially but may prolong as the QRS complex widens. The QRS complex may widen when the external potassium concentration exceeds 6.5 mEq/L; about 7.0 mEq/L, P wave amplitude diminishes, and P wave and PR interval duration are prolonged. About 8.0 to 9.0 mEq/L, the P wave frequently disappears. Sometimes ST segment deviation, both elevated and depressed, occurs and simulates an injury pattern. Clinically occurring potassium alterations do not correlate as well as during these experimental changes in animals, probably because the patient has multiple abnormalities that may influence the ECG differently. For example, in some studies less than 25% of patients with hyperkalemia developed the characteristic tall, narrow, peaked T waves. It is believed that extracellular potassium concentration accounts for the ECG patterns rather than changes in total body potassium or intracellular potassium concentration.

During hypokalemic states the ST segment becomes depressed, the U wave is exaggerated, and the T wave amplitude is decreased without changing the actual duration of QT interval (as long as it can be measured accurately). Actually, it is the QU interval that becomes prolonged. The P and QRS amplitude and duration may increase, and the PR interval may be prolonged. Clinical hypokalemia does not normally slow AV conduction significantly; however, isolated cases have been reported demonstrating varying degrees of PR prolongation. Intraventricular conduction in adults seldom lengthens by more than 20 msec, but it may be more prolonged in children.

Spontaneous hyperkalemia rarely, if ever, produces more advanced AV block than simple PR prolongation; large doses of potassium administered rapidly may produce further advanced forms of AV block, however. Often the P wave disappears, which precludes the diagnosis of AV block. As the plasma potassium level continues to rise above 6.5 and 7.0 mEq/L, slowed intraventricular conduction results, manifested by uniform widening of the QRS complex. Areas of intraventricular block may occur and lead to ventricular fibrillation.

Potassium may potentiate the slowing effects of digitalis on AV conduction, particularly if plasma potassium level rises rapidly. However, if AV conduction is also hampered by a rapid atrial rate, slowing the atrial rate with potassium actually may improve AV conduction and offset any direct depressing effects of potassium. Fortunately, potassium administration to patients with digitalis-induced arrhythmias suppresses ectopic discharge at a much lower blood potassium level than that which further depresses AV conduction.

Low blood potassium levels encourage spontaneous ectopic pacemaker discharge, presumably by enhancing automaticity and also possibly by slowing dominant pacemakers or producing conduction defects. Low potassium levels may initiate ventricular fibrillation in humans. Reduced potassium concentration may precipitate arrhythmias in animals and humans receiving digitalis at plasma

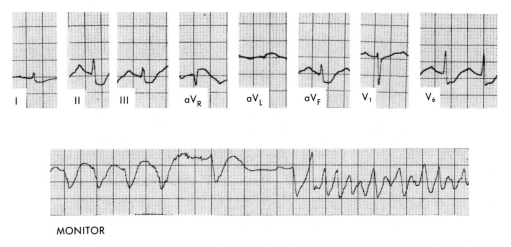

MONITOR

FIG. 8-87. Hypokalemia-induced ventricular tachycardia and fibrillation. The ECG demonstrates the characteristic changes of hypokalemia: depressed ST segment, low-amplitude T wave, and large U wave, blending into the following P wave. In the monitor lead a ventricular tachycardia briefly stops and then degenerates into ventricular fibrillation that was reversed with DC shock.

potassium levels that ordinarily do not produce ectopic beating in the absence of digitalis. Possibly the synergistic effects of digitalis and reduced potassium on automaticity and conduction make animals and humans receiving digitalis particularly prone to arrhythmias precipitated by hypokalemia.

The antiarrhythmic effects of potassium administration may suppress varied rhythms, regardless of cause and whether or not hypokalemia exists. Digitalis-induced ectopic discharge generally responds to potassium therapy at sufficiently low doses to avoid further AV conduction delay. Many believe that potassium remains the drug of choice for ectopic rhythms produced by excessive digitalis. Animals and humans with elevated potassium levels may tolerate large doses of digitalis without developing ectopic arrhythmias, whereas reduced potassium level predisposes to ectopic activity in digitalized animals or patients. Also, a low level of potassium may worsen the depression of AV conduction produced by digitalis.

Sodium

In general the magnitude of sodium change necessary to produce ECG alterations is not compatible with life, making clinical electrocardiographic manifestations of sodium derangements rarely seen, if ever.

Calcium (Fig. 8-88)

In the ECG, low calcium level prolongs the duration of the ST segment and QT interval without prolonging the duration of the T wave, although the T wave may reverse polarity. Elevated calcium level shortens the ST segment and QT interval; the QRS duration may be prolonged during severe hypercalcemia, and AV block may develop. High calcium level opposes the effects of high potassium level, whereas low calcium level opposes the effects of low potassium. If the calcium level varies in a direction opposite that of potassium level, the effects of the latter are enhanced.

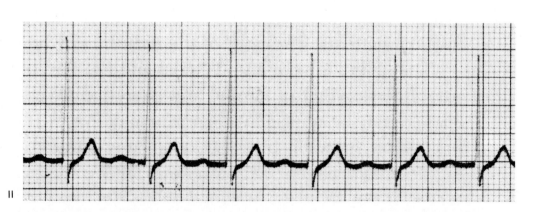

FIG. 8-88. The effects of hypercalcemia on the ECG. Serum calcium level, 14.0/100 ml. The ST segment and QT interval are shortened, and the PR interval is slightly prolonged (0.22 second).

INVASIVE ELECTROPHYSIOLOGIC STUDIES[22] (Figs. 8-89 to 8-92)

The technique to record His bundle activation involves passing an electrode catheter that is introduced percutaneously into the femoral vein, in a cephalad direction up the inferior vena cava, and positioning the catheter tip near the septal leaflet of the tricuspid valve. The His bundle potential (H) appears as a well-defined, most often bipolar spike between the low right atrial (A) and ventricular (V) electrograms. The interval between the earliest onset of the surface P wave or a high right atrial deflection (P) and the low right atrial deflection (PA interval) is a measure of intraatrial conduction. The AH interval is a measurement of the conduction across the AV node and varies in duration from 55 to 130 msec, depending on the cycle length and autonomic influences. The interval from H to V (HV interval) is determined by the interval between the His bundle deflection and the earliest ventricular activity recorded in any lead. The HV interval is a measure of conduction through the His bundle distal to the recording electrode, the bundle branches, and the Purkinje system up to the point of ventricular activation. In contrast to a relatively wide range of values for the AH interval, the HV interval is fairly constant, measuring 30 to 55 msec, with an average value of 45 msec. In some patients, discharge of the right bundle branch may be recorded.

The ability to separate AV nodal and His-Purkinje conduction has enhanced our understanding of normal and abnormal AV conduction. Abnormal AV conduction may be caused by prolongation of P-A, A-H, or H-V intervals or all three. In addition, intra-His block has been demonstrated. During type I (Wenckebach) AV block in a patient with a normal QRS complex the conduction disturbance occurs at the AV node, proximal to the His bundle (Fig. 8-89). Type II AV block in a patient with a bundle branch block virtually always results distal to the His bundle (Fig. 8-90). Thus in type I AV block the blocked P wave is not followed by a His spike, whereas in type II AV block the blocked P wave is followed by a His spike.

Insertion of several electrode catheters (2 to 5) permits recording and stimulating from multiple atrial and ventricular sites and has been useful in differentiating ventricular tachycardia and aberrant ventricular conduction, in understanding the nature of many supraventricular and ventricular tachycardias and other arrhythmias, in evaluating patients with the preexcitation syndrome or AV block, and in other areas as well, such as in initiating tachyarrhythmias in susceptible patients (Figs. 8-91 and 8-92). Significantly, adequacy of therapy can be judged by precipitating the patient's tachycardia in a control state and then attempting to restart it during therapy. Further, most recently catheters have been used for therapy (to ablate sites important for the genesis and/or maintenance of the arrhythmia) as well as for diagnostic purposes. Although areas of application of these electrophysiologic studies are still evolving, fairly definitive indications can be stated.[29]

Further discussion is beyond the scope of this text and the reader is referred to other sources.

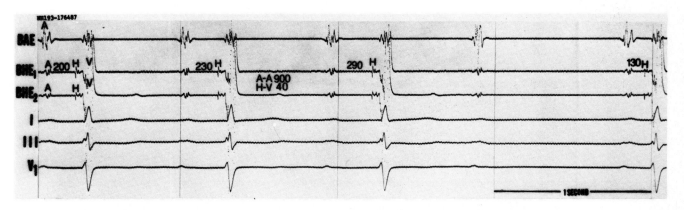

FIG. 8-89.   Type I (Wenckebach) AV nodal block. Simultaneous recordings of electrograms from the high right atrium *(BAE)* and His bundle *(BHE₁, BHE₂)* and scalar leads I, III, and V₁ are displayed during normal sinus rhythm. The PR interval progressively lengthens until the fourth P wave fails to conduct. The conduction delay is caused by AH prolongation that increases from 200 msec in the first beat shown (not the first beat in this Wenckebach series) to 290 msec just before the block. The AH interval then shortens to 130 msec in the first beat of the next Wenckebach series. The nonconducted P wave blocks proximal to the His bundle.

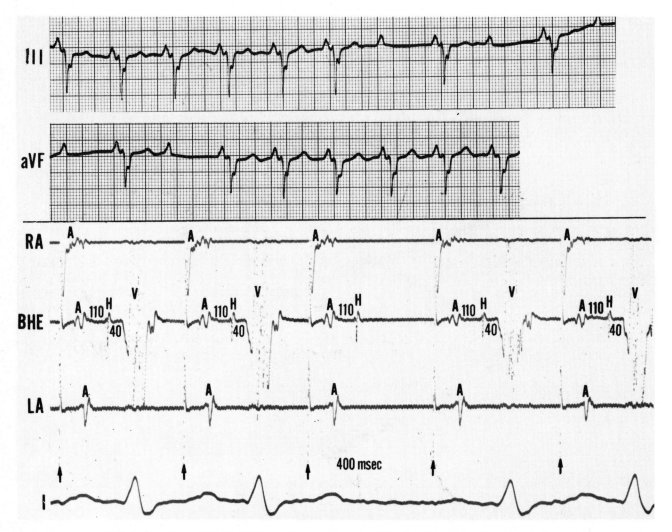

FIG. 8-90. Type II AV block. The scalar recordings in the top portion of the figure (leads III and AV_F) demonstrate type II AV block characterized by a fixed PR interval preceding the nonconducted P wave. During the electrophysiologic study *(bottom)*, right atrial pacing at a cycle length of 400 msec resulted in a fixed AH interval of 110 msec and HV interval of 40 msec. The third P wave *(A)* blocked distal to the His bundle recording site, characteristic of type II AV block. *LA,* Left atrial electrogram. Arrows point to stimuli delivered to right atrium.

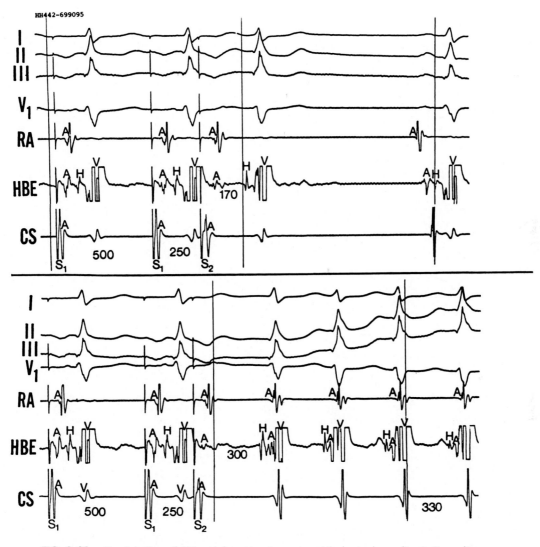

FIG. 8-91.   Precipitation of AV nodal reentrant, supraventricular tachycardia. A, Recordings were obtained simultaneously from scalar leads I, II, III, and V_1 and intracavitary recordings from the right atrium *(RA)*, His bundle area *(HBE)*, and coronary sinus *(CS)*. The coronary sinus was stimulated at a fixed cycle length of 500 msec (S_1 to S_1) and then stimulated prematurely (S_2) at a cycle length of 250 msec. The AH interval lengthened slightly to 170 msec, but tachycardia did not result. B, Premature stimulation at the same coupling interval produced an AH interval of 300 msec and precipitation of a supraventricular tachycardia caused by AV nodal reentry at a cycle length of 330 msec (rate: 182 beats/minute). Findings are consistent with "dual AV nodal" pathways.

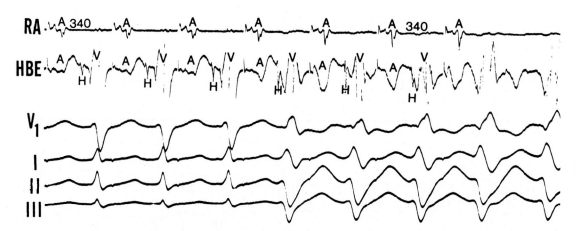

FIG. 8-92. Precipitation of ventricular tachycardia during right atrial pacing. In the left portion of the tracing the right atrium was paced at a cycle length of 340 msec. After the third normally conducted QRS complex, ventricular conduction becomes abnormally prolonged. The HV interval shortens, AV dissociation results, and the ventricular tachycardia continues, following cessation of atrial pacing *(top right)*. These findings are consistent with a ventricular tachycardia initiated during atrial stimulation. The tracing was recorded in an 18-year-old man who had exercise-induced ventricular tachycardia.

ARTIFACTS (Figs. 8-93 and 8-94)

Electronic instrumentation has provided vast dividends to the care of patients with heart disease. However, because we now rely so heavily on various types of monitoring devices, one must constantly be alert and recognize artifacts that mimic arrhythmias. A tracing that resembles ventricular fibrillation *must* be artifactual if the patient is found sitting up in bed in no distress, reading a newspaper! The cardinal rule is to treat the patient and not the monitor.

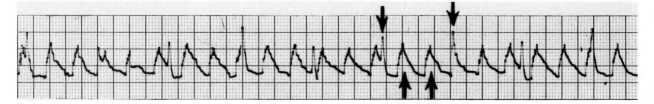

FIG. 8-93. Toothbrush tachycardia. This tracing was recorded from a patient brushing his teeth with an electric toothbrush at a rate of 188 brushes/minute. Note the regularly occurring artifacts *(upright arrows)* that do not influence the QRS complexes *(inverted arrows)*.

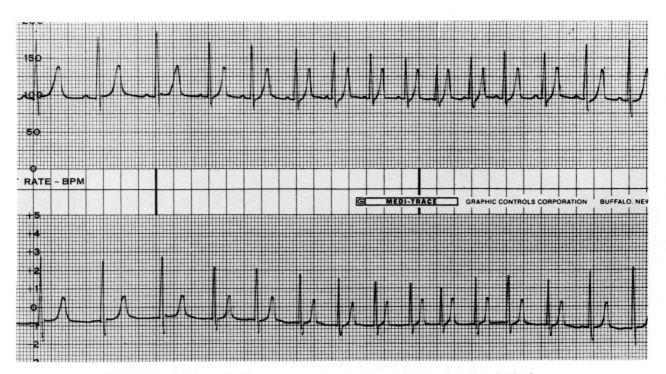

FIG. 8-94. Artifact simulating onset of supraventricular tachycardia. During playback of a tape-recorded ECG rhythm, the rate of revolutions per minute of the tape slowed and simulated the onset of a supraventricular tachycardia. The diagnosis of artifact is easily made, since, in addition to shortening of the RR interval, the PR, QRS, and QT intervals all decrease markedly. Both leads recorded simultaneously.

Arrhythmia Test Section

It is suggested that the reader use this section to test his knowledge of arrhythmias. Cover the interpretations in each legend, calculate intervals and irregularities as previously discussed, and determine the diagnosis. Consider also the significance of each arrhythmia and what form of treatment would most likely be employed. There may be disagreements in interpretation of rhythm strips, but the essential point is to make your diagnosis by using the analytic method described in this chapter. This approach offers a justification for your interpretation.

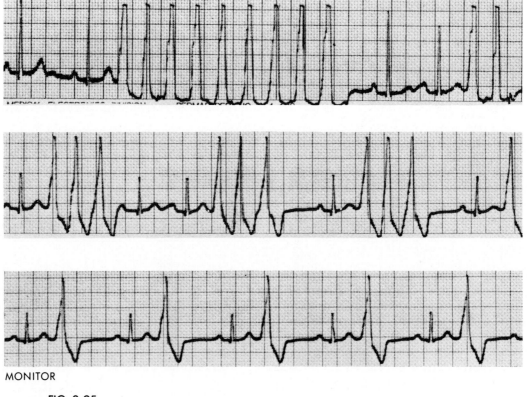

MONITOR

FIG. 8-95

Rate:	Atrial	60 to 75 beats/minute.
	Ventricular	170 to 210 beats/minute.
Rhythm:	Atrial	Slightly irregular.
	Ventricular	Irregular because of bursts of ventricular ectopy.
P waves:		Normal for the sinus-initiated QRS complexes.
PR interval:		Normal for the sinus-initiated QRS complexes, 0.16 second.
QRS:		Normal for the sinus-initiated complexes; wide, bizarre, prolonged (0.12 second) for the ventricular ectopy.
Arrhythmia:		Paroxysmal ventricular tachycardia gradually decreasing in frequency to bigeminy and then complete disappearance. This result followed administration of lidocaine, 50 mg IV in a patient with an acute myocardial infarction.

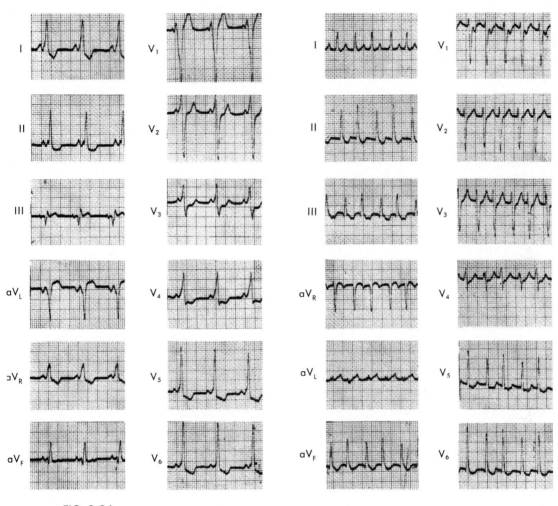

FIG. 8-96

Rate:	A, 82 beats/minute; B, varying between 150 and 180 beats/minute.
Rhythm:	A, Regular; B, slight variation in RR intervals with long cycles alternating with short cycles.
P waves:	A, Normal; B, retrograde; see V_1.
PR interval:	A, 0.08 second; B, RP interval 0.12 second.
QRS:	A, Prolonged, 0.12 second; B, normal, 0.08 second.
Arrhythmia:	A, Normal sinus rhythm during preexcitation syndrome; B, AVRT in the same patient.

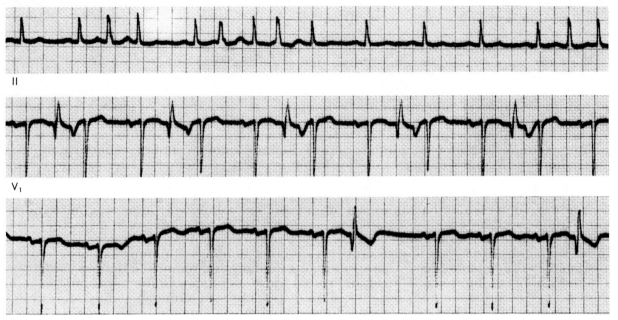

II

V₁

V₁

FIG. 8-97

Rate: 75 beats/minute, with premature complexes.
Rhythm: Irregular because of premature complexes.
P waves: Normal and precede each of the normal QRS complexes.
PR inverval: Prolonged following the premature complexes.
QRS: Normal for the sinus-initiated complexes; prolonged to almost 0.12 second for the premature complexes.
Arrhythmia: Interpolated premature ventricular complexes in the top and middle tracings. In the bottom tracing, premature ventricular complexes produce a compensatory pause and are therefore no longer interpolated.

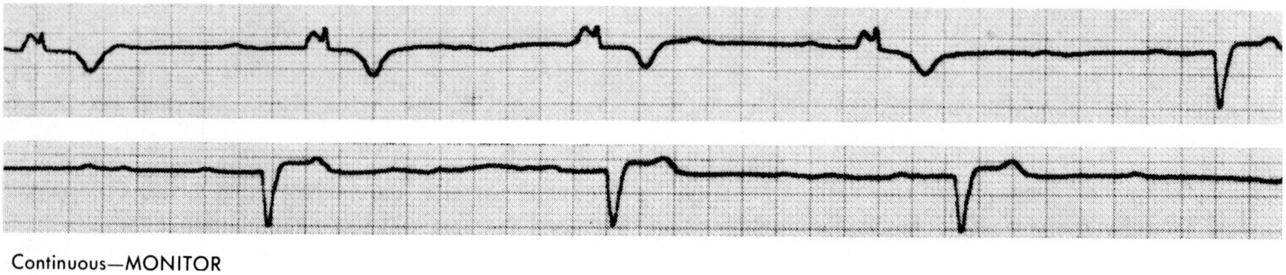

Continuous—MONITOR

FIG. 8-98

Rate: Atrial   86 beats/minute.
            Ventricular   Upright complexes 38 beats/minute; negative complexes 28 beats/minute.
Rhythm: Atrial   Regular.
            Ventricular   Fairly regular.
P waves: Normal and have no relationship to the QRS complexes. Clear P waves cannot be seen throughout the entire tracing.
PR interval: Not measurable.
QRS: Abnormal; upright complexes 0.14 second, negative complexes 0.12 second.
Arrhythmia: Complete AV block with a ventricular escape rhythm. The simultaneous change in ventricular contour and rate probably indicates a shift in the ventricular escape focus site.

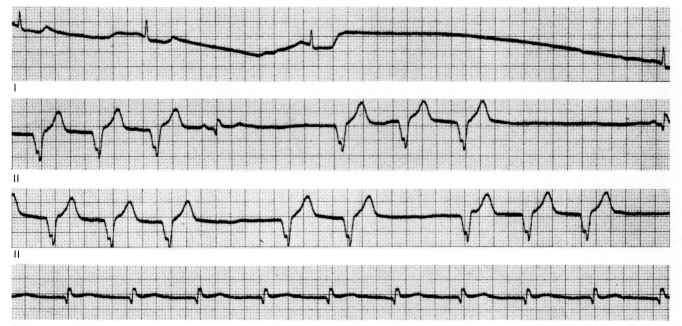

I

II

II

II Atropine, 0.75 mg IV

FIG. 8-99

Rate:	Top tracing, slow with periods of asystole. Middle two tracings, 75 beats/minute with periods of asystole. Bottom tracing, 65 beats/minute.
Rhythm:	Top three tracings, irregular; bottom tracing, regular.
P waves:	Normal contour, preceding the sinus-initiated QRS complexes in lead II but are hard to see in lead I.
PR interval:	Normal for the sinus-initiated P waves, not present for the other QRS complexes. In the bottom tracing no P wave or PR interval is apparent.
QRS:	Normal for the sinus-initiated QRS complexes, prolonged (0.13 second) for the ventricular ectopic beats.
Arrhythmia:	Various arrhytmias recorded in a patient with an acute inferior myocardial infarction. Top tracing, marked sinus bradycardia and periods of sinus arrest. Middle two tracings, an accelerated idioventricular rhythm, slightly irregular. The duration of the pauses in the third strip appears to be a multiple of the basic idioventricular cycle length, thus suggesting the possible presence of an intermittent exit block. Bottom tracing, a junctional rhythm following atropine administration suppresses the ventricular ectopy.

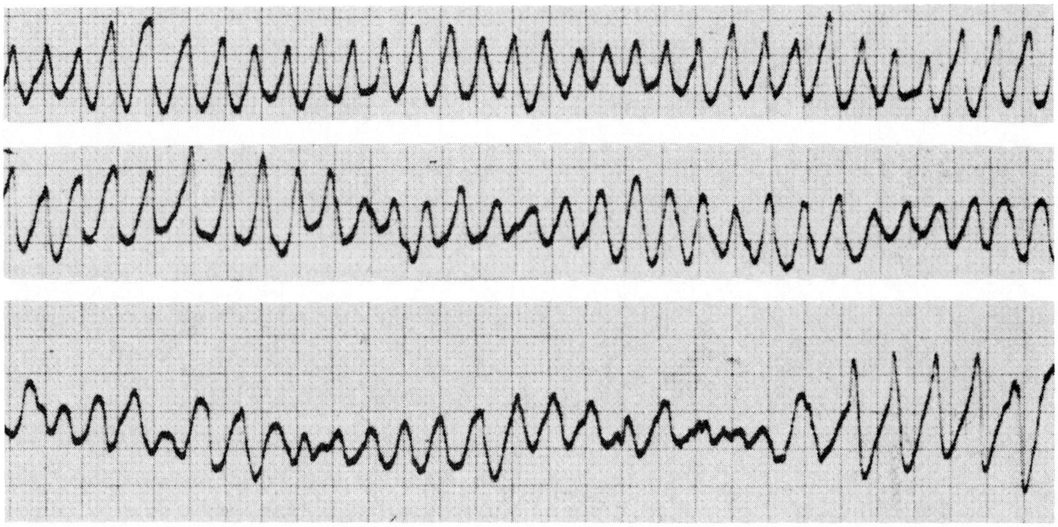

MONITOR

FIG. 8-100

Rate:	300 to 500 beats/minute.
Rhythm:	Grossly irregular.
P waves:	None seen.
PR interval:	Not measurable.
QRS:	Wide, bizarre, irregular.
Arrhythmia:	Ventricular flutter that becomes ventricular fibrillation in the bottom tracing. The ventricular fibrillation then seems to organize and merge into ventricular flutter or possibly ventricular tachycardia in the terminal portion of the tracing.

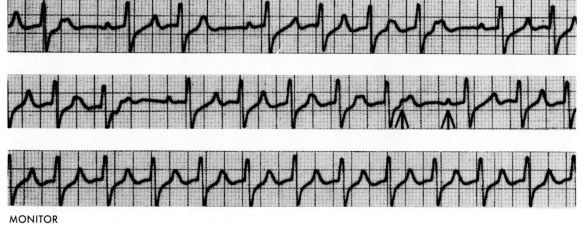

MONITOR

FIG. 8-101

Rate:	Atrial	115 beats/minute.
	Ventricular	Varying, depending on the degree of block.
Rhythm:	Atrial	Regular.
	Ventricular	Irregular.
P waves:		Precede each of the QRS complexes *(arrows)*.
PR interval:		Progressively lengthens until one P wave fails to conduct (Wenckebach AV block)
QRS:		Normal (0.08 second).
Arrhythmia:		Atrial tachycardia with varying block. Note the varying T wave contour as P waves fall during portions of the antecedent T wave. In the bottom tracing 1:1 AV conduction occurs.

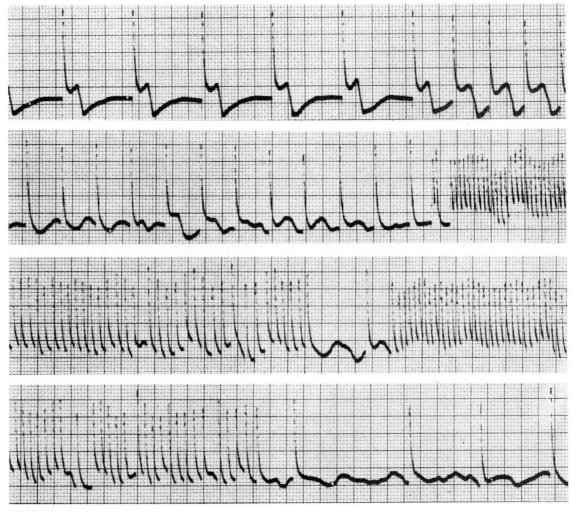

MONITOR

FIG. 8-102

Rate:	Ventricular	74 beats/minute to very rapid rates.
Rhythm:	Ventricular	Periods of regularity replaced by gross irregularity.
P waves:		None seen.
PR interval:		Not measurable.
QRS:		Wide, distorted, initiated by pacemaker spikes.
Arrhythmia:		Runaway pacemaker discharging at irregular and extremely rapid rates and finally initiating ventricular fibrillation. The pacemaker rate sped from 71 beats/minute to approximately 145 beats/minute and then greater than 1000 stimuli/minute.

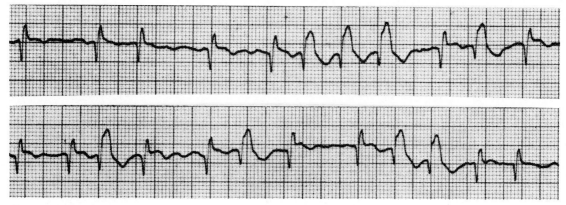

V_1

FIG. 8-103

Rate:	Ventricular	73 to 180 beats/minute.
Rhythm:	Ventricular	Grossly irregular.
P waves:		None seen.
PR interval:		Not measurable.
QRS:		Normal (0.08 second) and abnormal (0.12 second) with a right bundle branch block contour.
Arrhythmia:		Atrial fibrillation with a rapid ventricular response. QRS complexes, which demonstrate a right bundle branch block, terminate a short cycle (or a series of short cycles) that follows a long preceding cycle. The development of functional right bundle branch block caused by cycle length changes in this fashion is called the *Ashman phenomenon.*

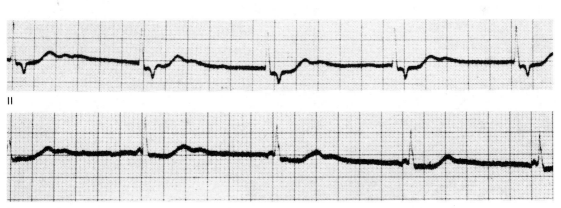

II

II

FIG. 8-104

Rate:	*Top,* 52 beats/minute; *bottom,* 48 beats/minute.
Rhythm:	Regular.
P waves:	Retrograde.
PR interval:	*Bottom,* 0.06 second.
RP interval:	*Top,* 0.08 second.
QRS:	Normal (0.06 second).
Arrhythmia:	AV junctional rhythm recorded on two occasions in the same patient. In the top tracing, retrograde P waves followed the QRS complex; in the bottom tracing, retrograde P waves preceded the QRS complex.

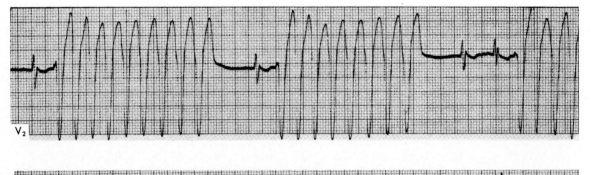

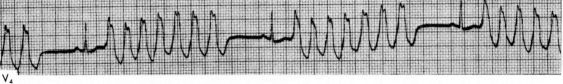

FIG. 8-105

Rate:	Ventricular	250 beats/minute.
Rhythm:	Ventricular	Regular in a recurrent paroxysmal fashion.
P waves:		Precede the normally conducted QRS complexes.
PR interval:		Normal for the normally conducted QRS complexes.
QRS:		Normal for the sinus-initiated QRS complexes, QRS prolonged for the ventricular ectopic systoles (0.14 seconds).
Arrhythmia:		Repetitive monomorphic ventricular tachycardia. The lack of fusion or capture beats and precise determination of atrial activity during the tachycardia prevent an unequivocal diagnosis of ventricular tachycardia from this tracing, although the diagnosis is highly suggestive.

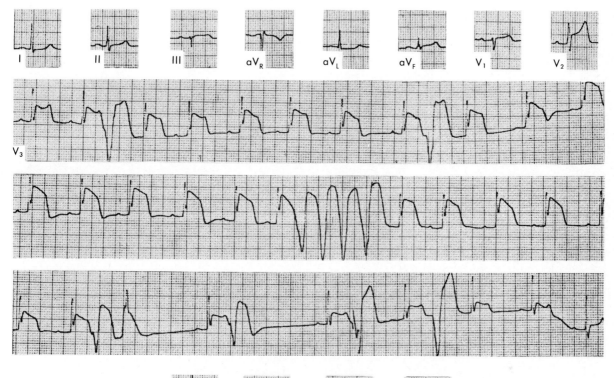

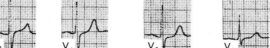

FIG. 8-106

Rate: During V_3, approximately 75 beats/minute, interrupted by ventricular ectopy.

Rhythm: Fairly regular except when interrupted by ventricular ectopy.

P waves: Normal and precede each of the normally conducted QRS complexes.

PR interval: Normal (0.16 second) and constant.

QRS: Note abrupt ST segment elevation between V_1 and V_2 and during the V_3 rhythm strip. The V_3 at the bottom shows a normal ST segment. Abnormal complexes have a QRS duration greater than 0.12 second.

Arrhythmia: Atypical (Prinzmetal) angina pectoris characterized by ST segment *elevation* probably a result of coronary artery bypass. Premature ventricular complexes trigger a short run of ventricular tachycardia in the midportion of the tracing. ST segments return to the baseline as the chest pain abates and the ectopic ventricular activity ceases.

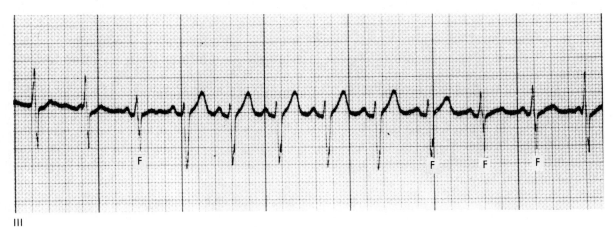

III

FIG. 8-107

Rate:	107 beats/minute.
Rhythm:	Regular.
P waves:	Normal and precede each of the QRS complexes in the midportion of the tracing.
PR interval:	Constant (0.16 second) for the QRS complexes in the midportion of the tracing.
QRS:	Normal duration (0.08 second) for both types of QRS complexes. Fusion QRS complexes indicated by F.
Arrhythmia:	Ventricular tachycardia at beginning and end of tracing, which generates QRS complexes with a slightly different contour than during sinus tachycardia that occurs in the midportion of the tracing. The supraventricular origin of the tachycardia is suggested by the QRS duration (<0.12 second). However, recent data suggest that such a tachycardia actually may be ventricular, originating in the upper portions of the fascicular system and generating a QRS complex with a duration *less* than 0.12 second. The presence of fusion beats *(F)* supports this conclusion. In any event, during the tachycardia at the beginning and end of the ECG, QRS complexes are not related to atrial activity. Thus AV dissociation is present because of ventricular tachycardia. In the midportion of the tracing, slight acceleration of the sinus rate allows the sinus node to regain capture of the ventricles, suppress the tachycardia, and eliminate the periods of AV dissociation.

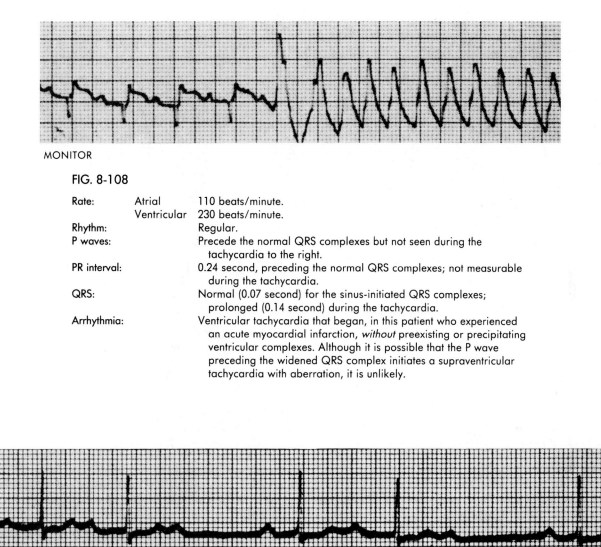

MONITOR

FIG. 8-108

Rate:	Atrial	110 beats/minute.
	Ventricular	230 beats/minute.
Rhythm:		Regular.
P waves:		Precede the normal QRS complexes but not seen during the tachycardia to the right.
PR interval:		0.24 second, preceding the normal QRS complexes; not measurable during the tachycardia.
QRS:		Normal (0.07 second) for the sinus-initiated QRS complexes; prolonged (0.14 second) during the tachycardia.
Arrhythmia:		Ventricular tachycardia that began, in this patient who experienced an acute myocardial infarction, *without* preexisting or precipitating ventricular complexes. Although it is possible that the P wave preceding the widened QRS complex initiates a supraventricular tachycardia with aberration, it is unlikely.

II

FIG. 8-109

Rate:	Atrial	75 beats/minute.
	Ventricular	3:2 conduction, average 50 beats/minute.
Rhythm:	Atrial	Regular
	Ventricular	Irregular
P waves:		Normal and precede each QRS complex.
PR interval:		Progressively lengthens before the nonconducted P wave.
QRS:		Normal (0.06 second).
Arrhythmia:		Second-degree AV block, type I (Wenckebach).

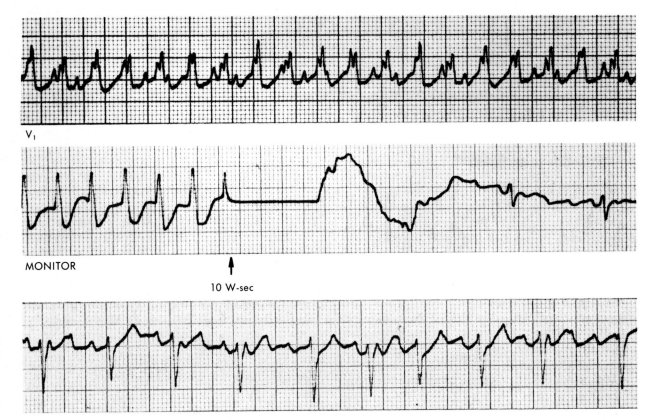

V₁

MONITOR

↑
10 W-sec

V₁

FIG. 8-110

Rate:	Atrial	300 beats/minute (top panel).
	Ventricular	200 beats/minute (top panel).
Rhythm:	Atrial	Regular.
	Ventricular	Regular.
P waves:		Atrial flutter.
PR interval:		Completely variable.
QRS:		Wide, prolonged (0.12 second)
Arrhythmia:		Atrial flutter and ventricular tachycardia in top tracing. Thus complete AV dissociation is present. In the monitor recording (middle tracing) the left portion reflects the same activity seen in V₁ above. However, the particular monitor lead fails to reveal the atrial flutter waves. Direct current cardioversion (*arrow*, 10 watt-seconds) terminates the ventricular tachycardia but allows the atrial flutter to persist, seen more clearly in V₁ below. The atrial flutter at this point is not as precisely regular as it was before the cardioversion.

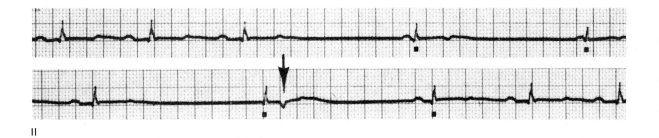

II

FIG. 8-111

Rate:	30 to 50 beats/minute.
Rhythm:	Fairly irregular.
P waves:	Precede and conduct to the QRS complexes that do not have dots beneath them. Those with dots beneath them are junctional escape beats.
PR interval:	Prolonged (0.26 second) and constant for the QRS complexes that do not have a dot beneath them.
QRS:	Normal duration and contour (0.08 second). Dots indicate AV junctional escape beats. The third AV junctional escape beat (lower tracing) retrogradely activates the atrium *(arrow)*.
Arrhythmia:	Sinus bradycardia with intermittent sinus arrest and AV junctional escape beats, the "sick sinus syndrome."

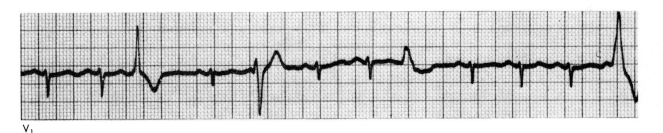

V₁

FIG. 8-112

Rate:	98 beats/minute.
Rhythm:	Irregular because of premature ventricular systoles.
P waves:	Normal and precede each sinus-initiated QRS complex.
PR interval:	Normal for the sinus-initiated QRS complexes (0.14 second).
QRS:	Normal for the sinus-initiated QRS complexes (0.08 second). Premature systoles are characterized by varied contour and a duration greater than 0.12 second.
Arrhythmia:	Multiform premature ventricular complexes with four different contours.

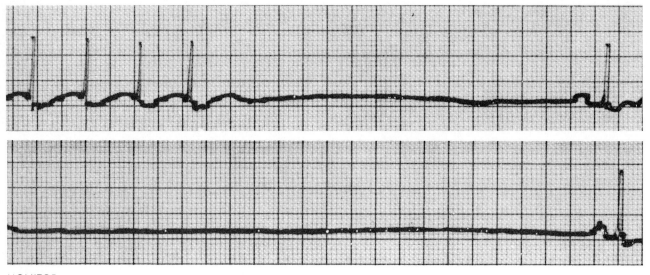

MONITOR

FIG. 8-113

Rate:　　　　140 beats/minute, abruptly slowing following carotid sinus massage. Two periods of asystole are finally terminated by sinus rhythm.

Rhythm:　　　Regular, followed by asystole, an atrial escape beat, and then sinus rhythm.

P waves:　　　Can be seen when tachycardia terminates.

PR interval:　Normal (0.18 sec) in those beats preceded by P waves.

QRS:　　　　Normal.

Arrhythmia:　Abrupt termination of paroxysmal supraventricular tachycardia by carotid sinus massage (at beginning of recording). A lengthy period of asystole results when the tachycardia stops, before sinus rhythm resumes.

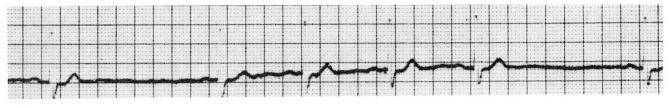

II

FIG. 8-114

Rate:　　　　33 to 66 beats/minute.

Rhythm:　　　Irregular.

P waves:　　　Normal contour. Long PP cycles are exactly twice the short PP cycles.

PR interval:　Normal (0.20 second).

QRS:　　　　Normal (0.08 second).

Arrhythmia:　2:1 sinus exit block

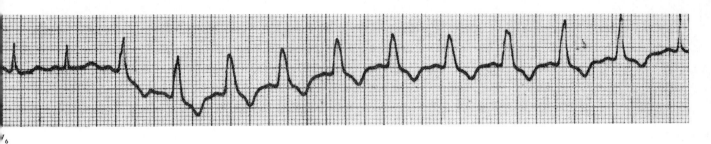

V_6

FIG. 8-115

Rate: Gradually accelerates from 105 to 115 beats/minute.
Rhythm: Fairly regular.
P waves: Normal and precede each QRS complex.
PR interval: Normal (0.14 second) and constant.
QRS: Normal at the slower rates; left bundle branch block (0.12 second) at the faster
                 rates.
Arrhythmia: Rate-dependent aberration with functional left bundle branch block.

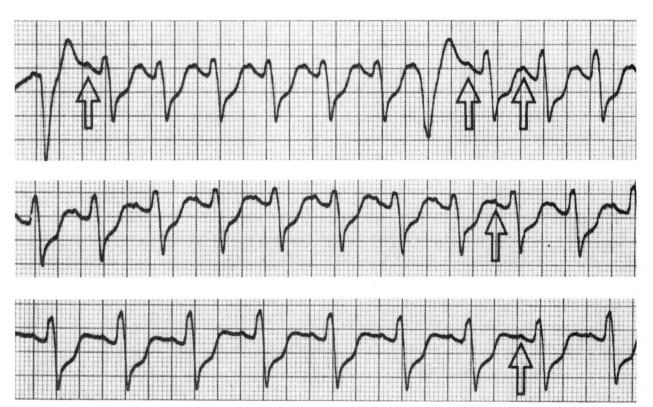

II—noncontinuous

FIG. 8-116

Rate: 125 beats/minute in top tracing; gradually slows to 100 beats/minute in bottom
                 tracing.
Rhythm: Regular.
P waves: Normal, but hidden by preceding T waves *(arrows)*.
PR interval: 0.16 second.
QRS: Abnormal, prolonged (0.14 second) because of the presence of a preexisting left
                 bundle branch block.
Arrhythmia: Sinus tachycardia. Patient has a preexisting bundle branch block. Clear P waves
                 (arrows) can be seen in the pause that follows the two premature ventricular
                 complexes (top tracing). The heart rate gradually slowed following edrophonium
                 (Tensilon) administration (middle and bottom tracings).

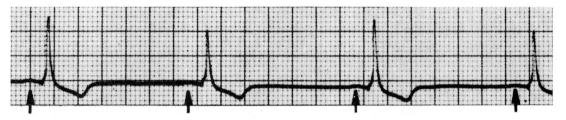

II

FIG. 8-117

Rate: 41 beats/minute.
Rhythm: Fairly regular.
P waves: Precede each QRS with a normal contour.
PR interval: 0.16 second.
QRS: Borderline prolonged (0.11 second).
Arrhythmia: Sinus bradycardia. Patient is receiving methyldopa for hypertension. Normal rate
             was restored following discontinuation of methyldopa therapy. Low-amplitude P
             waves indicated by arrows.

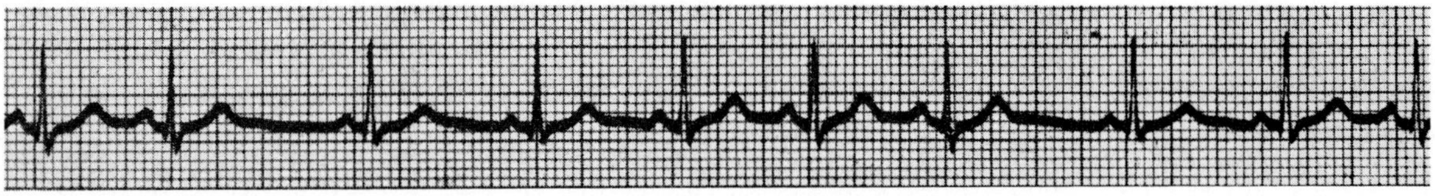

II

FIG. 8-118

Rate: Sinus rate increases with inspiration and decreases with expiration (70 to 110
             beats/minute).
Rhythm: Irregular with a repetitive phasic variation in cycle length according to respiratory
             cycles. Cycle lengths vary by more than 0.16 second. Breath-holding eliminates
             the rate variations.
P waves: Precede each QRS with a normal, fairly constant contour.
PR interval: 0.12 second.
QRS: Normal (0.08 second).
Arrhythmia: Respiratory sinus arrhythmia. The phasic variation corresponds to a respiratory
             rate of approximately 18 breaths/minute.

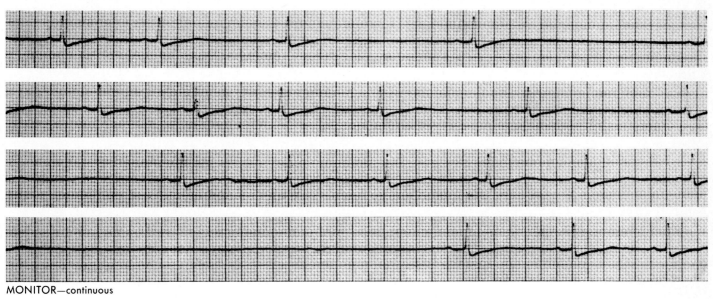

MONITOR—continuous

FIG. 8-119

Rate:	Varying, slow (maximum rate of 5 beats/minute).
Rhythm:	Irregular; periods of asystole not a multiple of basic sinus cycle length.
P waves:	Precede each QRS with a normal contour; may be altered by escape beats.
PR interval:	Slightly prolonged (0.21 second).
QRS:	Normal (0.09 secnd).
Arrhythmia:	Sinus arrest. Patient also has an acute inferior myocardial infarction. Asystolic intervals are not interrupted by escape beats.

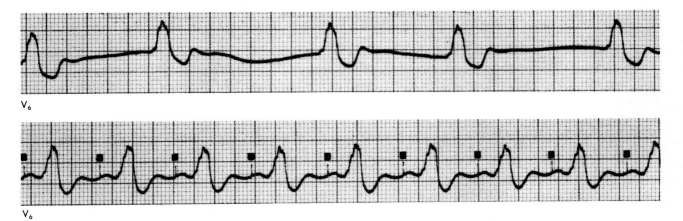

V₆

V₆

FIG. 8-120

Rate:	Varying, slow (36 to 50 beats/minute) *(top)*; normal (81 beats/minute) *(bottom)*.
Rhythm:	Irregular *(top)*; regular *(bottom)*.
P waves:	Not seen *(top)*; follows pacemaker stimulus *(bottom)*.
PR interval:	Not measurable *(top)*; 0.16 second *(bottom)*.
QRS:	Left bundle branch block (0.20 second).
Arrhythmia:	Sinus arrest *(top)* and right atrial pacing *(bottom)*. Patient also has a left bundle branch block. A supraventricular escape focus controls the rhythm in the top panel, but atrial activity is not apparent. Atrial pacing (stimuli indicated by filled squares, bottom tracing) results in atrial capture, producing a P wave and an unchanged QRS contour.

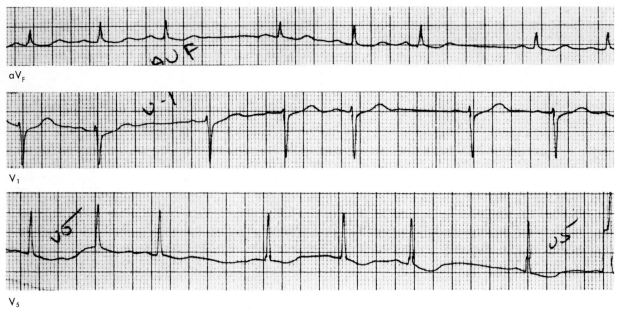

aV_F

V₁

V₅

FIG. 8-121

Rate:	Varying, slow (50 to 88 beats/minute).
Rhythm:	(1) A pause in atrial activity occurs. (2) The PP interval progressively shortens up until the pause. (3) The duration of the pause is less than twice the shortest PP interval. (4) The PP interval following the pause exceeds the PP interval preceding the pause.
P waves:	Contour normal, precede each QRS complex; intermittent loss of P wave.
PR interval:	Normal, constant (0.20 second).
QRS:	Normal (0.08 second).
Arrhythmia:	Sinus exit block (type I or Wenckebach). The four characteristic rhythm changes of this tracing allow the diagnosis of a Wenckebach exit block from the sinus node.

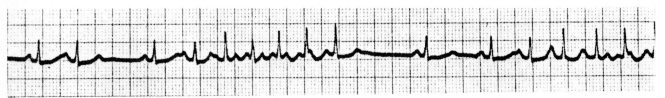

II

FIG. 8-122

Rate:	Varying.
Rhythm:	Irregular because of premature atrial complexes.
P waves:	Premature atrial complexes have different contour; some are buried in preceding T wave.
PR interval (of atrial systole):	0.14 second.
QRS:	Generally normal; may be aberrantly conducted (normal, 0.08 second).
Arrhythmia:	Single and multiple premature atrial complexes can be seen hidden within preceding T waves and appear to initiate short bursts of an atrial tachyarrhythmia, probably atrial flutter-fibrillation.

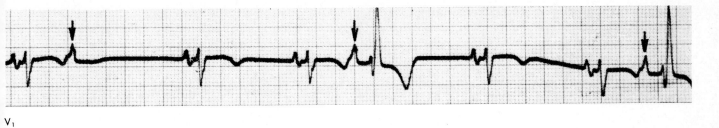

V_1

FIG. 8-123

Rate:	Slow, because of nonconducted premature atrial complexes.
Rhythm:	Irregular.
P waves:	Premature atrial complexes have different contour and are buried in preceding T wave *(arrows)*.
PR interval (of premature atrial systoles):	First two premature atrial complexes are completely blocked; third and fourth premature atrial systoles conduct with a prolonged PR interval 0.21 second.
QRS:	Third and fourth premature atrial complexes initiate aberrantly conducted QRS complex with a right bundle block pattern.
Arrhythmia:	Nonconducted premature atrial complexes and premature atrial complexes initiating functional right bundle branch block. Sinus-initiated P waves are abnormal and suggest left atrial enlargement. Premature atrial complexes *(arrows)* can be seen hidden in the preceding T waves. The first two premature atrial complexes are blocked and generate a pause in the ventricular rhythm. The second two premature atrial complexes conduct to the ventricle with a prolonged PR interval and initiate a functional right bundle branch block.

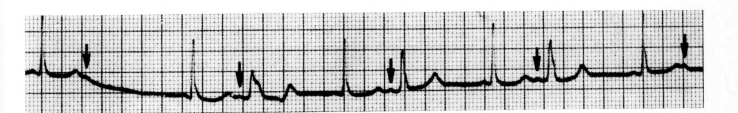

V_6

FIG. 8-124

Rate:	Varying.
Rhythm:	Irregular because of premature atrial complexes.
P waves:	Premature atrial complexes have different contour and look like U waves *(arrows)*.
PR interval (of premature atrial complexes):	Later premature atrial complexes (second, third, and fourth) conduct whereas early premature atrial complexes (first, fifth, and sixth) fail to reach the ventricles.
QRS:	Second, third, and fourth premature atrial complexes produce varying degrees of left bundle branch block.
Arrhythmia:	Nonconducted premature atrial complexes and premature atrial complexes that produce a functional left bundle branch block. Premature atrial complexes can be seen in the terminal portion of the preceding T waves and look like a U wave *(arrows)*. Fairly early premature atrial complexes block whereas slightly later premature atrial complexes conduct to the ventricles with an increase in PR interval and varying degrees of left bundle branch block.

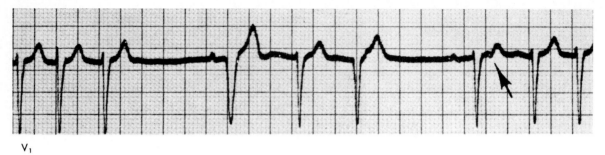

V₁

FIG. 8-125

Rate:	150 beats/minute.
Rhythm:	Varying.
P waves:	Not seen consistently.
PR interval:	Cannot determine.
QRS:	0.08 second.
Arrhythmia:	Paroxysmal supraventricular tachycardia. Paroxysmal supraventricular tachycardia suddenly terminates, begins briefly, stops, and then restarts again following a premature atrial complex *(arrow)* that conducts with a prolonged PR interval.

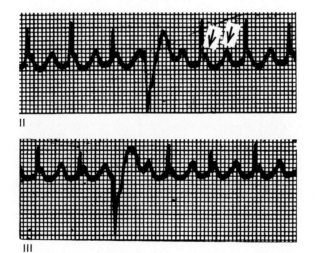

II

III

FIG. 8-126

Rate:	Atrial	280 beats/minute.
	Ventricular	140 beats/minute.
Rhythm:	Atrial	Regular
	Ventricular	2:1.
P waves:		Flutter waves with regular oscillations resembling a sawtooth pattern.
PR interval:		Flutter-R interval is constant.
QRS:		Normal (0.08 second).
Arrhythmia:		Uncommon form of atrial flutter. Flutter waves indicated by arrows. A single premature ventricular complex occurs in each lead. The conduction ratio is 2:1; that is, flutter waves are conducted alternately to the ventricle.

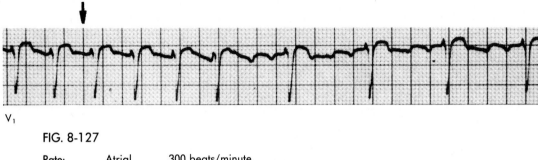

V₁

FIG. 8-127

Rate:	Atrial	300 beats/minute.
	Ventricular	150 beats/minute decreasing to 75 beats/minute.
Rhythm:	Atrial	Regular.
	Ventricular	Regular.
P waves:		Flutter waves clearly seen after carotid sinus massage *(arrows)* decreases the ventricular response.
PR interval:		Flutter-R interval fairly constant.
QRS:		Normal (0.08 second).
Arrhythmia:		Atrial flutter. Atrial flutter with a 2:1 ventricular response is present in the left portion of the tracing but cannot be clearly diagnosed from this lead. At the arrow, carotid sinus massage increases the degree of AV block to 4:1 and clearly exposes the atrial flutter waves.

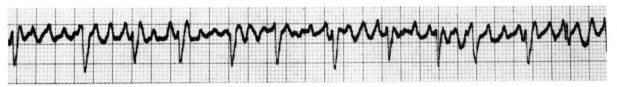

V₁

FIG. 8-128

Rate:	Atrial	300 to 500 beats/minute.
	Ventricular	72 to 150 beats/minute.
Rhythm:	Atrial	Irregular.
	Ventricular	Irregular.
P waves:		Variability in the contour and spacing of the flutter-fibrillation waves.
PR interval:		Nonmeasurable.
QRS:		Normal (0.09 second).
Arrhythmia:		Impure atrial flutter (coarse atrial flutter or flutter-fibrillation). Impure atrial flutter is characterized by a faster atrial rate than pure atrial flutter, and more variability shows in the contour and spacing of the flutter waves.

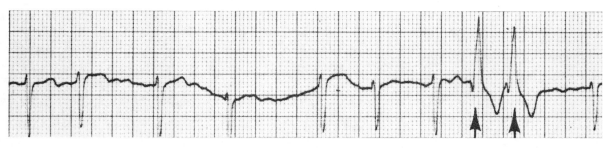

V₁

FIG. 8-129

Rate:	Atrial	350 to 600 beats/minute.
	Ventricular	65 to 160 beats/minute.
Rhythm:	Atrial	Irregularly irregular.
	Ventricular	Irregularly irregular.
P waves:		Irregular rapid baseline undulations indicate fibrillatory atrial activity.
PR interval:		Not measurable.
QRS:		0.08 second; two complexes indicated by arrows are functional right bundle branch block QRS complexes with a duration of 0.13 second.
Arrhythmia:		Atrial fibrillation. A long ventricular pause followed by a short ventricular pause precedes the QRS complex with a right bundle branch block contour *(arrow)*; this QRS complex is followed after a short interval by a second QRS complex, also with right bundle branch block *(arrow)*. The aberrant QRS pattern indicates functional right bundle branch block (Ashman phenomenon).

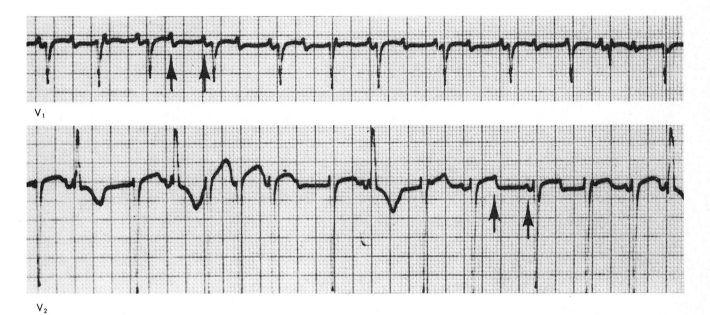

V₁

V₂

FIG. 8-130

Rate:	Atrial	167 beats/minute.
	Ventricular	Varies according to the degree of AV block (83 to 120 beats/minute).
Rhythm:	Atrial	Regular.
	Ventricular	Irregular (2:1, 3:2, and 4:3).
P waves:		Contour differs from sinus-initiated P waves.
PR interval:		Wenckebach cycles.
QRS:		0.08 second; functional right bundle branch block in lower tracing with a duration of 0.12 second.
Arrhythmia:		Atrial tachycardia with AV block. In the lower tracing, long-short QRS intervals, which follow longer intervals, set the stage for aberrant ventricular conduction that is manifest as a functional right bundle branch block. Arrows indicate P waves.

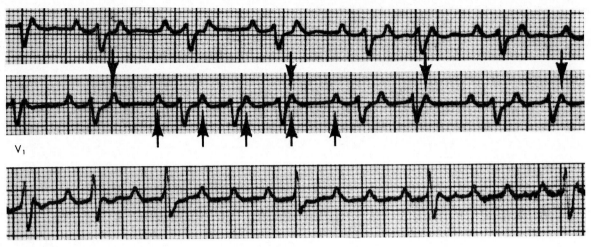

V₁

MONITOR

FIG. 8-131

Rate:	Atrial	150 beats/minute, *top;* 193 beats/minute, *bottom.*
	Ventricular	83 to 125 beats/minute, *top;* 50 to 94 beats/minute, *bottom.*
Rhythm:	Atrial	Regular.
	Ventricular	Irregular (2:1, 3:1, 4:1, 4:3, etc.)
P waves:		Contour differs from sinus-initiated P waves.
PR interval:		Wenckebach cycles.
QRS:		0.09 second.
Arrhythmia:		Atrial tachycardia with AV block caused by digitalis toxicity. Top two tracings recorded on admission. In the bottom tracing, continued digitalis administration increased the atrial rate to 193 beats/minute and increased the degree of AV block. Upright arrows indicate P waves; inverted arrows indicate nonconducted P waves.

II

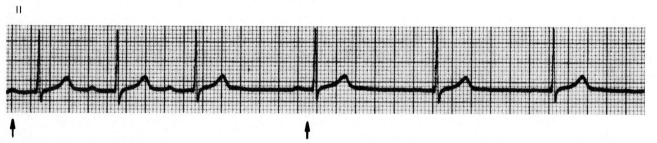

CSM

FIG. 8-132

Rate:	Atrial	75 beats/minute initially; atrial activity not apparent during the junctional rhythm.
	Ventricular	48 to 50 beats/minute during the junctional rhythm.
Rhythm:		Ventricular, generally regular.
P waves and PR interval:		Relationship between P and QRS as explained under premature AV junctional complexes. (P waves not apparent.) PR interval not determinable during junctional rhythm.
QRS:		Normal (0.08 second); may be conducted with slight aberration.
Arrhythmia:		AV junctional rhythm. Carotid sinus massage *(CSM,* between arrows) produces significant sinus slowing to allow the escape of an AV junctional rhythm (fifth QRS). Note unchanged QRS complexes. Atrial activity to the right of the last arrow is not apparent and may be caused by the AV junctional rhythm with retrograde capture of the P wave, lost within the QRS complex.

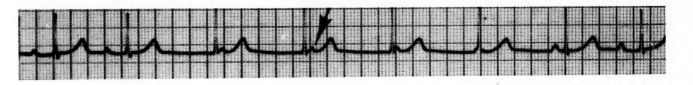

II

FIG. 8-133

Rate:	Atrial	45 to 70 beats/minute.
	Ventricular	58 to 70 beats/minute.
Rhythm:	Atrial	Slowing.
	Ventricular	Slowing but fairly regular.
P waves:		Normal.
PR interval:		See premature AV junctional complexes (AV dissociation in this tracing).
QRS:		Normal (0.08 second).
Arrhythmia:		AV junctional rhythm. Transient, spontaneous sinus slowing allows the escape of an AV junctional rhythm. P waves can be seen to occur just after the onset of the QRS complex *(arrow)* and represent normal sinus-initiated P waves. Gradual acceleration of the sinus rate reestablishes sinus control to the ventricular activity at the end of the tracing and thus terminates the period of AV dissociation in the midportion of the tracing. The PR interval is prolonged.

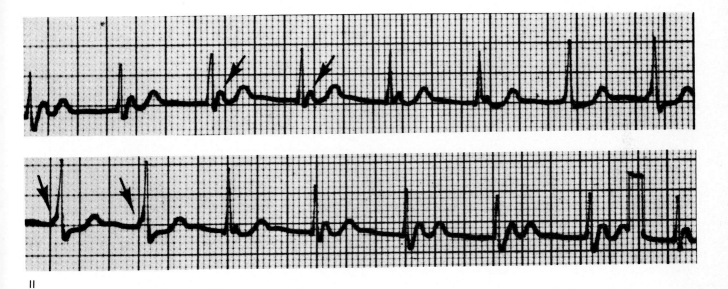

II

FIG. 8-134

Rate:	Atrial	100 beats/minute.
	Ventricular	100 beats/minute.
Rhythm:	Atrial	Reglular
	Ventricular	Fairly regular.
P waves:		Normal.
PR interval:		Varying.
QRS:		0.08 second.
Arrhythmia:		Nonparoxysmal AV junctional tachycardia. Atrial activity *(arrows)* follows, then slightly precedes, and then once again follows the inscription of the QRS complex. Therefore AV dissociation is present because of the accelerated AV junctional discharge. This type of AV dissociation is called *isorhythmic.*

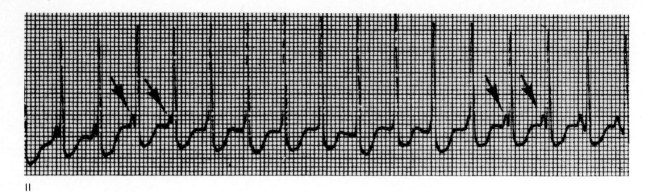

II

FIG. 8-135

Rate:	Atrial	166 beats/minute.
	Ventricular	166 beats/minute.
Rhythm:	Atrial	Regular.
	Ventricular	Regular.
P waves:		Normal.
PR interval:		Varying.
QRS:		0.06 second.
Arrhythmia:		Nonparoxysmal AV junctional tachycardia. Atrial activity *(arrows)* at a very similar rate and rhythm to the QRS can be seen to precede, then occur simultaneously with, and once again precede the onset of the QRS complex. This type of AV dissociation is called *isorhythmic.*

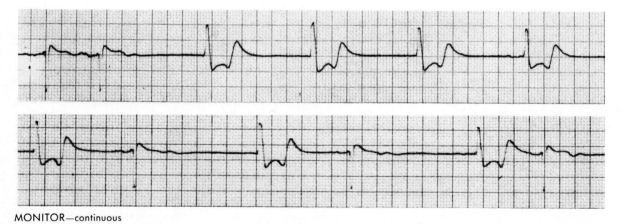

MONITOR—continuous

FIG. 8-136

Rate:	Atrial	Intermittent sinus arrest.
	Ventricular	43 beats/minute.
Rhythm:	Atrial	Irregular.
	Ventricular	Regular.
P waves:		Normal.
PR interval		Varying.
QRS (of ventricular escape rhythm):		0.13 second.
Arrhythmia:		Ventricular escape beats. Intermittent sinus arrest produced periods of asystole terminated by ventricular escape beats that are characterized by a prolonged, abnormal QRS complex. Intermittent return of sinus node activity establishes periods of supraventricular capture. The reason why AV junctional escape beats did not terminate the asystolic periods is not known.

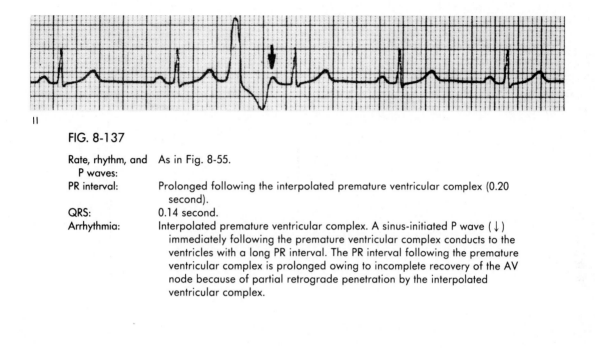

II

FIG. 8-137

Rate, rhythm, and P waves:	As in Fig. 8-55.
PR interval:	Prolonged following the interpolated premature ventricular complex (0.20 second).
QRS:	0.14 second.
Arrhythmia:	Interpolated premature ventricular complex. A sinus-initiated P wave (↓) immediately following the premature ventricular complex conducts to the ventricles with a long PR interval. The PR interval following the premature ventricular complex is prolonged owing to incomplete recovery of the AV node because of partial retrograde penetration by the interpolated ventricular complex.

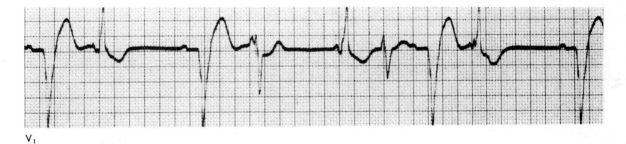

V₁

FIG. 8-138

Rate, rhythm, P waves, and PR interval:	As in Fig. 8-54.
QRS:	Wide, bizarre, greater than 0.12 second with varying contours and coupling intervals.
Arrhythmia:	Multiform premature ventricular complexes. The normally conducted QRS complexes have a left bundle branch block morphology. The PR interval is slightly prolonged (0.24 second). Premature QRS complexes with varying contours and coupling intervals are present and called *multiform ventricular complexes*.

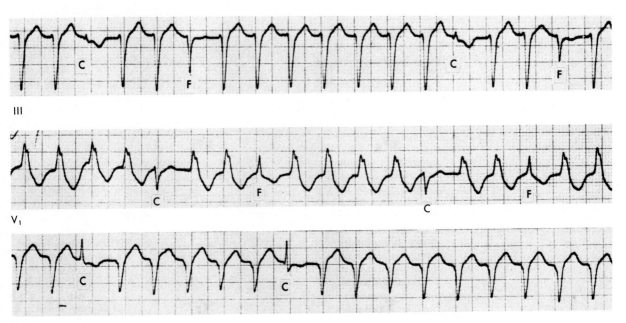

III

V₁

V₆

FIG. 8-139

Rate:	Atrial	Clear P waves not seen.
	Ventricular	150 beats/minute.
Rhythm:	Atrial	Regular.
	Ventricular	Regular.
P waves:		Atrial activity is probably under independent control of sinus node.
PR interval:		Not measurable.
QRS:		0.14 second.
Arrhythmia:		Ventricular tachycardia. QRS complexes with a prolonged duration and a right bundle branch block morphology occur at a regular interval and are occasionally interrupted by QRS complexes with a normal contour (*C*, capture) or QRS complexes with an intermediate contour. (*F*, fusion). Atrial activity cannot be seen; most likely, the atria are discharging independently to produce intermittent QRS captures and fusion beats. Therefore the most reasonable diagnosis is a ventricular tachycardia with AV dissociation.

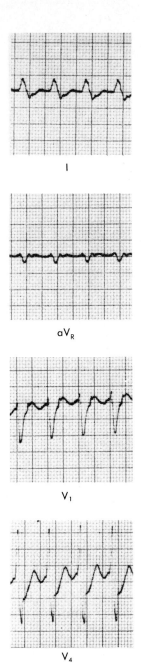
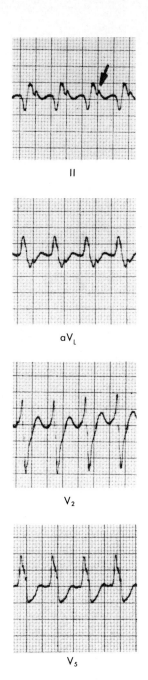
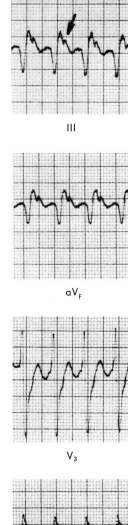
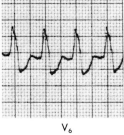

I

II

III

aV_R

aV_L

aV_F

V₁

V₂

V₃

V₄

V₅

V₆

FIG. 8-140

Rate:	Atrial	150 beats/minute.
	Ventricular	150 beats/minute.
Rhythm:	Atrial	Regular.
	Ventricular	Regular.
P waves:		Retrograde P waves inverted in 2, 3 *(arrows),* and aVF.
RP interval:		0.16 second.
QRS:		0.12 second.
Arrhythmia:		Ventricular tachycardia with retrograde atrial capture. Ventricular tachycardia cannot be diagnosed with certainty from this surface ECG because all the features of this arrhythmia can be mimicked by a supraventricular tachycardia with aberrant ventricular conduction of a left bundle branch block type. Electrophysiologic study proved that this was a ventricular tachycardia, however. The importance of the illustration lies in demonstrating 1:1 retrograde conduction to the atrium. Retrograde atrial activity is indicated by arrows. Thus AV dissociation is *not* present during this ventricular tachycardia.

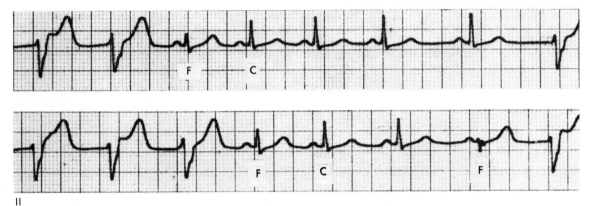

II

FIG. 8-141

Rate:	Atrial	70 to 90 beats/minute.
	Ventricular	72 beats/minute.
Rhythm:	Atrial	Regular.
	Ventricular	Regular.
P waves:		Independent.
PR interval:		Not measurable during accelerated idioventricular rhythm.
QRS:		0.14 second; fusion beats and capture bears often present (labeled *F* and *C*).
Arrhythmia:		Accelerated idioventricular rhythm. An accelerated idioventricular rhythm is present at the beginning and termination of the top and bottom strips. In the midportion of each tracing, slight sinus node acceleration reestablishes sinus node control by capturing the ventricles *(C)* and suppresses the accelerated idioventricular rhythm. When the sinus node slows, the accelerated idioventricular rhythm escapes. Fusion beats *(F)* may occur in the beginning and end of such arrhythmias because sinus and ventricular foci have similar rates.

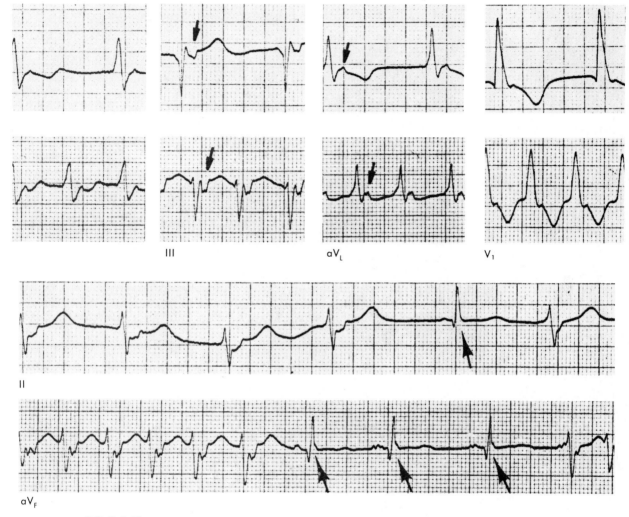

III aV$_L$ V$_1$

II

aV$_F$

FIG. 8-142

Rate: Accelerated idioventricular rhythm (60 beats/minute). Ventricular tachycardia
            (varying slight, 150 beats/minute).
Rhythm: Accelerated idioventricular rhythm (regular). Ventricular tachycardia (regular).
P waves: Retrogradely captured.
PR interval: 0.14 second.
QRS: 0.14 second.
Arrhythmia: Accelerated idioventricular rhythm and ventricular tachycardia. An accelerated
            idioventricular rhythm and a ventricular tachycardia occurred at different times
            in this patient. A illustrates leads, I, III, aV$_L$, V$_1$, and V$_6$ during the accelerated
            ventricular rhythm, whereas C (lead II) illustrates the onset of the accelerated
            idioventricular rhythm. B illustrates the ventricular tachycardia in leads I, III, aV$_L$,
            V$_1$, and V$_6$, whereas D (aV$_F$) illustrates the onset and termination of the
            ventricular tachycardia. Retrograde atrial capture (↓) occurred during both
            tachycardias. Normally conducted QRS complexes present in C and D (↑). Note
            identical QRS contours for both tachycardias (aV$_L$, V$_1$, and V$_6$ in A were recorded
            at different standardization), indicating that they arose at same or similar areas
            of the ventricle.

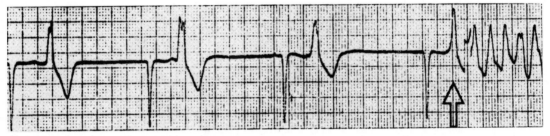

V_1

FIG. 8-143

Rate:	Atrial	60 to 100 beats/minute; any independent atrial arrhythmia may exist or the atria captured retrogradely.
	Ventricular	400 to 600 beats/minute.
Rhythm:	Atrial	Regular; may be irregular if the atria are retrogradely captured.
	Ventricular	Grossly irregular.
P waves:		Generally cannot be seen.
PR interval:		Generally not measurable.
QRS:		Baseline undulations without distinct QRS contours.
Arrhythmia:		Ventricular fibrillation. Premature ventricular complexes occurred in a bigeminal pattern with a decreasing coupling interval. The fourth premature ventricular complex discharged during the vulnerable period of the antecedent T wave and precipitated ventricular fibrillation *(arrow)*.

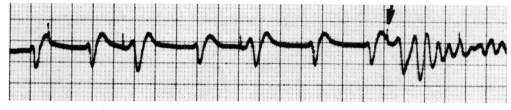

MONITOR

FIG. 8-144

Rate, rhythm, P waves, PR interval and QRS:	As in Fig. 8-143.
Arrhythmia:	Ventricular fibrillation. Pacemaker spikes *(arrow)* from a malfunctioning pacemaker fall randomly throughout the cardiac cycle at a slightly irregular interval. When the pacemaker spike discharged during the vulnerable period of the antecedent T wave *(arrow)*, it precipitated ventricular fibrillation. Ventricular rhythm preceding onset of ventricular fibrillation is probably slightly irregular, accelerated idioventricular rhythm.

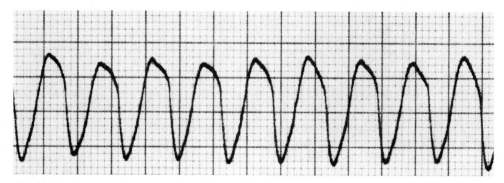

MONITOR

FIG. 8-145

Rate:	Atrial	P waves not seen.
	Ventricular	195 beats/minute.
Rhythm:	Ventricular	Regular.
P waves:		Cannot be seen.
PR interval:		Not measurable.
QRS:		0.16 second.
Arrhythmia:		Ventricular flutter. Sine wave with regular large oscillations. The QRS complex cannot be definitely distinguished from the ST segment or T wave.

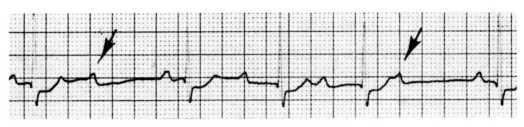

II

FIG. 8-146

Rate:	Atrial	Normal (83 beats/minute).
	Ventricular	Depends on degree of AV block, which may vary between 2:1, 3:2, 4:3, 5:3, 5:3, etc.
Rhythm:	Atrial	Regular.
	Ventricular	Varying, depending on the degree of AV block.
P waves:		More numerous than QRS complexes but are related to ventricular beats in a consistent, repetitive fashion.
PR interval:		Progressive PR prolongation preceding the nonconducted P wave. Finally, one P wave is blocked, and the cycle then repeats.
QRS:		Normal; RR interval gradually shortens until the blocked P wave occurs; the cycle then repeats.
Arrhythmia:		Second-degree AV heart block (type I Wenckebach). AV Wenckebach is characterized by progressive PR prolongation preceding the nonconducted P wave. Wenckebach AV block, in the presence of a normal QRS complex, is virtually always at the level of the AV node. Conduction ratios (that is, the number of P waves to the number of QRS complexes) are 2:1, 4:3, and 3:2 in this tracing. Because the increment in conduction time is greatest in the second cycle of the Wenckebach group and then decreases progressively over succeeding cycles, the following characteristics are also present: (1) the interval between successive RR cycles before the nonconducted P wave progressively decreases; (2) the duration of the pause produced by the nonconducted P wave is less than twice the shortest cycle, which is generally the cycle immediately preceding the pause; (3) the duration of the RR cycle following the pause exceeds the duration of the RR cycle preceding the pause. These features can be seen in the middle 4:3 grouping. Blocked P waves indicated by arrows.

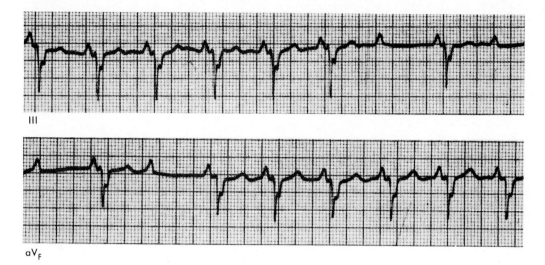

III

aV_F

FIG. 8-147

Rate:		86 beats/minute.
Rhythm:	Atrial	Regular.
	Ventricular	Varying, depending upon the degree of AV block.
P waves:		Normal.
PR interval:		Normal, constant (0.12 second) with sudden failure of conduction.
QRS:		Prolonged; right bundle branch block and left anterior hemiblock (0.12 second)
Arrhythmia:		Second-degree AV heart block, type II. Right bundle branch block (not readily apparent in leads III and aV_F) along with left anterior fascicular block is present in this patient. Sudden failure of AV conduction results without antecedent PR prolongation. The PR interval for the conducted beats is normal, as it often is during type II second-degree AV heart block.

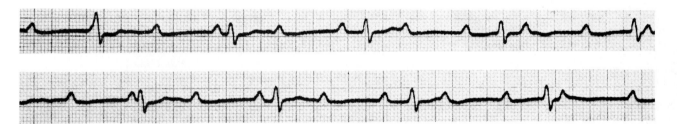

II

FIG. 8-148

Rate:	Atrial	85 beats/minute.
	Ventricular	38 beats/minute.
Rhythm:	Atrial	Regular.
	Ventricular	Regular.
P waves:		Normal.
PR interval:		Completely variable.
QRS:		Prolonged (0.12 second)
Arrhythmia:		Third-degree (complete) AV heart block. Complete AV dissociation is present *resulting from* complete heart block. The abnormal QRS complexes (prolonged duration) indicate a ventricular origin for the escape rhythm.

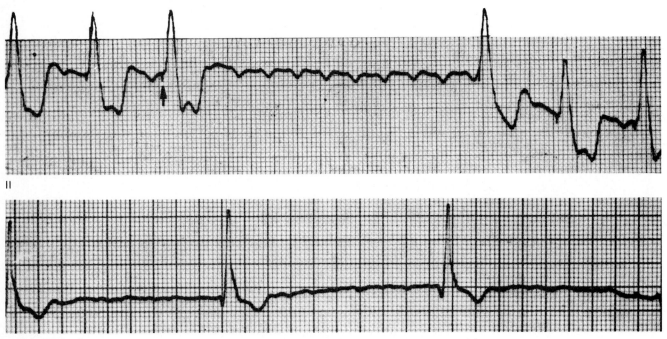

II

MONITOR lead

FIG. 8-149

Rate:	Atrial	*Top,* 250 beats/minute; *bottom,* 400 to 600 beats/minute.
	Ventricular	*Top,* 100 beats/minute; *bottom,* 32 beats/minute.
Rhythm:	Atrial	*Top,* regular; *bottom,* irregular.
	Ventricular	*Top,* regular; *bottom,* regular.
P waves:		*Top,* atrial flutter; *bottom,* atrial fibrillation.
PR interval:		Totally variable or nonmeasurable.
QRS:		*Top,* ventricular paced beats (0.16 second); *bottom,* 0.14 second.
Arrhythmia:		Complete (third-degree) AV heart block during atrial flutter and atrial fibrillation. In the top tracing a ventricular pacemaker controls ventricular activity (arrow indicates pacemaker artifact). In the midportion of the tracing the ventricular pacing was temporarily discontinued, and one can easily see the atrial flutter waves that fail to conduct to the ventricle. In the terminal portion of the tracing the ventricular pacemaker was turned on once again. In the bottom tracing the undulating baseline indicates the presence of atrial fibrillation. The regular ventricular rhythm establishes that none of the atrial fibrillatory impulses conduct to the ventricles; thus complete AV block is present during atrial fibrillation.

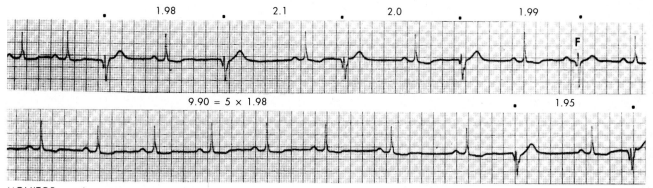

1.98 2.1 2.0 1.99

F

9.90 = 5 × 1.98 1.95

MONITOR—continuous

FIG. 8-150

Rate:	Atrial	Approximately 60 beats/minute.
	Ventricular parasystole	30 beats/minute.
Rhythm:	Atrial	Regular.
	Ventricular parasystole	Regular; interrupted by exit block or ventricular refractoriness.
P waves:		Normal.
PR interval:		During normally conducted beats, normal.
QRS (of ventricular parasystole):		Prolonged (0.13 second).
Arrhythmia:		Ventricular parasystole. The interval between ectopic ventricular systoles ranges between 1.98 and 2.1 seconds. The coupling interval varies between the sinus-initiated QRS complex and the parasystole complex. A ventricular fusion beat is labeled F. Ventricular refractoriness prevents the emergence of the ventricular parasystole during the long interval in which it is absent. This interectopic interval equals 9.90 seconds and is five times the normal interectopic interval. The dark marks above the tracing indicate the parasystolic ventricular systoles.

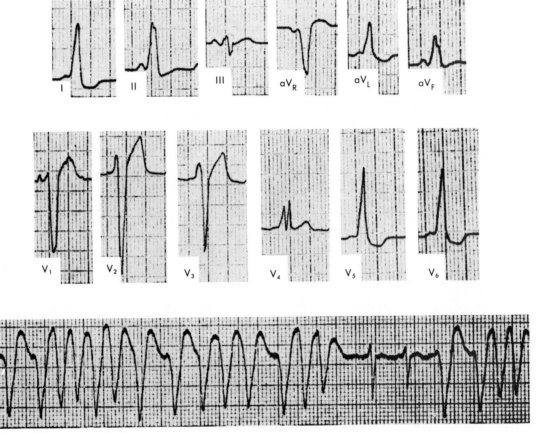

FIG. 8-151. Arrhythmia: twelve-lead ECG illustrating the preexcitation (Wolff-Parkinson-White) syndrome with a right anterior or paraseptal pathway. The lower recording (V₁ half standard) demonstrates an extremely rapid ventricular rate during atrial fibrillation in this same patient. The grossly irregular ventricular rhythm, extremely rapid rate, and gradations in QRS contour from normal to prolonged (as conduction changes from the normal AV nodal pathway to the anomalous route) help distinguish this arrhythmia from ventricular tachycardia. Bypass of the safety valve features provided by normal AV nodal delay accounts for the rapid ventricular rate that less commonly may actually cause the ventricles to fibrillate and result in sudden death.

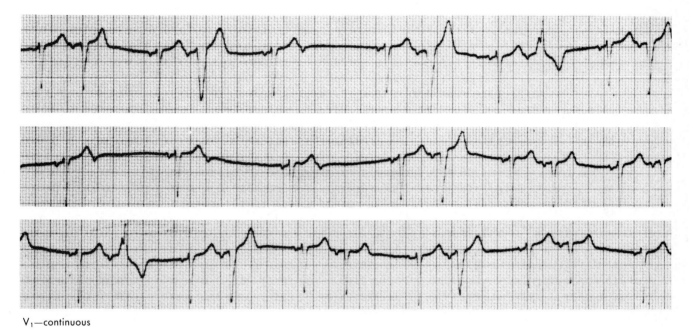

V₁—continuous

FIG. 8-152

Rate:	Determined by the number of premature atrial complexes.
Rhythm:	Irregular because of premature atrial complexes.
P waves:	Both sinus-initiated and premature atrial P waves are abnormal.
PR interval:	Normal (0.12 second) for the sinus-initiated P waves; prolonged following the premature atrial complexes. Some premature atrial complexes failed to conduct to the ventricle.
QRS:	Normal, following the sinus-initiated P waves; functional left bundle and functional right bundle branch block following the premature atrial complexes.
Arrhythmia:	Functional right and left bundle branch block following atrial premature complexes. Premature atrial complexes occur at varying coupling intervals. When they occur with a very short RP interval, they fail to reach the ventricle and are therefore nonconducted atrial complexes. At slightly longer RP intervals, they conduct with both functional right and functional left bundle block. Differences in the duration of the preceding long cycle and in the duration of the short cycle account for whether functional right or left bundle branch block results.

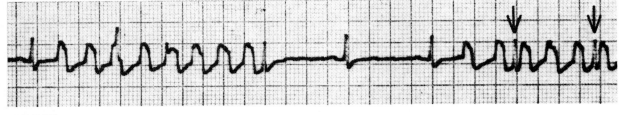

MONITOR

FIG. 8-153.   Artifact. Regularly moving a loose electrode creates an artifact that mimics ventricular tachycardia. However, careful scrutiny uncovers the fairly regularly occurring normal QRS complexes *(arrows)*, each preceded by a P wave. The question of ventricular tachycardia may be eliminated and the diagnosis of artifact established by observing that the QRS complexes continue uninterrupted and unaffected by the apparent ventricular tachycardia.

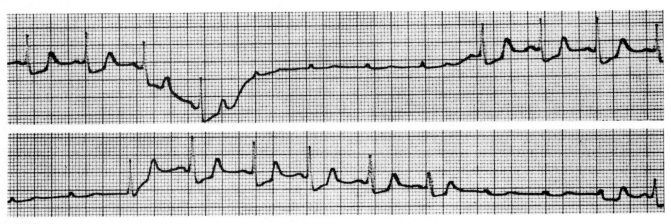

MONITOR

FIG. 8-154.   Artifact simulating AV block. These tracings were recorded in a patient who presented with an acute anteroseptal myocardial infarction and 1 day later developed left anterior fascicular block. The monitored recording was interpreted as illustrating the development of advanced AV block with sequentially blocked P waves. Temporary transvenous pacemaker insertion was deemed immediately necessary. However, careful observation of the tracing reveals that the nonconducted P waves are artifactual in origin. In reality the "nonconducted P waves" are QRS complexes with a grossly diminished amplitude caused by intermittent poor ECG lead contact. The diagnosis is established by noting QRS complexes with intermediate amplitudes, by noting T waves that follow the diminutive QRS complexes, and by "marching out" the QRS complexes and finding that they occur at the same time as the apparent P waves.

Electrocardiogram Test Section

The following section provides a series of ECG tracings of various conditions that have been discussed throughout this text. It is suggested that the reader cover the interpretations given at the end of each legend and attempt to identify the abnormal patterns that are found in each ECG.

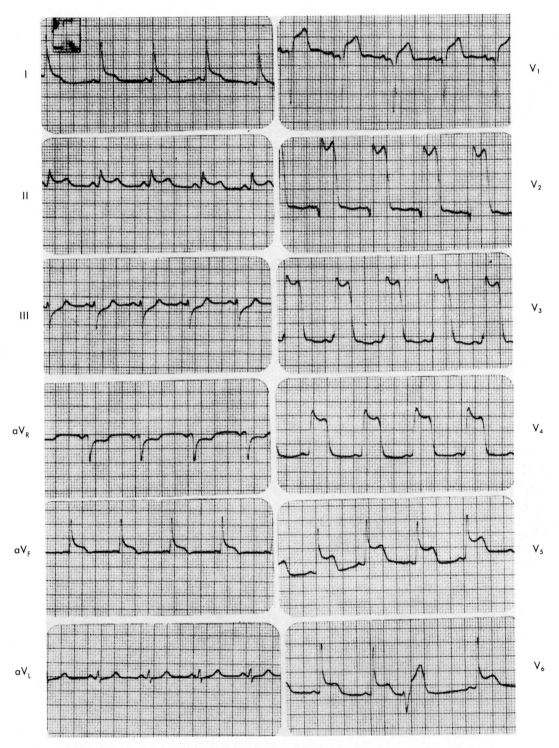

I

II

III

aV$_R$

aV$_F$

aV$_L$

V$_1$

V$_2$

V$_3$

V$_4$

V$_5$

V$_6$

FIG. 8-155. Normal sinus rhythm, Q waves in V$_1$ and V$_2$. Marked ST segment elevation in leads I, II, aV$_1$, and V$_1$ through V$_6$. T waves have not yet inverted.

Electrocardiogram: *Hyperacute anterolateral, possibly apical, myocardial infarction.*

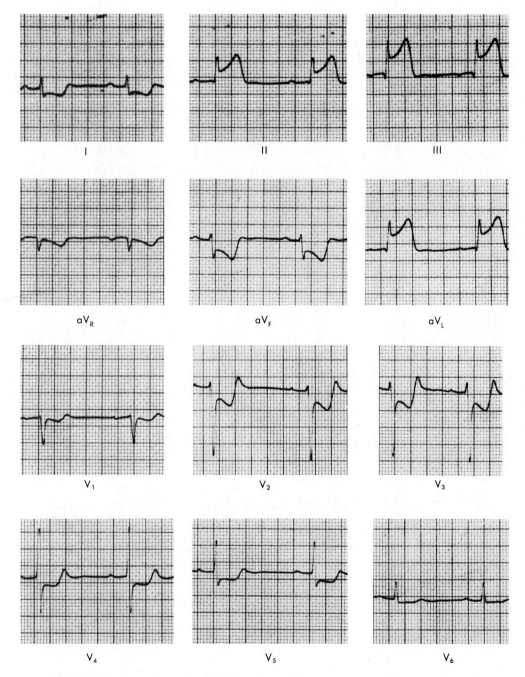

FIG. 8-156. Normal sinus rhythm. No pathologic Q waves have developed. Marked ST segment elevation in leads II, III, and aV_F, with reciprocal depression in leads I, aV_L and the anterior precordium. T waves are still upright.

Electrocardiogram: *Hyperacute inferior (diaphragmatic) myocardial infarction.*

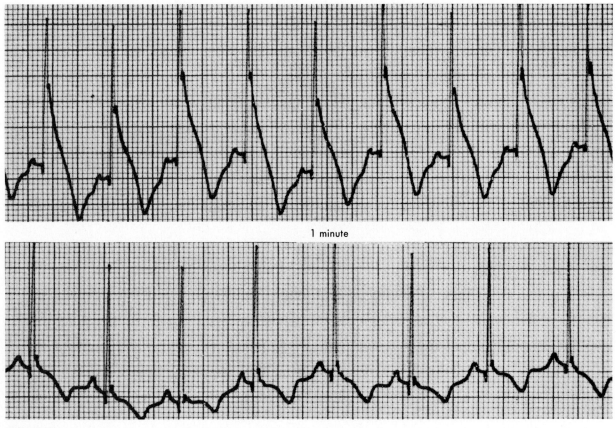

1 minute

MONITOR

FIG. 8-157. Top tracing demonstrates marked ST segment elevation and T wave inversion. One minute later (bottom tracing) the ST segments have returned to baseline. The T waves are still inverted.

Electrocardiogram: *The rapid ST changes from elevation to normal are characteristic of atypical (Prinzmetal) angina pectoris.*

9:30 AM   11:45 AM

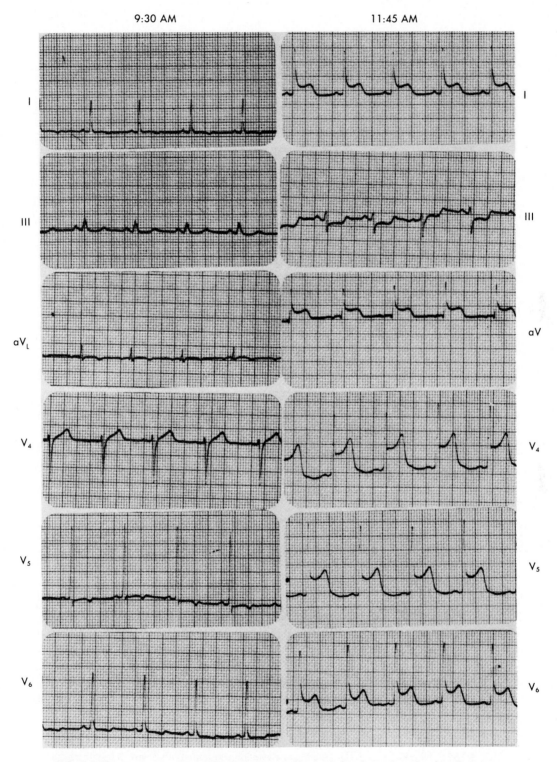

FIG. 8-158. Normal sinus rhythm. Tracing at 9:30 AM, (after the patient developed more chest pain) demonstrates ST segment elevation in leads I, aV$_L$, and V$_4$ through V$_6$. The T waves are still upright, and no pathologic Q waves have developed.

Electrocardiogram: *Hyperacute lateral myocardial infarction.*

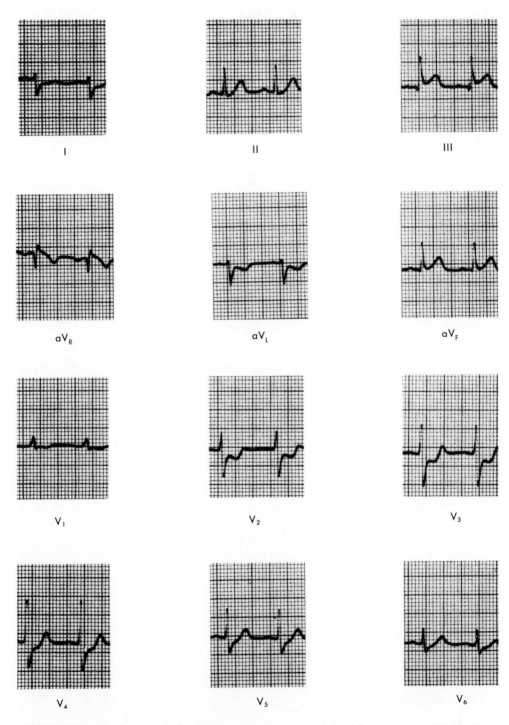

FIG. 8-159. Normal sinus rhythm. Right axis deviation suggesting left posterior hemiblock. ST segment elevation in lead III and slight ST segment elevation in lead aV$_F$. Large R wave in V$_1$, with slight ST segment depression in V$_1$, more marked in V$_2$ and V$_3$. T waves are still upright except for diphasic T waves in leads V$_1$ and V$_2$.

Electrocardiogram: *Acute posteroinferior myocardial infarction.*

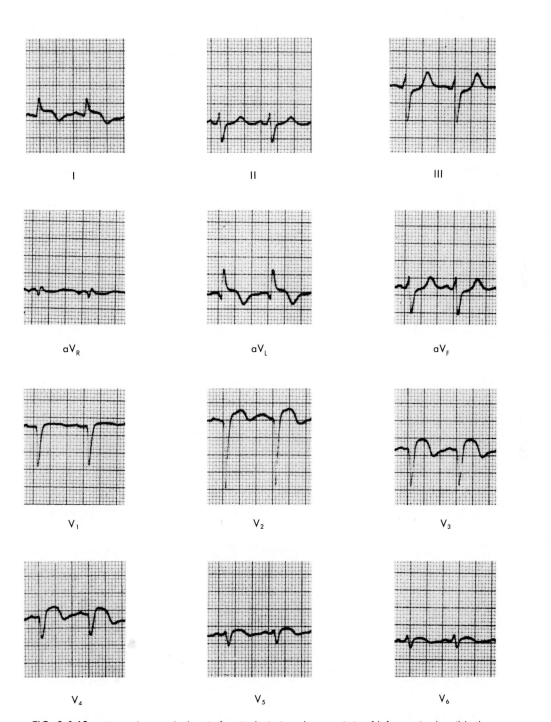

FIG. 8-160.   Normal sinus rhythm. Left axis deviation characteristic of left anterior hemiblock. ST segment elevation in leads I, aV$_L$, and V$_2$ through V$_6$. Abnormal Q wave in V$_1$ through V$_4$, with small R waves in V$_5$ and V$_6$. T wave inversion in leads 1 and aV$_L$ and terminal T wave inversion in V$_2$ through V$_5$.

Impression: *Acute anterolateral myocardial infarction and left anterior hemiblock.*

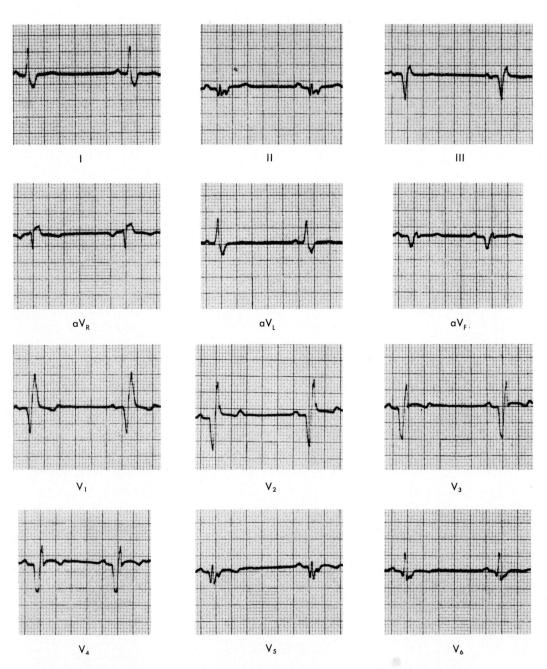

FIG. 8-161.   Normal sinus rhythm, right bundle branch block, and left axis deviation characteristic of left anterior hemiblock. ST segments are normal. There are nonspecific T wave changes. A pathologic Q wave is present in leads II, III, aV_F, and V_1 through V_4 and makes the diagnosis of left anterior hemiblock difficult.

Electrocardiogram: *Right bundle branch block, possible left anterior hemiblock, and anteroinferior myocardial infarction, probably old.*

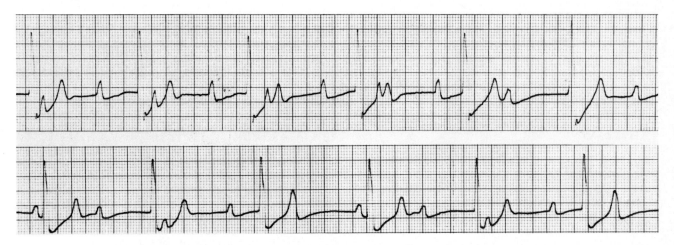

FIG. 8-162.   Third-degree (complete) AV heart block. Complete AV dissociation is present caused by complete AV heart block. Atria and ventricles are under control of separate pacemakers, and the sinus node and an idioventricular escape rhythm, respectively. Monitor lead.

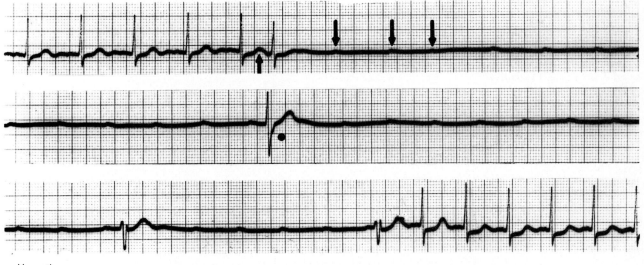

V₄ continuous

FIG. 8-163.   Paroxysmal AV block. Periods of complete AV block interrupted only by an occasional escape beat occurred in this patient who had recurrent syncope. Each episode of AV block was always introduced by a premature atrial complex *(upright arrow)* which then resulted in a series of successive nonconducted P waves *(inverted arrows)*. Finally, an escape beat occurred and restored conduction (bottom strip of this continuous recording of V₄). Electrophysiologic mechanism responsible for this form of paroxysmal AV block is not clear.

REFERENCES

1. Zipes, D.P.: Genesis of cardiac arrhythmias: electrophysiological considerations. In Braunwald, E., editor: Heart disease: a textbook of cardiovascular medicine, ed. 3, Philadelphia, 1984, W.B. Saunders Co.
2. Rosenbaum, M.B.: The hemiblocks: diagnostic criteria and clinical significance, Mod. Concepts Cardiovasc. Dis. **39**:141, 1970.
3. Jalife, J., and Moe, G.K.: A biologic model of parasystole, Am. J. Cardiol. **43**:761, 1979.
4. Anzelovitch, C., Jalife, J., and Moe, G.K.: Characteristics of reflection as a mechanism of reentrant arrhythmias and its relationship to parasystole. Circulation **61**:182, 1980.
5. Zipes, D.P.: A consideration of antiarrhythmic therapy (editorial), Circulation **72**:949, 1985.
6. Zipes, D.P., Bailey, J.C., and Elharrar, V.: The slow inward current and cardiac arrhythmias, The Hague, 1980, Martinus Nijhoff.
7. Zipes, D.P.: Management of cardiac arrhythmias. In Braunwald, E., editor: Heart disease: a textbook of cardiovascular medicine, Philadelphia, 1984, W.B. Saunders Co., p. 648.
8. Zipes, D.P.: Specific arrhythmias: diagnosis and treatment. In Braunwald, E., editor: Heart disease: a textbook of cardiovascular medicine, Philadelphia, 1984, W.B. Saunders Co., p. 683.
9. Prystowsky, E.N., and Zipes, D.P.: Treatment of tachycardia. In Rakel, R.E., editor: Conn's current therapy, Philadelphia, W.B. Saunders Co., p. 188.
10. Zipes, D.P., editor: Symposium on cardiac arrhythmias, Cardiology Clinics, vol. 1, 1983.
11. Zipes, D.P., editor: Symposium on cardiac arrhythmias, Medical Clinics of North America, vol. 68, 1984.
12. Pick, A., and Langendorf, R.: Interpretation of complex arrhythmias, Philadelphia, 1979, Lea & Febiger.
13. Josephson, M.E., and Seides, S.F.: Clinical cardiac electrophysiology, Philadelphia, 1979, Lea & Febiger.
14. Nattel, S., and Zipes, D.P.: Clinical pharmacology of old and new antiarrhythmic drugs, Cardiovasc. Clin. **11**:221, 1980.
15. Rinkenberger, R.L., and others: Effects of intravenous and chronic oral verapamil administration in patients with supraventricular tachyarrhythmias, Circulation **62**:996, 1980.
16. Arcebal, A., and Lemberg, L.: Mechanisms of supraventricular tachycardia, Heart Lung **13**:205, 1984.
17. Prystowsky, E.N., and others: Preexcitation syndromes: mechanisms and management, Med. Clin. North Am. **68**:831, 1984.
18. Huerta, B., and Lemberg, L.: Anticoagulation in atrial fibrillation, Heart Lung **14**:521, 1985.
19. Zipes, D.P., and others: Development of the implantable transvenous cardioverter, Am. J. Cardiol. **54**:670, 1984.
20. Kienzle, M., and others: Antiarrhythmic drug therapy for sustained ventricular tachycardia, Heart Lung **13**:614, 1984.
21. Markmann, P., and Chellemi, J.: Surgical management of ventricular tachycardia, Heart Lung **13**:622, 1984.
22. Rahimtoola, S., and others: Consensus statement of the conference on the state of the art of electrophysiological testing in the diagnosis and treatment of patients with cardiac arrhythmias, Circulation, April 1987.
23. Zipes, D.P.: Second-degree atrioventricular block, Circulation **60**:465, 1979.
24. Hindman, M.C., and others: The clinical significance of bundle branch block complicating acute myocardial infarction, Circulation **58**:689, 1978.
25. Miles, W.M., and others: Evaluation of the patient with wide QRS tachycardia, Med. Clin. North Am. **68**:1015, 1984.
26. Wellens, H.J.J., Bärf, W.H.M., and Lie, K.I.: The value of the electrocardiogram in the differential diagnosis of a tachycardia with a widened QRS complex, Am. J. Med. **64**:27, 1978.
27. Green, M., and others: Value of QRS alternation in determining the site of origin of narrow QRS synaventricular tachycardia, Circulation **68**:368, 1983.
28. Commerford, P.J., and Lloyd, E.A.: Arrhythmias in patients with drug toxicity, electrolyte and endocrine disturbances, Med. Clin. North Am. **68**:1051, 1984.
29. Akhtar, M., and others: NASPE Ad Hoc Committee on Guidelines for Cardiac Electrophysiological Studies, PACE **8**:611, 1985.

SUGGESTED READINGS

Josephson, M.E., and Wellens, H.J., editors: Tachycardias: mechanisms, diagnosis, treatment, Philadelphia, 1984, Lea & Febiger.
Kennedy, H.L.: Ambulatory electrocardiography, Philadelphia, 1981, Lea & Febiger.
Mandel, W.J., editor: Cardiac arrhythmias, ed. 2, Philadelphia, 1987, J.B. Lippincott Co.
Marriott, H.J.L.: Practical electrocardiography, ed. 6, Baltimore, 1977, The Williams & Wilkins Co.
Surawicz, B., Reddy, C.P., and Prystowsky, E.N., editors: Tachycardias, Boston, 1984, Martinus Nijhoff.
Zipes, D.P., and Jalife, J., editors: Cardiac electophysiology and arrhythmias, Orlando, Fla., 1985, Grune & Stratton, Inc.

CHAPTER 9

Sudden cardiac death is the loss of life occurring within 1 hour of the onset of cardiovascular symptoms in a patient previously free of symptoms who has not suffered circulatory collapse during the preceding 24 hours, and in whom no other cause of death is identified either by history or by autopsy.[1] Sudden cardiac death accounts for approximately 1000 deaths in the United States every day.[2] Since postmortems[3-5] and catheterization data[6] reveal that most victims have significant coronary artery disease, the ideal epidemiologic approach to prevent sudden death would be to decrease the incidence of atherosclerosis. In this regard, physicians and other health care personnel should instruct patients to stop smoking cigarettes and to maintain normal systemic arterial blood pressure, normal body weight, and normal plasma lipids. Moreover, prevention of atherosclerotic heart disease must start at a young age, and children and adolescents must be taught the value of an appropriate diet and life-style (see Chapter 3).

The wide-scale prevention of atherosclerotic heart disease will take years to accomplish, and until then alternative methods must be sought to decrease the frequency of sudden cardiac death. One way is to teach cardiopulmonary resuscitation techniques to emergency personnel and to the general public. In Seattle, Washington, Cobb and others[7] in association with the Seattle Fire Department have developed an emergency care system with various levels of medical expertise that has provided data on sudden death and the effects of resuscitation. Patient survival depends on the rapidity with which cardiopulmonary resuscitation is initiated. In this program the average response time from dispatch until the first unit arrives is 2.9 minutes,[7] and often a bystander may begin cardiopulmonary resuscitation before the arrival of the emergency care team.

Early results from emergency care systems were not promising; only approximately 15% of sudden death victims were resuscitated successfully and discharged from the hospital.[7,8] However, later data from Seattle demonstrate improved survival statistics.[7] In 1978, 60% of 290 patients were successfully resuscitated from out-of-hospital ventricular fibrillation and about half of these patients (30% of the total group) were discharged; still the majority of patients did not survive. Furthermore, about 80% of patients who have out-of-hospital ventricular fibrillation do not have associated acute myocardial infarction; the 1-year risk of recurrent sudden death is 22% in these patients.[9] It is therefore important to develop a means of identifying patients who are at risk for sudden death in the hope that appropriate therapy can prevent its occurrence. This chapter deals with the pathophysiology and risk factors of sudden death as well as the use of electrophysiologic testing to determine the efficacy of antiarrhythmic drug therapy.

PATHOPHYSIOLOGY OF SUDDEN CARDIAC DEATH

Ventricular fibrillation is the most common arrhythmia recorded at the onset of cardiopulmonary resuscitation in patients who have out-of-hospital cardiac arrest or in patients who die suddenly.[7,8,10,11] In one study[10] bradyarrhythmias were present in nearly one third of the patients, a frequency that is much higher than that found in other studies.[7,8,11] Since bradyarrhythmias commonly occur when there has been delay in initiating emergency care,[7] it is unclear how often they actually cause sudden death. For example, combined data from eight monitored patients who did not have evidence of acute myocardial infarction showed that ventricular fibrillation caused sudden death in seven patients and severe bradyarrhythmias in only one patient.[12-14] An example of cardiac arrest caused by the spontaneous onset of rapid ventricular tachycardia that degenerated into ventricular fibrillation is shown in Fig. 9-1. More research needs to be done to define the role of bradyarrhythmias in sudden death.

In contrast, ample data exist in support of ventricular tachyarrhythmias as the cause of sudden cardiac death.[11-16] Lie and others[15] continuously monitored 262 patients who had an acute myocardial infarction (excluding patients with congestive heart failure or shock). All 20 patients requiring resuscitation had ventricular fibrillation, and in four patients ventricular tachycardia preceded ventricular fibrillation (Fig. 9-2). In another study Lie and others[16] continuously monitored for 6 weeks 47 patients who had had a recent myocardial infarction associated with bundle branch block. Of the 47, 17 had cardiac arrest, and in all

This study was supported in part by the Herman C. Krannert Fund; by Grants HL-06308 and HL-07182 from the National Heart, Lung, and Blood Institute of the National Institutes of Health; by the American Heart Association, Indiana affiliate, and by the Veterans Administration.

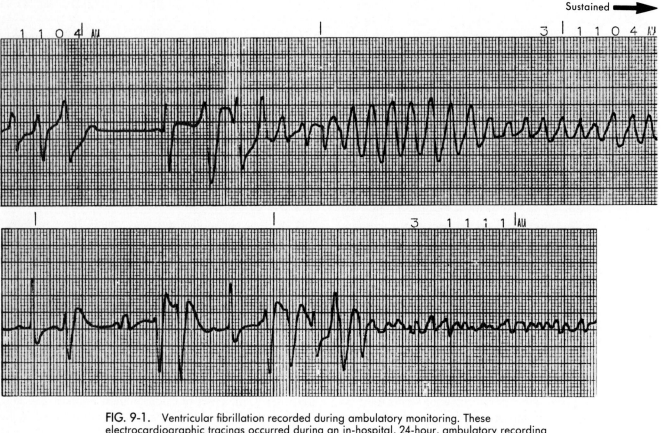

FIG. 9-1.   Ventricular fibrillation recorded during ambulatory monitoring. These electrocardiographic tracings occurred during an in-hospital, 24-hour, ambulatory recording on a patient who had a previous out-of-hospital cardiac arrest. A shows the onset of rapid (approximately 300 beats/minute) ventricular tachycardia that degenerated into ventricular fibrillation; the patient was successfully defibrillated to sinus rhythm. Seven minutes later (B) a second episode of ventricular fibrillation occurred after a short run of ventricular tachycardia; defibrillation again restored sinus rhythm.

patients the arrhythmia was ventricular fibrillation. In this group, 14 of 17 episodes of ventricular fibrillation were preceded by ventricular tachycardia. In both these studies ventricular tachyarrhythmias were the cause of sudden death in the majority of patients who had a recent myocardial infarction and lived long enough to be admitted to the hospital. Although not proved, ventricular arrhythmias are the most likely cause of sudden death in patients who have an acute myocardial infarction but die before being hospitalized.

Most patients who have coronary artery disease and develop sudden cardiac death demonstrate no recent thrombi in the coronary arteries at postmortem examination.[17,18] Moreover, the majority of patients successfully resuscitated from sudden death do not have an acute myocardial infarction.[19] In patients who are resuscitated from out-of-hospital sudden death, the presence of an acute myocardial infarction has important prognostic significance: of 424 survivors of ventricular fibrillation, the 1-year mortality in patients who had an acute myocardial

infarction was 2%, and in patients who did not have an infarction the mortality was 22%.[9] These data confirm the observation that the occurrence of ventricular fibrillation in the coronary care unit in patients who have an acute myocardial infarction does not increase the risk of sudden death in these patients after hospital discharge.[20]

The difference in long-term survival after resuscitation for a patient who had and one who did not have an acute myocardial infarction may be partially explained by the fact that the transient electrophysiologic and biochemical alterations that occur in the ventricle during an acute myocardial infarction may result in ventricular fibrillation.[21,22] When the acute phase of the infarction resolves, such patients have a low recurrence rate of ventricular fibrillation most likely because their hearts no longer have the electrophysiologic/anatomic capability to develop and/or sustain ventricular arrhythmias. In contrast, patients who have ventricular fibrillation without infarction have a relatively high risk of recurrent ventricular fibrillation. The high recurrence rate in these patients may be related to the fact

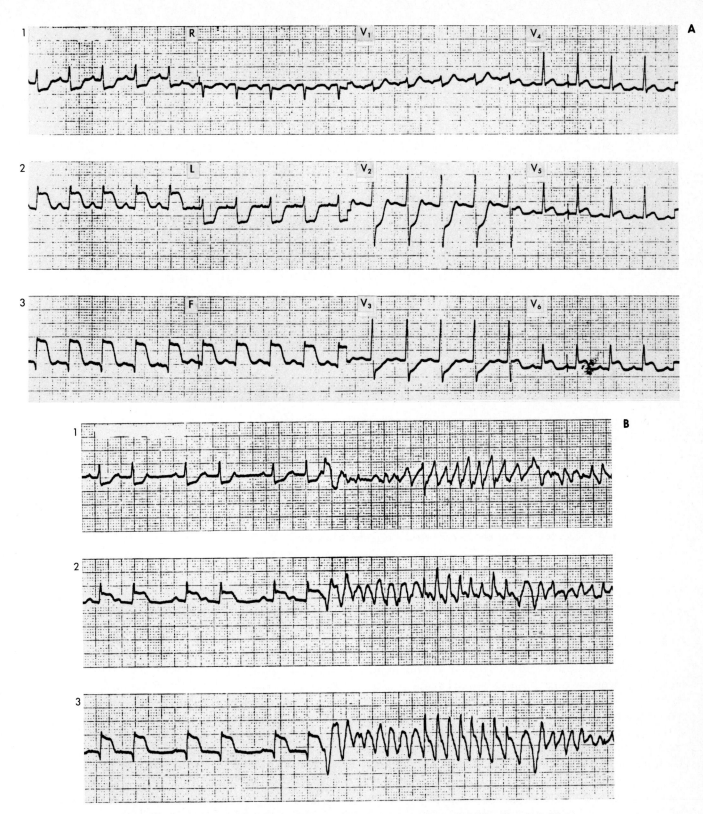

FIG. 9-2. Ventricular fibrillation in the presence of an acute myocardial infarction. A, A 12-lead ECG demonstrating a current of injury pattern (that is, ST elevations) in leads II, III aV_F, and V_4 to V_6. This patient later developed Q waves in these leads. In both A and B the three leads arranged vertically were recorded simultaneously (e.g., I, II, and III). B, A rhythm strip taken simultaneously for leads I, II, and III. Wenckebach AV block occurs on the left, and rapid ventricular tachycardia that degenerates into ventricular fibrillation is seen on the right.

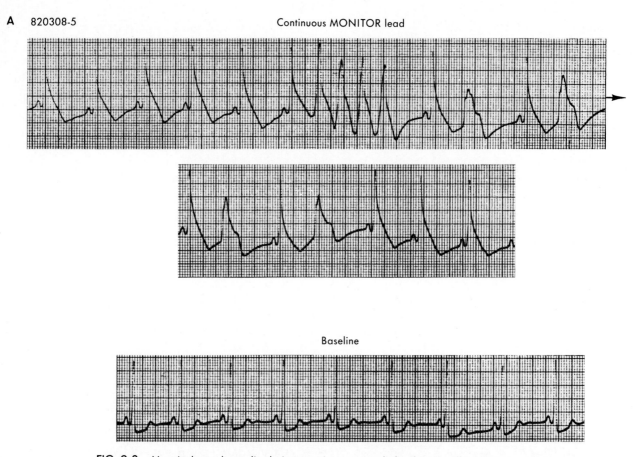

A 820308-5   Continuous MONITOR lead

Baseline

FIG. 9-3. Ventricular tachycardia during transient myocardial ischemia. All tracings are taken from the same patient. In the top of A the monitor lead recording shows ST elevations associated with a short run of nonsustained ventricular tachycardia. The lower tracing demonstrates the baseline QRS complex. In B the nonsustained run of ventricular tachycardia occurred *after* the elevated ST segment returned to baseline.

that the "arrhythmogenic" area of the ventricle does not become infarcted and remains capable of initiating or sustaining ventricular arrhythmias, although the actual cause of ventricular fibrillation in those patients is quite complex and probably multifactorial.[23]

Although an acute myocardial infarction does not occur in most patients who have out-of-hospital ventricular fibrillation, acute myocardial ischemia may still be an important factor in the genesis of ventricular arrhythmias. Recently during continuous ECG monitoring of a patient with a history of angina pectoris, the patient experienced chest pain associated with ST segment elevation and nonsustained ventricular tachycardia with an episode of ischemia (Fig. 9-3). Subsequent coronary angiography demonstrated that diffuse vasospasm was the cause for the angina. Since few patients have had ECG recordings during out-of-hospital ventricular fibrillation, the frequency of ventricular arrhythmias induced by ischemia versus other causes has not yet been defined. It will be interesting

to note whether the widespread use of percutaneous transluminal coronary angioplasty will decrease the incidence of sudden death.

Although sudden cardiac death occurs most often in patients who have coronary artery disease, it also occurs in patients with a variety of other cardiac conditions.[1,24-31] In a report on sudden death in 29 young athletes, 14 had hypertrophic cardiomyopathy and five had concentric hypertrophy; only three had obstructive coronary artery disease; three others had an anomalous origin of the left anterior descending coronary artery.[25] In one study[1] of 62 survivors of cardiac arrest not related to an acute myocardial infarction, drug toxicity or electrolyte imbalance, coronary artery disease occurred in 35 (55%) patients (Table 9-1). Of these, four patients had primary electrical disease, which is the presence of cardiac arrhythmias but with no other cardiac abnormalities found during physical examination, echocardiography, or cardiac catheterization.

Patients who have an increased risk of sudden death are

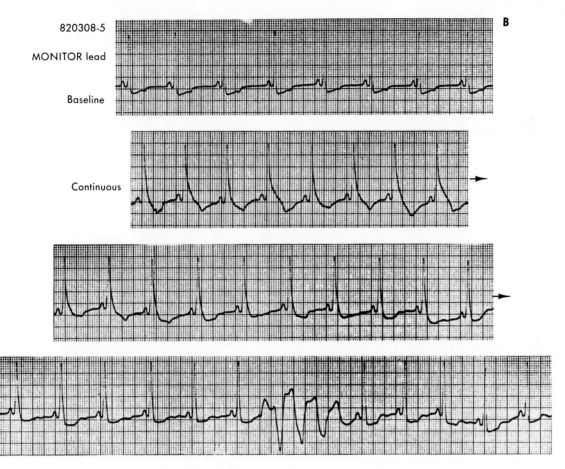

FIG. 9-3, cont'd.   For legend see opposite page.

those with prolonged QT entity.[26] The upper limit for QT duration corrected for heart rate (QTc) is usually given as 0.44 seconds. Although a QTc interval ≥0.44 seconds can occur in patients without arrhythmias, there is a congenital disorder called prolonged QT syndrome that occurs in patients with[27] or without deafness[28,29]; this disorder is associated with a predisposition to develop ventricular tachycardia or ventricular fibrillation. It has been suggested that ventricular arrhythmias may result from abnormalities in ventricular repolarization.[32] A study by Crampton[33] proposes that prolonged QT intervals in some of these patients result from excess activity of the left stellate ganglion, subnormal activity of the right stellate ganglion that creates "unopposed" left stellate ganglion activity, or both. Inflammation of epicardial ganglia has been reported in several patients who had QT prolongation syndrome and sudden death.[34]

Sudden cardiac death in patients with an acquired prolonged QT interval may be caused by hypokalemia and quinidine-like antiarrhythmic drugs. A connection between prolonged QT interval and sudden death has been dramatically demonstrated in patients receiving a liquid protein diet.[30,31] Singh and others[30] described three young women who had lost 36 to 41 kg of body weight in 3 to 5 months. All had prolonged QT intervals and syncope caused by ventricular tachycardia; only one patient survived. Isner and co-workers[31] reported clinical and pathologic data in 17 patients who died suddenly while taking this diet. Twelve patients had ECGs recorded during dieting, and in nine patients the corrected QT interval was prolonged. Four of these nine patients had an ECG done before dieting, and the corrected QT interval was normal in three. Ventricular tachycardia was documented in all 11 patients who died in hospital. Pathologic examination of 16 patients demonstrated no significant coronary artery disease; nor were myocardial abnormalities found by visual inspection. Some patients showed thinned left ventricular myocardial fibers consistent with starvation, but only one

TABLE 9-1. Heart disease in a cardiac arrest patient population (N = 62)

Disease Type	N
Coronary artery disease	35
Dilated cardiomyopathy	14
Asymmetric hypertrophic cardiomyopathy	3
Mitral valve regurgitation without prolapse	2
Mitral valve prolapse	2
Prolonged QT syndrome	2
Primary electrical disease	4

TABLE 9-2. Lown grading system for ventricular arrhythmias[51]

Lown Grade	Definition
0	No PVC
1	Occasional isolated PVC
2	>1 PVC per min or 30 PVCs per hour
3	Multiform PVC
4A	2 consecutive PVCs
4B	≥3 consecutive PVCs
5	R on T

patient had any histologic evidence of myocarditis. The cause for QT interval prolongation in these patients is unknown, but its frequent association with ventricular tachycardia suggests that if ventricular tachycardia occurs in patients taking the liquid protein diet, it may be caused by abnormalities of ventricular repolarization. Whether the QT prolongation in this group of patients, in the group receiving various drugs, or in the congenital group was caused by the same or different electrophysiologic factors is not known.

RISK FACTORS FOR SUDDEN DEATH
Premature Ventricular Complexes

Premature ventricular complexes (PVCs) are ubiquitous. In patients who have no structural heart disease, PVCs occur commonly and do not seem to predict subsequent sudden death. In a group of apparently healthy medical students, 50% had isolated PVCs, 12% had multiform PVCs, 6% had R-on-T phenomenon, and one patient had nonsustained ventricular tachycardia.[35] In another study,[36] 25 patients who had no evidence of coronary artery disease demonstrated frequent PVCs during continuous ECG recording. The mean PVC frequency was 559 per hour, and approximately 60% of the patients had couplets, although no ventricular tachycardia occurred. In fact, ventricular tachycardia occurred only after quinidine therapy in one patient who had no previous history of ventricular tachycardia. Hinkle and others[37] showed that PVCs existed in patients whether or not they had heart disease, but they were associated with an apparent increased risk of sudden death only in heart disease patients. Finally, Kostis and others[38] studied 101 patients who had normal hearts as determined by both noninvasive and invasive testing. During a 24-hour ambulatory ECG recording, 39 patients demonstrated at least one PVC. Thirty patients had their heart rhythms recorded for 72 hours, and only five (17%) of those thirty had no PVCs noted at the end of the record-

ing period. Since this sample excluded patients who were referred for PVCs or palpitations, it is likely that the study underestimated the incidence of PVCs in patients who have no structural heart disease.

Many investigators have studied the association between PVCs and the risk of subsequent sudden death in patients who have coronary artery disease.[39-50] Unfortunately, large differences in experimental design preclude accurate comparisons between studies. For example, although there appears to be a relatively high frequency of sudden death within the first 2 months after myocardial infarction,[45] in the study conducted by Ruberman and others,[44] 50% of the patients were entered into the study at least 3 months after suffering myocardial infarction. Drug administration, which conceivably could alter the incidence of sudden death, was not controlled for in the majority of the studies.

Earlier studies[39-41] did not differentiate types of PVCs, but most of the later studies[42-50] used the Lown modified grading system[51] to classify PVCs as complex or simple (Table 9-2). Minor differences in PVC classification occurred, but most often simple PVCs were defined as uniform PVCs that occurred infrequently, and complex PVCs generally included those that occurred frequently and were multiform, bigeminal, paired, and early-cycle (that is, R-on-T phenomenon). Recent data have shown that the detection of high PVC rates or complex PVCs varies logarithmically with the duration of the ECG recording,[52] and that although 95% of high PVC rates were detected during 12 hours of recording, recording for 18 hours was necessary to detect at least 95% of couplets or ventricular tachycardia. In another study the maximal PVC grade (Lown classification) in patients who had coronary artery disease was recorded in 74% of patients during 24 hours of ECG recording but required 36 hours of recording to document maximal PVC grade in 95% of patients.[53]

Despite the necessity for prolonged ECG recording

times to detect complex PVCs, most of the studies employed short recording periods. For example, duration of ECG recording used to detect arrhythmias included a single 12-lead ECG[34-41] and continuous ECG recording for 1 hour,[43,49,50] 6 hours,[45,46] and 8 to 12 hours.[47,48] Only two studies used recording times of 24 hours.[42,43] Thus in some studies with short ECG recording times, the increased frequency of sudden death in patients who had complex versus simple PVCs may be more apparent than real, since the patients who had simple PVCs might have demonstrated complex PVCs if longer ECG recording times had been used.

Most of the studies state the highest Lown PVC grade detection in a patient and do not examine whether more than one type of PVC grade exists. Bigger and Weld[54] have shown that this hierarchical type of PVC grading system has shortcomings regarding stratification of patients at risk for death after myocardial infarction. They studied 400 patients who were treated for acute myocardial infarction. All patients had a 24-hour ECG recording between 10 and 20 days after hospital admission, and the average follow-up was 30 months. Seventy-eight patients died during follow-up (the authors do not distinguish between patients who suffered sudden deaths from those who suffered nonsudden deaths). The authors found that the occurrence of paired PVCs and ventricular tachycardia led to a greater risk for subsequent cardiac death than R-on-T PVCs. Furthermore, the frequency of PVCs was a significant additional risk factor for cardiac death in patients who had repetitive PVCs or R-on-T PVCs. More research is required to corroborate these findings.

A more important issue is whether there is any value in subdividing PVCs into simple and complex forms. The premise for this subdivision appears to have originated during the early years of coronary care units when higher grades of PVCs were thought to represent "warning arrhythmias," that is, rhythms that presaged the occurrence of ventricular tachycardia and/or ventricular fibrillation.[51] However, in a later study of 262 patients who had an acute myocardial infarction, Lie and others[15] showed that many patients have ventricular fibrillation without warning arrhythmias, and many patients who have warning arrhythmias do not have ventricular tachyarrhythmias. Thus there seems to be no reason to grade PVC severity in patients who have acute myocardial infarction.

In patients who have angina but no history of myocardial infarction, PVCs are associated with an increased risk of sudden death, but there is no difference in risk between simple and complex PVCs.[49] After myocardial infarction, patients who have complex PVCs appear to have a greater risk of subsequent sudden death than patients who have simple PVCs or no PVCs.[42-45,47,48] The presence of complex PVCs is also associated with an increased risk of nonsudden

cardiac death,[44] and the prevalence of complex PVCs varies directly with the severity of coronary artery disease and left ventricular dysfunction.[43,55-57] In one study patients who had an elevated left ventricular end-diastolic pressure and multiple zones of asynergy demonstrated by cardiac catheterization had the largest yield of high-grade complex PVCs.[55] Thus patients who have advanced atherosclerotic heart disease tend to have a higher frequency of complex PVCs; whether the PVCs are merely associated with sudden death or actually cause it is unclear. If a causal relationship can be established, hope for decreasing sudden death by prophylactically treating patients who have PVCs becomes more realistic.

Lown assigned the highest PVC grade to those PVCs that interrupt the T wave of the previous QRS complex, that is, R-on-T phenomenon.[51] Repolarization of the ventricles accounts for the T wave on the surface ECG, and experimental work has shown that stimulation of the heart during early repolarization appears to be arrhythmogenic.[58,59] For example, in 1921 de Boef[58] demonstrated in the frog heart that a stimulus applied near the end of ventricular refractoriness could cause ventricular fibrillation. This observation was confirmed by Wiggers and Wegria[59] in a 1940 study conducted on dogs. These authors demonstrated that electrical stimuli of equal strength produced ventricular fibrillation when applied during the time of the T wave but induced only premature ventricular complexes when the stimuli occurred late in diastole. In 1960 Smirk and Palmer[60] reported a high occurrence of sudden death in patients who had R-on-T PVCs recorded on a 12-lead ECG. However, approximately 90% of these patients had significant heart disease and 25% had congestive heart failure.

Although there is no question that R-on-T PVCs can initiate ventricular fibrillation,[61] most recorded episodes of ventricular tachyarrhythmias result from midcycle rather than R-on-T PVCs.[15,62-66] In 52 patients who had acute myocardial infarction, 27 had a total of 131 episodes of paroxysmal ventricular tachycardia; early PVCs initiated only 12% of these episodes.[63] Furthermore, in 25 patients who did not have ventricular tachycardia, 13% of the PVCs were of the R-on-T variety. Winkle and co-workers[64] recorded 94 episodes of ventricular tachycardia during ambulatory ECG recording in 23 patients, and only 14 episodes of ventricular tachycardia were induced by an early PVC. In another study 339 patients had 24-hour ECG recordings, and only 5.6% of the PVCs recorded were early PVCs.[65] Forty-five episodes of ventricular tachycardia occurred, but only 16% of the patients who had early PVCs had ventricular tachycardia.[65] Finally, in a study by Follansbee and co-workers[66] only 7 of 37 patients had ventricular tachycardia initiated by early PVCs. From all these data it seems that R-on-T PVCs occur infrequently, and that in most patients do not induce ventricular tachycardia or fibrillation, and that most episodes of ventricular tachycardia or fibrillation are not initiated by early PVCs.

To summarize, simple and complex PVCs commonly occur in patients who have coronary artery disease. The prevalence of complex PVCs increases directly with the number of diseased coronary arteries and with the severity of left ventricular dysfunction.[43,55,57] Although complex PVCs increase the risk of subsequent sudden death, most patients who have complex PVCs do not die suddenly.

Ventricular Tachycardia

Ventricular tachycardia probably should be placed in a class by itself, although Lown[51] has considered it part of a general classification of PVCs. A small subset of patients who have ventricular tachycardia and no apparent structural heart disease are not at increased risk for subsequent sudden death.[67] However, our experience with over 600 patients who were treated for control of ventricular tachycardia or ventricular fibrillation as well as in recent studies,[11,12,15,16] it was found that ventricular fibrillation is often preceded by ventricular tachycardia (Figs. 9-1 and 9-2), but it is not known how frequently ventricular tachycardia degenerates into ventricular fibrillation.

Sudden death occurs in patients who have nonsustained ventricular tachycardia that can be associated with few or no symptoms.[68,69] In some cases nonsustained ventricular tachycardia may progress to sustained ventricular tachy-

cardia (Fig. 9-4), and this may lead to the development of ventricular fibrillation. The occurrence of a sustained ventricular tachycardia may depend on multiple factors such as myocardial ischemia, increased left ventricular dimension, electrolyte disorders, or autonomic perturbations. The rate of nonsustained and sustained ventricular tachycardia may be quite different in the same patient, and a relatively slow ($\leq$150/min) nonsustained ventricular tachycardia often occurs in patients with rapid ($\geq$200/min) sustained ventricular tachycardias.[70] Thus the decision to treat patients with nonsustained ventricular tachycardia should not be based on a rate criterion only.

In a retrospective study Lie and others[16] identified patients at high risk for the development of late in-hospital ventricular fibrillation after myocardial infarction. The authors demonstrated that the high-risk patients were those who had an anteroseptal myocardial infarction complicated by right or left bundle branch block. In a prospective study this same group[16] continuously monitored 47 high-risk post-myocardial infarction patients in the hospital for 6 weeks. Of these, 17 (36%) developed ventricular fibrillation, and in 14 of these, ventricular tachycardia preceded ventricular fibrillation. In our experience, ventricular tachycardia often precedes by seconds or even minutes almost all episodes of ventricular fibrillation induced in the electrophysiology laboratory (Fig. 9-5). Thus patients who have ventricular tachycardia appear to have a significant risk of sudden death, although the prevalence and natural

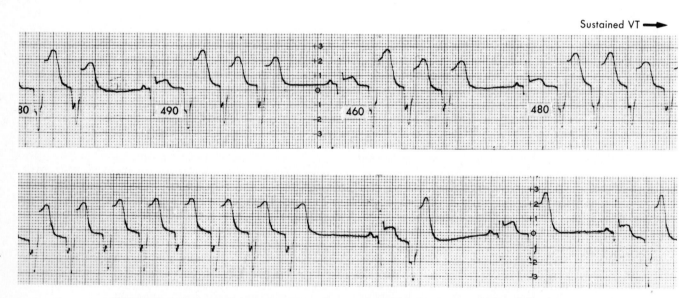

Sustained VT ➡

FIG. 9-4. Nonsustained ventricular tachycardia preceding the onset of sustained ventricular tachycardia. Tracings A and B were recorded during ambulatory monitoring and are not continuous. In A there are two episodes of nonsustained ventricular tachycardia followed by sustained tachycardia. The coupling interval between the sinus complex and the first complex of ventricular tachycardia is variable, and the shortest coupling interval, 460 msec, does not induce sustained tachycardia. B demonstrates the termination of the sustained ventricular tachycardia.

history of asymptomatic ventricular tachycardia in the general population remain unknown.

Left Ventricular Dysfunction and Other Risk Factors. Patients who have coronary artery disease and left ventricular dysfunction demonstrate an increased risk of sudden cardiac death.* In 425 survivors of out-of-hospital ventricular fibrillation, 340 had no acute transmural myocardial infarction, and 169 of these had no evidence of remote myocardial infarction.[9] In these 169 patients the 1-year risk for subsequent sudden death was 30% (7 out

*References 6, 9, 20, 43, 44, 46, 56, 57, 71, 72.

of 23) for patients who had congestive heart failure and 11% (16 out of 46) for those who did not have heart failure.[9] Patients who have an acute myocardial infarction are at increased risk of developing subsequent sudden death if they have congestive heart failure while still in the coronary care unit[20,72] or have a low cardiac ejection fraction (determined by radionuclide angiography) prior to hospital discharge.[43] As noted in the previous section, complex PVCs commonly occur in patients who have myocardial dysfunction, and the two abnormalities compound the risk for sudden death.[44,73] This risk is greatest in patients who have congestive heart failure and complex PVCs but is

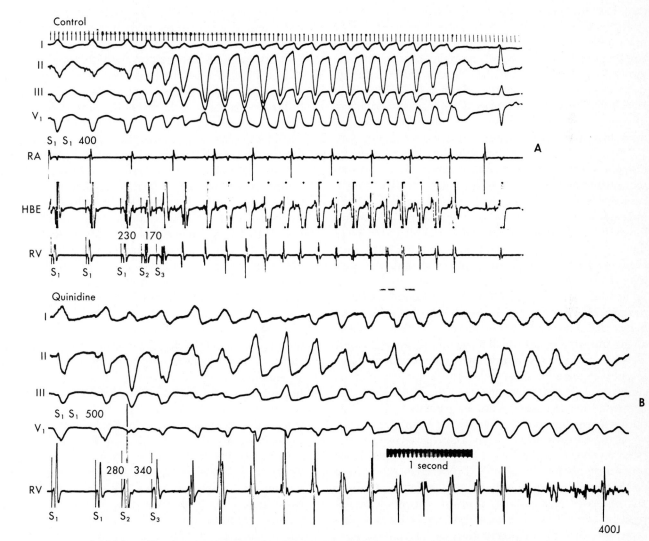

FIG. 9-5. Induction of nonsustained and sustained ventricular tachycardia during programmed ventricular stimulation. For both panels the top four tracings are ECG leads I, II, III, and V₁. Intracardiac electrograms were recorded from the right atrium *(RA)*, right ventricle *(RV)*, and His bundle area *(HBE)*. During control study, nonsustained ventricular tachycardia *(VT)* was induced by two premature stimuli introduced during ventricular pacing (panel A). A repeat electrophysiology study (panel B) was performed while the patient was receiving oral quinidine. Ventricular tachycardia was initiated, and within 5 seconds the VT degenerated into ventricular fibrillation.

lower for patients who have only congestive heart failure or complex PVCs.[44]

Many varied and seemingly unrelated factors appear to increase the risk of sudden death. Weinblatt and others[74] reported that in men who had similar traditional risk factors and similar arrhythmias there was a relationship between a low educational level and subsequent sudden death in the posthospitalization period following myocardial infarction. The authors noted that patients with less than 8 years of schooling had a threefold increase in risk of sudden death as compared with better-educated men. It is unclear why patients who had less formal education were at increased risk for sudden death, but the availability of medical care does not appear to be a major factor.[74]

Bigger and others[20] analyzed multiple variables in postmyocardial infarction patients. At 6- and 12-month intervals there was a 15% and 19% mortality respectively, and most of the deaths were sudden. Serum BUN ($\geq$20 mg/dl), creatinine ($\geq$1.4 mg/dl), and uric acid ($\geq$7.0 mg/dl) levels were higher risk factors for death than the occurrence of congestive heart failure in the coronary care unit, and more than one variable increased the risk for death.

There has been recent interest in the role of repolarization abnormalities recorded on the surface ECG and subsequent sudden death.[75-77] In 55 patients who had a myocardial infarction 2 months to 6 years in the past, the QT interval (heart rate corrected by Bazett's formula) was prolonged in 5 of the 27 patients who survived and in 16 of the 28 patients who died suddenly; this suggests that patients who survive myocardial infarction and have prolonged QT intervals may be at risk for subsequent development of sudden death.[75] Kentala and Repo[76] measured the corrected QT interval in patients 6 to 8 weeks after myocardial infarction and correlated these data with data about subsequent sudden death. The QT intervals were measured from ECGs recorded when the patient was resting in the supine position before and 5 minutes after exercise, and when the patient was in the upright position before starting exercise. Twenty-one patients died suddenly during follow-up, and in this group the mean QTc interval when the patients were upright before exercise was significantly longer than the resting supine QTc value. There was no significant change in QTc values in the upright versus the supine position for the nonsudden death group and survivors. Furthermore, when the patients were upright before exercise, the mean QTc interval was significantly longer in the sudden death group than in the nonsudden death group and survivors. Thus although the supine resting QT interval did not differentiate patients at risk for subsequent sudden death a prolonged ($\geq$440 msec), corrected QT interval recorded in the upright position occurred more frequently in patients who had subsequent sudden, as opposed to nonsudden, death. The

abnormally prolonged QT intervals recorded from patients in an upright position may reflect the inability of the patient's autonomic nervous system to respond normally to changes in cardiovascular tone. Since abnormalities of the autonomic nervous system may cause QT prolongation and may increase the risk for subsequent sudden death, future efforts to decrease the incidence of sudden death should include more detailed research on the autonomic nervous system and other factors that influence ventricular repolarization.[32] It is of particular interest that practolol,[78] alprenolol,[79] timolol,[80] and metoprolol[81] appear to decrease the risk of sudden death after myocardial infarction; these results may be explained in part by the effects of the drugs on the autonomic nervous system. A recent study[82] demonstrates a decrease in the mortality of patients receiving propranolol.

Treatment of Ventricular Arrhythmias. Ventricular tachyarrhythmias may be controlled by a variety of therapies that include drugs, pacemakers, cardioverter/defibrillators, and surgery. Probably the most difficult task in caring for patients who have ventricular arrhythmias is deciding *whether* to treat them rather than which treatment modality to use. Since the risk of sudden death is not the same for all ventricular arrhythmias, treatment to suppress ventricular arrhythmias should be guided by the relative risks of sudden death in a particular arrhythmia. The assumption, although often difficult to prove, is that abolition of the arrhythmia will prevent death; obviously, the decision to treat a patient must be made from the data obtained on the patient and sound clinical judgment. Of the ventricular arrhythmias, the lowest risk of sudden death occurs in patients who have PVCs but no structural heart disease, and the highest risk occurs in patients who have sustained ventricular tachycardia and severe congestive heart failure; as a rule, the former group should not receive antiarrhythmic therapy (assuming that the patient is asymptomatic), whereas the latter group requires therapy. In general, we do not recommend drug therapy for any patient with asymptomatic PVCs, but patients who have sustained ventricular tachycardia should be treated. If nonsustained ventricular tachycardia causes substantial symptoms in patients with or without structural heart disease, it may be desirable to suppress the arrhythmia; if the arrhythmia is asymptomatic and occurs in otherwise healthy individuals, treatment may not be necessary, but careful follow-up of these patients is suggested. It is still uncertain which patients with heart disease and asymptomatic nonsustained ventricular arrhythmias (VT) require therapy. These broad guidelines must be interpreted according to specific clinical situations.

Patients who do not appear to require therapy if they are asymptomatic and have no structural heart disease are those who have repetitive monomorphic ventricular tachy-

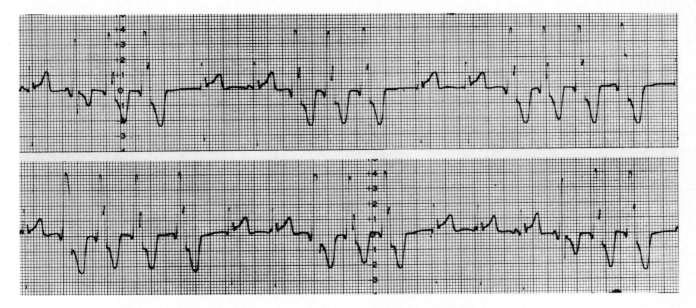

FIG. 9-6. Repetitive monomorphic ventricular tachycardia. The electrocardiographic tracings are not continuous. Note the recurrence of short episodes of nonsustained ventricular tachycardia with a uniform morphology and the normal intervening sinus complexes.

cardia (RMVT).[67] This is identified on the ECG by frequent, recurrent bursts of ventricular tachycardia exhibiting uniform contour and separated by sinus complexes that conduct with a normal QRS contour (Fig. 9-6). Of 18 patients who had RMVT documented for 1 month to 16 years (mean 5.3 years), seven who were asymptomatic were not treated and have remained asymptomatic during follow-up. Five of 6 untreated patients who had a 24-hour ambulatory ECG obtained a mean of 3.6 years after initial evaluation demonstrated no VT. Only 2 out of 9 patients had their arrhythmia induced during the electrophysiologic study, which suggests but does not prove that the mechanism responsible for the arrhythmia might be automaticity rather than reentry.

The largest group of patients who have ventricular arrhythmias are those who have heart disease and PVCs; it is this group of patients for whom treatment is the most controversial. For example, the risk of sudden death in these patients is greater than in patients who do not have heart disease but do have PVCs, and the risk of sudden death increases with decreasing myocardial function.[44] However, the overall risk of sudden death does not appear to be great, and there are no controlled studies to suggest that treating these patients with antiarrhythmic therapy decreases the incidence of sudden death. In fact, prospective studies of patients after myocardial infarction show that neither phenytoin,[83] procainamide,[84] nor aprindine[85] significantly decreases the incidence of sudden death as compared with control groups, although patients treated with aprindine and procainamide had fewer ventricular arrhythmias than the placebo-treated groups. The nonsignificant decrease in the incidence of sudden death in patients treated with procainamide may be related to the low dosage of procainamide (500 mg every 6 to 8 hours) prescribed.[84] In studies testing the effectiveness of therapy with beta-blocking drugs,[78-81] a significant decrease in sudden death occurred in patients treated with alprenolol, practolol, timolol, and metoprolol compared with control patients. The apparent benefits of beta blockers may be caused by their antisympathetic effects, membrane-active properties, their antiischemic effects, or a combination of multiple actions. A decrease in sudden death after myocardial infarction can also be achieved with high thoracic left sympathectomy.[86]

If antiarrhythmic drugs caused minimal side effects and had a high therapeutic-to-toxic ratio, their use to prevent sudden death, albeit unproven, would not be unreasonable. However, antiarrhythmic drugs commonly cause side effects[84] and in some patients can cause ventricular tachycardia and sudden death.[87-91] For example, in a 1980 study[88] 71 patients who had atrial fibrillation or flutter but no history of ventricular arrhythmias were given quinidine sulfate. Four patients developed ventricular fibrillation and two developed ventricular tachycardia, and there was no significant difference in the degree of QT prolongation or serum quinidine concentration between these patients and the patients who did not develop ventricular arrhythmias. Minardo and others[91] were also unable to detect a relationship between the amount of QT prolongation during drug therapy and the occurrence of drug-related ventricular

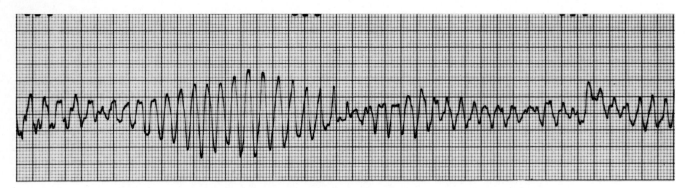

FIG. 9-7.   Torsades de pointes. This specific type of ventricular tachycardia usually occurs in the presence of a prolonged QT interval and is characterized by a QRS morphology that appears repeatedly to change its axis by 180 degrees.

fibrillation in patients treated primarily for nonsustained ventricular arrhythmias. In other patients administration of type I antiarrhythmic drugs (for example, quinidine, procainamide, or disopyramide) may cause marked prolongation of the QT interval and result in a specific form of ventricular tachycardia, know as *torsade de pointes*[89,90] (Fig. 9-7).

Because of the known adverse effects of antiarrhythmic drugs, and because a decrease in the incidence of sudden death in treated patients has not been demonstrated, antiarrhythmic drug therapy for all patients who have coronary artery disease and complex or simple PVCs appears unwarranted at this time. A prospective controlled study is needed to determine if antiarrhythmic drugs administered in doses that result in reasonable serum drug levels can prevent sudden death in patients who have coronary artery disease. According to Prineas,[92] as many as 2000 patients may be necessary for the study, thus requiring a multicenter cooperative effort.

Some physicians may think it unethical to initiate such a trial, since they believe that after myocardial infarction patients who have complex PVCs benefit from antiarrhythmic therapy. However, most believe that the efficacy of treating these patients has not been adequately tested. Knowledge of the total PVC count in such a trial would be of interest although one must remember that daily PVC counts vary considerably,[93] and, more importantly, the ability to suppress PVCs may not accurately predict the future occurrence of ventricular tachycardia or ventricular fibrillation.[85,94-97] Myerburg and others [94] studied survivors of out-of-hospital cardiac arrest.[94] Sixteen patients were treated with procainamide or quinidine and followed up after hospital discharge. All eight patients who died within 1 year of follow-up had unstable drug plasma levels that were often subtherapeutic, and only two of the survivors had unstable subtherapeutic plasma drug levels. It is noteworthy that no significant difference in PVC counts occurred between patients who survived and those who had

recurrent sudden death. In 1981, Myerburg and others[98] demonstrated in the same patients that suppression of spontaneous ventricular tachycardia requires significantly lower doses of procainamide than suppression of 85% of PVCs does. However, follow-up time was short, and these data should be considered preliminary at this time.

Electrophysiologic Testing. One method employed to assess the efficacy of drug therapy in the suppression of spontaneous ventricular tachycardia/fibrillation is to monitor for variable time periods the patient's heart rhythm during therapy under normal activity and during stress testing.[99] If ventricular arrhythmias are markedly suppressed during the monitoring period, the patient is discharged and further follow-up is done out-of-hospital. In many patients ventricular tachyarrhythmias are episodic, which precludes accurate assessment of drug efficacy by noninvasive monitoring techniques only; unfortunately, out-of-hospital sudden death is not an uncommon sequela in these patients.

Electrophysiologic testing with programmed electrical stimulation to induce ventricular tachycardia has been used to judge the ability of drugs to prevent ventricular arrhythmias.[1,100-109]

Thus patients who have ventricular tachycardia induced before but not after drug therapy usually have no recurrence of ventricular tachycardia if they continue to take the dosage of the antiarrhythmic drug that prevented induction of ventricular tachycardia at electrophysiologic study. We routinely use electrophysiologic testing as part of our treatment protocol (Fig. 9-8), and find that combined use of continuous ECG monitoring and electrophysiologic testing makes it possible to detect ventricular tachycardia in almost all patients referred for evaluation. For example, of 46 patients who had a history of ventricular tachycardia, in the drug-free control period 32 had ventricular tachycardia induced during electrophysiologic study and 33 had ventricular tachycardia detected during prolonged continuous ECG recording[105]; only two patients did not dem-

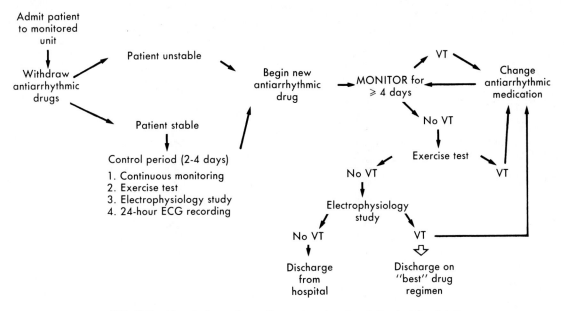

FIG. 9-8. Ventricular tachycardia treatment protocol. See text for details.

onstrate ventricular tachycardia during either ECG monitoring or electrophysiologic testing.

Fig. 9-8 outlines our current method of treating ventricular tachycardia. Patients are admitted to an intensive care unit, and all antiarrhythmic drugs are withheld. If the patient's condition is stable, he is monitored continuously for 48 to 96 hours, and during this time a 24-hour ECG recording, a baseline electrophysiologic study and, often, a treadmill exercise test are performed. To induce ventricular tachycardia during electrophysiologic testing the following protocol is used[108]:

1. Incremental (at progressively faster rates) left and/or right atrial pacing starting at rates just faster than the spontaneous sinus rate and progressing until AV block occurs.
2. Premature left and/or right atrial stimulation during sinus rhythm and atrial pacing.
3. Incremental right ventricular pacing to rates ≥240 msec until ventriculoatrial block occurs or until limited by patient symptoms.
4. Premature right ventricular stimulation during sinus rhythm and during right ventricular pacing (S_1), with induction of one (S_2), two (S_2, S_3), and, if needed, three (S_2, S_3, S_4) premature stimuli. Premature ventricular stimulation is performed at three pacing cycle lengths (usually 600, 500, and 400 msec, that is, 100, 120, and 150 per minute, respectively) and at two right ventricular sites (usually the apex and outflow tract) until ventricular tachycardia is reproducibly induced.
5. In selected patients, programmed electrical stimulation of the left ventricle is performed.

Fig. 9-9 shows the influence of the type of heart disease and clinical arrhythmia on induction of ventricular tachycardia during programmed ventricular stimulation using only right ventricular stimulation and two or fewer extra stimuli. Use of three extrastimuli and left ventricular pacing will increase the sensitivity of the test. The highest (92%) yield occurred in patients with coronary artery disease and sustained ventricular tachycardia, and the lowest (30%) induction was in those patients with primary electrical disease and cardiac arrest.

The majority of patients referred to us have ventricular tachycardia that was not controlled by conventional antiarrhythmic drugs. Often the patient is intolerant of the drugs; thus most patients are treated with an investigational drug. If the patient spontaneously develops ventricular tachycardia during drug therapy while being monitored continuously (Fig. 9-8), a new drug is tried. When a drug results in total suppression of ventricular tachycardia during continuous ECG monitoring, treadmill stress testing, and a 24-hour ECG recording, a repeat electrophysiologic study is performed. If programmed electrical stimulation does not induce ventricular tachycardia, the patient is discharged and followed up closely in an outpatient arrhythmia clinic. Many patients who have no ventricular tachycardia observed during noninvasive testing still have ventricular tachycardia induced during electrophysiologic testing[105] (Fig. 9-10). When tachycardia is induced, the antiarrhythmic drug is changed and this process is continued until either no ventricular tachycardia is induced during electrophysiologic testing or a drug or drug combination that can markedly alter the ventricular tachycardia is found, for example if no spontaneous ventricular tachy-

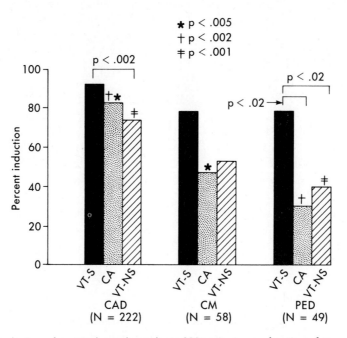

FIG. 9-9. Induction of ventricular tachycardia in 329 patients as a function of type of arrhythmia and heart disease. *CA,* Cardiac arrest; *CAD,* coronary artery disease; *CM,* cardiomyopathy; *PED,* primary electrical disease; *VT-NS,* nonsustained ventricular tachycardia; *VT-S,* sustained ventricular tachycardia. (With permission of the American Heart Association.)

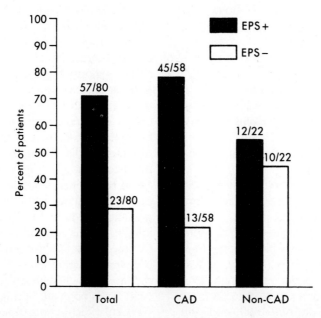

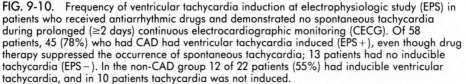

FIG. 9-10. Frequency of ventricular tachycardia induction at electrophysiologic study (EPS) in patients who received antiarrhythmic drugs and demonstrated no spontaneous tachycardia during prolonged (≥2 days) continuous electrocardiographic monitoring (CECG). Of 58 patients, 45 (78%) who had CAD had ventricular tachycardia induced (EPS+), even though drug therapy suppressed the occurrence of spontaneous tachycardia; 13 patients had no inducible tachycardia (EPS−). In the non-CAD group 12 of 22 patients (55%) had inducible ventricular tachycardia, and in 10 patients tachycardia was not induced.

cardia is noted during noninvasive testing and if the induction of a ventricular tachycardia is markedly slower than the tachycardia induced prior to drug therapy. When discharged, the patient receives the drug(s) that prevented or altered ventricular tachycardia and then is followed up closely in the outpatient arrhythmia clinic.

Many patients sent to tertiary referral centers undergo multiple drug trials over a period of 3 to 4 weeks and a drug regimen that prevents ventricular tachycardia initiation during programmed ventricular stimulation cannot be identified. Some of these patients are candidates for nonpharmacologic therapy such as surgery or implantable electrical devices. Several investigators[110-112] have tried to determine which patients might benefit most from serial electrophysiologic-pharmacologic testing. Clinical and electrophysiologic data were analyzed in 197 patients[112] to determine whether baseline variables identified patients most likely to experience VT suppression at drug study. Patients with primary electrical disease or cardiomyopathy—regardless of the clinical arrhythmia group studied (that is, sustained VT, nonsustained VT or cardiac arrest)—and younger patients with faster VT rates induced at predrug electrophysiologic study were most likely to have drug suppression of VT during serial drug testing. If certain patient groups have a very low frequency of success during serial drug studies, then individuals within these groups who are good candidates for nonpharmacologic therapy might undergo only two or three drug trials before the physician considers other forms of treatment; patients in high-success groups would undergo several pharmacologic trials before alternative therapeutic approaches are tried.

Electrophysiologic testing offers the additional advantage of enabling the physician to determine the patient's hemodynamic response to the ventricular arrhythmia that might recur, since the arrhythmia induced in the electrophysiology laboratory is usually what develops during follow-up if that patient has recurrent tachyarrhythmias. For example, in 11 patients in whom drug therapy suppressed ventricular tachycardia as judged by noninvasive tests, sustained ventricular tachycardia often causing severe hypotension was induced during repeat electrophysiologic testing.[113] If the patients had been discharged receiving the drugs associated with induction of sustained ventricular tachycardia, it is possible that in some patients a recurrent episode of ventricular tachycardia might have resulted in sudden death.

The sudden appearance of a cardiac arrhythmia, especially one that is life-threatening, is often devastating to patients and frequently produces feeling of anger, anxiety, and depression. The thought of undergoing an invasive procedure can only magnify these emotions. Darling and Faust[114] evaluated a group of patients before and after electrophysiologic testing and found that although anxiety decreased after testing, there was no significant change in the level of anger. The intensity of both anger and anxiety was higher in patients aged 18 to 31 years than in those 60 to 72 years old. Younger patients frequently also suffered more depression than older ones.

It is very important for nurses and physicians to realize the emotional upheaval that occurs in patients with arrhythmias and make attempts to help them cope with their feelings. Although patients may use a variety of coping mechanisms on their own,[114] attempts should be made to make their environment calm, in or out of the electrophysiology laboratory. It is useful to bring patients to the laboratory on the day prior to the study to familiarize them with the surroundings. Patients often cannot remember what was explained to them in the laboratory at the end of the procedure, possibly because of their heightened emotional state, and therefore it is helpful to go over the study results with them routinely shortly after they have been retuned to their room. Other helpful measures like these should be undertaken to provide a better psychologic climate for the patient.

Many questions remain unanswered. For example, in patients who have frequent episodes of ventricular tachycardia prior to drug therapy but who have no ventricular tachycardia during drug therapy, it is not known whether the drugs should be discontinued because ventricular tachycardia is induced during electrophysiologic testing. It is also not clearly established which patients with ventricular tachycardia should have electrophysiologic testing. Patients usually undergo electrophysiologic testing if (1) they have a history of syncope and/or out-of-hospital ventricular fibrillation, (2) ventricular tachycardia results in substantial hemodynamic compromise, (3) ventricular tachycardia has not been controlled by multiple antiarrhythmic drug trials, and (4) the patient's arrhythmia does not occur often enough to evaluate drug efficacy, which is frequently the case.

In summary, electrophysiologic testing in selected patients who have ventricular tachycardia/fibrillation is an important adjunct to testing drug efficacy. Ideally, the patient should be discharged while receiving the antiarrhythmic drug (or drugs) that totally suppresses ventricular tachycardia/fibrillation during electrophysiologic testing. Practically, however, the total suppression of ventricular tachycardia during electrophysiologic testing is not accomplished in many cases, and nonsustained or sustained ventricular tachycardia can still be induced. If patients continue to have hemodynamically unstable ventricular arrhythmias with all drug combinations, they should be considered for alternative therapy such as surgery or the implantation of pacemakers or other electrical devices.[115-121]

REFERENCES

1. Skale, B.T., and others: Survivors of cardiac arrest: prevention of recurrence by drug therapy as predicted by electrophysiologic testing versus ECG monitoring, Am. J. Cardiol. 57:113, 1986.
2. Lown, B.: Sudden cardiac death: the major challenge confronting contemporary cardiology, Am. J. Cardiol. 43:313, 1979.
3. Kuller, L., Lilienfeld, A., and Fisher, R.: Epidemiological study of sudden and unexpected deaths due to arteriosclerotic heart disease, Circulation 34:1056, 1966.
4. Liberthson, R.R., and others: Pathophysiologic observations in prehospital ventricular fibrillation and sudden cardiac death, Circulation 49:790, 1974.
5. Reichenbach, D.D., Moss, N.S., and Meyer, E.: Pathology of the heart in sudden cardiac death, Am. J. Cardiol. 39:865, 1977.
6. Weaver, W.D., and others: Angiographic findings and prognostic indicators in patients resuscitated from sudden cardiac death, Circulation 54:895, 1976.
7. Cobb, L.A., Werner, J.A., and Trobaugh, G.B.: Sudden cardiac death. I. A decade's experience with out-of-hospital resuscitation, Mod. Concepts Cardiovasc. Dis. 49:31,1980.
8. Liberthson, R.R, and others: Prehospital ventricular defibrillation: prognosis and follow-up course, N. Engl. J. Med. 291:317, 1974.
9. Cobb, L.A., Werner, J.A., and Trobaugh, G.B.: Sudden cardiac death. II. Outcome of resuscitation; management, and future directions, Mod. Concepts Cardiovasc. Dis. 49:37, 1980.
10. Myerburg, R.J., and others: Clinical, electrophysiologic, and hemodynamic profile of patients resuscitated from prehospital cardiac arrest, Am J. Med. 68:568, 1980.
11. Pratt, C.M, and others: Analysis of ambulatory electrocardiograms in 15 patients during spontaneous ventricular fibrillation with special reference to preceding arrhythmia events, J. Am. Coll. Cardiol. 2:789, 1983.
12. Lahiri, A., Balasubramanian, V., and Raftery, E.B.: Sudden death during ambulatory monitoring, Br. Med. J. 1:1676, 1979.
13. Gradman, A.H., Bell, P.A., and DeBusk, R.F.: Sudden death during ambulatory monitoring: clinical and electrocardiographic correlations: report of a case, Circulation 55:210, 1977.
14. Denes, P., and others: Sudden death in patients with chronic bifascicular block, Arch. Intern. Med. 137:1005, 1977.
15. Lie, K.I., and others: Observations on patients with primary ventricular fibrillation complicating acute myocardial infarction, Circulation 52:755, 1975.
16. Lie, K.I., and others: Early identification of patients developing late in-hospital ventricular fibrillation after discharge from the coronary care unit: a 5½ year retrospective and prospective study of 1,897 patients, Am. J. Cardiol. 41:674, 1978.
17. Spain, D.M., and Bradess, V.A.: The relationship of coronary thrombosis to coronary atherosclerosis and ischemic heart disease (a necropsy study covering a period of 25 years), Am. J. Med. Sci. 240:701, 1960.
18. Myers, A., and Dewar, H.A.: Circumstances attending 100 sudden deaths from coronary artery disease with coroner's necropsies, Br. Heart J. 37:1133, 1975.
19. Braum, R.S., Alvarez, H., III, and Cobb, L.A.: Survival after resuscitation from out-of-hospital ventricular fibrillation, Circulation 50:1231, 1974.
20. Bigger, J.T., and others: Risk stratification after acute myocardial infarction, Am. J. Cardiol. 42:202, 1978.
21. Elharrar, V., and Zipes, D.P.: Cardiac electrophysiologic alterations during myocardial ischemia, Am. J. Physiol 233:H329, 1977.
22. Opie, L.H., Nathan, D., and Lubbe, W.F.: Biochemical aspects of arrhythmogeneisis and ventricular fibrillation, Am. J. Cardiol. 43:131, 1979.
23. Warren, J.V.: Di si dolce morte: it may be safer to be dead than alive, Circulation, 50:415, 1974.
24. Pedersen, D.H., and others: Ventricular tachycardia and ventricular fibrillation in a young population, Circulation, 60:988, 1979.
25. Maron, B.J., and others: Sudden death in young athletes, Circulation 62:218, 1980.
26. Moss, A.J., and Schwartz, P.J.: Sudden death and the idiopathic long QT syndrome, Am. J. Med. 66:6, 1979.
27. Jervell, A., and Lange-Nielsen, F.: Congenital deaf-mutism, functional heart disease with prolongation of the QT interval, and sudden death, Am. Heart J. 54:59, 1957.
28. Romano, C., Gemme, G., and Pongiglione, R.: Aritimie cardiache rare dell'eta pediatrica, Clin. Pediatr. (Bologna) 45:656, 1963.
29. Ward, O.: A new familial cardiac syndrome in children, J. Irish Med. Assoc. 54:103, 1964.
30. Singh, B.N., and others: Liquid protein diets and torsade de pointes, JAMA 240:115, 1978.
31. Isner, J.M., and others: Sudden, unexpected death in avid dieters using the liquid-protein modified-fast diet: observations in 17 patients and the role of the prolonged QT interval, Circulation 60:1401, 1979.
32. Zipes, D.P., and others: Roles of autonomic innervation in the genesis of ventricular arrhythmias. In Abboud, F.M, and others, editors: Disturbances in neurogenic control of the circulation, Baltimore, 1981, Williams & Wilkins Co.
33. Crampton, R.: Preeminence of the left stellate ganglion in the long QT syndrome, Circulation 59:769, 1979.
34. James, T.N., and others: Cardiac ganglionitis associated with sudden unexpected death, Ann. Intern. Med. 91:727, 1979.
35. Brodsky, M., and others: Arrhythmias documented by 24-hour continuous electrocardiographic monitoring in 50 male medical students without apparent heart disease, Am. J. Cardiol. 39:390, 1977.
36. Kennedy, H.L., and Underhill, S.J.: Frequent or complex ventricular ectopy in apparently healthy subjects: a clinical study of 25 cases, Am. J. Cardiol. 38:141, 1976.
37. Hinkle, L.E., Jr., Carver, S.T., and Stevens, M.: The frequency of asymptomatic disturbances of cardiac rhythm and conduction in middle-aged men, Am. J. Cardiol. 24:629, 1969.
38. Kostis, J.B., and others: Premature ventricular complexes in the absence of identifiable heart disease, Circulation 63:1351, 1981.
39. Chiang, B.N., and others: Relationship of premature systoles to coronary heart disease and sudden death in the Tecumseh epidemiologic study, Ann. Intern. Med. 70:1159, 1969.
40. The Coronary Drug Project Research Group: Prognostic importance of premature beats following myocardial infarction: experience in the Coronary Drug Project, JAMA 223:116, 1973.
41. Fisher, F.D., and Tyroler, H.A.: Relationship between ventricular premature contractions on routine electrocardiography and subsequent sudden death from coronary heart disease, Circulation 47:712, 1973.
42. Vismara, L.A., Amsterdam, E.A., and Mason, D.T.: Relation of ventricular arrhythmias in the late hospital phase of acute myocardial infarction to sudden death after hospital discharge, Am. J. Med. 59:6, 1975.
43. Schulze, R.A., Strauss, H.W., and Pitt, B.: Sudden death in the year following myocardial infarction: relation to ventricular premature contractions in the late hospital phase and left ventricular ejection fraction, Am. J. Med. 62:192, 1977.
44. Ruberman, W., and others: Ventricular premature beats and mortality after myocardial infarction, N. Engl. J. Med. 297:750, 1977.
45. Moss, A.J., and others: Ventricular ectopic beats and their relation to sudden and nonsudden cardiac death after myocardial infarction, Circulation 60:998, 1979.

46. Moss, A.J., and others: The early posthospital phase of myocardial infarction: prognostic stratification, Circulation 54:58, 1976.

47. Kotler, M.N., and others: Prognostic significance of ventricular ectopic beats with respect to sudden death in the late postinfarction period, Circulation 47:959, 1973.

48. Vismara, L.A., and others: Identification of sudden death risk factors in acute and chronic coronary artery disease, Am. J. Cardiol. 39:821, 1977.

49. Ruberman, W., and others: Ventricular premature complexes in prognosis of angina, Circulation 61:1172, 1980.

50. Ruberman, W., and others: Ventricular premature complexes and sudden death after myocardial infarction, Circulation 64:297, 1981.

51. Lown, B., and Wolf, M.: Approaches to sudden death from coronary heart disease, Circulation 44:130, 1971.

52. Thanavaro, S., and others: Effect of electrocardiographic recording duration on ventricular dysrhythmia detection after myocardial infarction, Circulation 62:262, 1980.

53. Kennedy, H.L., and others: Effectiveness of increasing hours of continuous ambulatory electrocardiography in detecting maximal ventricular ectopy, Am. J. Cardiol. 42:925, 1978.

54. Bigger, J.T., and Weld, F.M.: Analysis of prognostic significance of ventricular arrhythmias after myocardial infaction: shortcomings of Lown grading system, Br. Heart J. 45:717, 1981.

55. Calvert, A., Lown, B., and Gorlin, R.: Ventricular premature beats and anatomically defined coronary heart disease, Am. J. Cardiol. 39:627, 1977.

56. Schulze, R.A., Jr., and others: Ventricular arrhythmias in the late hospital phase of acute myocardial infarction: relation to left ventricular function detected by gated cardiac blood pool scanning, Circulation 52:1006, 1975.

57. Schulze, R.A., Jr., and others: Left ventricular and coronary angiographic anatomy: relationship to ventricular irritability in the late hospital phase of acute myocardial infarction, Circulation 55:839, 1977.

58. deBoer, S.: On the fibrillation of the heart, J. Physiol. (London) 54:400, 1921.

59. Wiggers, C.J., and Wegria, R.: Ventricular fibrillation due to single, localized induction and condenser shocks applied during the vulnerable phase of ventricular systole, Am. J. Physiol. 128:500, 1940.

60. Smirk, F.H., and Palmer, D.G.: A myocardial syndrome—with particular reference to the occurrence of sudden death and of premature systoles interrupting antecedent T waves, Am. J. Cardiol. 6:621, 1960.

61. Hinkle, L.E., Jr., and others: Pathogenesis of an unexpected sudden death: role of early cycle ventricular premature contractions, Am. J. Cardiol. 39:873, 1977.

62. Engel, T.R., Meister, S.G., and Frankl, W.S.: The R-on-T phenomenon: an update and critical review, Ann. Intern. Med. 88:221, 1978.

63. DeSoyza, N., and others: Ectopic ventricular prematurity and its relationship to ventricular tachycardia in acute myocardial infarction in man, Circulation 50:529, 1974.

64. Winkle, R.A., Derrington, D.C., and Schroeda, J.S.: Characteristics of ventricular tachycardia in ambulatory patients, Am. J. Cardiol. 39:487, 1977.

65. Boudoulas, H., and others: Malignant premature ventricular beats in ambulatory patients, Ann. Intern. Med. 91:723, 1979.

66. Follansbee, W.P., Michelson, E.L., and Morganroth, J.: Nonsustained ventricular tachycardia in ambulatory patients: characteristics of association with sudden cardiac death, Ann. Intern. Med. 92:741, 1980.

67. Rahilly, G.T., and others: Clinical and electrophysiologic findings in patients with repetitive monomorphic ventricular tachycardia and otherwise normal electrograms, Am. J. Cardiol. 50:459, 1982.

68. Meinertz, T., and others: Significance of ventricular arrhythmias in idiopathic dilated cardiomyopathy, Am. J. Cardiol. 53:902, 1984.

69. Miles, W.M., and others: Management of patients with asymptomatic nonsustained ventricular tachycardia directed by electrophysiologic study, Clin. Res. 34(2):326A, 1986.

70. Kammerling, J.M., and others: Characteristics of spontaneous nonsustained ventricular tachycardia poorly predict rate of sustained ventricular tachycardia, Clin. Res. 34(2):312A, 1986.

71. Oberman, A., and others: Sudden death in patients evaluated for ischemic heart disease, Circulation 51-52(III):170, 1975.

72. Christensen, D., and others: Sudden death in the late hospital phase of acute myocardial infarction, Arch. Intern. Med. 137:1675, 1977.

73. Bigger, J.T., and others, and Multicenter Post-Infarction Research Group: The relationships among ventricular arrhythmias, left ventricular dysfunction, and mortality in the 2 years after myocardial infarction, Circulation 69:250, 1984.

74. Weinblatt, E., and others: Relation of education to sudden death after myocardial infarction, N. Engl. J. Med. 299:60, 1978.

75. Schwartz, P.J., and Wolf, S.: QT interval prolongation as predictor of sudden death in patients with myocardial infarction, Circulation 57:1074, 1978.

76. Kentala, E., and Repo, U.K.: QT interval prolongation during somatomotor activation as predictor of sudden death after myocardial infarction, Ann. Clin. Res. 11:42, 1979.

77. Haynes, R.E., Hallstrom, A.P., and Cobb, L.A.: Repolarization abnormalities in survivors of out-of-hospital ventricular fibrillation, Circulation 57:654, 1978.

78. Green, K.G., and others: Improvement in the prognosis of myocardial infarction by long-term beta-adrenoreceptor blockade using practolol, Br. Med. J. 3:735, 1975.

79. Wilhelmsson, C., and others: Reduction of sudden deaths after myocardial infarction by treatment with alprenolol: preliminary results, Lancet 2:1157, 1974.

80. The Norwegian Multicenter Study Group: Timolol-induced reduction in mortality and reinfarction in patients surviving acute myocardial infarction, N. Engl. J. Med. 304(14):801, 1981.

81. Olsson, G., and others: Long-term treatment with metoprolol after myocardial infarction: effect on 3-year mortality and morbidity, J. Am. Coll. Cardiol. 5:1428, 1985.

82. National Heart, Lung, and Blood Institute of Bethesda, Maryland: the β-blocker heart attack trial, JAMA 246:2073, 1981.

83. Lovell, R.R.H.: Arrhythmia prophylaxis: long-term suppressive medication, Circulation 51-52(III):236, 1975.

84. Kosowsky, B.D., and others: Long-term use of procainamide following acute myocardial infarction, Circulation 47:1204, 1973.

85. Hugenholtz, P.G., and others: One year follow-up in patients with persistent ventricular dysrhythmias after myocardial infarction treated with aprindine or placebo. In Sando, E., Julian, D.G., and Bell, J.W., editors: Management of ventricular tachycardia—role of mexiletine, Amsterdam, 1978, Excerpta Medica.

86. Schwartz, P.J., and others, and the Sudden Death Italian Prevention Group: surgical and pharmacological antiadrenergic interventions in the prevention of sudden death after a first myocardial infarction, Circulation 72(III):385, 1985.

87. Selzer, A., and Wray, H.W.: Quinidine syncope: paroxysmal ventricular fibrillation occurring during treatment of chronic atrial arrhythmias, Circulation 30:17, 1964.

88. Ejvinsson, G., and Orinius, E.: Prodromal ventricular premature beats preceded by a diastolic wave, Acta Med. Scand. 208: 445, 1980.

89. Dessertenne, F.: La tachycardie ventriculaire à deux foyers opposeś variable, Arch. Mal. Coeur 59:263, 1966.

90. Smith, W.M., and Gallagher, J.J.: "Les Torsades de Pointes": an unusual ventricular arrhythmia, Ann. Intern. Med. 93:578, 1980.

91. Minardo, J.D., and others: Drug associated ventricular fibrillation: analysis of clinical features and QTc prolongation, J. Am. Coll. Cardiol. 7:158A, 1986.

92. Prineas, R.J.: Problems in design and evaluation of antiarrhythmia trials, Circulation 51-52(III):249, 1975.

93. Morganroth, J., and others: Limitations of routine long-term electrocardiographic monitoring to assess ventricular ectopic frequency, Circulation 58:408, 1978.

94. Myerburg, R.J., and others: Antiarrhythmic drug therapy in survivors of prehospital cardiac arrest: comparison of effects on chronic ventricular arrhythmias and recurrent cardiac arrest, Circulation 59:855, 1979.

95. Herling, I.M., Horowitz, L.N., and Josephson, M.E.: Ventricular ectopic activity after medical and surgical treatment for recurrent sustained ventricular tachycardia, Am. J. Cardiol. 45:633, 1980.

96. Krone, R.J., and others: The effectiveness of antiarrhythmic agents on early-cycle premature ventricular complexes, Circulation 63:664, 1981.

97. Naccarelli, G.V., and others: Amiodarone: risk factors for recurrence of symptomatic ventricular tachycardia identified at electrophysiologic study, J. Am. Coll. Cardiol. 6:814, 1985.

98. Myerburg, R.J., and others: Relationship between plasma levels of procainamide, suppression of premature ventricular complexes, and prevention of recurrent ventricular tachycardia, Circulation 64:280, 1981.

99. Graboys, T.B., and others: Long-term survival of patients with malignant ventricular arrhythmia treated with antiarrhythmic drugs, Am. J. Cardiol. 50:437, 1982.

100. Naccarelli, G.V., and others: Role of electrophysiologic testing in managing patients who have ventricular tachycardia unrelated to coronary artery disease, Am. J. Cardiol. 50:165, 1982.

101. Fisher, J.D., and others: Serial electrophysiologic-pharmacologic testing for control of recurrent tachyarrhythmias, Am. Heart J. 93:658, 1977.

102. Mason, J.W., and Winkle, R.H.: Electrode-catheter arrhythmia induction in the selection and assessment of antiarrhythmic drug therapy in recurrent ventricular tachycardia, Circulation 58:971, 1978.

103. Horowitz, L.N., and others: Recurrent sustained ventricular tachycardia. III. Role of the electrophysiologic study in selection of antiarrhythmic regimens, Circulation 58:986, 1978.

104. Ruskin, J.N., DiMarco, J.P., and Garan, H.: Out-of-hospital cardiac arrest: electrophysiologic observations and selection of long-term antiarrhythmic therapy, N. Engl. J. Med. 303:607, 1980.

105. Heger, J.J., and others: Comparison between results obtained from electrophysiology testing, exercise testing, and ambulatory ECG recording. In Wenger, N.K., Mock, M.B., and Ringquist, II, editors: Ambulatory electrocardiographic recording, Chicago, 1981, Year Book Medical Publishers, Inc.

106. Prystowsky, E.N.: Selection of antiarrhythmic drugs based on electrophysiologic studies. In Dreifus, L., editor: Cardiac arrhythmias: electrophysiologic techniques and management, Cardiovascular Clinica, Philadelphia, 1985, F.A. Davis Co., p. 239-259.

107. Heger, J.J., and others: Amiodarone: clinical efficacy and electrophysiology during long-term therapy for recurrent ventricular tachycardia, N. Engl. J. Med. 305:539, 1981.

108. Prystowsky, E.N., and others: Induction of ventricular tachycardia during programmed electrical stimulation: analysis of pacing methods, Circulation 73(2):32, 1986.

109. Prystowsky, E.N.: Electrophysiologic testing in patients with ventricular tachycardia: past performance and future expectations, J. Am. Coll. Cardiol. 1(2):558, 1983.

110. Spielman, S., and others: Predictors of the success or failure of medical therapy in patients with chronic recurrent sustained ventricular tachycardia: a discriminant analysis, J. Am. Coll. Cardiol. 1:401, 1983.

111. Swerdlow, C.D., and others: Clinical factors predicting successful electrophysiologic-pharmacologic study in patients with ventricular tachycardia, J. Am. Coll. Cardiol. 1:409, 1983.

112. Prystowsky, E.N., and others: Factors associated with ventricular tachycardia suppression at electrophysiologic study during drug therapy, Circulation 70(2):2-56, 1984.

113. Rinkenberger, R.L., and others: Drug conversion of nonsustained ventricular tachycardia to sustained ventricular tachycardia during serial electrophysiological studies: identification of drugs that exacerbate tachycardia and potential mechanisms, Am. Heart J. 103:117, 1982.

114. Darling, E., and Faust, B.: Interrelationships between concerns, selected emotions, and coping in patients undergoing electrophysiologic testing, master's thesis.

115. Gallagher, J.J.: Surgical treatment of arrhythmias: current status and future directions, Am. J. Cardiol. 41:1035, 1979.

116. Guiraudon, G., and others: Encircling endocardial ventriculotomy: a new surgical treatment for life-threatening ventricular tachycardias resistant to medical treatment following myocardial infarction, Ann. Thorac. Surg. 26:438, 1978.

117. Josephson, M.E., Harken, A.H., and Horowitz, L.N.: Endocardial excision: a new surgical technique for the treatment of recurrent ventricular tachycardia, Circulation 60:1430, 1979.

118. Mirowski, M., and others: Clinical treatment of life-threatening ventricular tachyarrhythmias with the automatic implantable defibrillator, Am. Heart J. 102:265, 1981.

119. Fisher, J.D., Mehra, R., and Furman, S.: Termination of ventricular tachycardia with bursts of rapid ventricular pacing, Am. J. Cardiol. 41:94, 1978.

120. Zipes, D.P., and others: Clinical transvenous cardioversion of recurrent life-threatening ventricular tachyarrhythmias: low energy synchronized cardioversion of ventricular tachycardia and termination of ventricular fibrillation in patients using a catheter electrode, Am. Heart J. 103:789, 1982.

121. Zipes, D.P., and others: Early experience with the implantable cardioverter, N. Engl. J. Med. 311:485, 1984.

The drugs available to treat cardiovascular disease continue to multiply in number and complexity. As more is learned about the physiology and pathophysiology of cardiovascular disorders, new strategies for drug therapy are developed. As yet, however, there are few "magic bullets," drugs that are exact, precise, and specific in their action. For these reasons much of drug therapy remains an art in which guidelines must be specifically tailored to meet the needs of an individual patient. In this chapter selected pharmacologic aspects of drugs used to treat cardiovascular disorders are outlined. Although some overlap is evident, the agents are grouped in general classifications according to their clinical use.[4]

Clinical pharmacology, the study of drugs in man, is often divided into pharmacokinetics and pharmacodynamics. Pharmacokinetics deals with the processes of drug absorption, distribution, metabolism, and excretion. Pharmacodynamics is concerned with the mechanisms and effects of drug action in the body. It includes such areas as analysis of the structure-activity relationship and toxicology, or the study of adverse effects of drugs. This chapter consists of a brief review of general pharmacokinetics principles and discusses various aspects of pharmacodynamics in the clinical setting.

CLINICAL PHARMACOKINETICS[5]

A drug exerts its pharmacologic effects when it reaches a critical concentration at a specific site of action. Factors that determine drug concentration include the processes of drug absorption, distribution, biotransformation, and elimination. *Pharmacokinetics,* the quantitative study of these processes, provides a rational basis to determine the method of administration, dose strength, and dose timing.

Several mathematical models may be employed to describe drug pharmacokinetics in humans, but the simplest and most applicable are the one-compartment and two-compartment models depicted in Fig. 10-1. The one-compartment model assumes that a drug has rapid and homogeneous distribution throughout the body. Although such an assumption is an oversimplification, this model is useful in describing the pharmacokinetics of some orally administered drugs during chronic dosing. The two-compartment model consists of a smaller central compartment, which represents blood volume in highly perfused tissues, and a larger peripheral compartment with a slower rate of perfusion. The drug is administered into and eliminated from the central compartment, which also reaches equilibrium with the peripheral compartment.

The rates at which the drug moves to and from the central and peripheral compartments and the rate at which it is eliminated from this central compartment are the kinetics of drug action. Most drugs exhibit "first-order kinetics" (Fig. 10-2), which means that the rate at which a drug leaves a compartment is proportional to the amount of drug present in that compartment. Therefore over a given time period a larger quantity of drug is eliminated if the initial amount of drug is large rather than small.

Elimination half-life ($T_{1/2}$) is an important concept in pharmacokinetics; it refers to the amount of time required to eliminate one half of the drug load from a given compartment (Fig. 10-2). Because most cardiac drugs have a narrow toxic-therapeutic ratio, it is desirable to maintain a narrow range of drug concentrations. In most cases this is best accomplished by timing each dose administration to approximate the half-life of the drug.

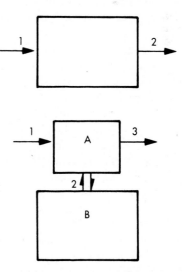

FIG. 10-1. *Top,* One-compartment model of drug pharmacokinetics. Drug is administered *(step 1)* and eliminated *(step 2)* from a large single compartment. Drug concentration in the single compartment is homogenous. *Bottom,* Two-compartment model of drug pharmacokinetics. Drug is administered *(step 1)* and eliminated *(step 3)* from a small central compartment *(A).* The small central compartment reaches an equilibrium *(step 2)* with the larger peripheral compartment *(B).*

297

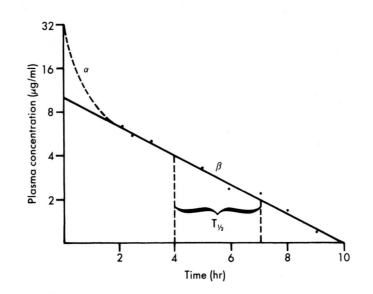

FIG. 10-2. Plasma concentration plotted over time following administration of a single dose of a drug exhibiting "first order" elimination kinetics. Distribution phase *(A)* is followed by elimination phase *(B)*. The time required to eliminate half of a given amount of drug is termed the *elimination half-life* ($T_{1/2}$).

Loading dose refers to the drug dose required to reach a desired concentration. As illustrated in Fig. 10-3, if a drug is begun by administering the usual maintenance dose, steady state conditions will be reached after 4 to 5 elimination half-lives, which in this example would require 12 to 15 hours. Steady state conditions are achieved more rapidly if an initial loading dose is given. Similarly, following an increase in a drug dose, the time required to reach a new steady state level will be 4 to 5 elimination half-lives. The new steady state and the new concentration are achieved more rapidly if an additional loading dose is given. *Maintenance dose* is the amount of drug administered to maintain the body load over a given time interval during steady state conditions.

Each drug used in cardiac therapy has unique pharmacokinetics. However, a number of common variables modify therapy by affecting the relationship between drug dose and drug effects. These include age, weight, sex, nature of heart disease, route of administration of drug, patient tolerance, physiologic milieu (e.g., acid-base balance, electrolytes, hypoxia), and concurrent medications.

Plasma drug concentrations are often used to guide therapy, but this method must be interpreted and used according to the individual clinical situation. Plasma drug concentrations are especially useful to ascertain whether a toxic concentration is present and to determine whether an apparent drug failure may be caused by unexpectedly low plasma levels. However, for a given patient, drug toxicity may occur at a drug concentration usually considered to be therapeutic and a subtherapeutic effect of a drug may

occur at a drug concentration considered to be toxic. In addition, measurement of plasma drug concentration does not consider the contribution of metabolites or changes in protein binding, which may contribute to overall drug effect. Therefore plasma drug concentrations must be approached as any other laboratory test, that is, in light of the entire clinical picture of the patient.

DRUGS THAT INCREASE CARDIAC CONTRACTILITY[1,9]
Digitalis

Digitalis preparations are the oldest and most widely used drugs in the treatment of heart disease. Many forms of digitalis are available, but at present digoxin and digitoxin are most often employed. The major uses of digitalis are to treat congestive heart failure and supraventricular arrhythmias, especially atrial fibrillation.

Digitalis increases myocardial contractility, a positive inotropic effect. The mechanism by which digitalis increases myocardial contractility appears to involve an increase in intracellular calcium. It is postulated that by inhibition of the NA^+-K^+ membrane pump, digitalis increases the intracellular pool of calcium ions available for excitation-contraction coupling.[12] Catecholamines (epinephrine, norepinephrine) also increase myocardial contractility, but their mechanism of action is different from that of digitalis, as evidenced by the finding that the effects of digitalis on contractility are not inhibited by beta-adrenergic blocking drugs.

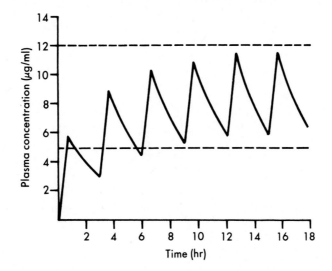

FIG. 10-3. Plasma concentration of a hypothetical drug administered at dosing intervals equal to an elimination half-life of 3 hours .Five half-lives are required to reach a steady-state level. A hypothetical range of effective plasma concentration is illustrated by hash lines.

The positive inotropic effects of digitalis are evident in normal and failing hearts; however, the net effect on myocardial oxygen consumption differs in these two conditions. Digitalis increases oxygen consumption in the normal, nonfailing ventricle, whereas in the failing myocardium, the net effect of digitalis is to decrease ventricular size and reduce wall tension, changes that decrease myocardial oxygen consumption. An additional factor that decreases myocardial oxygen consumption is the decrease in heart rate produced by digitalis, particularly in patients with atrial fibrillation.

Digitalis produces cardiac electrophysiologic effects by direct cellular actions and indirect actions mediated by the parasympathetic nervous system. One major clinically important antiarrhythmic action of digitalis is to prolong A-V nodal refractoriness and conduction time. Digitalis also shortens atrial and ventricular refractoriness, generally depresses normal automaticity in Purkinje fibers but may produce abnormal forms of automaticity.

Digitalis has actions on the central nervous system and autonomic nervous system. Through direct vascular and sympathetic neural actions, digitalis produces vasoconstriction, but in patients treated with digitalis for heart failure, the increased cardiac output and reflex vasodilatation usually outweigh the direct effects of vasoconstriction.

Clinical Uses (Table 10-1). The fact that digitalis increases the contractility of the heart makes it useful in treating congestive heart failure and low cardiac output. Clinical experience suggests that some forms of congestive heart failure respond well to digitalis while others do not.

Thus digitalis seems most likely to improve cardiac function in the clinical setting of cardiac dilatation, and especially when heart failure is accompanied by atrial fibrillation and a rapid ventricular response. Increase in myocardial contractility from digitalis may aggravate hypertrophic cardiomyopathy with obstruction by producing an increase in left ventricular outflow obstruction.

Digitalis is the drug of choice as an antiarrhythmic agent, and it is often the sole agent required to treat and prevent recurrences of paroxysmal supraventricular tachycardia and to control ventricular rate in atrial fibrillation or atrial flutter.

Precautions

1. Each digitalis preparation has unique pharmacokinetics (Table 10-1). Route of administration, loading dose, and maintenance dose must be determined for the individual patient and clinical situation.
2. Loading doses of digitalis are often not required for treatment of mild heart failure because smaller amounts of the drug will produce a positive inotropic effect in an incremental manner.
3. Digoxin is excreted primarily by the kidneys so dosage must be adjusted during renal insufficiency.
4. Digitoxin is metabolized primarily by the liver, so dosage must be adjusted in patients who have liver dysfunction.
5. Electrolyte disorders, especially hypokalemia, sensitize the myocardium to development of digitalis toxicity.

TABLE 10-1. Digitalis preparations

	INTRAVENOUS USE				
Agent	Initial Dose	Subsequent Dose	Onset of Action	Peak Effect	Elimination Half-Life
Ouabain (G-Strophanthin)	0.25-0.5 mg	0.1 mg every 30 to 60 min for total dose ≤1 mg/24	5 min	30-60 min	21 hr
Lanatoside C (Cedilanid)	0.8-1.0 mg	0.4 mg every 2 to 4 hr for total dose ≤2 mg/24 mg	5-10 min	30-120 min	
Digoxin (Lanoxin)	0.5-1.0 mg	0.25 mg every 2 to 4 hr for total dose ≤1.5 mg/24 hr	10-15 min	30 min-4 hr	36 hr

	ORAL USE				
Agent	Loading Dose in 24 Hr	Maintenance Dose in 24 Hr	Elimination Half-Life $T_{1/2}$	Principal Route of Elimination	Therapeutic Serum Levels
Digitoxin	0.7-1.2 mg	0.05-0.15 mg	4-5 days	Enterohepatic	14-24 ng/ml
Digoxin	1.0-1.5 mg	0.125-0.5 mg	36 hr	Renal	0.7-2.0 ng/ml

6. Thyroid status. Patients who have hyperthyroidism require large doses of digitalis to achieve clinical effects such as a decrease in the ventricular rate during atrial fibrillation and they frequently require combined therapy with beta-adrenergic receptor blockers. Patients who have hypothyroidism may require less than average doses of digitalis to achieve clinical response.

7. Drug interactions. Quinidine, verapamil, and amiodarone have significant interactions with digoxin to elevate serum digoxin levels. In many instances the dose of digoxin should be decreased by up to 50%.

8. Pulmonary disease. Arrhythmias in the setting of pulmonary disease are often difficult to control, and patients may exhibit increased sensitivity to digitalis toxicity.

9. The serum digitalis level does not define toxicity or efficacy. Digitalis serum levels may be useful as a guide, as discussed in the section on drug levels, but efficacy and toxicity are defined by total clinical assessment of the patient.

10. ECG effects of digitalis on the ST-T segment and QT interval should not be confused with ECG manifestations of digitalis toxicity (Fig. 10-4).

11. The toxic manifestations of digitalis therapy, listed in the box on p. 302, must be correctly identified.

Dopamine (Intropin)

Dopamine, an endogenous catecholamine, is the immediate precursor in the synthesis of norepinephrine. The cardiovascular effects of dopamine result from actions mediated through dopamine-specific receptors and alpha and beta-adrenergic receptors.[1]

Actions

1. The predominant cardiovascular effects of dopamine depend upon the dose administered.

2. At doses less than 7 μg/kg/min dopamine-specific and beta-adrenergic effects predominate. These effects include increases in myocardial contractility, cardiac output, and renal blood flow but little or no peripheral vasoconstriction.

3. At doses greater than 7 μg/kg/min alpha-adrenergic effects predominate, leading to peripheral vasoconstriction and an increase in mean arterial pressure.

4. Additional dopamine-specific effects include dilatation of mesenteric and renal vessels that results in an increased blood flow to these organs.

Clinical Uses

1. The unique hemodynamic effects of dopamine make it an important agent in the treatment of cardiogenic, septic, or traumatic shock because it directly increases cardiac output and increases renal blood flow.

2. Low dose (0.5 to 2.0 μg/kg/min) dopamine is used to treat chronic congestive heart failure that has been refractory to treatment with diuretics and digitalis. Such therapy, of course, is temporary and used only until more definitive long-term treatment can be formulated.

3. Dopamine is administered intravenously, preferably through a central venous line because tissue necrosis may occur if there is local extravasation.

4. The dose is best administered by infusion pump to ensure precision.

5. Usual dosage is 0.5 to 20 μg/kg/min, although up to 50 μg/kg/min is occasionally required.

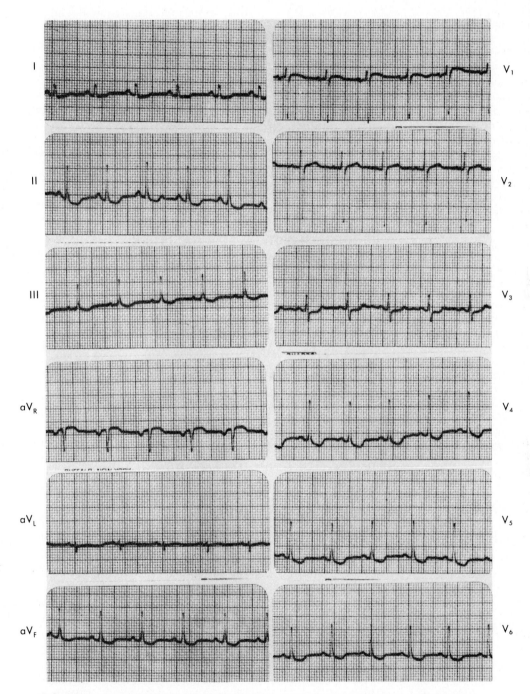

FIG. 10-4. Digitalis effect on the ECG. ST segment depression and shortened QT interval commonly occur with digitalization. This event should not be equated with digitalis intoxication. ST segment depression is present in lead I, II III, aVF$_F$ and V$_3$ to V$_6$. Note characteristic "sagging" of ST depression.

DIGITALIS INTOXICATION

Cardiac

1. Changes in rhythm (effects on cardiac automaticity and conduction)
   a. Ventricular premature contractions, coupled rhythm (bigeminy)
   b. Ventricular tachycardia; precursor of ventricular fibrillation; may be mechanism of sudden death in digitalis intoxication
   c. Nonparoxysmal AV junctional tachycardia with or without AV block
   d. Atrial tachycardia with or without block; most frequently seen in patients with associated potassium deficiency caused by concurrent use of thiazide diuretics
   e. Virtually any arrhythmia may be produced by digitalis excess
2. Effect on conduction system
   a. Prolonged PR interval
   b. Slow heart rates including sinus bradycardia and first-, second- (type I Wenckebach), and third-degree AV block
3. Cardiac failure

Neurologic

1. Mental depression and personality changes
2. Abnormal visual sensations
   a. Color (especially brown, yellow, and green)
   b. Scotoma
   c. Blurred or dimmed vision
   d. Photophobia
3. Cerebral excitation manifested as headache, vertigo, increased irritability, convulsions
4. Peripheral neuritis
5. Generalized muscular weakness

Gastrointestinal

1. Anorexia
2. Nausea
3. Vomiting
4. Diarrhea

Other

1. Gynecomastia
2. Allergic manifestations such as skin rash

Contraindications and Precautions

1. As with all inotropic agents, dopamine should be administered only after central blood volume and cardiac filling pressures are adequate.
2. Dopamine is contraindicated in the presence of uncontrolled arrhythmia and pheochromocytoma.

3. Effects of dopamine may be increased in the presence of monoamine oxidase inhibitors so dosage of dopamine must be reduced.
4. Dopamine is inactivated in alkaline solutions.

Adverse Side Effects and Toxicity

1. Most serious adverse side effect of dopamine is the genesis or exacerbation of arrhythmia.
2. Dopamine, especially in higher doses, may increase the demand for myocardial oxygen and cause further myocardial ischemia in the presence of coronary artery disease. Thus dopamine may precipitate angina pectoris
3. Occasionally, vasodilator effects of dopamine may produce hypotension.
4. Other side effects of dopamine include nausea, vomiting, and headache.

Nursing Implications. Intensive nursing care is required with special attention to proper solution strength, infusion rate, monitoring of vital signs, cardiac rhythm, and signs of toxicity. Frequent dose adjustments may be needed based on these assessments.

Dobutamine (Dobutrex)

Dobutamine is a synthetic catecholamine designed to achieve positive inotropic effects without the chronotropic and peripheral vasoconstriction of other sympathomimetic agents.[1]

Actions

1. Dobutamine, by direct beta-adrenergic agonist effects, increases myocardial contractility and cardiac output.
2. At equivalent dosages, dobutamine produces a greater increase in cardiac output, less increase in heart rate, less increase in peripheral vascular resistance, and less cardiac arrhythmia than dopamine.
3. These differences in actions are even more pronounced when dobutamine is compared with norepinephrine or isoproterenol.
4. Dobutamine increases peripheral and renal blood flow as a result of increased cardiac output and direct vasodilatation effects.

Clinical Uses

1. Dobutamine is the agent of choice for emergency treatment of severe heart failure by various causes, especially in shock states caused by direct myocardial decompensation.
2. When shock is caused by vascular collapse and marked vasodilatation, as in anaphylactic shock, the absence of vasoconstrictor effects argues against the use of dobutamine.

Administration

1. Dobutamine is only effective as an I.V. preparation.
2. The usual dosage is from 2.5 to 10.0 μg/kg/min, but rarely up to 40 μg/kg/min may be needed to achieve desired effects.

Side Effects and Toxicity

1. Dobutamine may increase heart rate, blood pressure, and the development of arrhythmia, so constant monitoring of these parameters and prompt dosage reductions, if these effects occur, is mandatory.
2. Occasionally nausea, headache, angina pectoris, and dyspnea may occur.

Nursing Implications. Same as for dopamine.

Amrinone

Amrinone increases myocardial contractility by a mechanism that is distinct from digitalis or catecholamines.[2]

Actions

1. A potential mechanism by which amrinone increases contractility is inhibition of the intracellular enzyme phosphodiesterase III. This action leads to an increase in cyclic AMP in the cell which, in turn, promotes an increase in intracellular calcium to participate in cardiac contraction.
2. Amrinone increases myocardial contractility directly without having any direct effect on heart rate.
3. Amrinone also has vasodilating properties.

Clinical Uses

1. Amrinone is used as an intravenous agent to treat congestive heart failure and cardiogenic shock.
2. Since its mechanism of action differs, amrinone may have additive effects with dobutamine.

Administration

1. Amrinone is administered intravenously with a loading dose of 0.75 to 1.5 μg/kg over 3 to 5 minutes, followed by a maintenance infusion of 5 to 10 μg/kg/min. Dosage of 18 mg/kg/24 hours is the maximum recommended.
2. Amrinone is not approved for oral use.
3. Other agents currently under investigation, such as milrinone, have an action similar to that of amrinone and may be useful for chronic oral therapy of heart failure.

Side Effects and Toxicity

1. Decreases in platelet counts to less than 100,00/mm³ are observed in 2% to 3% of patients.
2. Amrinone may cause supraventricular or ventricular arrhythmias and hypotension.

3. Less common effects may include nausea, vomiting, abdominal pain, liver toxicity, and fever.

Nitrates

This category includes nitroglycerin and isosorbide dinitrate. Their pharmacologic actions are caused by the property of nitrate to relax smooth muscle, especially in vascular beds.

Nitroglycerin. Nitroglycerin produces venodilatation, which decreases venous return to the heart and reduces ventricular filling pressure. Nitroglycerin also produces arteriolar dilatation, but its effects on systemic arterial resistance are less marked than the effects of other vasodilators. Coronary artery dilatation is also seen after nitroglycerin.

CLINICAL USES

1. Nitroglycerin is the preferred drug in the treatment of acute episodes of angina pectoris because of the rapid onset of its action and its ability to decrease cardiac oxygen demands and dilate coronary vessels. Sublingual doses of 0.2 to 0.6 mg (usually 0.4 mg) terminate typical anginal episodes.
2. A recently released preparation delivers nitroglycerin as a lingual aerosol in metered doses of 0.4 mg. It is used for the same indications as sublingual nitroglycerin tablets.
3. Transdermal nitroglycerin, usually 1 to 2 inches of 2% nitroglycerin ointment, may be used to prevent angina; its effects last from 4 to 6 hours. There are several controlled-release transdermal nitroglycerin compounds in current use. Although they are recommended for a single daily application, there is considerable controversy about whether these agents maintain efficacy over a 24-hour period.
4. Controlled-release capsules containing 2.5 mg, 6.5 mg, or 9 mg of nitroglycerin may be effective in preventing angina and are administered every 12 hours.
5. Intravenous nitroglycerin makes it possible to continually administer a titratable dose of nitroglycerin. It is especially useful in treating unstable angina pectoris. The initial dosage is usually 10 μg/min titrated to achieve desired results.
6. The hemodynamic effects of nitroglycerin produce a decrease in left ventricular filling pressure and little change in systemic vascular resistance. Nitroglycerin preparations thus tend to reduce pulmonary congestion associated with heart failure without major effects on systemic blood pressure.
7. Drug tolerance refers to loss of or decrease in a specific pharmacologic effect during repeated drug exposure. Nitrate tolerance occurs during long-term drug exposure. It develops to some of the effects of the nitrate, such as headache. It is not clear whether

or to what extent tolerance develops to the therapeutic effects of nitrates, although some degree of tolerance for therapeutic effects may occur during chronic nitrate adminstration.

Isosorbide Dinitrate (Sorbitrate, Isordil). Antianginal and hemodynamic effects of isosorbide dinitrate are similar to those of nitroglycerin, but duration of action is longer. The efficacy of oral nitrates has long been questioned because first-pass hepatic metabolism deactivates a large amount of the orally administered dose. However, when given in sufficient doses to prevent complete degradation, oral doses have effects similar to those of sublingual doses.

CLINICAL USES

1. Sublingual isosorbide may be effective in terminating acute episodes of angina, but nitroglycerin is usually the preferred drug.
2. Onset of action of sublingual isosorbide is 2 to 5 minutes, whereas duration of action ranges from 1 to 2 hours.
3. Oral isosorbide has a duration of action from 1 to 4 hours.
4. Sustained release preparations, designed to last 6 to 12 hours, are available but have not been completely studied.
5. Sublingual or oral isosorbide is generally used as a prophylactic for angina pectoris and to maintain hemodynamic effects for a longer duration than obtainable with nitroglycerin.
6. Doses—sublingual: 2.5, 5, and 10 mg every 2 to 3 hours; oral: 10 to 40 mg every 3 to 4 hours.

SIDE EFFECTS AND TOXICITY

1. Nitrate therapy may cause postural hypotension, syncope, dizziness, headaches, nausea, and rarely, drug rash.
2. Abrupt withdrawal of chronic nitrate therapy may precipitate myocardial ischemia.

NURSING IMPLICATIONS OF NITRATE THERAPY

1. Patients with angina pectoris are taught to keep nitroglycerin readily accessible and to use it quickly to relieve angina attacks.
2. Patients are instructed to store tablets in a cool, dark place, and to remove any cotton from the bottle because this may absorb the drug.
3. Patients are taught to expect the burning under the tongue that occurs as the tablet dissolves. Nitroglycerin should relieve angina episodes within 2 to 5 minutes. If three or four doses of nitroglycerin are ineffective in relieving an episode, patients are usually instructed to seek medical attention.

4. The potential for orthostatic hypotension should be emphasized. Concurrent use of alcohol should be avoided.
5. If transdermal nitroglycerin is used, techniques of application, avoidance of coarsely-haired regions, maintenance of an occlusive dressing, and rotation of application sites may need to be emphasized.

Sodium Nitroprusside (Nipride). Sodium nitroprusside is a vasodilating agent that acts directly on vascular smooth muscle independent of autonomic innervation. Nitroprusside has an immediate onset and termination of action, and it has a balanced effect to dilate arterioles and venules equivalently, thus decreasing both preload and afterload of the heart. In the failing heart, afterload reduction increases the cardiac output either with a minimal decrease in mean arterial blood pressure or with none. Heart rate tends to remain unchanged or to increase slightly. Decreased preload, resulting from venodilatation, decreases pulmonary capillary wedge pressure. Beneficial hemodynamic effects are observed when the filling pressure and systemic resistance are elevated initially and cardiac output is depressed, as happens in the failing myocardium. In normal hearts, however, or when left ventricular filling pressure is normal or low, nitroprusside produces hypotension and tachycardia with little change in cardiac output.

CLINICAL USES

1. Nitroprusside is employed in the acute treatment of low cardiac output states and congestive heart failure, especially during acute myocardial infarction and following cardiac surgery.
2. Because of the potent and potentially harmful effects of nitroprusside, all patients should have hemodynamic monitoring of pulmonary artery and intra-arterial pressures.
3. Nitroprusside is infused intravenously, beginning at 10 μg/min and increased until desired effects are obtained.
4. Therapy is usually guided by the level of the pulmonary wedge pressure or pulmonary end-diastolic pressure and the systemic arterial pressure.

SIDE EFFECTS AND TOXICITY

1. Hypotension caused by excessive vasodilation is treated by decreasing the dosage or by stopping the infusion.
2. Nitroprusside is metabolized to thiocyanate, which may produce fatigue, nausea, muscle spasm, psychotic behavior, and hypothyroidism. Thiocyanate level should be measured if large amounts of nitroprusside (100 μg/min) are infused for more than 48 hours.

NURSING IMPLICATIONS

1. Carefully attending to vital signs and hemodynamic parameters includes recording baseline values before therapy, establishing desired endpoints for therapy, and frequently recording changes in any parameters during treatment.
2. Nitroprusside is light-sensitive so the solution bottle and infusion line must be covered with light-occlusive material, usually an aluminum foil wrap. A fresh, potent solution has a brownish tint.

Hydralazine (Apresoline)

Hydralazine directly relaxes vascular smooth muscle more so in arterioles than in veins. As a result of vasodilatation, systemic vascular resistance decreases and renal, splanchnic, and hepatic blood flow increases. Peripheral vasodilatation recruits a reflex increase in heart rate but hydralazine also may have a slight degree of direct cardiac stimulation. Reflex tachycardia may be prevented by beta-adrenergic blocking agents such as propranolol.

Clinical Uses and Administration

1. Originally introduced and widely used as an antihypertensive agent, hydralazine is also employed as an oral vasodilator to treat congestive heart failure and low cardiac output states.
2. Hydralazine is administered orally in doses of 40 to 400 mg/day in two to four divided doses.
3. For chronic treatment, dosage less than 200 mg/day are recommended to minimize toxicity, particularly drug-induced lupus erythematosus.

Side Effects and Toxicity

1. Reflex tachycardia may precipitate myocardial ischemia and angina pectoris. In some instances of congestive heart failure where the beta-adrenergic reflex responses are blunted, reflex tachycardia may not occur.
2. More importantly, chronic hydralazine therapy may induce a syndrome of systemic lupus erythematosus, possibly caused by an immunologic response to a metabolite of hydralazine.
3. Other side effects include headache, nausea, drug fever, urticaria, skin rash, neuritis, gastrointestinal hemorrhage, anemia, and pancytopenia.

Nursing Implications

1. Patients should be instructed about the signs and symptoms of orthostatic hypotension and how to minimize these effects.
2. Absorption of hydralazine is increased if given with meals. The increase in vasodilating effects combined with the known tendency in some patients for postprandial orthostatic hypotension may produce significant adverse effects.

Prazosin (Minipress)

Prazosin is an orally effective alpha-adrenergic blocking agent with clinical applications similar to the other vasodilators mentioned. It selectively blocks $alpha_1$-L adrenergic receptors to reduce peripheral vascular resistance. The net effect of prazosin is the dilatation of both arterioles and venules equally, which is similar to the effect of nitroprusside. The cardiac acceleration following vasodilatation with hydralazine or after nonselective alpha receptor blockade with phentolamine does not occur with prazosin. As a result of decreased systemic resistance, cardiac output increases and blood pressure falls, both in hypertensive patients and in patients with congestive heart failure. The improvement in cardiac output, however, may not be maintained during chronic therapy as tolerance to the effects of prazosin seems to develop.

Clinical Uses

1. Prazosin is employed as an oral vasodilator to treat congestive heart failure and low cardiac output states.
2. Prazosin is also an antihypertensive agent.
3. By plasma concentration measurements, prazosin has a half-life of 3 to 4 hours, although its vasodilating effects persist considerably longer.
4. Dosage of prazosin is 1 mg initially and up to 28 mg/day in two or three divided doses.

Side Effects and Toxicity

1. Excessive hypotension may occur, especially following the initial dose of prazosin.
2. Other side effects are uncommon or mild. Syncope caused by postural hypotension may occur, especially if nitrates are coadministered. Headache, drowsiness, nausea, lethargy, fluid retention, skin rash, urinary incontinence, and polyarthralgia may also occur.

Nursing Implications. Since the first dose of prazosin is most likely to induce hypotension, patients should remain supine or seated and be warned of the possibility of dizziness or weakness.

Electrolytes

Potassium. Potassium is a major intracellular cation found principally in muscle, including cardiac tissue. The most total body potassium is located within the cells, and intracellular concentration is approximately 30 times the extracellular concentration. Despite this, extracellular or serum potassium concentration usually correlates well with total body potassium in stable, steady-state conditions. Renal function provides the major regulation of body potassium. Certain metabolic diseases, kidney diseases, diarrhea, vomiting, diuretic therapy or infusions of potassium-free fluids that increase extracellular fluid volume may all reduce serum levels of potassium. Elevated serum levels of potassium are caused by acidosis, renal failure, massive tissue necrosis, major catabolic states, and the inadvertent administration of potassium.

ACTIONS. Potassium plays a major role in the maintenance of normal cellular excitability and conduction. Hypokalemia prolongs the recovery of excitability, manifested as a prolonged QU interval on the ECG, and slows atrioventricular and intraventricular conduction time. Premature ventricular complexes and disorders of atrioventricular conduction may occur. Hyperkalemia increases the rate of repolarization (shortened QT interval on the ECG) and at progressively high levels first increases and then decreases excitability and conduction velocity. Therefore potassium administration may initially facilitate conduction but later produce AV conduction delay and slow intraventricular conduction.

Factors other than the serum concentration of potassium influence its cardiac effects. Slow increases in potassium depress automaticity and lead to asystole, whereas rapid increases of potassium may transiently increase automaticity and lead to ventricular ectopy and ventricular fibrillation. Associated electrolyte and acid-base disturbances are important because acidosis and hyponatremia augment the changes produced by hyperkalemia. Hypokalemia is synergistic with digitalis in producing arrhythmias. Elevated levels of calcium concentration mitigate the effects of hyperkalemia, whereas reduced levels of calcium concentration enhance it. Conversely, reduced calcium levels mitigate the effects of hypokalemia, whereas elevated calcium levels enhance it.

CLINICAL USES AND ADMINISTRATION. Maintenance of potassium balance during diuretic and digitalis therapy involves the use of potassium salts and dietary adjustments. For severe potassium deficiency or treatment of arrhythmia secondary to digitalis toxicity, intravenous potassium may be required.

1. For patients receiving digitalis and diuretics, the routine prophylactic administration of 30 to 60 milliequivalents (mEq) of potassium chloride is recommended (10 mEq kcal = 750 mg kcal).
2. Since potassium loss in the urine parallels sodium loss to some degree, the restriction of dietary sodium will help mitigate potassium loss.
3. Potassium chloride, which also replenishes chloride ions lost during diuresis and sodium chloride restriction, is the preferred salt for oral administration.
4. Potassium supplements are also found in some "salt substitutes" and in bananas and citrus fruits.
5. Intravenous potassium is administered at a dose of 30 to 60 mEq kcal in 500 to 1000 ml D5W and at a rate no more than 30 to 40 mEq/hour.

SIDE EFFECTS AND TOXICITY

1. Rapid potassium infusion produces sinus bradycardia, depression of intrinsic pacemakers, and slowing of AV conduction to the point of block.
2. Adverse symptoms reported with potassium therapy are nausea, vomiting, diarrhea and abdominal discomfort.
3. Hyperkalemia may occur following administration of potassium, especially in the presence of impaired renal function. Hyperkalemia may manifest as weakness, paresthesias, decreased blood pressure, and ECG changes. Cardiac arrhythmias ranging from heart block to cardiac arrest caused by ventricular fibrillation or ventricular asystole may occur.
4. ECG manifestations of hyperkalemia include a peaked, narrowed T wave and shortened QT interval. As toxicity increases, the QRS complex widens, the PR interval lengthens, and the P wave may diminish in size or disappear.
5. ECG manifestations of hypokalemia are decreased T wave amplitude, depression of the ST segment, appearance of prominent U waves, and a prolonged QU interval. Symptoms of hypokalemia include muscular weakness, lassitude, and emotional lability.

PRECAUTIONS

1. In the presence of potassium depletion, the myocardium is sensitive to sudden increase in potassium concentration and appropriate precautions should be taken.
2. Potassium administration to control arrhythmias in the presence of normal serum potassium concentrations may lead to potassium excess and intoxication.
3. Intravenous infusion of potassium chloride may cause burning or pain at the infusion site.
4. In the presence of known or expected cardiac toxicity of potassium, ECG monitoring is mandatory.
5. Some potassium tablet formulations may cause intestinal ulceration and gastrointestinal bleeding.
6. If patients have any esophageal pathologic condition, tablet forms of potassium may cause ulcerations. Liquid potassium is the preferred form of administration.

CONTRAINDICATIONS

1. The presence of second-degree AV block is generally a contraindication to the use of potassium. However, in the case of digitalis-induced atrial tachycardia with AV block, potassium administration may slow the atrial rate and restore sinus rhythm without worsening the AV block.
2. Potassium is contraindicated in patients who have severe renal impairment, untreated Addison's dis-

ease, acute dehydration, heat cramps, acidosis, and preexisting hyperkalemia of any cause.

NURSING IMPLICATIONS

1. Nursing attention to conditions and drugs that may contribute to hypokalemia or hyperkalemia is important. Thus potassium supplements are usually necessary in patients receiving digitalis and diuretics but may not be needed if potassium-sparing diuretics are used and may be dangerous in patients with renal insufficiency.
2. In any patient receiving potassium, consideration should be given to renal function, urine flow, and serum potassium levels.
3. Potassium is given either orally or by slow intravenous infusion. There is potential for phlebitis and local tissue necrosis during parenteral administration. Rapid infusion may cause potentially fatal hyperkalemia.
4. There are multiple forms and preparations of oral potassium. Care should be taken that the proper amount of potassium is administered if different products are employed.
5. A sugar-free form of liquid potassium (Kaochlor S-F 10%) may be useful for some diabetic patients.
6. Factors that may assist patient tolerance of oral potassium liquids include administration with or after meals, use of water or fruit juice, and instructing the patient to take small amounts at a time.

Calcium. Calcium is a major body cation of prime importance in bone metabolism, muscle contraction, and many cellular membrane actions. Since over 90% of the body stores of calcium are in bone structures, changes in serum calcium concentration often do not reflect changes in total body calcium. Nevertheless, changes in serum calcium concentration may have profound electrical and mechanical effects on the heart.

ACTIONS

1. Calcium flow into the myocardial cell during systole accounts for a portion of phase II or plateau phase of the cardiac action potential. This slow inward calcium current plays an important physiologic role in impulse formation and conduction in SA nodal and AV nodal cells and in other cells under pathologic conditions.
2. Calcium directly increases myocardial contractility by interacting with the myofibrillar proteins in the coupling of excitation with muscle contraction.
3. Hypercalcemia shortens the plateau phase of the action potential, which is reflected as shortened QT interval, primarily by the shortening of the ST segment on the ECG.
4. Hypocalcemia produces opposite effects and pro-

longs the interval from the Q wave to the onset of the T wave with flattening and prolongation of the ST segment.
5. Calcium excess may result in sinus bradycardia, AV conduction block, and ectopic arrhythmias. These are usually seen only when digitalis is also present.

CLINICAL USES. In cardiovascular therapy calcium administration has been most commonly employed in the setting of cardiac arrest. If ventricular fibrillation has not responded to one or more electrical countershocks, initial CPR measures have not restored circulation and ventilation, and epinephrine infusion has not been effective, intravenous calcium may be indicated. A dose of 3 to 5 ml of 10% calcium chloride (3.4 to 6.8 mEq calcium) is employed. Stated but undocumented effects of calcium in this setting are an increase in myocardial tone, conversion from fine fibrillation to coarse fibrillation, and an increase in the success of electrical countershock. Currently, the role of calcium administration during cardiopulmonary resuscitation is being questioned, and it is quite possible that future guidelines may not include the use of calcium.

PREPARATION AND PRECAUTIONS

1. Calcium chloride is usually given intravenously in a concentration of 5% to 10%. Injection rate should be slow (not to exceed 1 to 2 ml/minute). This drug is irritating to tissue and will cause painful necrosis if extravasation occurs during intravenous therapy.
2. Calcium gluconate can be given intramuscularly or intravenously. Calcium gluconate has less ionized calcium and is less irritating to subcutaneous tissue than the chloride salt. For parenteral use calcium gluconate is administered as a 10% solution intravenously (5 to 30 ml).
3. Calcium injection may produce a moderate fall in blood pressure caused by peripheral vasodilatation.
4. Calcium administration may aggravate digitalis toxicity.

Sodium Bicarbonate. Sodium bicarbonate is a major extracellular buffer that acts to provide the physiologic control of acid-base balance. Bicarbonate metabolism is regulated primarily by the kidney, and the bicarbonate system is one of many acid-base buffer systems.

CLINICAL USES

1. Sodium bicarbonate is employed to correct metabolic acidosis, especially lactic acidosis, and is specifically indicated to treat acidosis caused by cardiogenic shock or ventricular fibrillation.
2. Sodium bicarbonate is administered at a dosage of 1 mEq/kg every 10 minutes during cardiopulmonary resuscitation until circulation is restored. When possible, administration should be guided by repeated measurements of arterial blood pH.

PRECAUTIONS

1. Treating acidosis with bicarbonate does not alter the underlying defect that caused the acidosis such as cardiogenic shock.
2. Overdosage of bicarbonate will produce a metabolic alkalosis.
3. The large sodium load administered with sodium bicarbonate may worsen preexisting congestive heart failure.

NURSING IMPLICATIONS

Sodium bicarbonate may inactivate many drugs if mixed in intravenous solutions. For example calcium will precipitate and catecholamines will be inactivated if mixed with bicarbonate.

Atropine

Atropine blocks activity in portions of the parasympathetic nervous system by inhibiting the action of acetylcholine. In the heart, atropine principally increases the rate of the automatic discharge of the SA node and shortens the refractory period and conduction time of the AV node. These effects lead to an increase in the ventricular rate during sinus mechanisms or many supraventricular rhythms. A lesser effect, particularly in the atria, may be to increase contractility.

Clinical Uses and Dosage

1. Atropine is indicated to block unwanted effects of vagal tone such as symptomatic sinus bradycardia, sinus bradycardia associated with increased ventricular ectopy during acute myocardial infarction, or AV block caused by increased vagal tone.
2. Atropine is administered intravenously, usually in an initial dose of 0.5 to 0.8 mg by rapid injection. Additional increments of 0.3 to 0.5 mg are administered until desired effects, unwanted side effects, or a total dose of 2.0 to 2.5 mg is reached.
3. Smaller doses or slower administration of atropine may evoke a vagomimetic effect that produces sinus node slowing and AV conduction delay.
4. Intramuscular atropine may be effective but since absorption is slow compared to intravenous doses, drug concentrations in the serum and at the site of action are low. Thus larger doses, usually twice the intravenous dose, are required.
5. The cardiac effects of intravenous atropine persist for about 2 hours and systemic effects may last up to 24 hours; therefore chronic therapy with intravenous atropine is usually not indicated.

Side Effects and Toxicity

1. Adverse side effects of atropine are usually caused by the effects of acetylcholine inhibition in extracar-diac organs and are related to the total dose of atropine.
2. Usual side effects are urinary retention, dryness of skin and of mucous membranes, and bronchial secretions, pupillary dilatation, acute glaucoma, mental confusion, and delirium.
3. Atropine-induced sinus node acceleration during acute myocardial infarction may precipitate further ischemia, and atropine may have direct effects on ventricular myocardium. Either one or both of these factors may lead to the emergence of a ventricular arrhythmia and ventricular fibrillation following atropine administration during acute myocardial infarction.

Nursing Implications

1. Atropine should be given as a rapid intravenous bolus.
2. Blood pressure and heart rate need careful monitoring following atropine.
3. Many of the side effects of atropine, such as urinary retention or visual blurring, which represent extensions of the pharmacologic effects, may persist for several hours after drug administration.

Edrophonium (Tensilon)

Edrophonium is a cholinergic drug that acts by inhibiting the action of acetylcholinesterase, the enzyme that degrades acetylcholine. Cardiac effects of edrophonium are similar to those produced by enhanced vagal tone. Edrophonium decreases sinus nodal discharge rate, increases refractoriness and conduction time of AV node, and decreases myocardial contractility.

Clinical Uses and Dosage

1. Edrophonium is primarily used to terminate episodes of paroxysmal supraventricular tachycardia (PSVT) when other vagal maneuvers such as carotid sinus massage or Valsalva maneuver are ineffective.
2. Edrophonium is administered as a 5 or 10 mg intravenous bolus. A test dose of 1 to 2 mg may be given initially.
3. Effects of edrophonium begin within 30 to 60 seconds after administration and may last as long as 10 minutes.
4. A continuous infusion of 0.25 to 2.0 mg/minute may be used if longer lasting effects are desired.

Side Effects and Toxicity

1. Enhanced vagal tone may aggravate preexisting conditions of intestinal obstruction, bronchial asthma, or urinary obstruction; edrophonium should be avoided in these circumstances.
2. Side effects relate mainly to results of vagal overac-

tivity and may include nausea, perspiration, salivation, bronchial spasm, slow pulse, and hypotension.

3. To counteract any potential life-threatening complications, atropine should be immediately available when edrophonium is used.

Nursing Implications
1. Monitoring of vital signs, especially respiratory rate and pattern, is needed.
2. Atropine should be immediately available at a dose of 0.5 to 1.0 mg.
3. Edrophonium is usually in a concentration of 10 mg/ml; the usual dose then is 1 ml.

ADRENERGIC PHARMACOLOGY

Adrenergic pharmacology includes the study of the sympathetic nervous system with its principal neurotransmitter, norepinephrine, the naturally occurring catecholamines, epinephrine and norepinephrine secreted by the adrenal medulla, and the effects of drugs that stimulate (agonist) or block (antagonist) the sympathetic receptors. The pharmacologic effects of neurotransmitters, hormones, or drugs are mediated by the interaction of the agent with specific receptors on all membranes. Adrenergic receptors are classified into two major subgroups of alpha receptors and beta receptors based upon the differences in the physiologic actions and relative potency of different catecholamines.

For the cardiovascular system, stimulation of alpha receptors located in the heart and smooth muscle of arterioles results in increased myocardial contractility and arteriolar constriction. Beta receptors are located in the heart, arterioles (primarily skeletal muscle arterioles), and lungs. Stimulation of beta receptors increases heart rate and contractility, decreases AV nodal conduction time and refractoriness, dilates arterioles of skeletal muscle beds, and dilates bronchioles.

Subclassification of Beta-Adrenergic Receptors

The response of beta-adrenergic stimulation or inhibition may be further subclassified into $beta_1$ and $beta_2$ action. This division is not complete because there is overlap in activity of drugs on $beta_1$ and $beta_2$ receptors. However, differences in the relative potency of drugs to stimulate (agonist activity) or inhibit (antagonist activity) either beta receptor subtype allows more selective use of drugs.

$Beta_1$ receptors are the predominant receptors in myocardium where stimulation increases heart rate and contractility and shortens AV nodal conduction time and refractoriness. $Beta_2$ receptors predominate in blood vessels and lungs where stimulation dilates arterioles and bronchioles.

Subclassification of Alpha-Adrenergic Receptors

The alpha-adrenergic receptors have also been subclassified into $alpha_1$ and $alpha_2$ receptors. Although subpopulations of beta receptors appear to be relatively tissue-specific in that $beta_1$ receptors are present in the heart and $beta_2$ receptors are present in arterioles and lungs, the situation is different for alpha receptors whose subclassification is not analagous to that of beta receptors.

As depicted in Fig. 10-5, the adrenergic neural terminal is composed of the presynaptic sympathetic neuron, the synaptic cleft, and the postsynaptic effector cell. Alpha- and beta-adrenergic receptors are located on the membrane of the effector cell and the sympathetic neuron. Alpha receptors, located on the effector cell, are termed *postsynaptic receptors* or *alpha₁ receptors,* whereas receptors on the nerve terminal are *presynaptic* or *alpha₂ receptors.*

Stimulation of the $alpha_1$ (postsynaptic) receptor mimics the effects of norepinephrine on the effector cell, whereas inhibition of the $alpha_1$ receptor antagonizes these effects. On the other hand, the $alpha_2$ receptor serves an autoregulatory function. Stimulation of the $alpha_2$ (presynaptic) receptor inhibits norepinephrine release from the nerve terminal, thus diminishing the effects of norepinephrine on the effector cell while inhibition of the $alpha_2$ receptor stimulates release of norepinephrine.

Drugs that are alpha-adrenergic agonists or antagonists may affect $alpha_1$ or $alpha_2$ receptors. Furthermore, clinical effects may not be identical to the effects determined in isolated tissue preparations.

Alpha- and Beta-Adrenergic Receptor Stimulating Drugs

Dopamine and Dobutamine. Both these agents stimulate cardiac beta receptors and peripheral alpha receptors. Dopamine and dobutamine are discussed in an earlier section because they are employed primarily as positive inotropic agents.

Epinephrine (Adrenalin)
ACTION. Epinephrine acts directly on $beta_1$ (cardiac) receptors to increase heart rate and contractility. In the peripheral circulation, epinephrine in lower doses produces $beta_2$ receptor stimulation that results in vasodilatation of skeletal muscle vessels while larger doses activate both $alpha_1$- and $alpha_2$-adrenergic receptors to elevate peripheral resistance and blood pressure.

CARDIOVASCULAR USES
1. Epinephrine is most often employed clinically during cardiac arrest to stimulate cardiac pacemaker activity and increase contractility. It is stated to render the fibrillating heart more responsive to DC electrical shock.

PRESYNAPTIC   POSTSYNAPTIC

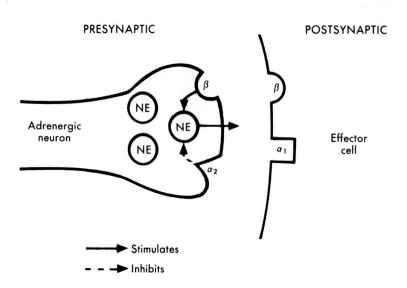

→ Stimulates

- - → Inhibits

FIG. 10-5. Diagram of the adrenergic nerve terminal illustrating alpha₁-, alpha₂-, and beta-adrenergic receptors in presynaptic and postsynaptic postions. The effector cell contains alpha₁- and beta-adrenergic receptors, which interact with norepinephrine to produce end organ effects. The presynaptic alpha₂- and beta-adrenergic receptors interact with norepinephrine to stimulate (beta receptor) or inhibit (alpha₂ receptor) further norepinephrine release.

2. Epinephrine is often the drug of choice in the immediate treatment of anaphylaxis.

ADMINISTRATION. The usual dose of epinephrine is 0.5 to 1.0 ml of 1:1000 solution or 5 to 10 ml of 1:10,000 solution administered by intravenous or intracardiac injection.

SIDE EFFECTS
1. Epinephrine may exacerbate ventricular arrhythmia.
2. Disturbing reactions of fear, anxiety, and tension may occur.
3. Epinephrine may precipitate myocardial ischemia because of the inability of coronary blood flow to meet increased myocardial oxygen requirements.
4. Epinephrine may produce headache, tremor, and weakness.
5. Renal blood flow, glomerular filtration rate, and sodium excretion are usually reduced after admission of epinephrine.

NURSING IMPLICATIONS
1. Epinephrine solutions deteriorate quickly and should be used within 24 hours of mixing. Avoid use if solution is dissolved or has a precipitate.
2. Avoid mixing in alkaline solutions; may be dissolved in dextrose or saline solutions.
3. Vasoconstriction may occur at site of injection.

Norepinephrine (Levarterenol)/(Levophed)
ACTIONS. Norepinephrine exerts a greater alpha-adrenergic stimulating effect (alpha₁ and alpha₂) than does epi-

nephrine, but its cardiac (beta₁) stimulating effect is approximately equivalent. Norepinephrine increases systolic and diastolic arterial pressure and total peripheral resistance. Cardiac output usually remains unchanged or decreased because of the increased peripheral resistance and slowed heart rate that result from reflex vagal activation. Coronary blood flow increases while renal, cerebral, visceral, and skeletal muscle blood flow diminishes.

CLINICAL USES. Norepinephrine is used to treat hypotension and shock, but it has largely been replaced in clinical practice by the newer agents dopamine and dobutamine. Norepinephrine may be especially useful when hypotensive states are accompanied by low peripheral vascular resistance and normal or slightly elevated cardiac output.

ADMINISTRATION. Dose requirements vary widely and require careful titration. The usual dosage ranges from 2 to 20 μg/min administered by intravenous infusion. A solution containing 4 to 8 mg of norepinephrine per 1000 ml of 5% dextrose and water is administered with an infusion pump.

SIDE EFFECTS AND TOXICITY
1. Anxiety, respiratory difficulty, and transient headaches may result.
2. Overdosage may cause severe hypertension with headache, photophobia, angina, intensive sweating, and vomiting.
3. Cardiac arrhythmias may be produced or exacerbated.

PRECAUTIONS

1. Blood pressure should be monitored frequently, ideally by intraarterial pressure recording.
2. Norepinephrine is best administered by infusion into a large central vein. If peripheral vein administration is employed, the site of administration should be observed frequently. Extravasation of drug at the infusion site may cause tissue sloughing as a result of local vasoconstriction. Local phentolamine (Regitine 10 mg) infiltration may prevent tissue loss should extravasation occur.

NURSING IMPLICATIONS

1. Careful dose titration with an infusion pump and intraarterial blood pressure monitoring are required.
2. Abrupt discontinuation may result in severe depression of blood pressure; the dose should be slowly decreased.

Beta-Adrenergic Stimulating Drugs
Isoproterenol (Isuprel)

ACTIONS. Isoproterenol has nearly exclusive beta-adrenergic receptor stimulating activity and acts on beta$_2$ (smooth muscle, bronchioles) and beta$_1$ (heart) receptors. Isoproterenol relaxes smooth muscle of bronchi, skeletal muscle vasculature, and alimentary tract. In the heart, isoproterenol increases heart rate and contractility. Isoproterenol lowers peripheral vascular resistance and decreases diastolic arterial pressure. The net hemodynamic effect is to elevate cardiac output and systolic pressure and to decrease mean and diastolic arterial pressure. In addition, myocardial oxygen consumption rises with isoproterenol administration. In conditions of hypovolemia, isoproterenol may also decrease systolic pressure.

CARDIOVASCULAR USES

1. Isoproterenol is most often used to enhance pacemaker activity and improve AV conduction during episodes of sinus bradycardia or AV block.
2. In certain cardiogenic shock states, isoproterenol may be used to increase cardiac output and decrease peripheral vasoconstriction. Isoproterenol is not indicated to treat cardiogenic shock caused by acute myocardial infarction.
3. In bronchospastic lung disease isoproterenol may be used to produce bronchodilatation but is nearly always employed as a local inhalant for this purpose.

ADMINISTRATION. In emergency situations, isoproterenol is usually administered by intravenous injection of 0.02 µg to 0.06 µg. Intravenous infusion of 0.5 µg/min to 4.0 mcg/min is used to achieve the clinical response.

SIDE EFFECTS

1. Isoproterenol increases myocardial oxygen consumption and may precipitate myocardial ischemia.
2. Cardiac arrhythmias, including sinus tachycardia, premature ventricular complexes, ventricular tachycardia, or ventricular fibrillation, may result.
3. In the presence of hypovolemia, the vasodilating effects of isoproterenol may produce hypotension.
4. Headache, flushing of the skin, angina, nausea, tremor, dizziness, weakness, and sweating may result.

NURSING IMPLICATIONS

Patients with symptomatic coronary artery disease, hypertrophic cardiomyopathy, and cardiac arrhythmias are particularly susceptible to adverse cardiac effects from isoproterenol.

Alpha-Adrenergic Receptor Stimulating Drugs
Phenylephrine (Neo-Synephrine) and Methoxamine (Vasoxyl)

ACTIONS. Phenylephrine and methoxamine are noncatecholamine drugs that have alpha$_1$-adrenergic receptor stimulating properties. They vasoconstrict renal, splanchnic, cutaneous, and muscular vascular beds but generally do not change or only slightly increase coronary blood flow. The increased mean arterial pressure produced by these drugs causes a reflex increase in vagal tone, which then slows heart rate and AV nodal conduction. In addition, direct alpha-adrenergic receptor stimulating effects on the heart may slow sinus node discharge rate to a slight degree.

CLINICAL USES

1. Phenylephrine and methoxamine are most commonly employed to treat paroxysmal supraventricular tachycardia. The hypertensive response increases vagal tone and may terminate the arrhythmia.
2. Hypotension caused by peripheral vasodilatation, such as occurs with ganglionic blocking agents or spinal anesthesia, may be reversed by phenylephrine or methoxamine.
3. These agents are not indicated in the treatment of cardiogenic shock.

ADMINISTRATION

1. The doses of phenylephrine and methoxamine should be titrated by clinical response, and intravenous dosing is usually recommended.
2. Phenylephrine is administered as 0.5 mg to 1.0 mg intravenous or 5 mg to 10 mg intramuscular following an initial test dose of 0.1 mg.
3. Methoxamine is administered as 5 mg to 10 mg intravenous or 10 mg to 20 mg intramuscular.

SIDE EFFECTS AND TOXICITY. Excessive dosage may produce headache, excessive hypertension, marked bradycardia, and vomiting.

PRECAUTIONS
1. To reduce the risk of excessive hypertension, systolic blood pressure should be continuously monitored during drug administration.
2. These agents should not be administered to hypertensive patients for treatment of paroxysmal supraventricular tachycardia.
3. In most cases there are now safer and more effective methods, such as verapamil, for termination of paroxysmal supraventricular tachycardia.

Alpha-Adrenergic Blocking Agents

Alpha-adrenergic blocking agents directly and selectively block the stimulation of alpha-adrenergic receptors. Effects are most prominent in peripheral vascular beds when vasoconstrictor responses are inhibited and vasodilatation results. Alpha-adrenergic blocking agents may accelerate heart rate either by reflex effects from peripheral vasodilatation or direct effects resulting from cardiac alpha$_2$ receptor inhibition, which increases norepinephrine release. The alpha-adrenergic blocking agents discussed here are phenoxybenzamine (Dibenzyline) and phentolamine (Regitine Prazosin (Minipress), the most commonly used and perhaps the most potent oral alpha-adrenergic blocker, is discussed in the section on vasodilators. Phenoxybenzamine and prazosin inhibit alpha$_1$ receptors and phentolamine inhibits both alpha$_1$ and alpha$_2$ receptors.

Clinical Uses
1. Alpha-adrenergic blocking agents are indicated to inhibit excessive alpha-adrenergic stimulation that occurs either from an endogenous source, as during treatment of pheochromocytoma, or from an exogenous source, as when catecholamines are administered to treat shock.
2. Alpha-adrenergic blockers also have been used as direct vasodilators to reverse peripheral vasoconstriction that accompanies low cardiac output states, systemic hypertension, and peripheral vascular insufficiency.

Administration. Phenoxybenzamine, although poorly absorbed, is effective orally and usually administered at doses of 20 mg to 200 mg/day. Phenoxybenzamine and phentolamine may be used intravenously, phenoxybenzamine in a dose of 1.0 mg/kg, infused over 1 hour in a glucose or saline solution, and phentolamine in titrated doses of 5 mg.

Side Effects and Toxicity
1. As with all vasodilators, blood pressure may fall precipitously. Maintenance of adequate volume status minimizes part of this problem.
2. Other side effects of alpha-adrenergic blockers include acceleration of heart rate, miosis (constriction of pupil), nasal stuffiness, inhibition of ejaculation, sedation, nausea, and vomiting.
3. Phentolamine has direct gastrointestinal actions that may cause abdominal pain and exacerbation of peptic ulcer disease.

Beta-Adrenergic Blocking Agents

Beta-adrenergic blocking agents act by competitive inhibition of adrenergic neuronal or hormonal action at the beta receptor. As a result of specific receptor interaction in the heart, beta-adrenergic blocking agents inhibit the increases in heart rate, AV nodal conduction and myocardial contractility that result from beta-receptor stimulation. In addition, beta-adrenergic blocking agents inhibit bronchodilatation, peripheral vasodilatation, and renin release induced by adrenergic stimulation. Although these are their most common, clinically significant effects, beta-adrenergic blocking agents act in all organs to inhibit the effects of beta-receptor stimulation.

Propranolol was the first beta-adrenergic antagonist to achieve widespread clinical use, but there are now multiple agents available, all having the primary effect of blocking beta receptors. Difference in clinical pharmacologic effects of these agents may be categorized according to their relative selectivity for beta$_1$ receptors, intrinsic agonist activity, relative lipid solubility, and membrane-stabilizing effects. Each agent also has a unique pharmacokinetic profile and potency that determine dosage strength and administration schedule. These properties of the available beta-adrenergic blocking agents are listed in Table 10-2.

The term *cardioselectivity* is used to describe a beta blocker that has predominant effects on beta$_1$ receptors and therefore has its major effects on the heart. The most common clinical advantage of cardioselectivity is that there is less inhibition of bronchodilatation and vasodilatation, effects mediated primarily by beta$_2$ receptors. Therefore cardioselective agents may lower the potential for precipitation of bronchospasm in patients with chronic lung disease. A theoretic disadvantage of cardioselective agents is that catecholamine-induced potassium release from skeletal muscle and excretion is not blocked, and hypokalemia may be more frequent with these agents. The clinical significance of this effect has not been established firmly. Selectivity for beta$_1$- or beta$_2$-receptor inhibition is relative, and higher doses of cardioselective agents also produce inhibition at beta$_2$ receptor sites. In addition, there is not complete segregation or different beta-receptor subtypes in each organ; thus, for example, about 15%-20% of cardiac beta receptors are comprised of beta$_2$ receptors. The current cardioselective beta antagonists include atenolol, metoprolol, and acebutolol, and the nonselective antagonists include propranolol, nadolol, timolol, and pindolol.

TABLE 10-2. Clinical features of beta-adrenergic blocking drugs

Drug	Usual Dosage	Cardio-selective	Intrinsic Agonist Activity	Membrane Stabilizing Effects	Hydrophilic
Propranolol (Inderal)	Oral: 40-480 mg/day in 2 to 4 doses Intravenous: up to 0.10-0.15 mg/kg given as 1 mg increments at 3-5 minute intervals	−	−	+	−
Metoprolol (Lopressor)	Oral: 50-100 mg BID	+	−	−	−
Nadolol (Corgard)	Oral: 40-160 mg once a day	−	−	−	+
Atenolol (Tenormin)	Oral: 50-100 mg once a day	+	−	−	+
Timolol (Blocadren)	Oral: 10-20 mg BID	−	−	−	−
Pindolol (Visken)	Oral: 5-30 mg BID	−	+	−	−
Acebutolol (Sectral)	Oral: 200-600 mg BID	+	+	+	+

+ = present; − = absent

When a drug occupies a receptor site, thereby blocking that receptor site to its usual agonist, the drug itself may possess weak agonist activity. This feature, termed *intrinsic agonist activity,* occurs with pindolol and acebutolol. One example of the clinical effects of intrinsic agonist activity is that these agents inhibit an exercise-induced increase in heart rate but have a minimal effect on resting heart rate as compared to other beta-adrenergic antagonists, which do not possess this activity. This property may confer a slight advantage on these agents in some clinical situations such as the treatment of hypertension; however, intrinsic agonist activity appears to preclude the use of these agents for the treatment of angina pectoris and in prophylaxis following myocardial infarction.

Beta-adrenergic blocking agents may be classified as primarily lipid soluble (lipophilic) or water soluble (hydrophilic). The potential importance of this property derives from the suggestion that hydrophilic compounds are less able than lipophilic compounds to cross the blood-brain barrier and so have fewer side effects on the central nervous system. Lastly, propranolol and acebutolol appear to possess membrane-stabilizing effects, which are direct effects on membrane action potentials similar to those produced by quinidine or other local anesthetics. At best, these effects probably play a minor role in the antiarrhythmic potential of beta-adrenergic blocking agents. For example, in the case of propranolol, these effects are present only at very high drug concentrations.

Clinical Uses. Beta-adrenergic blocking agents are used most often in the treatment of angina pectoris, cardiac arrhythmias, systemic hypertension and as prophylactic agents to reduce mortality following myocardial infarction.

Additional uses include the treatment of hypertrophic cardiomyopathy, the cardiovascular manifestations of hyperthyroidism, and anxiety states.

1. *Angina pectoris:* The goal in treatment is to decrease myocardial oxygen demands. This is accomplished primarily by lowering heart rate but also by decreasing myocardial contractility. Clinical effects appear additive to those of nitrates. The usual goal is to lower resting heart rate to 50 to 60/minute and to blunt the heart rate response to exercise.
2. *Arrhythmias:* Usual indications are to control the ventricular response to atrial flutter or fibrillation and to terminate and prevent recurrences of paroxysmal supraventricular tachycardia. Beta blockers are useful in treating selected ventricular arrhythmias, such as some arrhythmias induced by exercise, and in some of the arrhythmias caused by digitalis toxicity.
3. *Post–myocardial infarction:* Some beta-adrenergic blockers reduce mortality for up to 3 years following myocardial infarction.[10] Currently available agents indicated for this use are timolol (Blocadren), metoprolol (Lopressor), and propranolol (Inderal).

Side Effects and Toxicity

1. The most prominent adverse side-effects of beta-adrenergic blocking therapy are decreased myocardial contractility, heart failure, sinus bradycardia, asystole, AV block, bronchospasm, fatigue, impotence, insomnia, nightmares, and hypoglycemia in patients with diabetes.
2. Rebound effect refers to a syndome of an apparent increased sensitivity to catecholamines that follows

the discontinuation of beta-adrenergic blocking drugs. In patients who have ischemic heart disease, abrupt cessation of beta-adrenergic blocker therapy may produce angina pectoris, myocardial infarction, and arrhythmias. It is unclear whether slowly decreasing the dose of beta blocker prior to discontinuation would completely obviate this rebound syndrome.

Nursing Implications

1. It is useful to instruct patients about the possible side effects of beta-blocking drugs.
2. Patients should be cautioned that discontinuing beta-blocking drugs abruptly can cause "rebound" syndrome.

ANTICOAGULANTS

Anticoagulants inhibit the action or formation of one or more of the clotting factors and are used to prevent and treat a variety of thromboembolic disorders. Heparin and warfarin sodium (Coumadin) are the most widely used anticoagulants.

Precise indications for anticoagulation are unclear in many clinical situations. For example it has been suggested that anticoagulant therapy has beneficial results during acute myocardial infarction, but to date no randomized, controlled study has shown an improvement in mortality with the use of anticoagulants. It is clear, however, that anticoagulation reduces the incidence of venous thromboembolism, especially in the presence of heart failure. Low-dose subcutaneous heparin (10,000 units/day), which does not prolong clotting time, appears to decrease the incidence of venous thromboembolism and is currently recommended for most patients during the initial days of infarction when bed rest is prescribed.

Anticoagulant therapy in doses sufficient to significantly affect clotting factors is generally recommended for (1) demonstrated thromboembolism, either venous or arterial, (2) prevention of thrombosis and thromboembolic events in some patients after prosthetic valve surgery or prior to elective cardioversion of atrial fibrillation, and (3) when chronic atrial fibrillation is accompanied by mitral valve disease or congestive heart failure.

Heparin

Heparin is a naturally occurring substance, but its physiologic role has not been completely elucidated. In pharmacologic doses, heparin predominantly affects blood coagulation and blood lipids. Heparin inhibits thrombin and fibrin formation by complex mechanisms and produces prolongation of clotting time, prothrombin time, and thrombin time. Heparin also inhibits platelet aggregation induced by thrombin. Heparin clears plasma lipids by ac-

tivating lipoprotein lipase, although the clinical significance of this action is not fully established.

Clinical Uses

1. Heparin is administered intravenously or subcutaneously. Oral administration is ineffective, and intramuscular administration is usually not recommended because it may produce local hemorrhage.
2. Anticoagulant doses of heparin are determined by clotting time or activated partial thromboplastin time, both of which are maintained at 1½ to 2½ times the control values. Continuous infusion of heparin is associated with fewer hemorrhagic side effects than intermittent injection, since with the former a more stable anticoagulant effect is maintained.

Administration

The dosage of heparin varies with the method of administration.

1. Continuous infusion: 20,000 to 40,000 units/day; infusion is begun after a loading dose of 5000 units, and an increase in dosage should be initiated by a loading dose.
2. Intermittent dosage 5000 to 10,000 units every 4 to 6 hours.
3. Low-dosage heparin: 5000 units subcutaneously every 12 hours.
4. Heparin disappearance rate is proportional to the dose administered as larger doses have a longer half-life. Anticoagulant effects of a single intravenous dose of heparin last an average of 3 to 4 hours.
5. Heparin is the preferred anticoagulant in pregnant or lactating women because it does not cross the placenta or appear in maternal milk.

Side Effects and Toxicity

1. Hemorrhage is the predominant side effect, and heparin is contraindicated in the presence of active bleeding or hemorrhagic tendencies. The occurrence of hemorrhage during heparin therapy should initiate a search for a pathologic bleeding site.
2. Other side effects include thrombocytopenia, and, rarely, hypersensitivity or anaphylactic reactions.
3. Long-term heparin therapy has been associated with alopecia, osteoporosis, neuropathy, and priapism.
4. Anticoagulant effects of heparin are reversible by the administration of protamine sulfate. Doses of 1.0 to 1.5 mg protamine antagonize each 100 units of heparin, but the dose requirements fall quickly with time after the last heparin dose. In most cases discontinuation of heparin is sufficient therapy to correct anticoagulant effects.

Nursing Implications

1. If administered by continuous infusion, an infusion

pump is required. Other drugs should not be given in the same intravenous tubing.

2. Sites of subcutaneous administration should be varied.

3. Patients receiving full anticoagulation require special care in phlebotomy or any other procedure to avoid excess hemorrhage.

Warfarin Sodium (Coumadin)

Warfarin acts in the liver to inhibit the synthesis of vitamin K–dependent clotting factors, especially prothrombin. Effects take 24 hours or more to occur and anticoagulant effects of a single dose usually are not complete until at least 48 to 72 hours have elapsed.

Clinical Uses and Administration

1. When anticoagulation is required beyond a few days, warfarin is the treatment of choice because it is effective orally. Warfarin and heparin are often begun simultaneously, and then heparin is stopped once warfarin becomes effective.

2. The dosage of warfarin is individually determined based on the results of prothrombin time, which should be stabilized at 1½ to 2½ times control value. Usual dosage ranges from 2 to 15 mg/day.

3. Currently it is recommended that warfarin be given in a daily dose of 10 to 15 mg/day until therapeutic prolongation of prothrombin time occurs, rather than administering a large initial loading dose.

4. Peak effects on prothrombin time require 36 to 72 hours and duration of effect is 4 to 5 days.

Precautions

1. Drug and disease interactions are important features of warfarin therapy.

2. Anticoagulant effects of warfarin are enhanced in the presence of hepatic disease, vitamin K deficiency, heart failure, broad-spectrum antibiotics, salicylates, quinidine, anabolic steroids, chloral hydrate, clofibrate, phenylbutazone, thyroxin, indomethacin, tolbutamide, methyldopa, diazoxide, alcohol, allopurinol, and amiodarone, to name a few.

3. Anticoagulant effects are decreased by glucocorticoids, vitamin K, barbiturates, oral contraceptives, antacids, antihistamines, and others.

4. Warfarin crosses the placenta and appears in maternal milk, so there is danger of hemorrhage in utero or in nursing infants.

Side Effects and Toxicity

1. Hemorrhage occurs in 2% to 4% of patients who receive warfarin anticoagulation and may be life-threatening. Hemorrhage from nearly any source is possible; cutaneous, oral, gastrointestinal, genitourinary, or central nervous system hemorrhages are the most common. All patients receiving Coumadin need frequent monitoring and close surveillance of prothrombin time to detect changes in hepatic function or drug therapy that may affect prothrombin time or influence the metabolism of warfarin.

2. Hemorrhage is treated by reduction or withdrawal of warfarin dose and, if necessary, reversal of anticoagulant effects by intravenous vitamin K or fresh frozen plasma.

3. The existence of a "rebound" hypercoagulable state after rapid reversal of warfarin is controversial but should argue against the routine use of vitamin K to dissipate effects.

Nursing Implications

1. It is mandatory that patients receiving oral anticoagulation be given careful instructions concerning the signs of hemorrhage, the potential drug interactions, limitations on alcohol use, dose information, and a plan for monitoring the prothrombin time.

2. Patient identification cards indicating use of an anticoagulant may be useful.

THROMBOLYTIC AGENTS

Anticoagulants prevent formation of new clots but do not dissolve formed thrombi. Thrombolytic agents act directly to lyse formed thrombi and offer therapeutic advantages in certain situations.[11] Two drugs are available: streptokinase, which is derived from enzymes of the streptococcus, and urokinase, a substance found in human urine. Both activate the fibrinolytic system. Urokinase is very expensive and for the most part its use is limited to patients who are hypersensitive or show intolerance to streptokinase. New thrombolytic agents are in various stages of clinical development. At present, the most prominent of these is tissue plasminogen activator (t-PA), which can be synthesized by techniques of human gene cloning. Tissue plasminogen activator has potential advantages over streptokinase and urokinase both in terms of efficacy and because t-PA does not produce a systemic thrombolytic state.

Thrombolytic therapy of acute myocardial infarction is a rapidly evolving area of clinical use and investigation. The rationale for thrombolytic treatment of acute myocardial infarction derives from observations that intracoronary thrombosis is a frequent event in totally occluded coronary arteries during the initial period of myocardial infarction. The basis of this therapy is the assumption that restoration of flow in a previously occluded coronary artery early enough in the course of myocardial infarction will salvage acutely ischemic myocardium before irreversible necrosis is complete. Thrombolytic therapy restores the patency of previously occluded coronary arteries, and although acutely ischemic myocardium may be salvaged in some cases, definite demonstration of a reduction in the size of the infarction or in mortality awaits further study.

Clinical Uses

1. At present, streptokinase is the thrombolytic agent employed most often. Urokinase is generally reserved for patients who have known antibodies or hypersensitivity to streptokinase. There are several newer agents, such as t-PA, which may provide useful alternatives to streptokinase.
2. Intracoronary thrombolytic therapy involves the infusion of a thrombolytic agent directly into the occluded coronary artery that results in an acute ischemic event. Coronary patency is restored in 80% to 90% of cases.
3. Intravenous streptokinase, particularly when given in high doses, reestablishes coronary artery patency in 50% to 80% of cases of acute myocardial infarction.
4. Two central factors in determining efficacy of thrombolytic treatment are the ability to restore patency and the time elapsed from onset of ischemia until restoration of patency. Intracoronary streptokinase more often restores patency but intravenous streptokinase can be administered more quickly without the need for complete cardiac catheterization laboratory facilities.
5. Other indications for streptokinase or urokinase are in treatment of acute pulmonary embolism, acute deep venous or arterial thrombosis and acute occlusion of arterial cannulae.

Administration

Use in Acute Myocardial Infarction

1. Intracoronary streptokinase: bolus infusion of 20,000 IU followed by 2000 IU/min maintenance for up to one hour or until patency is established.
2. Intravenous streptokinase: 500,000 to 1.7 million units over 30 to 60 minutes. Usual dose is 750,000 IU over 30 minutes.
3. Thrombolytic treatment of acute myocardial infarction should be instituted within 6, and preferably 4, hours of the onset of ischemia.

Other Indications

1. Streptokinase: loading dose of 250,000 IU over 30 minutes followed by 100,000 IU/hr.
2. Urokinase: loading dose 2000 IU/lb over 10 minutes followed by 2000 IU/lb/hr.

Adverse Effects and Toxicity

1. For all thrombolytic agents, bleeding is a potentially significant complication. Bleeding most often occurs from sites of recent thrombus formation and even "clot specific" agents such as t-PA have this hemodynamic potential.
2. Every precaution should be taken to screen for potential contraindication to thrombolytic therapy and to avoid the potential for hemorrhage complications.
3. Allergic reactions ranging from mild urticaria to potentially fatal anaphylaxis can occur with streptokinase.
4. Fever is common following streptokinase.

Precautions and Contraindications

1. Active or recent internal hemorrhage, recent surgery, recent cerebrovascular accident, recent CPR or trauma, intracranial neoplasm, and severe hypertension are some of the potential contraindications to thrombolytic treatment.
2. Precautions during thrombolytic therapy include the following:
   a. avoid arterial punctures
   b. minimize venipunctures; apply compressive dressings to venipuncture sites
   c. discontinue parenteral drug administration
   d. avoid concurrent anticoagulation or antiplatelet treatment

DRUGS AFFECTING PLATELET FUNCTION

Both the demonstrated and the hypothesized effects of platelets suggest that these blood elements play an important role in several cardiovascular disorders, including the genesis of atherosclerotic plaque, coronary artery thrombosis, coronary spasm, and arterial thromboembolism. Therefore drugs that interfere with platelet function are potentially valuable therapeutic agents. Antiplatelet drugs include aspirin, sulfinpyrazone (Anturane), and dipyridamole (Persantine).

These agents, in part, prolong platelet survival and interfere with the metabolism of prostaglandins and thromboxane, agents that affect the ability of platelets to "clump" and initiate thrombosis. Effects on the prostaglandins contained in vascular endothelium may also influence the net result of antiplatelet drugs.

Clinical Uses

1. Clinical observations and therapeutic trials have suggested that aspirin, sulfinpyrazone, and dipyridamole may have beneficial effects in certain arterial thromboembolic disorders.
2. Aspirin has decreased the incidence of thrombotic stroke in men who have carotid artery disease and is indicated to treat cerebral transient ischemic attacks.
3. Aspirin, at doses of 325 to 1300 mg/day (1 to 4

tablets) in patients with unstable angina syndromes decreased subsequent cardiac mortality, sudden cardiac death, and the incidence of acute myocardial infarction, for up to 2 years.

4. Aspirin and Persantine may be therapeutic in maintaining the patency of saphenous vein coronary artery bypass grafts.
5. The results of several large studies using aspirin, Persantine, sulfinpyrazone in post–myocardial infarction patients do not show a significant decrease in overall mortality for treatment groups.
6. Aspirin and Persantine may play an adjunctive role in decreasing the risk of thromboembolic events in patients with prosthetic cardiac valves.

Side Effects and Toxicity

1. These agents have a relatively high incidence of intolerable side effects, the most common of which are gastrointestinal distress and bleeding.
2. The presence of active peptic ulcer disease, gastrointestinal bleeding, or known hypersensitivity are contraindications for use of these agents.

ANTIARRHYTHMIC DRUGS

An increasing number of antiarrhythmic drugs have become available for general clinical or investigative use.[3,7] Specific electrophysiologic and pharmacologic features of these agents are presented in Tables 10-3 and 10-4. This discussion focuses on selected clinical aspects of the use of these agents.

Lidocaine

Ease of administration, a wide range of clinical efficacy, and the infrequency of major adverse side effects make lidocaine the first drug of choice for emergency treatment to terminate or prevent ventricular tachycardia or ventricular fibrillation. Lidocaine is especially useful in treating ventricular arrhythmia complicating acute myocardial infarction and digitalis toxicity.

Electrophysiologic Effects

1. Clinically used doses of lidocaine produce little or no effect on usual ECG or clinical electrophysiologic parameters.
2. Cellular electrophysiologic studies indicate that lidocaine inhibits the fast inward sodium current and thus decreases the maximum rate of depolarization. These effects are particularly noted in ischemic tissue or when the frequency of stimulation is increased while effects on normal, resting cells are minimal.
3. Lidocaine decreases action potential duration but prolongs the time to recovery of maximum rate of depolarization.

Pharmacokinetics

1. Lidocaine is metabolized in the liver and its rate of metabolism is dependent on hepatic blood flow. Therefore conditions like heart failure, which decreases hepatic blood flow, may significantly decrease metabolism.

TABLE 10-3. Clinical electrophysiologic effects of antiarrhythmic agents

	Sinus Rate	PR	QRS	QT	A-H	H-V	ERP AV Node	ERP His-Purkinje	ERP Atrium	ERP Ventricle
			Intervals							
Lidocaine	0	0	0	0	0, ↓	0	0, ↓	0, ↑	0	0
Quinidine	0, ↑	0, ↑	↑	↑	↓ ↑	0, ↑	↓ ↑	0, ↑	↑	↑
Procainamide	0	0, ↑	↑	↑	0, ↑	0, ↑	0, ↑	0, ↑	↑	↑
Disopyramide	0, ↑	0, ↑	↑	↑	↓ ↑	0, ↑	↓ ↑	0, ↑	↑	↑
Phenytoin	0	0	0	0, ↓	0	0	0, ↓	↓	0	0
Propranolol	↓	0, ↑	0	0, ↓	0, ↑	0	↑	0	0	0
Bretylium	0, ↑	0	0	0	0	0	↓	0,	0, ↓	0, ↓
Amiodarone	↓	↑	0, ↑	↑	↑	0, ↑	↑	↑	↑	↑
Flecainide	0	↑	↑	↑	↑	↑	0	0, ↑	0, ↑	
Encainide	0	↑	↑	↑	↑	↑	↑	↑	↑	↑
Mexiletine	0	0	0	0	0, ↑	0, ↑	0, ↑	0, ↑	0	0
Tocainide	0	0	0	0, ↓	0	0	0, ↓	0	↓	↓
Propafenone	0	↑	↑	0	↑	↑	↑	↑	↑	↑

ERP = effective refractory period; ↑ = increase; ↓ decrease; 0 = no change.

TABLE 10-4. Clinical pharmacology of antiarrhythmic drugs

Agent	Administration and Dosage	Elimination Half-Life (T½)	Usual Plasma Concentrations	Comments
Lidocaine	IV: Load: 2 mg/kg Maintenance: 1-4 mg/min	100 min	1.5-6 µg/ml	Clearance depends on hepatic perfusion
Quinidine	IV: Load: 0.5 mg/kg/min Average loading dose: 9 mg/kg Oral: 1200-2400 mg/day	6-11 hr	3-5 µg/ml	Active metabolites Anticholinergic effects
Procainamide	IV: Load: 10-15 mg/kg at 20-50 mg/min Maintenance: 2-6 mg/min Oral: 2-8 gm/day	3-4 hr 6 hr for sustained release form	4-8 µg/ml	Active metabolite, NAPA, accumulates in renal insufficiency
Disopyramide	Oral: 400-1200 mg/day	4-8 hr 8-12 hr for sustained release form	3-8 µg/ml	Anticholinergic effects
Tocainide	Oral: 1200-1800 mg/day	12 hr	6-12 µg/ml	Electrophysiologic effects similar to lidocaine
Propranolol	IV: 0.1 mg/kg in 1 mg increments Oral: 40-1000 mg/day	4 hr	>40 µg/ml	Beta-adrenergic antagonist
Verapamil	IV: 5-10 mg bolus Oral: 240-480 mg/day	3-7 hr	15-100 mg/ml	Ca^{++} channel antagonist alpha-adrenergic antagonist
Bretylium	IV: Load: 5-10 mg/kg Maintenance: 1-2 mg/min	8-10 hr	0.8-2.4 µg/ml	Biphasic adrenergic effects: initial adrenergic agonist effect followed by depressant effects
Phenytoin	IV: Load: 12 mg/kg at 20 mg/min Oral: Load: 900-1200 mg/24 hr Maintenance: 300-400 mg/day	24 hr	10-20 µg/ml	Nonlinear kinetics
Amiodarone	IV: 2.3 mg/kg × 12 hr, then 0.7 mg/min × 36 hr Oral: Load: 800-1600 mg/day × 7-10 days Maintenance: 200-400 mg/day	45-60 days during chronic therapy	1.5-3.5 µg/ml	Antiadrenergic effects
Flecainide	Oral: 200-600 mg/day	16-20 hr	0.2-1.0 µg/ml	New antiarrhythmic agent with "local anesthetic" effects
Mexiletine	Oral: 600-1200 mg/day	12 hr	0.5-2 µg/ml	Effects similar to lidocaine
Encainide	Oral: 100-240 mg/day	3-4 hr	variable	Active metabolites account for much of antiarrhythmic effects
Propafenone	Oral: 450-900 mg/day	3-6 hr	0.2-3.0 µg/ml	Nonlinear kinetics; has weak beta blocking effects

2. Plasma elimination half-life in normal averages 100 minutes is prolonged to 4 to 10 hours in heart failure or shock.
3. Usual effective plasma levels are 2 to 6 µg/ml; levels above 10 µg/ml usually produce toxicity.

Administration

1. The usual loading dose of 1.5 to 2.0 mg/kg is administered over 20 to 30 minutes followed by a maintenance infusion of 2 to 4 mg/min.
2. Dose requirements are decreased in elderly patients, and in patients suffering from heart failure, shock, and severe liver disease. Dose requirements are only minimally affected by renal function.

Side Effects and Toxicity

1. Neurologic side effects, which are related to dosage and plasma concentration, predominate. These include paresthesias, confusion, slurred speech, tremors, and convulsions.
2. The risk of neurologic toxicity appears additive with other agents such as procainamide or mexiletine, which have central nervous system effects.
3. Lidocaine may aggravate preexisting AV conduction or sinus node disorders. It may occasionally worsen preexisting heart failure.

Nursing Implications

1. Neurologic toxicity from lidocaine is relatively com-

mon, so nursing staff should be particularly alert for any change in neurologic status.

2. The neurologic effects of lidocaine may be subtle or incorrectly attributed to other causes in intensive care unit patients.

Quinidine

Quinidine is an effective agent for a variety of ventricular and supraventricular arrhythmias, including symptomatic premature ventricular complexes, recurrent ventricular tachycardia, recurrent atrial fibrillation or flutter, and recurrent paroxysmal supraventricular tachycardia.

Electrophysiologic Effects

1. Quinidine produces direct cardiac effects, similar to many other agents classified as "local anesthetic" agents; it also has indirect effects mediated through the autonomic nervous system.
2. Direct cellular electrophysiologic effects of quinidine include a decrease in the rate of the rise and amplitude of action potentials, increase in the action potential duration and effective refractory period, and a decrease in the rate of spontaneous depolarization.
3. On the ECG, quinidine mildly prolongs the QRS duration and prolongs QT interval. Clinical electrophysiologic effects include prolongation of HV interval and refractoriness of atrium and ventricle.
4. Indirect effects of quinidine include anticholinergic and alpha-adrenergic blocking properties, which may result in atropine-like effects on the sinus and AV node and produce peripheral vasodilatation.

Pharmacokinetics

1. Quinidine is primarily metabolized by the liver and has at least one active metabolite.
2. Different preparations of quinidine vary in the time of absorption and elimination. For quinidine sulfate the elimination half-life averages 6 hours but with wide variability (from 3 to 16 hours) among patients.
3. Although quinidine is minimally affected by changes in renal function, active metabolites accumulate in renal failure, so dose adjustments may be necessary.
4. The usual effective plasma concentrations of quinidine are from 3 to 6 μg/ml.

Administration (Table 10-5)

1. Quinidine is usually administered orally, and familiarity with its various formulations is important.
2. The usual oral dose of quinidine sulfate ranges from 200 to 600 mg every 6 hours.
3. The usual intravenous dose of quinidine gluconate is 9 mg/kg at a rate of 0.5 mg/kg/min.

TABLE 10-5. Quinidine preparations

Formulation	Dose (mg)	Quinidine Base (mg)
Quinidine sulfate	300	250
Quinidine gluconate	324	200
Quinidine polygalacturonate	275	200

Side Effects and Toxicity

1. Chronic quinidine treatment is associated with limiting side effects in 30% or more of patients. The most common side effects include nausea, diarrhea, headache, dizziness, ringing in the ears, fever, skin rash, thrombocytopenia, hemolytic anemia, and anaphylaxis.
2. Quinidine may induce or exacerbate ventricular arrhythmia despite low or "therapeutic" plasma levels. These drug-induced arrhythmias frequently appear as a polymorphic ventricular tachycardia termed *torsade de pointes,* which occurs in the setting of a prolonged QT interval.
3. At toxic doses, in the setting of elevated plasma quinidine concentrations, quinidine excessively prolongs QRS interval, may produce AV block and ventricular arrhythmias.
4. The alpha-adrenergic blocking effects of quinidine may result in hypotension, particularly in patients receiving nitrates, other vasodilators, or diuretics.
5. Intravenous quinidine has a significant potential to produce hypotension and possibly to aggravate arrhythmias.
6. Quinidine interacts with digoxin to elevate digoxin plasma concentrations and produce signs of digitalis toxicity.

Nursing Implications

1. The nursing staff must be alert to the particular forms of quinidine prescribed for each patient (Table 10-5).
2. Attention must be paid to concomitant medications such as digoxin, antacids, laxatives, nitrates, vasodilators, and diuretics.
3. The occurrence of new arrhythmias or excessive prolongation of QRS or QT interval may be signs of quinidine toxicity.

Procainamide

Procainamide is a versatile antiarrhythmic drug used intravenously for immediate treatment and orally for chronic treatment of supraventricular and ventricular arrhythmias. The electrophysiologic actions of procainamide are similar to those of quinidine, and indications for procainamide treatment likewise are identical to those of quinidine.

Pharmacokinetics

1. Renal excretion accounts for 40% to 60% of procainamide elimination with the remainder caused by liver metabolism and the formation of an active metabolite, *N*-acetyl procainamide (NAPA).
2. Plasma levels of procainamide and NAPA increase significantly with impairment of renal function.
3. The plasma elimination half-life of procainamide is 3 to 4 hours, and therapeutic plasma concentrations range from 4 to 10 µg/ml. Occasionally higher plasma concentrations are tolerated and effective.
4. Slow-release preparations of procainamide permit 6-hour dosing intervals.

Administration

1. Oral: 2 to 8 g/day in divided doses.
2. Intravenous: loading dose of 10 to 20 mg/kg at 20 to 50 mg/min.
Maintenance dose of 2 to 6 mg/min.

Side Effects and Toxicity

1. Chronic procainamide therapy is frequently associated with adverse side effects. These include gastrointestinal intolerance, skin rash, and, rarely, agranulocytosis.
2. Long-term treatment is associated with a positive antinuclear antibody titer in 70% to 80% of patients, and drug-induced lupus syndrome occurs in 10% to 20% of patients. This syndrome includes fever, arthralgia, and pleural pericarditis.
3. Procainamide may induce polymorphic ventricular tachycardia, similar to that occurring during quinidine treatment.
4. Procainamide may worsen congestive heart failure and in toxic doses may prolong or block atrioventricular and intraventricular conduction.
5. Intravenous procainamide administration may produce systemic hypotension that necessitates either slowing the rate of infusion or discontinuing it. Hypotension usually responds to saline infusion.

Disopyramide

Disopyramide is available as an oral antiarrhythmic drug for ventricular and supraventricular arrhythmias. It appears to be as effective as quinidine or procainamide.

Electrophysiologic Effects

1. Direct cellular electrophysiologic effects of disopyramide are similar to those of procainamide and quinidine.
2. In addition to direct effects, disopyramide has sig-nificant anticholinergic or atropine-like effects that may modify its clinical electrophysiologic profile. For example, the anticholinergic effects may result in the acceleration of the sinus rate or in the enhancement of AV node conduction.

Pharmacokinetics

1. Above 40% to 70% of a dose of disopyramide is excreted unchanged in urine, so dose adjustments are required during renal insufficiency.
2. The usual elimination half-life with normal renal function ranges from 6 to 9 hours.
3. Usual therapeutic plasma concentrations of disopyramide range from 2 to 4 µg/ml.
4. A controlled-release preparation of disopyramide that permits dosing at intervals of 8 to 12 hours is available.

Administration

1. Disopyramide is currently available only in the oral form.
2. The usual oral dosage ranges from 400 to 1200 mg/day administered every 6 to 8 hours for the standard form and every 8 to 12 hours for the controlled-release form.

Side Effects and Toxicity

1. Disopyramide has frequent, clinically significant, and potentially dangerous adverse effects.
2. The significant inotropic effect of disopyramide is a relative contraindication to its use in the presence of heart failure.
3. Disopyramide may aggravate ventricular arrhythmias in a manner similar to quinidine and procainamide.
4. The most frequent symptomatic side effects relate to the anticholinergic properties of disopyramide and include dry mouth, urinary hesitancy or retention, or constipation. Preliminary evidence suggests these side effects may be significantly diminished by the concurrent use of cholinesterase inhibitors, such as pyridostigmine.
5. In toxic doses, heart failure, electrical-mechanical association, excessive QRS and QT prolongation, and abnormalities of atrial ventricular and intraventricular conduction may occur.

Nursing Implications

1. QRS, QT intervals, and cardiac rhythms should be monitored for possible signs of disopyramide toxicity.
2. The anticholinergic effects of disopyramide, particularly urinary retention in elderly men, require careful monitoring.

Bretylium

Bretylium is an intravenous drug useful for the emergency treatment of recurrent ventricular tachycardia and ventricular fibrillation.

Electrophysiologic Effects

1. Bretylium has direct cellular electrophysiologic effects and complex, clinically significant interactions with the sympathetic nervous system.
2. Direct cellular electrophysiologic effects include a prolongation of action potential duration and effective refractory periods.
3. Interaction with the sympathetic nervous system appears to be twofold. Initially bretylium releases norepinephrine from adrenergic nerve endings, thereby producing effects similar to an adrenergic agonist. These effects last approximately 30 minutes.
4. The later effect is to block the uptake of release norepinephrine and to prevent the release of norepinephrine during sympathetic nerve depolarization. This later effect produces adrenergic blockade and accounts for the orthostatic hypotension that occurs with bretylium.

Pharmacokinetics

1. Bretylium is primarily excreted in kidneys so dose adjustments are required in the presence of renal insufficiency.
2. The plasma elimination half-life of bretylium averages 6 to 8 hours in patients with normal renal function.

Administration

1. Bretylium is administered intravenously with an initial dose of 5 to 10 mg/kg, repeated at 30 minute intervals up to a total dose of 30 mg/kg.
2. If maintenance therapy is required after the loading dose, an infusion rate of 1 to 2 mg/minute is administered.

Side Effects and Toxicity

1. Initially, bretylium may act as an adrenergic agonist producing increases in blood pressure, heart rate, and myocardial contractility.
2. More common during prolonged infusion are the effects secondary to adrenergic blockade, which include postural hypotension caused by peripheral vasodilatation. This effect may persist for hours or days after the discontinuation of bretylium.
3. Other side effects of bretylium include nausea, vomiting, and during prolonged therapy, severe parotid pain.

Nursing Implications. The severe orthostatic hypotension that usually accompanies chronic bretylium therapy often mandates complete bedrest. Syncope caused by hypotension may occur if patients sit or stand during bretylium treatment.

Flecainide

Flecainide has been approved recently as an antiarrhythmic drug for the treatment of ventricular arrhythmias.

Electrophysiologic Effects

1. The principal cellular effect of flecainide appears to be the slowing of the rate of rise of the cardiac action potential.
2. The most marked clinical electrophysiologic effect of flecainide is to slow atrial, AV nodal, His-Purkinje, and intraventricular conduction.
3. The usual ECG effects of flecainide are prolongation of the QRS interval and a slight prolongation of the PR interval.

Pharmacokinetics

1. Flecainide is principally eliminated by the kidneys. In patients who have heart disease, the elimination half-life averages 20 hours.
2. The average effective plasma concentration of flecainide is about 800 ng/ml with the usual therapeutic range from 300 to 1600 ng/ml. Adverse reactions seem more frequent as plasma concentrations are greater than 1000 ng/ml.

Clinical Uses

1. Flecainide is approved for use in the treatment of recurrent ventricular arrhythmias. It is useful for decreasing the number of ventricular extrasystoles and preventing the recurrence of ventricular tachycardia and ventricular fibrillation.
2. Although not approved for supraventricular arrhythmias, flecainide appears to be a very effective drug for treatment of Wolff-Parkinson-White syndrome. Flecainide often slows or blocks conduction in accessory pathways and slows atrioventricular conduction.
3. The usual dosage of flecainide is 100 to 200 mg taken orally twice a day.
4. Dosage of flecainide needs to be altered in patients who have renal insufficiency.

Side Effects and Toxicity

1. Flecainide decreases myocardial contractility and has significant potential to worsen congestive heart failure.
2. Flecainide also has significant potential to worsen preexisting arrhythmias or promote the appearance of new ventricular arrhythmias. In patients who have abnormal ventricular function and recurrent sus-

tained ventricular tachycardia, the incidence of these proarrhythmic effects of flecainide may approach 15%.

3. Other common side effects of flecainide include lightheadedness, blurred vision, dizziness, tremor, constipation, and pruritus. Usually these side effects are mild and resolve with reduction of dose or discontinuation of the drug.

Nursing Implications

1. Patients receiving flecainide should have continuous ECG monitoring during initiation of treatment. The QRS interval and PR interval should be measured regularly.

2. It is necessary to monitor patients carefully for potential proarrhythmic effects of flecainide. Increases in frequency of ventricular extrasystoles or new or more frequent appearance of episodes of ventricular tachycardia should raise questions of potential proarrhythmic effects of the drugs.

3. Patients should be observed for signs of worsening congestive heart failure while receiving flecainide.

Amiodarone (Cordarone)

Amiodarone has been recently approved for general use as an antiarrhythmic agent in the United States. During over 15 years of clinical experience, amiodarone has been found useful as an antiarrhythmic agent for the treatment of multiple supraventricular and ventricular arrhythmias, including recurrent paroxysmal atrial fibrillation, supraventricular arrhythmias associated with Wolff-Parkinson-White syndrome, as well as recurrent ventricular tachycardia and ventricular fibrillation.

Electrophysiology

1. The effects of amiodarone on cellular electrophysiology include prolongation of action potential duration and frequency-dependent decreases in the maximum rate of depolarization.

2. The clinical electrophysiologic effects include increased refractory periods of atria and ventricle, prolongation of AV nodal conduction time and refractory period and a decrease in spontaneous sinus node discharge rate. Amiodarone also increases refractory period and slows conduction in accessory pathways in patients with Wolff-Parkinson-White syndrome.

Pharmacokinetics

1. Amiodarone has unique pharmacokinetic properties. Early in its clinical use, it was noted to have a prolonged duration of action as well as a delayed onset of maximum antiarrhythmic effects.

2. After oral administration, 30% to 50% of a dose of amiodarone reaches the systemic circulation.

3. Amiodarone is metabolized in the liver and negli-

gible excretion is performed by the kidney. This suggests that its dose does not need to be altered in patients who have renal failure.

4. Amiodarone is eliminated very slowly with an elimination half-life that ranges from 30 to 60 days in most patients.

5. Measurement of amiodarone concentrations appears to be useful during chronic drug treatment. The usual effective plasma concentrations are from 1.5 to 3.5 $\mu g/ml$.

Administration

1. Because of its pharmacokinetic profile, it is recommended that amiodarone be dosed initially with a large loading phase lasting several days to weeks. The usual loading dose is from 800 to 1600 mg/day for 1 to 2 weeks.

2. Following the loading dose administration, the dosage of amiodarone is gradually decreased over the next month of treatment to establish a maintenance dosage that usually averages 400 mg/day.

3. Administration of maintenance dosages greater than 600 mg/day is often associated with drug toxicity. On the other hand, very low maintenance doses appear sufficient to maintain efficacy in some instances, and doses less than 200 mg/day or dosing for 5 of 7 days may be sufficient.

Side Effects and Toxicity

1. Amiodarone may produce a variety of adverse side effects, the most common of which are neurologic and gastrointestinal. These may include nausea, anorexia, tremor, ataxia, insomnia, weakness, and fatigue. Many are dose-related side effects that disappear upon dose reduction but rarely require drug discontinuation.

2. Pulmonary toxicity is a serious, life-threatening effect of amiodarone treatment. Estimates of the overall incidence of pulmonary toxicity have ranged from 2% to 15%. Pulmonary toxicity typically first appears as diffuse interstitial or alveolar infiltrates on chest radiography, accompanied by dyspnea, cough, fever, and malaise. Discontinuation of amiodarone is usually sufficient treatment. Although some patients have received glucocorticoids, the efficacy of these drugs is unproven.

3. Amiodarone has potentially adverse side effects on the heart which include the following:
   a. Administered orally, amiodarone may rarely produce a worsening of preexisting congestive heart failure.
   b. Amiodarone may worsen preexisting sinus node dysfunction or abnormalities of atrioventricular conduction.

c. Like other antiarrhythmic drugs, amiodarone may exacerbate ventricular arrhythmias and has been associated with the development of *torsade de pointes,* ventricular fibrillation, or incessant ventricular tachycardia.

4. A variety of other adverse effects, including hepatotoxicity, severe anorexia and weight loss, peripheral neuropathy, photosensitivity, blue skin discoloration, and abnormalities of thyroid function, may occur during amiodarone treatment.

5. Amiodarone interacts with many drugs, including digoxin, Coumadin, and other antiarrhythmic agents, doses of digoxin and Coumadin should be halved if they are administered with amiodarone. Reduction in doses of other concurrently administered antiarrhythmics may also be necessary to lower the risk of toxicity.

Nursing Implications

1. Patients should be informed of the potential toxicity of amiodarone. They should specifically be instructed to report any new symptoms and particularly any new pulmonary symptoms.

2. A well-defined follow-up program is necessary for patients receiving amiodarone. Frequent evaluations to determine optimum dose may be needed during the initial weeks or months of treatment. During follow-up patients should have regular chest x-rays to monitor for potential pulmonary toxicity.

3. Patients should be cautioned about concomitant use of digoxin, Coumadin, or other antiarrhythmic agents while taking amiodarone.

4. The potential for phototoxicity and blue skin discoloration appears greatest in lighter-skinned patients. Patients should be cautioned about sun exposure. The only method to completely prevent phototoxicity from amiodarone is to wear protective clothing or sun barriers such as zinc oxide.

Phenytoin (Dilantin)

Primarily an anticonvulsant agent, phenytoin has antiarrhythmic effects, especially in arrhythmias caused by digitalis toxicity and less commonly in arrhythmias associated with ischemic heart disease.

Electrophysiology

1. Phenytoin possesses direct cardiac cellular electrophysiologic effects similar to those of lidocaine.

2. Phenytoin also has indirect cardiac effects through its activity in the central nervous system, including a decrease in sympathetic nerve activity.

Pharmacokinetics

1. Phenytoin exhibits nonlinear plasma pharmacokinetics, that is, the relationship between plasma concentration and the administered dose is not linear, but the plasma concentration may rise disproportionately for a given increase in dose.

2. During long-term therapy it appears that single daily doses of phenytoin are adequate to maintain stable plasma levels. However, monitoring plasma drug levels is important, especially if dose adjustments are made.

3. Phenytoin is extensively metabolized by the liver. Its metabolism may be slowed significantly by liver disease or by drugs that compete with phenytoin for hepatic enzyme sites, such as phenothiazines or phenylbutazone. Phenytoin metabolism may be accelerated by agents such as barbituates, which induce hepatic microsomal enzymes.

4. The usual therapeutic plasma concentrations of phenytoin are from 10 to 20 μg/ml.

Administration. The usual oral dosage is 300 to 400 mg/day given as a single dose. For oral loading, the dosage is 300 mg/8 hours for three doses. Intravenously, the loading of phenytoin is 12 mg/kg infused at 20 mg/minute. The maintenance dose is 300 to 400 mg a day.

Side Effects and Toxicity

1. Phenytoin toxicity is usually manifested by central nervous system effects. Its severity usually correlates with plasma drug concentration.

2. Manifestations of toxicity include nystagmus, ataxia, drowsiness, lethargy, and coma.

3. Chronic phenytoin therapy has been associated with skin rash, megaloblastic anemia, lymphoid hyperplasia, gingival hyperplasia, and drug-induced systemic lupus erythematosis.

Nursing Implications

1. When administered intravenously, phenytoin should not be infused with 5% dextrose because crystalization occurs.

2. Patients receiving chronic phenytoin therapy should be instructed on how to maintain good oral hygiene.

3. Administration with food may lessen gastrointestinal distress associated with the drug.

Tocainide

Tocainide is a primary amine analog of lidocaine that is effective orally. Tocainide has recently been introduced for general clinical use in the United States for treatment of ventricular arrhythmias.

Electrophysiology

1. Clinical and experimental electrophysiologic effects of tocainide are very similar to those of lidocaine.

2. The electrophysiologic effects in man include shortening of refractory period of the atrium, AV node,

and right ventricle but minimum changes in AV conduction.

Clinical Pharmacokinetics

1. The elimination half-life of tocainide ranges from 10 to 17 hours with a mean of 13.5 hours. Therefore tocainide may be administered every 8 to 12 hours.
2. Approximately 60% of the drug undergoes hepatic metabolism, and 40% is excreted unchanged in the urine. Therefore some dose adjustment is required in renal insufficiency.
3. The report of range of therapeutic plasma concentrations are from 6 to 12 μg/ml which is usually achieved by total daily doses of 1200 to 1800 mg.

Clinical Use and Dosage

1. The usual starting dose for tocainide is 400 mg every 8 hours with the dose increased to 600 mg every 8 hours depending upon clinical response and patient tolerance. Daily doses greater than 1800 mg/day are occasionally effective.
2. Tocainide is indicated for treatment of ventricular arrhythmias. Tocainide has minimal, if any, efficacy in treatment of supraventricular arrhythmias or of arrhythmias associated with Wolff-Parkinson-White syndrome.
3. There is a reasonable correlation between the documented response of an arrhythmia to lidocaine and the response expected from tocainide.
4. The efficacy of tocainide in preventing recurrent ventricular tachycardia or ventricular fibrillation in the setting of chronic heart disease has been modest at best. It appears equally effective or slightly less effective than quinidine. Several studies have suggested that tocainide may add antiarrhythmic efficacy when used as a second antiarrhythmic drug.

Side Effects and Toxicity

1. Tocainide therapy has been associated with frequent adverse side effects that, although mild and reversible, may often limit therapy.
2. The most common side effects of tocainide include nausea, vomiting, anorexia, tremulousness, memory impairment, skin rash, sweating, paresthesias, diplopia, dizziness, anxiety, and tinnitus.
3. The side effects of tocainide are usually dose-related, often resolving with a decrease in tocainide dose.
4. Tocainide may be associated with occurrence of pulmonary alveolitis or with severe hematologic abnormalities, including granulocytopenia or aplastic anemia.

Nursing Implications. Patients should be monitored to detect the adverse effects of tocainide, which initially may be subtle.

Mexiletine (Mexitil)

Mexiletine has been introduced recently in oral form for general use in the United States. This antiarrhythmic agent is effective orally, although it has structural and pharmacologic properties resembling those of lidocaine. Mexiletine is indicated for the treatment of ventricular arrhythmias and appears to have an efficacy similar to that of quinidine, disopyramide, or procainamide.

Electrophysiology

1. The electrophysiologic properties of mexiletine resemble those of lidocaine. The major electrophysiologic action of mexiletine is to depress inward sodium current, which results in a decrease in the rate of the rise of the action potential.
2. Mexiletine produces minimum changes on the resting electrocardiogram as QRS duration and QT intervals remain unchanged.
3. Mexiletine may occasionally worsen preexisting sinus node dysfunction or preexisting atrioventricular conduction disturbances.

Pharmacokinetics

1. Mexiletine is eliminated primarily by hepatic metabolism; metabolites of mexiletine have only very slight electrophysiologic effects.
2. Mexiletine is effective orally with high oral bioavailability and very low first-pass hepatic extraction.
3. The elimination half-life of mexiletine in patients who have cardiac disease is about 12 hours during steady state conditions.
4. The usual therapeutic plasma concentrations of mexiletine range from 0.5 to 2.0 μg/ml.

Clinical Uses and Dosage

1. Mexiletine is indicated for the treatment of ventricular arrhythmias and appears to have limited use in the treatment of supraventricular arrhythmias.
2. The usual chronic maintenance dosage of mexiletine is 200 to 300 mg every 8 hours.
3. It is usual to initiate dosing at 200 mg every 8 hours with dose increments of 50 to 100 mg based on the response of the arrhythmia and tolerance.
4. If an oral loading dose of mexiletine is required for more rapid control of ventricular arrhythmias, an initial dose of 400 mg followed by 200 mg every 8 hours is usually administered.
5. In transferring from intravenous lidocaine to oral mexiletine therapy, mexiletine is introduced at maintenance levels and lidocaine is discontinued after the first mexiletine dose.

Side Effects and Toxicity

1. Side effects of mexiletine appear frequently and 30% to 40% of patients may require a dose change or

discontinuation of therapy because of drug toxicity.

2. The most common side effects are neurologic. These include tremor, dysarthria, dizziness, paresthesia, diplopia, nystagmus, mental confusion, and anxiety. Gastrointestinal side effects such as nausea, vomiting, and dyspepsia may also appear.

3. Significant cardiovascular adverse effects are uncommon with oral treatment, although a small incidence of exacerbation of ventricular arrhythmia has been noted.

4. Many of the adverse side effects of mexiletine are dose-related and appear at plasma concentrations that are often within the range of expected therapeutic levels. Therefore effective use of mexiletine requires careful titration of dose and monitoring of plasma concentration in the individual patient.

Encainide

Encainide is an antiarrhythmic agent currently undergoing clinical investigation in the United States. It is capable of significantly reducing ventricular extrasystole frequency and preventing recurrent ventricular tachyarrhythmias. It seems to be effective in a variety of supraventricular arrhythmias, particularly those associated with Wolff-Parkinson-White syndrome.

Electrophysiology

1. Many of the electrophysiologic effects are caused by active metabolites. Therefore the electrophysiologic effects of a single intravenous dose are quite different from those of chronic dosing.

2. Single intravenous doses of encainide prolong HV and QRS intervals, have variable effects on QT interval and do not significantly affect AH interval or the refractoriness of atrium, AV node or ventricle.

3. During oral encainide treatment, however, there is significant prolongation of atrial and ventricular refractoriness, AH interval, and AV nodal refractory periods. In addition, there are significant effects on accessory pathways with prolongation of refractory period and slowing of conduction. In many patients with Wolff-Parkinson-White syndrome, complete conduction block in the accessory pathway may be obtained during oral encainide treatment.

Pharmacokinetics

1. Encainide undergoes extensive hepatic metabolism with at least two active metabolites, 0-de-methyl encainide and 3 methoxy 0-de-methyl encainide.

2. In addition to differences in electrophysiologic effects, these metabolites have different pharmacokinetic parameters. Although the elimination half-life of encainide appears to be 3 to 4 hours, that of the metabolites is longer. Therefore during chronic ther-

apy, dosing intervals of 6 to 8 hours or longer may be effective.

3. The rate of encainide metabolism and accumulation of metabolite is determined by hepatic enzyme metabolism whose activity is genetically controlled. Approximately 10% of patients may be expected to be poor or slow metabolizers of encainide and thus will have relatively high plasma concentrations of encainide with low concentrations of metabolite.

4. Because of the variability in metabolite formation and the variable effects of parent compound and metabolite, the exact role of plasma concentration monitoring has not been determined for encainide.

Clinical Uses and Dosage

1. Encainide is currently undergoing investigation in the treatment of a variety of ventricular and supraventricular arrhythmias, including ventricular extrasystoles, recurrent ventricular tachycardia and ventricular fibrillation, paroxysmal supraventricular tachycardia caused by AV node reentry, or that associated with Wolff-Parkinson-White syndrome and recurrent paroxysmal atrial fibrillation.

2. The usual oral dosage for encainide is 100 to 240 mg/day. A daily dose may be given at 6- or 8-hour dose intervals.

Side Effects and Toxicity

1. The most common adverse side effects of encainide appear to include dizziness, diplopia, vertigo, paresthesia, leg cramps, headache, and metallic taste in the mouth.

2. Encainide may also have significant cardiovascular effects. Encainide prolongs PR, QRS, and QT intervals, may be associated with worsening of atrioventricular conduction, and most significantly, may result in exacerbation of ventricular arrhythmias. In patients who have left ventricular dysfunction and recurrent ventricular tachycardia or ventricular fibrillation, exacerbation of ventricular arrhythmias may occur in as many as 10% to 15% of patients. Encainide appears similar to flecainide in this regard.

Propafenone

Propafenone has been undergoing trials as an oral antiarrhythmic agent in the United States and has been used clinically in several European countries for the past decade. It has been examined as an agent for the treatment of both ventricular and supraventricular arrhythmias including those associated with Wolff-Parkinson-White syndrome.

Electrophysiology

1. The predominant cellular electrophysiologic effect of propafenone is to slow the rate of rise of the action

potential by blocking the fast inward sodium channel.

2. Clinical electrophysiologic effects in man include prolongation of PR and QRS intervals, prolongation of AV nodal conduction, ventricular refractory periods, and induced ventricular tachycardia cycle length.
3. Propafenone may have the clinical effect of mildly inhibiting response to beta-adrenergic stimulation.

Pharmacokinetics
1. Propafenone exhibits nonlinear pharmacokinetics, that is, for a given increase in dose, there is a disproportionate increase in plasma concentration. Thus greater than expected effects, either therapeutic or toxic, may occur after a given dose increase. Propafenone is extensively metabolized by the liver, and its rate of enzymatic disposition appears genetically determined in a manner similar to that of encainide.
2. There is extensive interpatient variability in pharmacokinetics of propafenone, with elimination half-lives ranging from 2 to 17 hours and averaging approximately 8 hours.
3. Propafenone appears to have an active metabolite.
4. Plasma concentrations of propafenone vary considerably with an average plasma concentration of 800 ng/ml.

Clinical Uses and Dosage
1. Propafenone is currently being tested in the treatment of a variety of supraventricular and ventricular arrhythmias.
2. Daily dosage of propafenone ranges from 300 to 900 mg/day administered in increments at dosing intervals of 8 or 12 hours.

Side Effects and Toxicity
1. The most common adverse reactions to propafenone are gastrointestinal or neurologic and include nausea, abdominal discomfort, altered taste, constipation, visual blurring, paresthesias, and dizziness.
2. Cardiovascular adverse side effects include exacerbation of ventricular arrhythmias with an incidence as high as 10% reported. Propafenone may also aggravate congestive heart failure or aggravate preexisting sinus node or AV conduction abnormalities.

SLOW-CHANNEL BLOCKERS (CALCIUM CHANNEL BLOCKERS)

Slow-channel blocking drugs or calcium antagonists represent an exciting new field of cardiovascular physiology and pharmacology. Slow-channel blocking drugs affect electrophysiologic and mechanical properties of the heart and have vasodilator effects mediated through actions on the vascular smooth muscle.[8] Electrophysiologic effects include decreased discharge rate of the sinus node and prolonged conduction and refractoriness of the AV node. These effects are manifested as an increase in the sinus node cycle length and prolongation of the PR interval. Slow-channel blockers have the potential to decrease myocardial contractility by interfering with the calcium flow into the cell and the inhibition of excitation-contraction coupling.

In cardiovascular therapy, slow-channel blocking agents have been used most commonly in the following ways:
1. As antiarrhythmic agents to terminate and prevent recurrences of PSVT and to control ventricular rate during atrial fibrillation or atrial flutter
2. As antianginal agents, particularly for treatment of coronary artery spasm
3. In treatment of systemic hypertension
4. In treatment of hypertrophic cardiomyopathy

Verapamil (Isoptin, Calan)

Verapamil possesses electrophysiologic, hemodynamic, and vasodilator effects at doses commonly employed in clinical practice.

Clinical Uses
1. Verapamil is the preferred agent for termination of acute episodes of paroxysmal supraventricular tachycardia.
2. In PSVT caused by AV nodal reentry or by AV reentry using an accessory pathway, 5 to 10 mg of intravenous verapamil is usually effective in terminating the arrhythmia.
3. Intravenous verapamil will also slow the ventricular response to atrial fibrillation by slowing conduction through the AV node.
4. On the other hand, atrial fibrillation associated with anterograde conduction through the accessory pathway is a relative contraindication to the use of verapamil.
5. Verapamil rarely terminates sustained ventricular tachycardia. Its usual effects, if administered during ventricular tachycardia, are to produce vasodilatation, and possibly negative inotropic effects resulting in hypotension and significant hemodynamic deterioration.
6. Oral verapamil has been effective in treatment of angina pectoris, coronary artery spasm, and hypertrophic cardiomyopathy.

Dosage
1. Verapamil is administered intravenously as boluses of 5 to 10 mg. The onset of action is within 2 minutes.
2. Since verapamil undergoes extensive first-pass he-

patic metabolism, oral doses are significantly higher than those administered intravenously. The usual oral dosage of verapamil is 80 to 160 mg given every 6 to 8 hours.

Side Effects and Toxicity

1. Verapamil may produce sinus bradycardia or arrest, AV nodal conduction block, negative inotropic effects, hypotension, edema, headache, and flushing.
2. The effects on AV conduction and myocardial contractility appear additive to those of beta-adrenergic blocking agents. Simultaneous intravenous administration of beta-blockers and verapamil is contraindicated. Concurrent administration in other circumstances requires careful monitoring.

Nifedipine (Procardia, Adalat)

Nifedipine acts by a different mechanism than verapamil to produce slow-channel blockade. At usual clinical doses, vasodilatation is the major effect with little, if any, prolongation of AV nodal conduction time or decrease in myocardial contractility.

Clinical Uses

1. Nifedipine is used as a vasodilator to treat coronary artery spasm, chronic stable angina pectoris, and systemic hypertension.
2. Nifedipine lacks the antiarrhythmic properties of verapamil.

Dosage

1. The oral dosage of nifedipine is 10 to 30 mg administered every 8 hours.
2. Nifedipine appears to be safe when combined with beta-adrenergic blocking agents or digitalis.

Side Effects and Toxicity. The usual adverse side effects of nifedipine include hypotension, headache, flushing, nausea, vomiting, and dizziness.

Diltiazem (Cardizem)

Diltiazem has properties similar to those of both verapamil and nifedipine; that is, it produces vasodilatation but also slows AV nodal conduction, although to a lesser extent than verapamil.

Clinical Uses

1. Diltiazem is currently indicated for treatment of coronary artery spasm and angina pectoris.
2. Diltiazem is undergoing investigation as an antiarrhythmic agent for treatment of paroxysmal supraventricular tachycardia.
3. The usual dosage of diltiazem is 30 to 90 mg/day administered every 8 hours.

Side Effects and Toxicity. Adverse side effects appear similar to those of nifedipine or verapamil although the risk of adverse cardiovascular effects is lower than that of verapamil.

REFERENCES

1. Collucci, W.S., Wright, R.F., and Braunwald, E.: New positive inotropic agents in the treatment of congestive heart failure: mechanisms of action and recent clinical developments, N. Engl. J. Med. 314:290, 1986.
2. Frishman, W.H.: B-adrenoceptor antagonists: new drugs and new indications, N. Engl. J. Med. 305:500, 1981.
3. Zipes, D.P.: A consideration of antiarrhythmic therapy, Circulation 72:949, 1985.
4. Gilman, A.G., Goodman, L.S., and Gilman, A., editors: The pharmacological basis of therapeutics, ed. 7, New York, 1986, Macmillan Publishers Limited.
5. Fenster, P.E.: Clinical pharmacology: clinical uses of pharmacokinetic principles in prescribing cardiac drugs, Med. Clin. North Am. 68:1281, 1984.
6. Heger, J.J., and others: Clinical use and pharmacology of amiodarone, Med. Clin. North Am. 68:1339, 1984.
7. Heger, J.J., Prystowsky, E.N., and Zipes, D.P.: Drug therapy of cardiac arrhythmias, Cardiol. Clin. 1:305, 1983.
8. Henry, P.D.: Comparative pharmacology of calcium antagonists: nifedipine, verapamil and diltiazem, Am. J. Cardiol. 46:1047, 1980.
9. McCall, D., and O'Rourke, R.A.: Congestive heart failure. II. Therapeutic options: old and new, Mod. Concepts Cardiovasc. Dis. 54:61, 1985.
10. Shand, D.G.: Beta-adrenergic blocking drugs after acute myocardial infarction, Mod. Concepts Cardiovasc. Dis. 51:109, 1982.
11. Sharma, G.V.R.K., and others: Thrombolytic therapy, N. Engl. J. Med. 306:1268, 1982.
12. Smith, T.W., editor: Digitalis glycosides, Orlando, Fla., 1986, Grune & Stratton, Inc.

CHAPTER 11

Artificial Cardiac Pacemakers

Edwin G. Duffin, Jr.
Nancy L. Stephenson
Douglas P. Zipes

The artificial cardiac pacemaker is an electronic stimulator used in place of the natural cardiac pacemaker, the SA node, and/or the specialized AV conducting system in the diseased, congenitally malformed, or iatrogenically damaged heart. The pacemaker system is comprised of a power source, usually a battery, electronic circuitry for generating appropriately timed stimuli, and an electrode/wire system ("lead") used to complete the electrical connection between the circuitry and the myocardium. Pacemakers may be packaged for implantation totally within the body (permanent pacemakers), or they may be configured so that the electronics and power source remain outside the body (temporary pacemakers). The first completely implantable devices were reported in the late 1950s.[1,2] Currently there are an estimated one million patients worldwide who have implanted pacemakers. Advances in technology have been rapidly applied to pacemaker systems, providing noninvasively programmable single- and dual-chamber pacemakers typically weighing 40 to 50 g and lasting an estimated 6 to 10 years. These highly reliable devices are dramatically different from the 250 g, asynchronous, 18-month devices of the early 1960s.

INDICATIONS
Permanent

The most common indications for permanent pacing are sinus node dysfunction and fixed or intermittent third-degree AV block,[3] their primary cause being fibrosis and sclerotic degeneration of the sinus nodal area and the AV conducting system. These indications account for 80% to 90% of all implants. Sick sinus syndrome may be manifested as sinus arrest or block, severe sinus bradycardia, or alternating periods of bradycardia and supraventricular tachycardia (bradycardia-tachycardia syndrome). Further indications for permanent pacing include the following:[4]

1. Mobitz type II second-degree AV block distal to the His bundle
2. Hypersensitive carotid sinus syndrome causing symptomatic severe slowing of sinus rate and/or AV block[5]
3. Chronic atrial fibrillation with a slow ventricular response that results in symptoms

4. Bifascicular block with prolonged His-ventricular (H-V) interval in patients who have syncope or presyncope and no other demonstrated cause of syncope (Bifascicular block with prolonged H-V interval in asymptomatic patients is generally accepted as not being an indication for permanent pacing, although the issue is not entirely resolved.)[4]
5. Termination or overdrive suppression of supraventricular and, less frequently, ventricular tachycardia resistant to drug therapy and not amenable to surgical correction[6,7,8]
6. Periods of bradycardia or asystole following abrupt termination (overdrive suppression) of supraventricular or ventricular tachycardia resistant to drug therapy and not amenable to surgical correction
7. Prophylactic implantation in patients after myocardial infarction complicated by advanced AV block during the acute stages of infarction; this indication also causes some controversy, and the issue is not completely settled
8. Prevention of tachyarrhythmia by providing rate maintenance in combination with drugs or by control of AV conduction through use of dual-chamber pacemakers

Temporary

Indications for temporary pacing include the following:[4,6,7]

1. Maintenance of adequate heart rate and rhythm in patients during a variety of circumstances, such as postoperatively, during cardiac catheterizations or surgery, during administration of some drugs that might inappropriately slow the rate, and prior to implantation of a permanent pacemaker
2. Prophylaxis following open heart surgery
3. Acute (generally anterior) myocardial infarction with type II second-degree or third-degree AV block
4. Acute (generally anterior) myocardial infarction with concurrent onset of right bundle branch block with left axis deviation or concurrent onset of left bundle branch block
5. Acute inferior myocardial infarction with third-degree AV block refractory to pharmacologic inter-

TABLE 11-1. Five-position pacemaker code (ICHD)

I. Chamber Paced	II. Chamber Sensed	III. Mode of Response	IV. Programmability	V. Tachyarrhythmia Functions
V = Ventricle A = Atrium D = Atrium and ventricle O = None		I = Inhibited T = Triggered D = Atrial triggered and ventricular inhibited O = None	P = Programmable rate and/or output M = Multiprogrammability O = None C = Programmable with telemetry	B = Burst N = Normal rate competition S = Scanning E = External

vention and producing ventricular dysrhythmias and/or hemodynamic compromise

6. Termination of AV nodal reentry or reciprocating tachycardia associated with Wolff-Parkinson-White syndrome (see p. 160), atrial flutter, or ventricular tachycardia
7. Suppression of ectopic activity, atrial or ventricular
8. Electrophysiologic studies to evaluate diagnoses, mechanisms, and therapy in patients who have a variety of bradyarrhythmias and tachyarrhythmias[9]

PACEMAKER MODALITIES
ICHD Code

The Inter-Society Commission for Heart Disease (ICHD) has devised a three-position code[10] designed as a shorthand notation to identify the many pacing modes (Table 11-1).

This table provides a shorthand description of pacemaker operation. Symbols placed in the first two positions indicate the chambers in which the pacemaker functions; in the third position, the mode of operation of the pacemaker; in the fourth position, its programmable characteristics; and in the fifth position, its antitachycardia features. For example, if the pacing lead is inserted into the ventricle and the pulse generator is a demand ventricular type, then the chamber paced is the ventricle, and the first letter in the five-position code is V. The chamber sensed is the ventricle and therefore the second letter in the five-position code also is V. The mode of response of the pacemaker is to inhibit a pacing spike when spontaneous electrical activity is sensed, and therefore I is in the third position. If only the rate and/or output of the pulse generator can be programmed externally, P is in the fourth position. If the pacemaker is used to treat tachycardias, then the tachyarrhythmia function is indicated in the fifth position.

Pulse generators that pace or sense in both the atrium and ventricle are indicated by the designation D, meaning dual. If the pacemaker does not have a function in one of the classifications, O is used. The different types of tachyarrhythmia functions are discussed in the chapter.

Atrial and Ventricular Asynchronous Pacemakers (AOO, VOO)

The first pacemakers simply stimulated the myocardium at a constant rate independent of any underlying cardiac rhythm; these pacemakers only paced and did not sense any spontaneous activity. If connected to the atrium the pacemaker was referred to as an asynchronous atrial pacemaker (AOO), and if applied to the ventricles it was referred to as a ventricular asynchronous pacemaker (VOO). Asynchronous pacemakers are rarely used today, since it is relatively simple to provide noncompetitive pacemakers that avoid the potential risks of pacing during spontaneous rhythms.

Atrial and Ventricular Demand Pacemakers (AAI, AAT, VVI, VVT)

In the early 1970s, sensing circuits were added to pacemakers so that they would stimulate only when there was no appropriate underlying spontaneous rhythm. These pacemakers paced and sensed spontaneous activity. This prevented competitive pacing and the attendant risk of inducing fibrillation. Demand pacemakers are supplied in two versions, inhibited and triggered. Inhibited devices withhold the stimulus and reset their timing on sensing spontaneous cardiac activity. Triggered devices are activated to deliver a stimulus just after spontaneous depolarization into the refractory tissue and reset their timing immediately on sensing spontaneous cardiac activity. Both types deliver a stimulus at the end of their timing cycle (pacemaker escape interval) if no spontaneous cardiac activity is detected. The triggered mode was invented to address concerns that unipolar inhibited devices might allow a patient to become asystolic if extracardiac signals (for example, pectoral muscle potentials, electrical signals from radio transmitters, or power lines) were sensed, erroneously interpreted to be cardiac signals, and permitted to inhibit pacemaker output. Modern circuitry has reduced the likelihood of such occurrences, and the disadvantages of stimulating when not really necessary with a triggered mode (ECG waveform distortion, high-power requirements for the pacemaker) have resulted in relatively little usage of this form of pacing. However, it can be of value to achieve termination of some tachycardias or to be certain diagnostically when or if the pacemaker sensed a spontaneous event; it is therefore generally available in modern pacemakers as an option. Block diagrams and typical ECGs for the ventricular demand inhibited (VVI), ventricular demand triggered (VVT), atrial demand inhibited (AAI), and atrial demand triggered (AAT) devices are shown in Fig. 11-1.

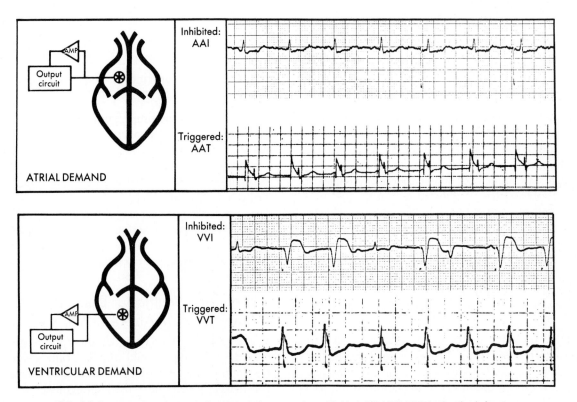

FIG. 11-1. Atrial and ventricular demand pacemakers (AAI, AAT, VVI, VVT). On the left are schematic diagrams of the heart; the right and left atria are in the top region of the diagrams, and the right and left ventricles are in the bottom portion. The names of the pacemakers are placed beneath the drawings of the heart, and the ICHD codes are given in the middle panel. The "output" circuit (the part of the pacemaker that creates the electrical stimulus), connected to the heart in the cardiac chamber marked with an *asterisk*, indicates the chamber *stimulated* by the pacemaker. The triangular element labelled *AMP* (represents the portion of the pacemaker that has an electrical amplifying circuit to enable sensing of cardiac activity), connected to the heart in the cardiac chamber marked with a *circle*, indicates the cardiac chamber that is *sensed* by the pacemaker. *Circled asterisk* indicates that both *sensing and stimulation* can be accomplished at the location marked.

In the top panel a circled asterisk indicates that atrial demand pacemakers sense and pace in the atrium. In the top ECG of the upper panel the action of an atrial inhibited (AAI) pacemaker is illustrated. Note that the pacing spike is inhibited from discharging until the fifth and seventh complexes, when atrial rhythm slows slightly and allows escape of the atrial demand pacemaker. In the second ECG example each sensed P wave elicits a pacing spike delivered within the P wave (third, fourth, and fifth P waves). A pacing spike initiates the first, second, sixth, and seventh P waves. This is an example of AAT pacing.

In the lower panel a circled asterisk indicates that ventricular demand pacemakers sense and pace in the ventricle. In the upper ECG of the bottom panel the action of a ventricular demand pacemaker (VVI) is illustrated. Note that spontaneous ventricular activity inhibits pacemaker discharge, and pacing spikes are delivered only when the ventricular rate becomes slower than the escape interval of the pacemaker. In the lower ECG, pacing spikes are delivered into each of the appropriately sensed QRS complexes; this is correct operation of the VVT pacemaker.

Atrial Synchronous Ventricular Pacemakers (VAT, VDD)

To approximate normal cardiac function more closely, sophisticated dual-chamber (atrium and ventricle) "physiologic" pacemakers were developed. The atrial synchronous ventricular pacemaker (VAT) was designed for use in patients with normal sinus function and impaired AV conduction.[11] This device senses atrial activity by means of an electrode in the atrium and, after a suitable delay, paces the ventricle, thereby providing an artificial AV node in lieu of the malfunctioning natural AV pathway. The VAT pacemaker does not pace the atrium. This method of atrial sensing and ventricular pacing preserves the atrial contribution to ventricular filling and maintains sinus control of ventricular rate. Rate limits are designed into the pacemaker so that during periods of atrial bradycardia at rates that are slower than the escape rate of the pacemaker, the unit paces as an asynchronous ventricular pacemaker at a predetermined backup rate. During atrial tachycardia the pacemaker paces no faster than its upper rate limit, yielding an AV response to sensed atrial activity that is similar to type I or type II AV block. The VAT device has been refined by the addition of circuitry that enables it to detect ventricular activity (ventricular sense amplifier). This modified pacemaker is called the atrial synchronous ventricular inhibited pacemaker (ASVIP), described in the ICHD

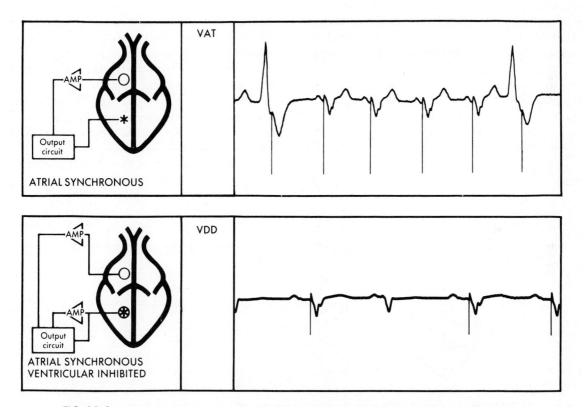

FIG. 11-2.   Atrial synchronous pacemakers (VAT, VDD). For the VAT pacemaker *(top panel)* the circle in the atrium and the asterisk in the ventricle indicate that the pacemaker senses atrial activity and paces the ventricle. In the lower panel the circle in the atrium and the circled asterisk in the ventricle indicate that the pacemaker senses both atrial and ventricular activity and paces the ventricle (VDD).

In the midportion of the top ECG the pacemaker delivers stimuli following each sensed P wave and produces a paced QRS complex. The first and last QRS complexes are spontaneous premature ventricular complexes (PVCs) that are *not* sensed by the pacemaker. The sinus P wave (hidden within the QRS complex) is sensed by the pacemaker and triggers it to deliver a pacing spike to the ventricle. Conceivably, such a response can deliver a stimulus into the T wave of the PVC. To avoid this problem, the VDD pacemaker has been equipped with a sensing circuit to sense spontaneous ventricular activity. Note in the lower ECG (VDD pacemaker) that the second P wave conducts to the ventricle with a PR interval shorter than the P-stimulus interval of the pacemaker. This conducted QRS complex is sensed by the pacemaker, and the pacing spike is inhibited, thus eliminating problems of pacemaker competition with spontaneous ventricular activity.

code as VDD.[12] (The VDD pacemaker, like the VAT pacemaker, does not have the ability to pace in the atrium, but it does sense in both the atrium and the ventricle and paces in the ventricle.) The VAT and VDD pacemakers are rapidly being displaced by the more flexible DDD pacemakers, which can stimulate and sense in both the atrium and the ventricle. Block diagrams and ECGs for the VAT and VDD devices are shown in Fig. 11-2.

AV Sequential Pacemakers (DVI)

In patients who have bradycardia in addition to impaired AV conduction, the atrial contribution to ventricular filling can be preserved by using an AV sequential pacemaker (DVI).[13] This pacemaker senses only ventricular activity but is capable of pacing both the atrium and the ventricle. Following sensed or paced ventricular events the DVI pacemaker monitors the ventricle for activity. If none is detected within a prescribed pacemaker escape interval, the pacemaker stimulates the atrium. It then waits long enough to allow passage of a normal AV interval and, if no ventricular activity occurs, paces the ventricle.* Sensed ventricular activity inhibits the ventricular stimulus and resets

---

*Some AV sequential pacemakers are of the committed type; that is, they do not wait for normal AV conduction to occur but, instead, always deliver a stimulus to the ventricle one AV interval after delivery of an atrial stimulus.

---

all pacemaker timing. If the ventricular rate is sufficiently rapid, atrial stimuli are also inhibited. It is important to emphasize that the DVI pacemaker does not sense spontaneous atrial activity. A variant of the DVI pacemaker, the DDI pacemaker, does sense atrial activity. This device inhibits the atrial stimulus to avoid competition between the pacemaker and an underlying atrial rhythm, but it does not provide atrial synchronous pacing. Fig. 11-3 contains the block diagram and representative ECG for the DVI pacemaker. Currently DVI pacing is most often obtained by programming a DDD pacemaker to the DVI mode rather than by implanting a purely DVI pulse generator.

Fully Automatic or Universal Stimulation (DDD)

In 1977 came the first clinical implants of the DDD pacemaker, a dual-chamber device that functions in the atrial synchronous mode during normal sinus activity and provides AV sequential pacing during periods of bradycardia.[14] Thus the DDD pacemaker senses and paces the atrium and the ventricle. This pacemaker operates in four modes, adapting automatically to the patient's underlying rhythm according to the schema in Table 11-2. Fig. 11-4 shows a block diagram and representative ECGs for the DDD pacemaker.

A summary of each of the pacemaker modes described is presented in Table 11-3.

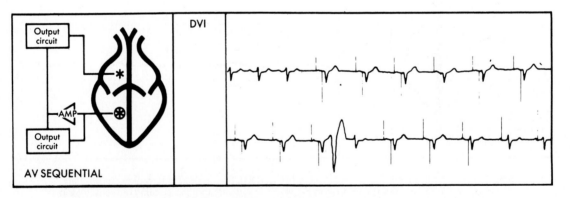

FIG. 11-3. AV sequential pacemaker (DVI). In the diagram the asterisk in the atrium and the circled asterisk in the ventricle indicate that the pacemaker paces the atrium, paces the ventricle, and senses spontaneous activity in the ventricle. The ECG example demonstrates this operation. The first three sinus-initiated QRS complexes occur at a rate faster than the escape rate of the pacemaker, and the pacemaker is completely inhibited. At this point, SA node discharge rate slows and the pacemaker delivers a stimulus *(upper spike)* to the atrium. Because the paced P wave does not conduct to the ventricle within the escape interval of the pacemaker, the pacemaker then paces the ventricle *(downward directed spikes)*. This occurs for three beats. Then the PR interval shortens slightly, inhibiting ventricular pacemaker discharge. The last two beats in the top strip and first three beats in the lower strip indicate pacing in the atrium and ventricle. Then a PVC occurs and is sensed, and pacemaker activity is inhibited. The pacemaker then resumes delivery of spikes to atrium and ventricle. In the terminal portion of this ECG the atrial rate speeds slightly. Since atrial activity is *not* sensed, pacemaker spikes "march" through the P wave but ventricular spikes are inhibited.

Rate Responsive Devices

As the benefits of rate variability associated with atrial synchronous ventricular pacing became appreciated, it was recognized that similar advantages might be available to patients with impaired atrial function.[15] However, an appropriate physiologic parameter independent of sinus nodal function is needed to set the pacemaker's rate. Various approaches are being explored, though most remain investigational. These include central venous temperature sensing devices,[16] oxygen saturation sensing devices,[17] pH responsive systems,[18] stroke volume[19] and ventricular pressure controlled devices.[20] Substantial clinical experience does exist with three single-chamber ventricular pacemaker designs that vary pacing rate in response to changes in the QT interval,[21,22] changes in respiratory rate,[23] or sensed mechanical activity of the body.[24]

TABLE 11-2. Operating modes of DDD pacemakers

Underlying Rhythm	Pacemaker Function
Normally conducted sinus rhythm	Totally inhibited
Normally conducted sinus brady-cardia	Atrial pacing
Atrial bradycardia and prolonged or blocked AV conduction	AV sequential pacing
Normal sinus rhythm and prolonged or blocked AV conduction	Atrial synchronous ventricular pacing

TABLE 11-3. Summary of pacemaker modalities

Pacemaker Type	ICHD Code	Atrium	Ventricle
Atrial asynchronous	AOO	PACE	
Ventricular asynchronous	VOO		PACE
Atrial demand	AAI/AAT	PACE/SENSE	
Ventricular demand	VVI/VVT		PACE/SENSE
Atrial synchronous	VAT	SENSE	PACE
Atrial synchronous ventricular inhibited	VDD	SENSE	PACE/SENSE
AV sequential	DVI	PACE	PACE/SENSE
Fully automatic	DDD	PACE/SENSE	PACE/SENSE

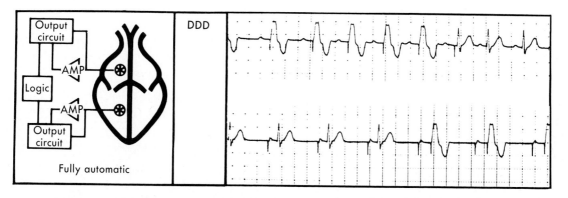

FIG. 11-4. Fully automatic sequential pacemaker (DDD). The diagram on the left indicates that the DDD pacemaker both senses and paces in the atrium and ventricle. The ECG on the right illustrates this feature. In the first five complete complexes, spontaneous atrial activity (P waves) is not followed by a spontaneous QRS complex within an appropriate PR interval. Therefore a pacemaker spike is delivered to the ventricle following each sensed P wave. The third QRS complex from the end occurs in time to be normally conducted from the P wave but not quite early enough to inhibit the pacemaker spike. The next QRS complexes follow a normal PR interval and thus inhibit pacemaker output. In the lower strip the development of sinus bradycardia triggers atrial pacemaker discharge, and pacemaker spikes precede the onset of P waves. Finally, in the bottom right portion, an atrial stimulus paces the atrium, and a ventricular stimulus paces the ventricle.

The QT sensing pacemaker uses a conventional electrode system to sense and pace, but it has circuitry designed to determine the interval between stimulation and the peak of the intracardiac T wave. Its operation is based on the physiologic concept that sympathetic tone increases in response to the body's need for an increased heart rate. Heightened sympathetic tone shortens the QT interval and shortening of this QT interval produces an increase in the pacemaker rate. An increase in QT interval slows the pacing rate. Advantages of this pacemaker include use of a stable rugged sensor (the standard pacing lead) that requires no change in implant technique, and the device responds to a parameter reflecting metabolic demand. Disadvantages include relatively slow response times, nonsustained rate changes, and some difficulty ensuring reliable T wave sensing without noise effects.

The respiratory-dependent pacemaker currently requires placement of two leads, a conventional cardiac pacing lead in the ventricle and an auxiliary lead in the subcutaneous tissue of the thorax. Variations in the electrical impedance between the thoracic electrode and the pacemaker's indifferent electrode (generator case) reflect the patient's respiratory rate, which is processed to control the pacemaker rate. This approach uses a simple reliable sensor and is responsive to exercise and metabolic needs. It does require placement of an extra lead (currently) and may not respond appropriately in patients with pulmonary disease or heart failure.

The activity sensing pacemaker uses a conventional lead system for sensing and pacing and incorporates a microphone-like sensor inside the pacemaker pulse generator. This sensor responds to mechanical vibrations of the body, producing electrical signals that are proportional to the patient's physical activity level. These "activity" signals are used to determine an appropriate pacing rate, an approach that affords a rapid response to patient needs, uses a sensor that is hermetically sealed within the pulse generator for reliable long-term service, and requires no change in implant technique. Its disadvantages are an inability to respond to nonexercise–induced metabolic demands and the potential for minor rate increases in the presence of infrasonic environmental noises.

Mode Selection

Selection of the optimum pacemaker modality for a given patient can be rather complex, requiring knowledge of the electrophysiologic performance of the SA node, AV conduction pathways, and hemodynamic status. A reasonable, though less rigorous, mode selection can be made by considering the patient's atrial rhythm and AV conduction status, as indicated in Table 11-4.

Patients who have normal atrial rhythms do not require a pacemaker if AV conduction is also normal. If AV function is interrupted, then atrial synchronous ventricular pacing (VDD, DDD) provides a means for maintaining sinus control of ventricular rate. However, in patients who have prolonged retrograde conduction time, atrial activation following ventricular stimulation may trigger an atrial synchronous device, producing a pacemaker-mediated tachycardia. If this cannot be prevented (e.g., by use of a long atrial refractory period in the pacemaker), then DVI or DDI pacing may be used. DVI pacemakers are not triggered by atrial signals; hence they cannot induce pacemaker-mediated tachycardias. However, a rate-responsive VVI or VVT pacemaker may be preferred to the DVI device because such pacemakers provide a varying ventricular rate as the patient's needs change.

Atrial pacing (AAI or AAT) is appropriate in patients who have atrial bradycardia and normal AV function, since it ensures the atrial contribution to ventricular filling. Rate-responsive atrial pacing is advantageous when available, since it provides additional compensation during exercise.

AV Conduction	Atrial Rhythm		
	Normal	Bradycardia	Brady/Tachy
Normal, no hypersensitive carotid sinus syndrome	None	AAI/AAT AAI/AAT-RR	AAI/AAT AAI/AAT-RR
Antegrade and retrograde block	VDD DDD	DDD DVI/DDI VVI/VVT-RR	DVI/DDI VVI/VVT VVI/VVT-RR
Antegrade block, prolonged retrograde conduction time	DVI VVI/VVT-RR	DVI/DDI VVI/VVT-RR	DVI/DDI VVI/VVT-RR

TABLE 11-4. A guide to pacemaker mode selection*

*By matching the patient's AV conduction and atrial rhythm to those in this table, an appropriate pacemaker mode can be determined. RR after an ICHD code indicates rate-responsive pacing.

Atrial pacing alone is not acceptable in patients who have impaired AV conduction. In these patients dual chamber pacing (DDD or DVI) provides atrial pacing for benefits already cited and ventricular stimulation to compensate for the lack of AV conduction. In these patients rate-responsive pacing (VVI or VVT) may be preferable to the fixed rate DVI devices, or to the DDD devices in patients who have prolonged retrograde conduction times.

Finally, in patients who have atrial bradycardia and tachycardia (bradycardia-tachycardia syndrome), atrial synchronous devices (other than those incorporating specific antitachycardia features) are inappropriate because they will accelerate ventricular rhythm during periods of atrial tachycardia. In all other respects mode selection factors are comparable to those cited for patients who have only atrial bradyarrhythmias.

Ultimately, selection from among the several possible modes depends on additional factors, such as pulse generator size and patient physique, availability and unique traits of specific devices, follow-up capabilities, patient age and hemodynamic needs, and economics (dual-chamber pacemaker/lead systems typically cost 35% more than comparably advanced single-chamber systems, which in turn may cost 60% more than single nonprogrammable single-chamber devices).

Antitachycardia Pacing[6-8,25]

Tachyarrhythmia control is achieved with pacemakers using one or more of three broad approaches: rate maintenance, termination of tachyarrhythmias, and prevention of onset of tachycardia.

Some therapeutic approaches to control tachyarrhythmias result in symptom-producing bradyarrhythmias. Pacing can be combined with drug therapy in such situations to prevent the bradycardia. For example, digitalis or propranolol, given to treat the tachycardia component of the tachycardia-bradycardia syndrome, may aggravate the bradycardia, establishing the need for pacemaker implantation. Similarly, surgery to interrupt the AV conducting system in a patient who has drug-refractory supraventricular tachycardia with a rapid ventricular rate results in a bradycardia (caused by the AV block) that needs to be treated by pacing.

Certain drug-refractory tachycardias, not amenable to surgical therapy, can sometimes be terminated by a pacemaker designed to produce an appropriate sequence of electrical stimuli. Some of the pacemakers are activated by the patient when perceiving the presence of a tachyarrhythmia, whereas other automatically discharge when the pacemaker senses that a tachycardia is present. Various cadences of stimuli can be delivered, including short bursts at high rates, stimuli that scan the cardiac cycle and automatically change rate or shift the timing of one or more premature stimuli,[26] and coupled or paired stimuli. A *dual-demand* pacemaker is one that automatically delivers stimuli at a fixed, but relatively slow, rate (for example, 70 beats/minute) when it senses the presence of a bradycardia (for example, rates less than 70 beats/minute) or a tachycardia (for example, rates greater than 150 beats/minute). The tachycardia is terminated when an appropriately timed stimulus occurs during a particular part of the tachycardia cycle; this is called *underdrive termination*. Dual-chamber (DVI) pacemakers can be made to operate in the dual-demand mode and pace with short AV intervals for patients who have accessory bypass tracts.[27] Unique custom-built devices with characteristics tailored for specific patients can also be applied. Investigational trials have begun on a low-energy transvenous cardioverter[28] designed to increase the safety and efficacy of chronic electrical control of ventricular tachycardia, and an implantable defibrillator[25] for automatic termination of ventricular fibrillation has been approved by the FDA and is now available in limited quantities.

The preferred therapeutic approach to tachyarrhythmias is prevention. In some cases simply improving the patient's hemodynamic status or restoring normal AV synchrony by means of an appropriate standard pacemaker prevents the development of tachycardia. Some patients have bradycardia-dependent tachycardias (for example, ventricular tachycardia associated with complete AV block), and pacing at normal rates eliminates the ventricular tachycardia. In others pacing at moderately elevated rates suppresses ectopy that might otherwise precipitate tachycardias. In patients with accessory AV pathways use of an atrial synchronous or DDD pacemaker with a suitably short AV interval may preclude development of a reciprocating tachycardia while preserving normal sinus control of ventricular rate.

Currently, pacing for tachyarrhythmia control accounts for less than 3% of all pacemaker implantations,[3] although it is anticipated that this indication will become increasingly frequent in the future.

PROGRAMMABILITY[29-32]

The vast majority of permanent pacemaker implants today employ a programmable pacemaker. *Programmability* can be defined as noninvasive, reversible alteration of the electronically controlled performance of an implantable device such as a pacemaker. Use of a simple magnet to convert a demand pacemaker to its asynchronous mode generally is excluded from this definition, although it is in reality a simple form of programming. In the most advanced pacemakers many performance characteristics are programmable, including rate, stimulus output amplitude or duration, amplifier sensitivity, amplifier refractory period, hysteresis, pacing mode (for example, unipolar/bipolar,

TABLE 11-5. Applications of programmable pacemaker parameters

Parameter	Patient/Pacemaker Optimization	Diagnostic Applications	Correction of Malfunctions
Rate	Improve cardiac output by allowing greater range of conducted sinus activity. Minimize angina by keeping the rate below that which produces pain. Suppress arrhythmias. Adapt pulse generator to pediatric needs (faster rates). Terminate tachycardias with short rapid bursts. Minimize "pacemaker syndrome" (caused by AV dissociation) by selecting low rate.	Suppress pacing to access underlying rhythm by ECG. Test AV conduction with an atrial pacemaker by determining rates at which AV nodal Wenckebach behavior occurs. Test sinus function with an atrial pacemaker by using bursts of rapid pacing to determine SA node recovery times. Confirm atrial capture by altering pacemaker rate and observing concomitant ventricular rate change.	
Output; amplitude, or duration	Maximize pulse generator longevity by selecting output energy that provides the minimal level of stimulation consistent with reliable maintenance of pacing. Provide increased energy for high threshold patients. Avoid extracardiac stimulation (pectoral muscle, phrenic nerve).	Evaluate pacing threshold.	Regain capture following threshold increases caused by infarcts, electrolyte disturbances, drugs. Eliminate diaphragmatic or pectoral muscle stimulation.
Amplifier sensitivity	Establish appropriate sensitivity to detect intracardiac electrogram while avoiding sensing of extraneous signals (pectoral muscle potentials, electromagnetic interference). Increase sensitivity for atrial sensing applications.	Alter sensitivity to evaluate possible sources of oversensing or undersensing.	Compensate for changes in intracardiac electrogram amplitude. Resolve oversensing of T waves, muscle potentials, electromagnetic interference.
Refractory period*	Extend duration for atrial applications to avoid sensing conducted R waves. Shorten duration in ventricular applications to detect closely coupled ectopic events.	Alter duration to evaluate possible causes of over- or undersensing.	Lengthen duration to avoid T wave sensing. Shorten duration to eliminate failure to sense closely coupled ectopic events.
Hysteresis	Minimize pacemaker syndrome by allowing sinus rhythm over widest possible rate range while establishing adequately high pacing rate when needed.		
Unipolar/bipolar		Evaluate lead fracture (bipolar → unipolar). Enhance stimulus artifact visibility on ECG (bipolar → unipolar).	Convert to unipolar operation to regain capture in case of lead fracture. Change mode to adapt to altered electrogram causing sensing failure.

*Refractory period: that portion of a pacemaker's timing cycle during which intrinsic cardiac activity will not be allowed to reset the pacemaker's lower rate escape. Upper rate limits, noise reversion timing, and other pacemaker timing sequences may or may not be reset during the refractory period depending upon the specific design.

TABLE 11-5. Applications of programmable pacemaker parameters—cont'd

Parameter	Patient/Pacemaker Optimization	Diagnostic Applications	Correction of Malfunctions
Unipolar/bipolar—cont'd		Evaluate oversensing (unipolar → bipolar).	Convert to bipolar to eliminate sensing of myopotentials. Convert to bipolar to avoid extracardiac stimulation.
Mode	Select optimum mode (e.g., VDD for patients who have normal sinus function and impaired AV conduction). Alter mode if patient's needs change (e.g., VDD → DVI if patient develops sinus bradycardia).	Establish triggered mode to enable external control of pacemaker from chest electrodes and external stimulator to perform noninvasive electrophysiologic studies of sinus function, AV conduction, efficacy of antiarrhythmic agents. Confirm oversensing signal source by selecting triggered mode.	Change to backup mode (e.g., VVI) if atrial portion of dual-chamber system is nonfunctional (e.g., lead displacement). Prevent oversensing by selecting asynchronous mode.
AV delay	Maximize hemodynamic efficacy. Control or prevent tachyarrhythmias.		
Atrial-rate–tracking limit	Maintain widest range of sinus rate control without incurring angina. Control ventricular response to atrial arrhythmias. Prevent rapid synchronization to dissociated atrial activity during ventricular escape pacing in VDD mode. Prevent occurrence of retrograde atrial activity that would result from a long delay between the triggering event in the atrium and the resultant stimulus in the ventricle. This retrograde activity can continuously trigger the pacemaker causing "pacemaker tachycardia."	Select high rate limit for stress testing.	Reduce tracking rate limit if pectoral muscle activity triggers rapid pacing.
Telemetry		Compare programmed settings to actual device operation. Use marker channel indicators to determine which events pacemaker is causing and which events are being sensed. Use electrogram to evaluate causes of under- or oversensing. Use electrogram to evaluate drug effects on myocardium.	

VVI/VVT/VOO), and operation of special information transfer channels (telemetry of intracardiac electrograms, programmed settings, and device operation indicators, such as "marker channel," battery status, and lead impedance). Furthermore, in dual-chamber pacemakers it is frequently possible to program AV intervals, atrial rate tracking limits, and the pacing mode (for example, DDD to DVI or VVI).

Programmability is of benefit to the clinician and patient in that it allows optimizing pacemaker function for specific patient needs, minimizes the need for invasive procedures to correct malfunctions or to revise the system to meet changing patient needs, and facilitates troubleshooting procedures. Table 11-5 indicates applications for many of the commonly available programmable parameters. It should be emphasized that programmability must be used with care, since it presents the risk of establishing inappropriate parameter settings (for example, insufficient output energy to maintain capture, dangerously high or low rates) and imposes a greater need for maintaining accurate records to prevent erroneous decisions based on lack of knowledge about the rationale for the current status of the programmed settings in a given patient. Thus it is essential to document the rationale for program changes at the time at which they are made.

Many programming devices available today produce printed records of the parameter settings of the implanted pacemaker. Some printers are activated automatically when the programmers are turned on, although others require specific activation. Whenever possible, it is advisable to include the printouts in the patient's records. It is also advisable to routinely determine and record all programmed parameters as a first step in each patient follow-up session and as a final step. This ensures that spontaneous reprogramming of the implanted device, a rare phenomenon, can be correctly identified if it should occur.

POWER SOURCES[33,34]

Nearly all pacemakers are battery-powered. External pacemakers typically use standard alkaline or mercury batteries of the type found in common household appliances (such as transistor radios and flashlights), although an occasional external device uses a rechargeable or lithium battery.

Virtually all current implantable pacemakers are powered by one of the many varieties of lithium batteries. These batteries share certain characteristics that make them especially suitable for implantation, yet they are also significantly different. Each of the lithium systems offers high-energy density and a low self-discharge characteristic that ensures the delivery of maximum energy where it is needed and minimizes wasted energy. Most of the systems can be hermetically sealed to prevent ingress of body fluids and egress of tissue-damaging battery materials. Each system offers unique electrical characteristics and varying degrees of reliability.[34,35] The most commonly used lithium batteries are the lithium iodide and lithium cupric sulfide batteries.

Reported performances of the major power sources clearly show the substantial progress made toward creating a pacemaker that will have sufficient longevity to curtail the need for replacement in the majority of patients. In 1985 survival probabilities were reported for large groups of pacemakers using lithium power sources.[35] A total of 6853 lithium *iodide* powered pacemakers showed a cumulative survival probability of 68% of an 8-year longevity; 2856 lithium *cupric sulfide* powered pacemakers showed a survival probability of 70% at a longevity of 8.8 years. These data reflect actual clinical results and clearly demonstrate the success of lithium power sources.

A very small group of special-purpose antitachycardia pacemakers is powered by radio frequency energy transmitted through the body to the implanted pulse generator. This is practical because these pacemakers are not required to pace constantly but are used to generate short bursts of rapid asynchronous stimuli to terminate episodes of tachycardia.

PACEMAKER ELECTRODE SYSTEMS ("LEADS")[36,37]

The pulse generator is electrically connected to the heart by means of a wire and electrode system referred to as a *lead*. The electrodes may be unipolar or bipolar. In bipolar systems the positive and negative electrodes both are located within the cardiac chamber and are in contact with the endocardium or are on the heart. Unipolar systems place only the negative electrode at the heart and use a large area anode electrode, usually the metallic housing of the pulse generator, at a remote location. Either approach is clinically acceptable. Bipolar systems are less susceptible to extraneous electromagnetic interference (such as electrical signals generated by nearby power lines, automobile spark plugs, and radio transmitters), extracardiac myopotential interference, unwanted extracardiac stimulation, or threshold changes caused by defibrillatory currents.

At the time of initial implantation of a pacemaker system, and at the time of each replacement of a pacemaker or a lead, electrical measurements must be made to ensure that the system will function correctly. The *stimulation threshold* is the minimum amount of energy necessary to capture the chamber of the heart to be paced; output of the pacing device must therefore be higher than this amount. Measurement of *cardiac signal amplitudes* (intracardiac electrogram) ensures that these signals are large enough to be sensed by the pacing device to enable it to respond appropriately to spontaneous cardiac electrical activity. These measurements are typically made using a pacing system analyzer (PSA).

Transvenous

Permanent pacing leads are designed for either transvenous or epicardial placement. Transvenous leads are usually implanted within the right ventricular apex for ventricular pacing and in the right atrial appendage or coronary sinus for atrial applications. The leads are typically inserted via the cephalic, subclavian, or external jugular veins, using fluoroscopy for visualization and stiff wires (stylets) inserted within the lumen of the lead for control during positioning. (The stylets must be removed following lead placement to avoid damaging the lead.) A rapid technique for lead placement in the subclavian vein with minimal trauma employs a simple venipuncture using a special percutaneous lead introducer.[38] This approach is gaining favor and involves minimal risk, although there is the possibility of inadvertently entering the pleural cavity or the arterial system. The urethane-insulated leads have reduced diam-

eters and a decreased coefficient of friction, making it possible to pass an atrial and a ventricular lead through a single vein, and facilitating use of dual-chamber pacemakers.[39,40]

Transvenous leads come in a variety of designs, each purporting to ensure stable permanent positioning of the electrodes. Fig. 11-5 includes examples of ventricular and atrial leads with flanges, tines, barbs, and screws for fixation. Many atrial leads also incorporate a J shape to aid in proper positioning within the atrial appendage. The transvenous approach is associated with very low morbidity and, with current lead designs, a very low rate of displacement.[41,42,43]

New designs in transvenous leads offer improvements in electrical efficiency. Electrodes made of carbon have been shown to result in improved stimulation thresholds.[44] In another design, grooves were cut in a standard ring electrode, and the surface was then coated with small particles of platinum. Again, improvements in stimulation thresholds were noted.[45] Introduced fairly recently for clinical study are atrial and ventricular leads that incorporate a

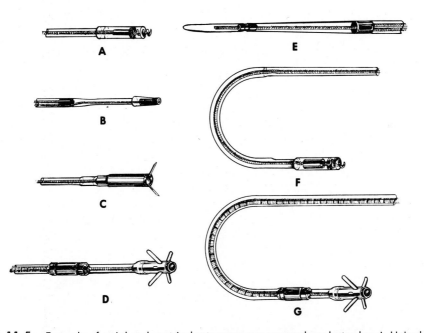

FIG. 11-5. Example of atrial and ventricular transvenous pacemaker electrodes. A, Unipolar endocardial urethane lead with screw-in tip electrode for active fixation to atrial or ventricular endocardial surface (Medtronic model 6957). B, Bipolar ventricular electrode utilizing flanged Silastic tip for positioning stability (Medtronic model 6901R). C, Unipolar ventricular electrode with extensible metallic barb that provides active fixation to the ventricular myocardium (Biotronic model IE 65-I). D, Bipolar urethane ventricular electrode with flexible tines adjacent to the target tip™ electrode. The tines provide passive lead fixation by lodging within the trabecular structure of the ventricle (Medtronic model 4012). E, Bipolar Silastic lead designed for stable placement in the coronary sinus; the electrodes are shaped for atrial pacing applications (Medtronic model 6992). F, Unipolar urethane lead with J shape and screw-in tip electrode for active fixation to the atrial endocardial surface (Medtronic model 6957J). G, Bipolar urethane atrial lead with J shape and flexible tines adjacent to the tip electrode The J shape and tines provide passive fixation of the electrode within the atrium (Medtronic model 4512).

steroid-containing pellet behind a porous electrode, permitting minute amounts of the steroid to be dissolved by body fluids and deposited into the tissues immediately surrounding the electrode. This design decreases stimulation thresholds and increases cardiac signal amplitudes both acutely and chronically.[46,47] This approach may offer significant benefits, particularly to those patients in whom high stimulation thresholds and low cardiac signal amplitudes have resulted in repeated clinical problems with their pacemaker systems, often necessitating use of short-lived high-output pulse generators. However, the mechanism responsible for these improved characteristics is as yet unknown.[48,49]

Epicardial

Epicardial leads are used less frequently than transvenous systems, but they are of particular benefit in problem patients who have smooth, dilated right ventricles and in patients who have truncated right atrial appendages. The placement approach depends on the type of epicardial electrode used. A transthoracic approach (thoracotomy) is used to apply electrodes that are sutured to the myocardium. More commonly, for ventricular applications a sutureless corkscrew electrode is used, since this device can be applied with a transmediastinal approach avoiding entrance into the pleural cavity and reducing morbidity and discomfort.[50] Fig. 11-6 shows examples of myocardial electrodes.

Temporary

Temporary pacing leads include transvenous catheter electrodes, wire electrodes, and, in extreme circumstance, precordial surface electrodes. Temporary transvenous catheter electrodes can be placed in a fashion similar to that used for permanent leads. Placement is facilitated by designing the catheters to be stiffer than would be acceptable for permanent use, and by sometimes incorporating additional aids such as inflatable balloons or cuffs that "float" the

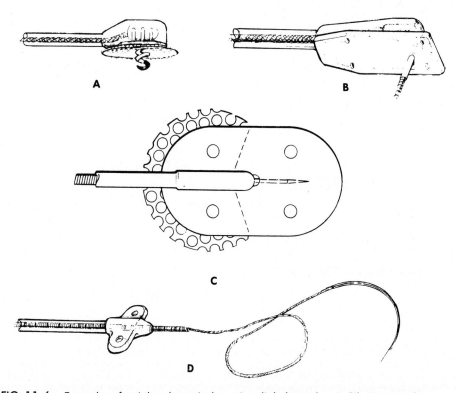

FIG. 11-6.   Examples of atrial and ventricular epicardial electrodes. A, Silastic sutureless unipolar ventricular electrode with corkscrew tip. Positive fixation is achieved by screwing the electrode into the myocardium (Medtronic model 6917A). B, Silastic unipolar epicardial electrode designed to be sutured to either the atrial or ventricular myocardium (Medtronic model 5815A). C, Urethane unipolar epicardial barbed-hook electrode providing positive fixation (without sutures) to either the atrial or ventricular myocardium (Medtronic model 4951). D, Silastic unipolar electrode for atrial or ventricular use. The needle and suture material extending from the exposed stainless steel electrode are used to fasten the electrode directly to the myocardium (Telectronics 030-170).

catheter in the bloodstream to the right ventricle. In the absence of fluoroscopy, ECG recordings from the catheter enable the user to determine the location of the electrodes (Fig. 11-7).

Heart wires are frequently placed in the atria and ventricles of patients at the time of open heart surgery. These stainless steel wires are used during the surgical procedure and during the postoperative recovery phase. In emergency situations wire electrodes can be inserted percutaneously into the heart by a pericardiocentesis (or similar) needle.

Similarly, during emergencies surface skin electrodes placed on the chest wall can be stimulated with very high voltages to achieve cardiac pacing transthoracically. Such an approach should be used only until a transvenous catheter electrode can be positioned. Recently an improved technique for noninvasive pacing has been reported to be of minimal discomfort and suitable for prolonged use. Special, large surface area electrodes and external pulse generators with very wide (about 40 msec) stimulus pulse widths are required.[51]

For temporary and permanent pacing it is important to place the electrodes in a position that provides acceptably low stimulation thresholds and sufficiently large intracardiac signals to be sensed by the pulse generator. Generally this implies acute thresholds of less than 2 mA and 1.25 V, with ventricular electrograms greater than 4mV or atrial electrograms in excess of 2mV. Thresholds generally rise following acute positioning, reaching a peak two to four times the acute values within the first 2 to 6 weeks and then falling to intermediate values.[52] The electrogram typically decreases in amplitude by 15%; its rate of rise with respect to time (slew rate) decreases as much as 50% with maturation of the implant.[53] These factors must be considered when evaluating the appropriateness of a given lead position.

POSTIMPLANTATION FOLLOW-UP

Despite the reliability demonstrated by current pacemakers, it is important to monitor the patient and the pacemaker system regularly after implantation. Such monitoring has four major goals: evaluate electrical function of the pacing system to detect malfunctions or imminent power-source depletion; evaluate the implant site for possible mechanical difficulties such as erosion or infection; detect progression of the patient's cardiac problems, which may necessitate reprogramming or revising the pacing system or accompanying drug regimen; and reassure patients that due concern and attention is being given their progress and offer opportunities to discuss concerns that may arise.

The follow-up schedule should be arranged to provide close monitoring during the immediate postimplantation period, moderately frequent observation during the routine service life of the system, and increased surveillance as the system nears completion of its service life. A suggested schedule is 6 weeks after implantation, twice annually beginning 6 months after implantation, and monthly once initial signs of power-source depletion are observed (in almost all pacemakers this appears as a rate decrease when monitored with a magnet over the pulse generator). Given the longevity of modern systems, it may be counter-pro-

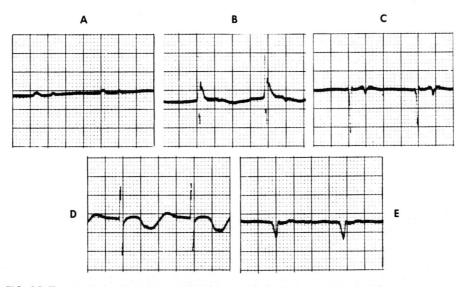

FIG. 11-7. Electrograms obtained when bipolar electrode is located in high superior vena cava (A), superior vena cava/right atrium (B), right atrium (C), right ventricle (D), and pulmonary artery (E). All tracings calibrated at 1 mV/cm except D, which is recorded at half standard.

ductive to attempt to stretch out the last few months of service by frequent monitoring since this will probably add but 5% to 10% to the total service life while increasing monitoring costs by 30% to 40%.

Follow-up visits should be scheduled in the physician's office or in a special pacemaker clinic where the patient can be seen in person. (Telephone monitoring of the patient's ECG, pacing rate, and pulse generator stimulus duration can be of value as a supplement between personal evaluations but should not replace office visits.) Each visit should include a recording of a 12-lead ECG with a rhythm strip showing that the pacemaker appropriately captures and senses, a measurement of pacemaker parameters with appropriate rate and pulse width measurement equipment, and a general physical examination including careful scrutiny of the pacemaker pocket. If a problem is evident or if the patient reports symptoms, an x-ray film may be obtained to evaluate the lead and its position, blood tests may help uncover threshold problems related to electrolyte imbalances, and long-term ambulatory monitoring may be indicated if intermittent failures are suspected. The results of the follow-up procedure should be carefully recorded,[54] since much of the required analysis depends on changes in operation rather than on absolute values of measured parameters. This record is especially important when following patients who have programmable pacemakers and for whom changes may be totally innocuous if intentional (such as a rate change programmed to improve cardiac output) or may signify device-performance problems (such as a rate decrease caused by battery depletion).

Care should be exercised in selecting follow-up equipment, and data must be analyzed with full understanding and knowledge of the idiosyncrasies of the equipment used. For example, digital monitoring and recording systems frequently do not register the pacemaker stimulus artifact reliably and reproducibly because of its extremely short duration. As a result, the pacemaker artifact may not always be recorded even if present, or its polarity and amplitude may vary markedly throughout the recording. On the other hand, such systems may substitute a standardized artifact for the real signal, eliminating diagnostic information in the process. As another example, some follow-up clinics perform waveform analysis using an oscilloscope or special ECG machine to display the waveshape of the pacemaker stimulus. One must be fully aware of the correct waveshape for each pacemaker to be evaluated. Modern pacemakers frequently produce much more complex stimulus pulse shapes than the traditional "square wave," and it is not unusual for such waveforms to be misread as signs of malfunction.

An often underestimated benefit of follow-up is a reduction in patient anxiety. A clear answer to a simple question can be extremely important to a patient's well-being.

In recognition of this, some clinics have formed pacemaker clubs which allow patients to meet periodically to compare notes and provide mutual support.

TROUBLESHOOTING[55-57]

Complex systems involving electrical, mechanical, and physiologic interactions will inevitably develop malfunctions, and pacemakers are no exception. Fortunately, the detection and correction of such problems are relatively straightforward for the knowledgeable user if appropriate equipment is available.

Equipment

The most useful troubleshooting tool is a *12-lead analog ECG machine*. This permits evaluation of pacemaker sensing, capture, and approximate rate, evaluation of electrode positioning (by vector analysis of ventricular activity), and confirmation of appropriate function for the mode of pacing employed. Multiple ECG leads are necessary for vector analysis of lead positioning and are frequently helpful in increasing visibility of small artifacts produced by bipolar systems or in evaluating atrial activity when dealing with dual-chamber or atrial demand pacemakers.

A *digital counter* is useful in obtaining accurate rate and pulse width information. These counters may be supplied as specialized patient monitors, built into pacemaker programmers, or purchased alone. Such devices are necessary when evaluating pacing rate and pulse width changes caused by battery depletion, component failure, or reprogramming.

A *magnet* should always be available for troubleshooting sessions. Nearly all pacemakers can be converted to asynchronous operation by the placement of a magnet over the generator site. This enables evaluation of capture when the patient's intrinsic rhythm inhibits the pacemaker and can be useful in diagnosing oversensing by disabling all sensing function. Magnet application should be used with care, since some pacemakers can be programmed by application of a suitable magnet, and there is always a definite but slight risk of inducing tachyarrhythmias when pacing asynchronously.

Carotid sinus massage or Valsalva maneuver may slow a patient's intrinsic rhythm and induce pacing. Such a procedure may be used to evaluate capture if a pacemaker fails to respond to magnet application because of either a component failure or a unique design having no asynchronous magnet mode.

Exercise may be used to speed the patient's spontaneous rate in the evaluation of sensing capability.

Chest wall stimulation with an external stimulator connected to precordial surface electrodes can be used to test sensing function and to determine rate tracking limits for atrial tracking pacemakers (VAT, VDD, DDD).

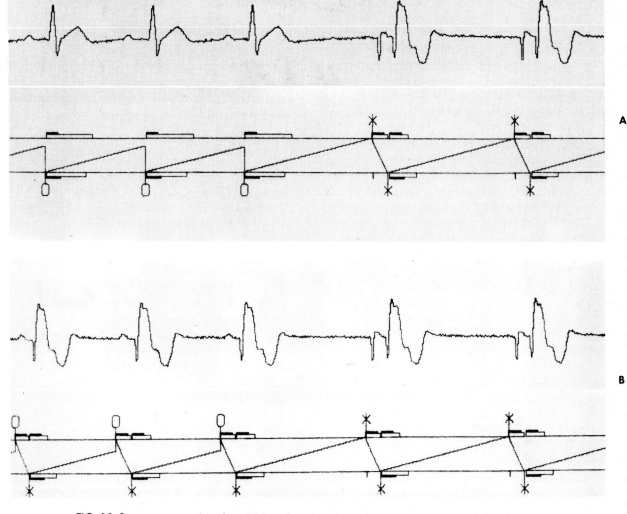

FIG. 11-8. *Upper panel;* surface ECG and marker channel generated diagnostic ladder diagram beneath, taken from a patient with an implanted DDD pacemaker. The surface ECG may appear to show normal inhibition of the pacemaker by three cycles of sinus rhythm after which a sinus pause elicits AV sequential pacing for two cycles. The diagram, however, reveals that the pacemaker is malfunctioning and is not sensing atrial activity. In the diagram *O* represents sensing; *, pacing; *white rectangular area,* pacemaker refractory periods; *solid rectangular area,* absolute refractory periods (blanking); sloping lines between the horizontal parallel lines indicate timing of AV (↘) and VA (↗) escape intervals. Atrial sensing, pacing, and refractory periods are marked above the top horizontal line, and ventricular events are marked beneath the lower line. The diagram in this upper panel shows *O* beneath the first three QRS complexes, indicating that the pacemaker correctly senses ventricular depolarization, and the upward sloping line following each O shows that the pacemaker is timing VA intervals appropriately. However, there is no O on the upper rung of the diagram beneath the sinus P waves. This indicates that the pacemaker is failing to sense atrial activity. During the last two complexes the diagram shows proper AV sequential pacing with asterisks beneath the paced P and QRS complexes to indicate stimulation.

Lower panel, same format as above. Records obtained after the atrial amplifier of the implanted pacemaker was programmed to increase its sensitivity. The pacemaker now clearly senses atrial activity during the first three cycles as evidenced by the sensing symbols *(O)* seen in the upper rung of the left portion of the ladder diagram and by the ventricular stimuli (indicated with * on the diagram) following the P waves one AV interval later. Pacemaker operation is now normal, with each P wave sensed, causing the pacemaker to deliver a ventricular stimulus one AV interval later.

Manipulation of the pulse generator in its pocket can sometimes elicit electrocardiographic signs of a loose connection or damaged lead close to the generator site.

X-ray examination or fluoroscopy of the chest and pacemaker system in multiple views helps determine lead position, gross lead fractures, and disconnections at the generator. A baseline x-ray film should be obtained before the patient is discharged, following implantation of the system.

An *oscilloscope* or special ECG recorder designed to display the waveshape of the pacemaker stimulus is used by some centers to evaluate lead problems or unusual component failures.

A pacemaker *programmer* is an extremely useful troubleshooting tool in dealing with a programmable pacemaker, allowing the user to vary stimulus strength, amplifier sensitivity, rates, refractory periods, and pacing modes. This permits noninvasive threshold evaluation and, in some of the newer systems, permits the user to obtain noninvasive intracardiac electrograms to evaluate sensing operation. Many systems include digital telemetry of the programmed settings of the pacemaker allowing actual performance to be compared to expected performance. The most sophisticated systems provide a *marker channel,* a noninvasively telemetered signal indicating pacemaker sensing and pacing, which in conjunction with a surface ECG clearly identifies pacemaker operation (Fig. 11-8).

Invasive procedures are necessary if noninvasive approaches fail. A *pacing system analyzer* is the primary tool for invasive troubleshooting. This instrument typically can analyze the implantable pulse generator function (sensitivities, refractory periods, rates, pulse widths, and amplitudes), evaluate lead integrity and positioning, and provide electrophysiologic patient data (stimulation thresholds, electrogram amplitudes, AV conduction, sinus function).

In addition to the troubleshooting hardware, it is equally important to have detailed patient records, including prior ECGs and x-ray films, and full information on the characteristics of the implanted system. Unfortunately, it is common for a normally functioning pacemaker to be diagnosed as malfunctioning simply because of inadequate understanding of proper device operation. Systems with hysteresis,* special antitachycardia pacemakers, and synchronous pacemakers are especially vulnerable to misdiagnosis.

Pacemaker-related problems fall into five broad categories: failure to pace, loss of sensing, oversensing, pacing at an altered rate, and undesirable patient/pacemaker interactions.

Failure to Pace

Failure to pace implies nondelivery of a stimulus or loss of capture (delivery of an ineffective stimulus that fails to depolarize the myocardium).

Failure to deliver a stimulus can result from various factors: improper connection of the lead to the generator (as when set screws are not tightened); broken lead wires with no insulation defect; "crosstalk" between atrial and ventricular portions of dual-chamber pacemakers so that the atrial stimulus is sensed by the ventricular amplifier, inhibiting the ventricular stimulus (caused by improper electrode placement or incorrect electrode types); pulse generator component failure; or power source depletion. Occasionally, a misdiagnosis of failure to pace is made when a normally functioning pacemaker is merely inhibited by the patient's intrinsic rhythm. This is especially common with programmable pacemakers set at relatively low rates. (Inappropriate nondelivery of a stimulus also may be caused by oversensing that is discussed later.)

Loss of capture may be caused by lead dislodgement

*Pacemakers with hysteresis are designed to work as follows: the escape interval (before pacing) following the last sensed spontaneous activity exceeds the interval between subsequent consecutive pacing artifacts. This allows maintenance of normal sinus rhythm over a wide range of rates (pacemaker-inhibited) while ensuring an adequate pacing rate when needed. This type of operation is diagrammed in Fig. 11-9.

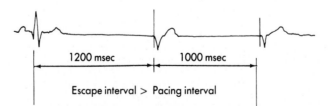

1200 msec   1000 msec

Escape interval > Pacing interval

FIG. 11-9. Diagrammatic representation of operation of a VVI pacemaker incorporating hysteresis. The last beat of the patient's sinus rhythm is shown as the first complex on the left. Spontaneous sinus bradycardia results, and the pacemaker "escapes" at an interval of 1200 msec. The subsequent pacing interval is 1000 msec, however; thus the escape interval of the pacemaker exceeds the pacing interval (in other words, the initial escape rate of pacemaker discharge is *slower* than the subsequent rate of pacing) to allow the patient to remain in a normally conducted rhythm for as much of the time as possible.

(the most common cause), myocardial perforation with lead migration to an extracardiac position, failure of lead insulation and/or wire fracture; increased stimulation threshold caused by infarction, drug effects, electrolyte imbalances, or fibrosis at the electrode site, or inappropriate programming of pacemaker stimulus strength. Lack of capture when a stimulus is delivered during the myocardial refractory period is a frequent source of misdiagnosis.

Loss of Sensing

A pacemaker may fail to sense intracardiac signals, resulting in competitive pacing or, in the case of atrial synchronous units, loss of AV synchrony. This may be caused by the following: lead dislodgement (the most common cause); inadequate amplitude or waveshape of the intracardiac electrogram caused by inappropriate lead placement, fibrosis, infarct, drugs, or electrolyte disturbances; inappropriate programming of amplifier sensitivity, refractory periods, or mode (for example, AOO, VOO); lead fracture or insulation defect; connector defect; or component failure (such as a stuck magnetic reedswitch).

Occasionally, a misdiagnosis of sensing failure is made when spontaneous activity occurs simultaneously with delivery of the pacemaker stimulus and results in fusion beats. This is because electrical activity may occur within the myocardium and be visible on the surface ECG record before it reaches the pacemaker electrode site. Concurrently, the pacemaker escape interval may elapse with resultant stimulation just before arrival of the spontaneous depolarization. This apparent failure to sense is, in fact, perfectly normal operation. Another cause of apparent sensing failure is reversion to asynchronous operation in the presence of electromagnetic interference—also a normal mode of operation for many pacemakers. Finally, closely coupled intracardiac signals may occur within the

pacemaker refractory period and not be sensed. This is frequently seen with certain AV sequential (DVI) pacemakers, which initiate the ventricular sensing amplifier refractory period upon stimulating in the atrium. If the atrial response propagates to the ventricles, the pacemaker will not sense this conducted ventricular activity but will stimulate into the refractory tissue. This is normal operation for such "committed" DVI devices (Fig. 11-10).

Oversensing

Occasionally a pacemaker will sense signals other than those cardiac signals that it is designed to detect, a phenomenon referred to as *oversensing*. Ventricular sensing pacemakers (DVI, VVI, VVT, VDD, DDD) may sense T waves if the amplifier is too sensitive or has too short a refractory period, or if the patient has unusually large or delayed intracardiac T waves. A dislodged ventricular lead resting near the right ventricular inflow tract may cause inappropriate sensing of atrial activity. Conversely, atrial sensing pacemakers (AAI, AAT, VAT, VDD, DDD) may inappropriately sense ventricular activity if the atrial amplifier refractory period is too short, or if the atrial signals are too small to be sensed with consequent failure to initiate appropriate atrial refractory periods. Some AV sequential pacemakers (DVI) may sense delivery of an atrial stimulus and inhibit the ventricular stimulus ("crosstalk") if they are used with incorrectly spaced bipolar electrodes, or if the atrial and ventricular electrodes are not separated by a suitable distance (typically a minimum of 4 cm).

Unipolar pacemakers may sense skeletal muscle potentials generated by contraction of the major pectoralis muscles, resulting in inappropriate inhibition (AAI, VVI, DVI, VDD, DDD) or triggering (AAT, VVT, VAT, VDD, DDD) of stimuli.

All pacemakers except asynchronous devices sense the

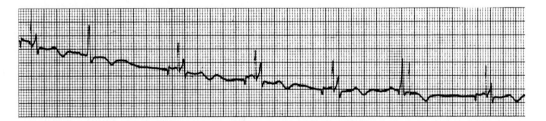

FIG. 11-10. Surface ECG (monitor lead) demonstrating an example of a "committed" mode DVI pacemaker. Note that the first, third, fourth, fifth, and seventh complexes are initiated by an atrial spike (small negative deflection) that paces the atrium and then a ventricular spike (large upright deflection) that paces the ventricle. The second QRS complex occurs sufficiently early to inhibit pacemaker discharge. However, the sixth QRS complex occurs early, but not early enough to inhibit the atrial discharge. Following the atrial spike (seen as the initial negative deflection preceding the onset of the QRS complex, after the P wave) a conducted QRS occurs. However, this QRS complex is not sensed by the pacemaker, which is committed to delivering a pacemaker spike (large upright spike following the QRS complex in the ST segment) regardless of spontaneous ventricular activity.

voltage changes produced when a lead with a hairline fracture or loose connection makes intermittent contact or when two endocardial leads come into contact. Electromagnetic interference from power lines, radio or television transmitters, and other electrical noise sources may occasionally be sensed, especially by unipolar pacemakers. Sometimes this may result in inhibition or triggering, but it more commonly produces reversion to the asynchronous mode that provides the patient with continued pacing support. Very rarely, a pacemaker may sense the afterpotentials remaining on a lead following delivery of a stimulus. This is most commonly the result of using very wide pulse widths or excessively short refractory periods.

In all cases of suspected oversensing, placing the pacemaker in an asynchronous mode (with application of a magnet if it is a permanent pacemaker, or turning off the sensitivity if it is an external pacemaker) will abolish the symptoms caused by the pacemaker malfunction and confirm the diagnosis.

Pacing at an Altered Rate

A fairly common cause for concern is apparent operation of a pacemaker at an unexpected rate. This can be an indication of a real problem with the pacemaker system but more frequently reflects a diagnostic error.

The possible true causes of unexpected pacing at an altered rate include the following: oversensing that induces rate slowing caused by inhibition, or rate acceleration caused by triggering; rate drift, a gradual benign shift of the pacing rate caused by component aging or temperature effects (most commonly found in older pacemakers that do not use digital timing circuits); rate slowdown built into most pacemakers to indicate approaching power source depletion; and component failure (usually causing either no stimulus output or a rapid stimulation rate typically limited to less than 150 beats/minute by "runaway" protection circuits).

Frequent causes of pacing at an altered rate when there is no system failure include the following: presence of a rate hysteresis that produces a long escape interval following sensed activity; reprogramming of a programmable pacemaker without proper recording of the change in the patient records; tracking of spontaneous intrinsic cardiac rate accelerations with VVT, AAT, VAT, VDD, or DDD pacemakers; failure of the reader to note a nearly isoelectric atrial or ventricular complex in a single-lead ECG tracing so that the pacemaker appears to have a prolonged stimulus-to-stimulus interval; misinterpretation of nonpacemaker artifacts such as rapid spike potentials generated by muscle fasciculation or electrical noise in the ECG recording system; lack of familiarity with device operation (such as a DVI pacemaker perceived to be pacing the ventricles at a rate equivalent to its VA interval when it is, in fact, pacing atrially and appropriately inhibiting the ventricular stimulus in response to conducted ventricular activity).

Undesirable Patient-Pacemaker Interactions

Occasionally, undesirable patient-pacemaker system interactions can develop. The pacemaker pocket may become infected or develop hematomas, or the generator may erode through the pocket site. These problems occur less frequently with the current small, lightweight generators. Some patients exhibit "twiddler's syndrome," playing with their pulse generators and rotating them in their pockets, retracting the lead and producing total system failure.

Extracardiac stimulation of the pectoralis muscles or diaphragm may be observed. These problems are generally restricted to unipolar pacemakers, although they have been reported, in rare instances, with bipolar systems. Decreasing the pulse width, voltage, or current of the stimulus can be useful in eliminating or reducing such extracardiac stimulation.

Incorrect pacing mode selection for a given patient or changes in a patient's postimplantation status can have serious consequences. For example, atrial tracking pacemakers (VAT, VDD, DDD) may detect slowly conducted retrograde atrial activity (long RP interval) following ventricular stimulation, inducing "pacemaker tachycardia" with a rate equal to the pacemaker's upper rate limit. Patients may respond poorly to other specific pacing modes depending on their underlying hemodynamic and electrophysiologic substrates. In many such cases, the use of multiprogrammable pacemakers allows the clinician to alter the pacing system characteristics without resorting to invasive procedures.

Table 11-6 summarizes various pacemaker problems and their likely causes.

An Illustrative Approach

The following hypothetical example demonstrates how one troubleshoots a pacemaker malfunction, in this case intermittent loss of capture and failure to sense spontaneous ventricular activity (Fig. 11-11). The patient has a ventricular demand (VVI) pacemaker implanted 1 year ago.

The first step in troubleshooting is to list the likely causes of the symptoms. Since there are two malfunctions in this example, it is highly probable, although not absolutely certain, that there is a common cause. The most likely causes are:

Lack of capture	Lack of sensing
Lead dislodgement, perforation	Lead dislodgement, perforation
Lead wire fracture	Lead wire fracture
Lead insulation failure	Lead insulation failure
Pulse generator failure	Pulse generator failure
Inappropriate programming of output energy	Inappropriate programming of amplifier sensitivity or refractory period

TABLE 11-6. Pacemaker system problems and etiologies*

	Nonpacing (NP) Noncapture (NC)	Non-sensing	Over-sensing	Altered Rate	Undesirable Patient/ IPG Interactions
ACTUAL MALFUNCTIONS					
Lead dislodged or perforated myocardium (possibly caused by twiddler's syndrome)	NC	X	X	X	X
Lead insulation failure	NC	X	X	X	X
Lead fracture with fluid in lumen	NC	X	X	X	
Skeletal muscle potentials, EMI, hairline lead fractures	NP	X	X	X	
Pulse generator failure	NP, NC	X	X	X	
Poor lead/IPG connection	NP	X	X	X	
Power source depletion	NC, NP	X	X		
Lead fracture with dry lumen	NP	X			
Electrical interference resulting in asynchronous pacing		X		X	
Cross-talk between atrial and ventricular channels			X	X	
Sensitivity too high			X	X	
Refractory period too short			X	X	
High threshold: fibrosis, infarct, drugs, electrolyte imbalance, lead position	NC				
Low output energy setting	NC				
Poor electrogram: fibrosis, infarct, drugs, electrolyte imbalance, lead position		X			
Sensitivity too low		X			
Refractory period too long		X			
Asynchronous mode: magnet or programmed		X			
End of service life indicator activated				X	
High output energy setting: extracardiac stimulation					X
Infection, hematoma, erosion					X
POTENTIAL MISDIAGNOSES					
Recording system masks ECG signal (e.g., lead switching)	NP, NC		X	X	
Recorder malfunction (e.g., paper speed error)		X	X	X	
Hysteresis mode			X	X	X
Fusion of activity from pacemaker and cardiac source	NC	X			
Artifacts from source other than IPG (e.g., muscle fasciculation)	NC			X	
Stimulus falls in tissue refractory period	NC				
Atrial stimulus misread as ventricular without capture or vice versa	NC				
Cardiac activity is within IPG refractory period (e.g., QRS within AV interval of committed DVI pacemaker)		X			
Rate responsive pacemaker changing rate in response to parameter not reflected in ECG record (e.g., activity)				X	

*The column headings are symptoms of a malfunctioning pacemaker system. The leftmost entries in each row are specific mechanisms that can produce those symptoms marked with an X, NC (noncapture = ineffective stimulus), or NP (nonpacing = no stimulus artifact). After determining the type and number of symptoms exhibited by a system, one can find a match to entries in this table, thereby determining the most probable cause of the malfunction. The lower half of the table links apparent symptoms with mechanisms that do not result from pacemaker malfunction.

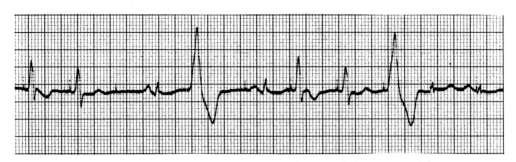

FIG. 11-11. Failure of a VVI pacemaker. Note that pacing stimuli occasionally fail to elicit a paced QRS complex and also occasionally fail to sense spontaneous electrical activity. Lead II.

Lack of capture	Lack of sensing
High threshold	Inadequate electrogram amplitude (caused by infarct, electrolyte disturbance, myocardial disease)
Misread ECG ("loss of capture" seen only when stimulus occurs during cardiac refractory period)	Electromagnetic interference-induced (EMI) reversion to asynchronous mode
	Stuck reed switch
	Misread ECG (fusion beats)

Analysis should begin by comparing a current 12-lead ECG to a baseline tracing predating occurrence of the problem. The current tracing should be carefully reviewed to prevent misinterpretation of fusion beats as sensing failure or pacing artifacts during the cardiac refractory period as lack of capture. EMI-induced reversion to the asynchronous mode can usually be eliminated as a cause if the problem of nonsensing persists in a 12-lead ECG that shows no signs of electrical interference. Comparison of the current and baseline ECGs establishes the presence or absence of lead position changes, including perforation, as evidenced by shifts in the paced QRS vector and pacing artifact vector.* An x-ray examination provides confirmation of significant dislodgements. Insulation defects in the lead will result in vector changes in the pacing artifact but usually not in the paced QRS complex.

Application of a magnet should result in pacing without sensing. In most pacemakers magnet application alters the pacing rate (sometimes by only a few milliseconds), confirming that the reed switch is functioning and allowing one to eliminate the possibility of nonsensing caused by a stuck reed switch.

If inappropriate programming is thought to be the problem, it is a simple matter to reprogram the amplifier sensitivity and refractory period to restore sensing and to increase the stimulus intensity to restore capture. If such reprogramming fails to resolve the problem or if the parameter settings required are not within normally accepted bounds, then inappropriate programming can be excluded.

*Digital ECG systems with low sampling rates cannot be used to determine the reliability of the vector of the pacemaker artifact.

Wire fracture can produce nonsensing and lack of capture, but it is generally accompanied by random resetting of the escape interval as the broken wire ends touch intermittently. An x-ray examination can sometimes be helpful in confirming wire fracture, but not all fractures are visible on the x-ray film. In this example the regularity of the escape intervals probably eliminates wire fracture as the cause of the problem.

At this point noninvasive procedures have been explored to evaluate the majority of potential causes for the reported malfunctions. Threshold elevation, inadequate electrogram characteristics, and pulse generator failure all require invasive evaluation, although some noninvasive determinations can be obtained if the patient has a sophisticated multiprogrammable pulse generator. Some of these devices can telemeter the intracardiac electrogram, facilitating evaluation of sensing problems. They also allow the user to obtain noninvasive threshold measurements. Nevertheless, correction of sensing and pacing failure caused by any of these factors will require invasive procedures.

In the example cited, ECG evidence, shown in Fig. 11-12, indicates a lead dislodgement. Note the axis shift in the pacemaker stimulus artifact and in the paced QRS complexes. Lead placement is the most common cause of sensing and capture failures.

NURSING CARE OF THE PACEMAKER PATIENT

Nursing care of pacemaker patients encompasses both patients and their families and begins the moment the need for a pacemaker is identified. Patients may have vastly different prior knowledge of such devices, ranging from having no knowledge at all to having a reasonably accurate understanding. But whatever their level of knowledge, thorough and accurate information presented in a clear and logical manner will help reassure the patient and stimulate acceptance of the need for a pacemaker, while letting the patient understand what life with a pacemaker will be like.

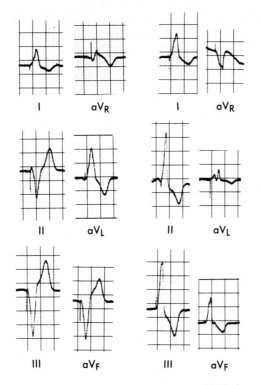

FIG. 11-12. ECG leads I, II, III, aV_R, aV_L, and aV_F were recorded before *(left panel)* and after *(right panel)* pacemaker malfunction. VVI pacemaker developed sensing and capture problems. Note that the vector and amplitude of the spikes are different in the two 12-lead ECGs and that the generated QRS complexes also are different. This ECG example is most consistent with migration of the pacing electrode from its initial appropriate location in the right ventricle apex to a different position in the ventricle. This was the case, and the lead was repositioned.

Preimplant, the use of charts, drawings or models help patients understand the parts of a pacemaker system and where they will be placed. Such visual aids also help patients understand how the heart functions and why a pacemaker is necessary. Showing patients a model of the actual pacemaker and lead to be implanted is often helpful, since patients may imagine the devices to be considerably larger than they actually are. These models, as well as the visual aids, are often available from various pacemaker manufacturers, sometimes at a nominal charge. Additional teaching aids such as slide series and materials written specifically for children are also usually available.

A patient booklet is usually packaged with each pacemaker, and extra copies can be obtained. Patients should be encouraged to read the booklet and to ask any questions they may have.

During the pacemaker implantation procedure, the implant team should be careful of what they are saying, since patients are often fully conscious or only minimally sedated. Patients should be told ahead of time if there are specific things they will be asked to do during the procedure, such as coughing or deep breathing to help ensure

that the lead has been securely stabilized. The absence of general anesthesia also means that patients should be told that they will be covered with surgical drapes, that their arms and legs will be secured, and that they should not move unless asked to do so. They should be told to indicate if they are in pain, such as when the pacemaker pocket is being created, so that additional local anesthesia can be given if necessary. In general, patients should be prepared for what they will see, feel, and hear, and medical and nursing personnel should be constantly attentive to minimize anxiety, to answer questions, and to reassure patients regarding the progress of the procedure.[58]

Postimplant nursing care is specific to the type of implant, the pacemaker system involved, the area where the patient is cared for, and the policies and procedures of the institution. Continuous ECG monitoring for a period of time helps ensure that the newly implanted pacemaker is pacing and sensing appropriately. In addition, a postoperative chest x-ray confirms proper positioning of the lead(s). The pacemaker implant site should also be checked to ensure that sutures are intact and drainage is not excessive. In some institutions restrictions are placed on body movement during the first several hours or days after implantation of a new lead system, and practices concerning length of hospitalization differ. Resumption of normal activities after pacemaker implantation varies from patient to patient, and depends to a large degree on the patient's state of health before the implant and the reason(s) a pacemaker was felt to be necessary. Patients should be encouraged to resume normal daily activities and recreational pursuits, gradually increasing the levels as their state of health permits.

Lifestyle adaptation, the most important aspect of which is regular follow-up care, should also be emphasized.[59] Patients should have a thorough knowledge of why they now need to be seen or heard from regularly, and the type of follow-up chosen for them (clinic visits, transtelephonic monitoring, or a combination of both) should be fully explained to them. This is also the time to discuss the safe use of common electrical devices such as microwave ovens, electric toothbrushes, and hair dryers (all properly functioning household electrical devices are generally considered safe to use), symptoms they might experience in the presence of strong continuous electrical interference (commonly a return of their preimplant symptoms), and what should be done if this occurs (move away from or stop using the device in question and then telephone their medical contact person). Patients who have previously been using or working with more complex electrical devices on the job or for leisure activities may need special information. Such devices might include welding equipment, automobile engines, or power tools. If a patient must continue using such equipment, the manufacturer of the patient's device can be asked to assess specific situations, determine if continued use of the equipment in question is safe or if it can be modified to ensure its safe use. In general, use of electrical devices by patients with pacemakers does not present problems unless the electrical signals generated by the equipment are interpreted by the pacemaker's sensing circuits as being generated by the heart. Depending on the type of pacemaker implanted, this could then result in inappropriate inhibition of the implanted device or inappropriate triggering, especially in antitachycardia pacemakers. But since pacemakers differ from one manufacturer to another, and since various electrical devices generate different signals, individual assessment of specific situations is essential, and it is important not to assume that patients with pacemakers are automatically restricted in their use of certain electrical devices.

Some patients may enjoy participating in clubs specifically designed for pacemaker recipients, or receiving newsletters and magazines designed for them. Medical and nursing personnel involved in caring for patients with pacemakers should therefore become familiar with what is available in their communities. Information can be obtained from local heart associations and from pacemaker manufacturers. Patients should also be encouraged to carry with them at all times the pacemaker identification card issued by the manufacturer of their devices, and other medical identification information if appropriate. This is particularly important when traveling, since implanted pacemakers can sometimes trigger airport security systems. In addition, should adjustment of pacemaker parameters become necessary for any reason, the pacemaker identification card will enable medical and nursing personnel to accurately identify the implanted device and quickly locate the appropriate equipment needed to reprogram it. If defibrillation is required, it is essential that defibrillation paddles not be placed directly over an implanted pacemaker, and that assessment of the pacing system be made as soon as possible after defibrillation has occurred. This includes verification of the device's programmed parameters, as well as verification of appropriate pacing and sensing, which in most cases should not be affected by the defibrillation.[60]

A useful book for patients desiring more detailed information about their pacemaker system is "Understanding Pacemakers" with a foreward by the late Henry Fonda, a notable pacemaker recipient. Written by a medical writer, an electrical engineer, and a physician, this paperback offers everything any patient would want to know about pacemakers, in a style that is easy to read and understand.[61] The book is also useful to medical and nursing personnel who may have had little previous experience with pacemaker systems.

REFERENCES

1. Elmquist, R., and Senning, A.: An implantable pacemaker for the heart, Proceedings of the second international conference of medical-electrical engineers, London, 1959, Iliffe & Sons Ltd.
2. Zoll, P., and Linenthal, A.: Long-term electrical pacemakers for Stokes-Adams disease, Circulation **22:**341, 1960.
3. Goldman, B.S., and Parsonnet, V.: World survey on cardiac pacing, PACE **2**(5):W1, 1979.
4. Zipes, D.P., and Duffin, E.: Cardiac pacemakers. In Braunwald, E., editor: Heart disease: a textbook of cardiovascular medicine, ed. 2, Philadelphia, 1984, W.B. Saunders Co.
5. Sutton, R., Perrins, J., and Citron, P.: Physiological cardiac pacing, PACE **3**(2):207, 1980.
6. Osborn, M.J., and Holmes, D.R.: Antitachycardia pacing, Clin. Prog. Electrophysiol. Pacing **3**(4):239, 1985.
7. Duffin, E., and Zipes, D.P.: Chronic electrical control of tachyarrhythmia. In Mandel, W.J.: Cardiac arrhythmias, their mechanisms, diagnosis and management, Philadelphia, 1987, J.B. Lippincott.
8. Zipes, D.P.: Electrical therapy of cardiac arrhythmias (editorial), N. Engl. J. Med. **309:**1179, 1983.
9. Akhtar, M., and others: NASPE ad hoc committee on guidelines for cardiac electrophysiological studies, PACE **8:**611, 1985.
10. Parsonnet, V., Furman, S., and Smyth, N.P.D.: A revised code for pacemaker identification, PACE **4**(4):400, 1981.
11. Nathan, D., Center, S., and Wu, C.: An implantable synchronous pacemaker for the long-term correction of complete heart block, Am. J. Cardiol. **11:**362, 1963.

12. Kruse, I., Ryden, L., and Duffin, E.: Clinical evaluation of atrial synchronous ventricular inhibited pacemakers, PACE **3**:641, 1980.

13. Berkovits, B., Castellanos, A., and Lemberg, L.: Bifocal demand pacing, Circulation **39**:44, 1969.

14. Funke, H.D.: Three years experience in optimized sequential cardiac pacing, Stimucoeur **9**(1):26, 1981.

15. Fananapazir, L., and others: Atrial synchronized ventricular pacing: contribution of the chronotropic response to improved exercise performance, PACE **6**(3):601, 1983.

16. Fearnot, N.E., and others: Increasing cardiac rate by measurement of right ventricular temperature, PACE **7**(6):1240, 1984.

17. Wirtzfeld, A., and others: Regulation of pacing rate by variations of mixed venous oxygen saturation, PACE **7**(6):1257, 1984.

18. Cammilli, L., and others: Results, problems, and perspectives with the autoregulating pacemaker, PACE **6**(2):488, 1983.

19. Salo, R.W., and others: Continuous ventricular volume assessment for diagnosis and pacemaker control, PACE **7**(6):1267, 1984.

20. Bennett, T., and others: Alternative modes for physiological pacing. In Gomez, F., editor: Cardiac pacing, Futura Media Services, Mount Kisco, N.Y., 1985.

21. Fananapazir, L., and others: Reliability of the evoked response in determining the paced ventricular rate and performance of the QT or rate responsive (TX) pacemaker, PACE **8**(5):701, 1985.

22. Goicolea de Ore, A., and others: Rate responsive pacing: clinical experience, PACE **8**(3):322, 1985.

23. Rossi, P., and others: Increasing cardiac rate by tracking the respiratory rate, PACE **7**(6):1246, 1984.

24. Humen, D., and others: Activity-sensing, rate-responsive pacing: improvement in myocardial performance with exercise, PACE **8**(1):52, 1985.

25. Mirowski, M., and others: Clinical performance of the implantable cardioverter-defibrillator, PACE **7**:1345, 1984.

26. Nathan, A.W., Spurrell, R.A.J., and Camm, A.J.: Steps towards the development of a safe and effective tachycardia terminating pacemaker, Eur. Heart J. **5**:993, 1984.

27. Portillo, B., and others: Treatment of drug-resistant A-V reciprocating tachycardias with multiprogrammable dual demand A-V sequential (DVI-MN) pacemakers, PACE **5**(6):814, 1982.

28. Zipes, D.P., and others: Early experience with the implantable cardioverter, N. Engl. J. Med. **311**:485, 1984.

29. Parsonnet, V., and Rodgers, T.: The present status of programmable pacemakers, Prog. Cardiovasc. Dis. **23**(6):401, 1981.

30. Furman, S., and Pannizzo, F.: Output programmability and reduction of secondary intervention after pacemaker implantation, J. Thorac. Cardiovasc. Surg. **81**(5):713, 1981.

31. Hayes, D.L., and others: Initial and early follow-up assessment of the clinical efficacy of a multiparameter-programmable pulse generator, PACE **4**(4):417, 1981.

32. Billhardt, R.A., and others: Successful management of pacing system malfunctions without surgery: the role of programmable pulse generators, PACE **5**(5):675, 1982.

33. Parsonnet, V.: Cardiac pacing and pacemakers. VII. Power sources for implantable pacemakers, part 1, Am. Heart J. **94**(4):517, 1977.

34. Brennen, K.R., and others: A capacity rating system for cardiac pacemaker batteries, J. Power Sources **5**:25, 1980.

35. Bilitch, M., and others: Performance of cardiac pacemaker pulse generators, PACE **8**(2):276, 1985.

36. Greatbatch, W.: Metal electrodes in bioengineering, CRC Crit. Rev. Bioeng. **5**(1):1, 1981.

37. Smyth, N.P.D.: Techniques of implantation: atrial and ventricular, thoracotomy and transvenous, Prog. Cardiovasc. Dis. **23**(6):435, 1981.

38. Littleford, P., Parsonnet, V., and Spector, S.: Method for the rapid and atraumatic insertion of permanent endocardial pacemaker electrodes through the subclavian vein, Am. J. Cardiol. **43**:980, 1979.

39. Parsonnet, V., and others: Transvenous insertion of double sets of permanent electrodes, JAMA **62**, 1980.

40. Parsonnet, V.: Routine implantation of permanent transvenous pacemaker electrodes in both chambers: a technique whose time has come, PACE **4**(1):109, 1981.

41. Furman, S., Pannizzo, F., and Campo, I.: Comparison of active and passive adhering leads for endocardial pacing, PACE **2**(4):417, 1979.

42. Furman, S., Pannizzo, F., and Campo, I.: Comparison of active and passive adhering leads for endocardial pacing, part 2, PACE **4**(1):78, 1981.

43. Kertes, P., and others: Comparison of lead complications with polyurethane tined, silicone rubber tined and wedge tip leads: clinical experience with 822 ventricular endocardial leads, PACE **6**(5):957, 1983.

44. Timmis, G.C., and others: The evolution of low threshold leads, Clin. Prog. Pacing Electrophysiol. **1**:313, 1983.

45. Heineman, F., David, M., and Helland, J.: Clinical performance of a pacing lead with a platinized "target tip" electrode (abstract), PACE **7**:471, 1984.

46. Timmis, G.C., and others: A new steroid-eluting low threshold pacemaker lead. In Steinbach, K., editor: Proceedings of the seventh world symposium on cardiac pacing, Vienna, 1983.

47. Kruse, I.M., and Terpstra, B.: Acute and long-term atrial and ventricular stimulation thresholds with a steroid-eluting electrode, PACE **8**:45, 1985.

48. Timmis, G.C., and others: Late effects of a steroid-eluting porous titanium pacemaker lead electrode in man (abstract), PACE **7**:479, 1984.

49. King, D.H., and others: A steroid-eluting endocardial pacing lead for treatment of exit block, Am. Heart J. **106**:1438, 1983.

50. deFeyter, P., and others: Permanent cardiac pacing with sutureless myocardial electrodes: experience in first one hundred patients, PACE **3**(2):144, 1980.

51. Zoll, P., Zoll, R., and Belgard, A.: External noninvasive electric stimulation of the heart, Crit. Care Med. **9**(5):393, 1981.

52. Furman, S., Hurzeler, P., and Mehra, R.: Cardiac pacing and pacemakers. IV. Threshold of cardiac stimulation, Am. Heart J. **94**(1):115, 1977.

53. Furman, S., Hurzeler, P., and DeCaprio, V.: Cardiac pacing and pacemakers. III. Sensing the cardiac electrogram, Am. Heart J. **93**(6):794, 1977.

54. MacGregor, D., and others: Computer assisted reporting system for the follow-up of patients with cardiac pacemakers, PACE **3**(5):568, 1980.

55. Furman, S.: Cardiac pacing and pacemakers. VI. Analysis of pacemaker malfunction, Am. Heart J. **94**(3):378, 1977.

56. Barold, S.: Modern cardiac pacing, Mt. Kisco, N.Y., 1985, Futura Publishing Co.

57. Mond, H.G.: The cardiac pacemaker: function and malfunction, N.Y., 1983, Grune & Stratton.

58. Krumbach, B., and Maran, J.: Pacemaker insertion: the perioperative role, Today's OR Nurse **6**(11):8, 1984.

59. Lasche, P.: Permanent cardiac pacing. Technology and follow-up, Focus Crit. Care **10**(5):28, 1983.

60. Owen, P.M.: Defibrillating pacemaker patients, Am. J. Nurs. **84**(9):1129, 1984.

61. Sonnenburg, D., Birnbaum, M., and Naclerio, E.: Understanding pacemakers, New York, 1982, Michael Kesend Publishing, Ltd.

CHAPTER 12

Care of the Cardiac Patient

Martha E. Branyon
Cynthia M. Schuch

Much has been learned about treating critical cardiac illnesses in the past three decades. Technology and aggressive therapy have become increasingly prominent in the cardiac care unit.

At a time when modern technology and scientific research are expanding the ability of health professionals to diagnose and treat patients with acute myocardial infarction, some investigators are questioning the necessity of admitting all patients with chest pain and possible diagnosis of myocardial infarction to the coronary care unit (CCU). As health care costs rise and private and governmental agencies investigate the validity of these rising costs, it is small wonder that research teams have questioned the value of managing all patients with suspected acute myocardial infarction in hospital CCUs. The basic premise for CCUs seems sound: the CCU has generally been considered an indispensable component of any acute care hospital. The introduction of the CCU coincided with a remarkable reduction in mortality from myocardial infarction (MI) in North America. The CCU has been credited with a major contribution to this reduced mortality; however, in recent years the validity of this claim has been questioned. Some studies have suggested that admission to a CCU favorably influenced the mortality rate; others have failed to show benefits.[1-8]

The belief that the survival rate of patients with pump failure can be greatly influenced by treatment may be arguable,[1] but there is general agreement that the procedures involved require a special care unit. The two activities most likely to positively influence myocardial infarction mortality are the prevention of ventricular fibrillation and its successful management when it does occur.

Ventricular fibrillation associated with myocardial infarction can occur early or late in the course of the illness. Early ventricular fibrillation is the greatest single cause of death in MI. It occurs most often during the first 4 hours after the commencement of the infarction,[9] and studies in animals suggest it may be caused by impaired conduction in ischemic subepicardial muscle.[10] In contrast, late ventricular fibrillation may occur any time after the completion of the infarction process and may be caused by patchy retardation of conduction and increased automaticity in the Purkinje system of the infarcted area.[11] Factors that predict the occurrence of late ventricular fibrillation will be discussed later in this chapter.

The CCU should be used to prevent or treat malignant arrhythmias associated with acute ischemia and early acute myocardial infarction.[1] The three categories of patients who would benefit most from treatment in a CCU are those who (1) have angina at rest, (2) have an MI in progress, or (3) have an extension of the infarction.

McGregor[1] concluded that a CCU is clearly desirable for the management of life threatening complications of MI. In addition, patients who have angina at rest should be managed in the CCU for 24 hours after the last ischemic episode and patients with uncomplicated MIs who are free of pain for 8 hours can be managed in general cardiology units. Mortality caused by myocardial infarction can be reduced if patients enter an emergency medical system and CCU as soon as possible after the onset of the illness.[1]

Scientific and technologic advances have created an increasingly complex environment for the care of the cardiac patient. In an effort to improve patient care services, new or more specialized health practitioners have been introduced into the milieu of coronary care. Many units now employ monitor and cardiovascular technicians whose primary responsibility is maintenance of the equipment used in patient care. Many of these technicians are also responsible for monitoring cardiac rhythms and initiating appropriate therapy. A variety of respiratory, physical, and occupational therapists are also involved. Dietitians and pharmacists are often employed solely for the hospital's cardiac patient population. Cardiovascular nurse clinicians and cardiovascular clinical nurse specialists are commonplace in many CCUs and have varying responsibilities related to patient care and staff development. Physicians seek consultation from specialists who have advanced knowledge and skill in cardiovascular nuclear radiology, electrocardiography, echocardiography, electrophysiology, and arteriography. Associated with these specialists are a variety of additional technicians who interact with the patient.

The proliferation of health practitioners in coronary care introduces the potential for fragmentation of patient care and loss of focus on the patient as a whole being. This concern led the NIH Consensus Conference on Critical Care to conclude in 1983 that "nurses are the key element in critical care."[12] To prevent fragmentation and to promote effective, efficient, and holistic care for the cardiac patient, collaboration and cooperation are essential among all care providers. The primary physician and nurse have the responsibility to seek advice and assistance as appropriate from other health practitioners, the patient, and the family, and to use their contributions as they make decisions concerning patient care. The physician and nurse together need to develop a comprehensive plan that encompasses the goals and activities of all who interact with the patient.

The environment in which the cardiac patient is managed has made the process of treating and caring for the patient complex; however, close networking among all health care providers can expedite decisions about the patient's needs. Priorities can be established more easily, and the process of providing care can be more rewarding for all involved.

The purpose of this chapter is to present a comprehensive approach to planning and implementing care based on the patient's individual needs from admission to discharge. Such an approach is important because patients are likely to be moved from one hospital area to another as their condition improves. Needs change as the patient and family adjust to the suddenness of admission to a CCU and as they plan for discharge and resumption of their normal activities. Of course, recovery is not always uneventful and the patient and family must address crises as they occur.

PRIORITIES IN ADMISSION TO THE CCU

Patients are admitted to a CCU for rapid management of existing problems, surveillance for and early management of arrhythmias, and initial rehabilitation. At the time of admission it is important to collect baseline data for initiating therapy and for comparison at later stages in the patient's course (Fig. 12-1).

Immediate Monitoring of Cardiac Rate and Rhythm

Because disturbances in cardiac rhythm occur frequently in the early course of acute myocardial infarction and because these arrhythmias may be lethal, it is essential that electrodes be applied immediately. A brief explanation of the purpose of the electrodes should be given to the patient at this time. As the patient becomes stabilized, the monitoring equipment can be discussed with the patient more thoroughly. *Rate meter alarms should always be set* to alert the staff to any tachyarrhythmia or bradyarrhythmia.

Establishment of a Patent Intravenous (IV) Line

An indwelling catheter is inserted and secured in place as a means of administering fluids and pain medication and emergency drugs, should they be required. Needles should never be used because they are easily dislodged from the vein.

Relief of Pain and Anxiety

Complaints of pain should be treated immediately with analgesic medication. Morphine sulfate is often the drug of choice, but may be contraindicated if second-degree AV block or sinus bradycardia is present. If morphine sulfate is given and the degree of AV block or sinus bradycardia worsens, atropine may be administered to counteract its effects. After morphine is given, it is important that blood pressure, heart rate, and respiratory rate be carefully monitored for any adverse effects. The effects of pain and anxiety may be synergistic and result in an increased myocardial oxygen demand by an already compromised heart. Therefore it is vital that both pain and anxiety be promptly alleviated. The physician will usually prescribe analgesics and nitrates for relief of pain, and these should be administered as needed. Brief explanations to the patient about activities and equipment may assist in relieving anxiety. A mild sedative such as diazepam may be prescribed to reduce anxiety and stress. Opiates and sedatives, however, should be given cautiously if at all to confused and restless patients suffering from shock or heart failure. Family visits may contribute to or mitigate against stress and anxiety and should be carefully monitored for these effects. A booklet about the CCU that is tailored to the individual is helpful to families in understanding what is being done and why (Fig. 12-2).

Supplemental Oxygen

Even in patients with uncomplicated infarctions, hypoxemia may be present and necessitate the use of oxygen. Most often a binasal cannula administering 1 to 2 L/min is sufficient. Application of a lubricant or emollient to the nares will help to prevent irritation and maintain skin integrity. Measurement of arterial blood gas levels 30 minutes after initiating oxygen therapy provides a baseline for arterial oxygenation; however, recent investigation suggests that only 10 minutes is required for equilibration.[13] Arterial blood gas levels are measured as necessary to guide oxygen administration and maintain acid-base balance.

Decrease in Myocardial Oxygen Consumption

Recovery of the myocardium requires that the workload and subsequent oxygen demand of the heart be reduced. This is accomplished generally through bed rest and assistance with activities of daily living. While complete bed rest for several weeks was once thought to be necessary for the healing of the infarction, current regimens are less restrictive. The concept of METs is frequently used to determine appropriate activity following myocardial infarction. A MET is an unit of measurement for oxygen uptake with 1 MET representing an oxygen uptake of 3.5 ml/kg of body weight per minute. Sitting quietly in a chair

---

Stamp here with patient's plate

_____

ADMISSION NOTE

Admission status: Clinic _____ ER _____ Date _____ Time _____
Married _____ Single _____ Widowed _____ Divorced _____
Race and nationality _____ Religion _____ Age _____

Patient history

Chest pain _____ Onset _____ Duration _____ Location _____
  Radiation _____ Subjective description _____
Associated acute events:
  Loss of consciousness _____ Duration _____ Cardiac arrest _____
  Palpitations _____ GI _____ Perspiration _____ Anxiety _____

  Dyspnea _____
Medications taken or administered and time _____
Medical history and risk factors (check those appropriate):
  Myocardial infarction _____ Angina _____ Obesity _____
  Weight loss _____ Cerebrovascular accident _____ Alcohol _____
  Respiratory _____ Hypertension _____ Glaucoma _____ Diabetes _____
  Smoking _____ Prostatic hypertrophy _____ Blood transfusion _____
  Gout _____ Surgery _____ Reaction to anesthesia _____
Postcardiopulmonary resuscitation _____ Contraindications to anticoagulation _____
Other _____

Personal information

  Height _____ Weight _____ Dentures _____ Glasses _____ Contacts _____
  Sleeping habits _____ Usual diet _____
  Food, medication, environmental allergies (especially to streptokinase) _____
  Prostheses _____ Family history _____

Physical examination

  General appearance _____ Mental status _____
  Vital signs: Temperature _____ Pulse _____ Respiration _____
  Blood pressure: Right _____ Left _____
  Lungs: Aeration _____ Wheezes _____ Crackles _____
  Cardiovascular: Heart sounds _____ Quality _____ Rhythm _____
    Lifts _____ Heaves _____ Thrills _____ Murmur _____ Rub _____
    Gallop _____
  Pulses (all extremities) _____ Neck Veins _____ Abdomen _____
  Skin: Color _____ Temperature _____ Cyanosis _____ Edema _____
  Clubbing _____ Other _____

Signature _____

Insert ECG strip here.

FIG. 12-1. Sample form for admission note to the CCU.

CORONARY CARE UNIT INFORMATION

While you, a family member, or friend are in the CCU, you may hear terms such as *coronary, electrocardiogram* (ECG), or *congestive heart failure* and be uncertain as to what they mean about the patient's condition. This may be a time when you have a lot of questions and anxieties.

The CCU staff understands this and has prepared this information sheet to help you understand what goes on in a CCU. If you want to know more about heart disease, there is literature available in our unit on request. Also we will be glad to try to answer any questions you may have.

Patient care

A CCU is for the "intensive" care of cardiac patients. This CCU has 16 beds and is attended 24 hours a day by registered nurses who are specially trained to read ECGs and recognize any early signs of complications. From the time a patient arrives in the unit until he is transferred to a room, there is a nurse near the bedside to render the care needed.

Because of the serious nature of heart disease, a patient is placed in the CCU during the critical phase of the heart's condition and remains there until this critical phase is over, usually 3 to 5 days. Progress is followed continuously with special monitoring equipment at each bedside and at the nurses' station to record the patient's ECGs, which indicate the heart rhythms.

While in the CCU, patients need only their necessary personal belongings. Shaving equipment (razor with nurse's approval), cosmetics, toilet articles, eyeglasses, and small change may be kept in the bedside drawer. Male patients may wear pajama bottoms. Female patients do not need their night gowns, since it is preferred that a hospital gown be worn. A small radio and reading materials are allowed if approved by the physician. Television, flowers, and suitcases are not allowed.

When the physician approves transfer out of the CCU, the patient is usually taken to a room on another floor. Transferring patients is usually done during the day, but if an emergency situation arises and a bed is needed in the unit during the night, a patient may have to be moved then.

Visiting is permitted from 10 AM to 8 PM for members of the patient's immediate family or significant others. Because of the nature of the patient's illness, no more than two visitors should be in the patient's room at one time. *If emergency situations exist, visitation may be refused.*

Phone

There is a pay phone available. Direct calls to the unit are not permitted. Families may leave their phone numbers at the desk in the CCU.

Chaplain

This service is available on request at any time by contacting a CCU nurse or the chaplain's office.

Waiting rooms

The waiting room is open only until 8:30 PM. Those who wish to stay during the night must use the waiting room in the emergency department.

If you have questions, please contact a CCU nurse.

The CCU Staff

FIG. 12-2.   Sample fact sheet given to families of patients in the CCU.

requires 1 MET, while slow walking requires 3 METs. In the CCU activities that require 1.5 to 2 METs are generally permitted. The process of progressively increasing activities is described later in this chapter. Other protocols for increasing activity may include gradually increasing exercise to a level that raises the heart rate 20 beats per minute or less above resting heart rate. The systolic blood pressure (SBP) also increases with exercise, and activity should be adjusted so that SBP does not increase by more than 30 mm Hg above resting pressure.[14]

Completion of Data Base

As soon as possible after admission, information necessary to complete the data base should be obtained. The patient history and physical examination should be completed (see Chapter 4), paying particular attention to the following:

A. Patient history (see Chapter 4)
B. Physical examination (see Chapter 4)
   1. Inspection of skin for color, diaphoresis, and other abnormalities.
   2. Palpation of chest area for unusual movements, excursion, cardiac enlargement, apical impulse, and other signs.
   3. Percussion of chest for areas of dullness and of liver for edge and size. Cardiac borders are seldom defined by percussion.
   4. Auscultation of blood pressure, carotid arteries (bruit), apical heart rate, heart sounds, pericardial friction rub, gallops, and murmurs. The murmur of papillary muscle dysfunction may occur in the acute phase of myocardial infarction as a result of ischemia and/or infarction of the papillary muscle. The murmur of mitral regurgitation results when the injured papillary muscle fails to contract properly, allowing blood to regurgitate into the left atrium during systole. The murmur is often transient, but it may be permanent if the papillary muscle does not heal completely. A ventricular septal defect murmur may also occur during the first 10 days after infarction and is a very loud grade 4 or 5 systolic murmur. There is usually an accompanying systolic thrill, and the murmur is best heard along the lower left sternal border. The appearance of this murmur is an ominous event prognostically, sudden in onset, and frequently accompanied by profound cardiogenic shock. (See Chapter 4 for complete description of murmurs.) It is also important to auscultate the lungs for crackles, rhonchi, wheezes, and increased or decreased breath sounds. Note the rate, character, and depth of respirations. These data are necessary to evaluate the presence or absence of congestive heart failure and are useful

for comparison should this be a consideration at a later date.
C. Supportive data
   1. Serum cardiac isoenzyme levels (see Chapter 5) should be measured initially and then daily for 3 days to document any abnormal increase in serum levels. Should the patient have a sudden exacerbation of pain with associated ECG changes, cardiac enzyme level measurements may be indicated to assist in determining whether the previous infarction has continued.
   2. Arterial blood gas levels may be measured initially and then as needed (depending on the patient's condition) to determine the adequacy of oxygenation and acid-base balance.
   3. Fluid and electrolyte balance should be monitored. It is imperative that fluid intake and output be accurately measured. Equally important is that an accurate daily weight of the patient be taken at the same time each day on the same scale. This can help to determine the minimum weight gain that occurs in the early stages of heart failure or when other indicators, such as the chest x-ray film, are still normal. Personnel must be reminded to actually measure rather than to estimate intake, just as all output is measured. It should also be remembered that fluids, such as tube feedings, those used to flush the Swan-Ganz catheter and arterial lines, and those from any other sources, must be included in the patient's total fluid intake measurement. Output should include bleeding and drainage from any site, as well as urine and stool. The patient's state of hydration may also be evaluated by the skin tone.
   4. Edema may be a late sign of congestive failure and should be added to the data base already gathered on the fluid balance of the patient. The extent of peripheral edema should be measured by palpation once it appears, and comparative evaluations should be performed frequently to determine changes in edema noted in the periphery. Edema in a bedridden cardiac patient is frequently noted in dependent areas such as the sacrum or genitalia.
   5. The dietary regimen, if different from the patient's usual diet, should be explained to the patient and family. Cardiac patients are usually placed on a low-sodium diet for several days. In some cardiac patients sodium restriction may be unnecessary or impractical; these patients are given food with the usual sodium content. A soft diet is usually prescribed with frequent small feedings, although some physicians prefer clear liquids on the first day, followed by full liquids on the second day. Since metabolic demands increase following ingestion of

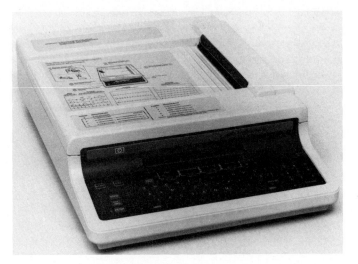

FIG. 12-3.   Computerized electrocardiograph machine showing components that provide for display of three leads simultaneously. (Reprinted with permission of Hewlett-Packard Co., Palo Alto, Calif.)

12-LEAD ECG PROCEDURE FOR CCU

A. Purpose: to record an ECG for diagnostic uses (An ECG is a graphic record registered by electrodes placed on the body surface of the electrical impulses that cause heart action)
B. Equipment (Equipment will vary among institutions; consult your individual procedure.)
   1. ECG machine with cable (see Fig. 12-3)
   2. Disposable electrodes for limbs and chest
   3. Cotton or gauze pads
   4. Alcohol sponges
C. Procedure
   1. Instruct patient regarding procedure and ensure that there is no associated discomfort.
   2. Place patient in a comfortable position on back with legs and arms adequately supported. Feet should not touch the footboard of the bed nor should arms touch the sides of the bed.
   3. Plug in ECG machine. Turn power switch to ON position.
   4. Plug in patient cable to top of recorder.
   5. Select site for limb electrode placement on each extremity. Electrodes may be placed anywhere on the extremities from shoulder to hand or hip to foot.
   6. Clean the skin area with alcohol; attempt to achieve a slight erythema by rubbing skin.
   7. Apply electrodes.
   8. Attach each of the lead wires to the appropriate limb electrode. The cables are color-coded and letter-labeled for easy identification.
   9. Before proceeding with recording, check the instrument controls.
      a. Check the grounding of the instrument by placing the lead selector on STD position. Using one finger, touch the top of the switch marked TEST. If the writing stylus vibrates, press the test button down. The test button is left in the position in which there is no vibration of the writing arm when the button is touched.
      b. Adjust the *position control* so that the writing is centered on the ECG paper.
      c. Adjust the *intensity control* to produce the necessary heat in the writing arm to give a firm, clear black line.

Continued.

12-LEAD ECG PROCEDURE FOR CCU—cont'd

    d. Turn the power switch to RUN and check the standardization of the machine. When the button marked STD (l MV, or 1 millivolt) is pressed, the writing arm should deflect exactly two large squares (10 mm) when the *sensitivity indicator* is on I (see Chapter 6). Accurate standardization is important, since some diagnostic and measurement criteria are meaningless without a point of reference.

      NOTE: ECGs are standardized before lead I. ECGs are routinely run at standard I.

10. All ECGs must be identified by labeling at the beginning of the tracing with patient's name, medical record number, date, and time.

11. A standard ECG consists of 12 separate leads. Each of these leads must be marked for the purposes of identification. This can be done by using the button labeled MARKER to create a mark in the upper margin of the paper. The following lead code is used for this purpose.

$$
\begin{array}{ll}
\text{I} \_ & \text{V}_1 \_\_\_\ \text{-} \\
\text{II} \_\_ & \text{V}_2 \_\_\_\ \text{- -} \\
\text{III} \_\_\_ & \text{V}_3 \_\_\_\ \text{- - -} \\
\text{aV}_R \_\_\_\_ & \text{V}_4 \_\_\_\ \text{- - - -} \\
\text{aV}_L \_\_\_\ \_\_ & \text{V}_5 \_\_\_\ \text{- - - - -} \\
\text{aV}_F \_\_\_\ \_\_\_\ \_\_\_ & \text{V}_6 \_\_\_\ \text{- - - - - -}
\end{array}
$$

12. To record the first 6 leads:
    a. Place the lead selector switch at I. Observe the writing arm; it should oscillate in the center of the strip.
    b. Turn the power switch to RUN.
    c. Push the STD (l MV) button once while the paper is running, and identify the lead by pushing the *lead marker button*. (Some machines mark automatically.)
    d. After recording 8 to 10 beats with a stable baseline, turn power button to ON position.
    e. Move the lead selector to lead II and proceed as above. Continue through the series and, including lead aV$_F$, move the lead selector to the next *dot position* on the lead selector dial. Some machines record 3 to 6 channels simultaneously.

13. To record the V leads of the ECG:
    a. Connect the electrode on the lead marked C (for "chest").
    b. Expose the patient's chest.
    c. Locate the electrode positions of leads V$_1$ through V$_6$. Cleanse the areas with alcohol sponge, rubbing to produce a slight erythema.
    d. Place the electrodes as follows:
        V$_1$—fourth intercostal space at right of sternal border
        V$_2$—same intercostal space at left of sternal border
        V$_3$—midway between position V$_2$ and V$_4$
        V$_4$—fifth interspace at midclavicular line
        V$_5$—same level as V$_4$ at anterior axillary line
        V$_6$—same level as V$_4$ at midaxillary line
    e. Turn lead selector to V position and power switch to RUN. Position stylus as necessary. Press *lead marker* to identify lead.
    f. Repeat the preceding step for each of the chest lead positions on chest.

14. Disconnect electrodes from the patient, and reposition the patient for comfort. Wipe electrode paste off chest and extremities.

15. Be sure ECG is correctly labeled. See that ECG is mounted on the patient's chart.

---

food, the quantity of food at each serving should be kept small. Studies show that hot and cold liquids are not detrimental, so their exclusion from diets is unnecessary. Decaffeinated coffee and tea are permitted. The relationship between caffeine intake and heart problems has not been clearly es-

tablished. Mathewson, for example, has concluded that there is no relationship between caffeine intake and MI but there is a relationship between caffeine intake and arrhythmias in the ischemic heart.[15]

6. A 12-lead ECG (see Chapter 6) should be performed initially in the emergency room or in the

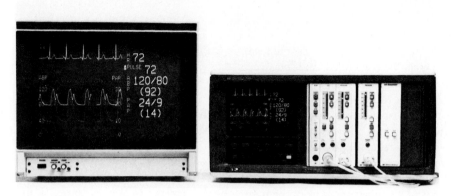

FIG. 12-4. Monitoring system shows oscilloscope, digital and numerical display and wave forms. (Reprinted with permission of Hewlett-Packard Co., Palo Alto, Calif.)

CCU. A copy should be maintained on the patient's chart for comparison with later tracings, which are performed daily for 3 days and with every exacerbation of chest pain, and/or developing arrhythmia. Personnel in the CCU should be adept at obtaining and interpreting the 12-lead ECG in a patient with myocardial infarction. (See box on pp. 357-358.)

Medical and nursing diagnoses are derived from the compiled data and serve as the basis for planning medical and nursing therapies.

EQUIPMENT
Monitoring System

In the CCU the first equipment with which the patient is likely to come in contact is the monitoring system. For a patient who has suffered a myocardial infarction or who has had a pacemaker implanted, careful monitoring of cardiac performance is the objective of preventive care. The cardiac monitor simplifies such care by continuously displaying the cardiac rhythm, blood pressure, and other parameters not readily followed by other means. Since most arrhythmias occur during the first 48 to 72 hours after infarction and 80% to 90% of patients who have myocardial infarctions experience arrhythmias, the need for constant surveillance is vital.

Components. The cardiac monitor is an instrument that displays electrical activity during the cardiac cycle as a wave pattern across a screen. Since the components of particular monitoring systems vary widely, the basic components of most cardiac monitors are shown in Fig. 12-4.

Oscilloscope. The screen on which the patient's electrocardiographic pattern appears is an oscilloscope.

Digital Display. An electronic mechanism averages the number of ventricular complexes per minute, and this rate is shown on the rate scale indicator. Also, each QRS complex is indicated by an audible beep and flashing light. If the pulse rate can be relayed to a console at the nursing station, the bedside monitor beep should be silenced so that the patient does not hear it.

Rate Meter. Integrated with the alarm system is the rate meter, which signals if the rate goes above or below predetermined limits. The limits vary according to the routine of a particular unit based on the sensitivity of the electrodes and monitoring system. For example, the alarm may be triggered to sound at either 25 beats above or below an individual patient's average heart rate, or it may be set to sound automatically at the high-low values of 150 beats/minute and 50 beats/minute.

Alarm Control System. When the heart rate falls below or rises above the preset levels, audio and visual alarms alert the staff. Each time an alarm is triggered, the staff must observe the patient and make a prompt decision regarding the cardiac rhythm.

When the CCU personnel depend on an alarm system for warning, the rate limit indicators and alarm system must be checked regularly—not only for accuracy but also to be sure that the system is operative. There are situations when the limit settings are temporarily turned off in the patient's room. At these times personnel must depend on visual observation of the oscilloscope and the related clinical picture. For instance, the limit settings are turned off to prevent false alarms from electrical interference resulting from the use of a high-power machine (e.g., a direct write-out ECG machine, or a portable x-ray machine). False alarms may also be triggered by manipulation of the chest electrodes when repositioning them to other sites on the chest or when bathing the patient. The patient's welfare is endangered if the alarm limit settings remain off; therefore it is essential to check these settings periodically.

When such an alarm system is not available, personnel must develop some other means of being alerted to changes in rhythm on the monitor oscilloscope. Only through an adequate method of observation can significant changes be identified and further rhythm disturbances prevented.

Sweep Speed. The rate at which the electronic beam sweeps across the screen can be controlled, and the sweep can be set at trace speeds of 25 mm/second (beam sweeps across standard screen in 6 seconds) or 50 mm/second (the 3-second sweep position). The 6-second position is generally used for routine monitoring. The 3-second position often provides for better interpretation of the rhythm or the pressure waveform by spreading the complexes.

Filter. The filter reduces extraneous muscular artifacts. However, when a 12-lead ECG is recorded from the monitor, the filter must be switched off, since it may distort the ST segment.

Central Console. Individual bedside monitors in a CCU are connected to a central console at the nursing station to permit continuous observation of the ECG patterns from all the monitors.

Additional Components. Complementary parts can be added to the basic monitoring system as necessary. For example, a direct write-out ECG machine can be located in the central station; this is triggered to record the cardiac rhythm automatically during alarm situations or on demand. Such recordings may be used to demonstrate the patient's response to antiarrhythmic therapy.

Some monitor systems have memory tapes that store a predetermined duration of the patient's ECG, which can then be recalled at will. This allows a printout of the cardiac rhythm recorded over the previous 60 seconds. At the time of alarm some monitors printout memory storage and then the current rhythm from the time of trigger. Memory mechanisms, however, erase after a period of time; therefore at the moment of an alarm personnel must decide whether to record the stored memory information or the current rhythm. Use of 24-hour tape monitoring simplifies this problem. The monitoring system may also include multichannel recorders to monitor central venous, pulmonary artery, pulmonary capillary wedge, and arterial pressures, and other physiologic parameters. In some centers this information can be stored and retrieved from a computer. Also many new monitoring systems use computer analysis for arrhythmia interpretation.

Electrodes

Topical electrode patches are commonly used for patient monitoring. The following steps are involved in preparing the skin and in applying the electrodes:

1. At the sites chosen for electrode placement, clean the skin thoroughly with alcohol to remove all residues. If necessary, shave the hair at these sites.

2. The skin of some patients may require abrasion at the electrode sites to obtain an adequate ECG signal. If this is the situation, abrade each site by rubbing the area with a gauze pad.

3. Apply adhesive electrode pads and press them against the skin at the prepared sites. For extra adhesion a strip of nonallergenic tape may be applied over electrodes.

Placement of Electrodes. The lead that best displays the QRS complexes and P waves (and pacing stimuli if pacing is used) is ideal for monitoring.

A positive electrode, a negative electrode, and a ground electrode are required to record one bipolar lead. The location for these electrodes determines the lead recorded by the monitor. For example, a modification of lead V_1 (MCL_1) is recorded by placing the negative electrode just under the outer quarter of the left shoulder and the ground electrode beneath the right clavicle, with the positive electrode being placed at the fourth right intercostal space at the right sternal border (the usual V_1 position).

Many of the computerized monitoring systems use lead II for interpretation. The negative electrode is placed just under the outer quarter of the right shoulder and the ground electrode is positioned in the left lower abdominal area (left leg position).

To prevent their interfering with the physical examination, the chest electrodes should be placed away from the area near the apex of the heart. Placement of the electrodes on the chest reduces motion and muscle artifacts and allows the patient more freedom of movement than does limb-lead monitoring. Electrodes should be repositioned daily to prevent local skin irritation caused by prolonged contact of the hypertonic electrode paste with one point of the skin surface.

The modified V_1 chest lead has the added advantage over the other chest leads (often haphazardly positioned on the chest) of giving a maximum amount of information about rhythm disturbances and conduction. The MCL_1 provides an easily recognized recording of the sequence of ventricular activation and therefore furnishes maximum information to discriminate between right and left bundle branch block and between PVCs and aberrant supraventricular complexes.

The electrode wires from the patient are attached to a connector unit pinned to the patient's gown. From this unit a cable leads to the monitor where the electrode wires are connected to their respective terminals: positive wire to positive terminal, negative wire to negative terminal, and ground wire to ground terminal. In certain machines the electrode terminals are specifically labeled. In other machines it is necessary to be familiar with the terminal connections. Incorrect matching of electrodes and terminals will change the lead that is to be monitored.

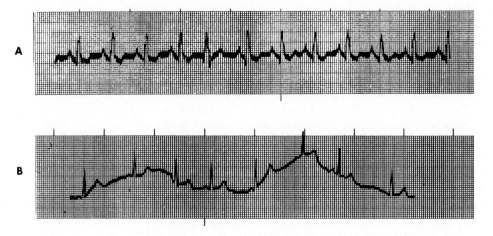

FIG. 12-5.   A, ECG tracing that shows external voltage interference (alternating 60-cycle current) appearing as a smooth thickening of the baseline as a result of the 60 tiny peaks per second. B, ECG tracing in which patient interference (coughing, turning, etc.) is shown by a wandering baseline.

Interference with Monitoring. Faulty techniques probably cause over 90% of the problems encountered in the course of cardiac monitoring. The common artifacts produced by electrical interferences can be prevented.

External voltage and patient movements generally are responsible for interference that occurs in a properly operating monitoring system. External voltage interference (alternating 60-cycle current) appears on the screen as a smooth thickening of the baseline resulting from the 60 tiny peaks/second (Fig. 12-5, *A*). Inadequate grounding of the monitor and other equipment or improper electrode placement and connection may produce this type of interference.

Since the cardiac monitor registers muscle potential, any sudden voluntary or involuntary movement by the patient can cause interference. For example, coughing or turning over in bed may precipitate a wandering baseline and erratic or irregular fluctuations on the oscilloscope (Fig. 12-5, *B*). Placing the electrodes in areas of limited muscular activity will reduce this problem.

In the tense, nervous, or cold patient, the monitor may display a harsh, jagged, uneven oscillation about the baseline. Personnel must be careful not to interpret these baseline undulations as signifying fibrillatory waves.

Computer Systems

During the past 20 years, computers have been developed and used primarily for acquiring, reporting, and storing electrocardiographic and hemodynamic data. This information can be used in the management of the critically ill patient. The role of the computer in the medical setting began with a few large, costly computers dedicated to physiological data acquisition. Soon thereafter computer-based

reports were obtained from clinical chemistry, pharmacy, and functional laboratories. Computers later were used for closed-loop control of fluid and drug therapy. Recent trends indicate that the medical decision-making process via computer has a bright future.[16] Extensive use of computers in most health care centers remains limited to admitting, billing, scientific, laboratory, and diagnostic applications.[17]

For computerization to become operational in institutions, two things must occur. First, personnel must be educated about the many capabilities of the computer and its applications to their area. Second, personnel must be able to communicate adequately with programmers to maximize the benefits of the computer for the institution's needs.

For computerization to be useful to the practitioner, a Hospital Information System (HIS) must be used. The HIS is composed of hardware and software. This system should provide *administration* with information about personnel records, staffing, patient acuity levels, supplies and equipment, communications, and reports needed for long-range planning and budgeting. In *clinical* application, the staff would use the HIS to transmit physician requests, schedule procedures, retrieve laboratory test results, order supplies, develop and maintain care plans, and provide selected patient care. Staff and patient *education* is facilitated because nurses can readily obtain information about diet, medications, laboratory tests, policies, procedures, and protocols. Instructions for patients can be written in layperson language, printed, and taken home by the patient. Individuals responsible for orientation and in-service education could use the HIS to disseminate announcements and keep continuing education records for each staff member. Research efforts are facilitated for the practitioner in the availability and access to stored data.[18]

Health personnel envision the potential benefits of computer usage in the CCU; however, they are often confronted with large differences between projected and actual computer performance. Systems that were thought to be laborsaving devices often are not. Computers may interfere with established staff procedures. Successful operation of a computer system may require employment of skilled technical personnel for programming and maintenance. Reliable computer systems have infrequent hardware and software failures, but when they do occur, catastrophic alterations in patient care patterns may ensue. Computer equipment is often declared obsolete shortly after purchase, particularly since the advent of microprocessor-based systems.[16]

Limitations of computer usage include downtime, response time, storage capacity, and interface. The factors that affect the functioning of a computer in a hospital environment are related both to the capacity of the technology and the professional's ability to control the technology.

For the professional to be able to use the information systems, knowledge is required in theory and hands-on application. A program must be available in the hospital for adequate training. Educational institutions are beginning to respond by preparing their graduates in computer proficiency.

Currently in some CCUs data can be entered into the HIS directly from the bedside, while in others this information is placed into the HIS from the mainframe outside the patient's room. Facilities with closed-loop systems obtain such physiologic data as heart rate, blood pressure, temperature, and urinary output, and these data are entered into the computer directly from the patient. In addition, these systems can also infuse and regulate the administration of drugs, fluids, and blood products according to preset parameters (Fig. 12-6).[19]

On the horizon are voice-activated terminals. Edmunds states that by 1990 these systems will have progressed to the point where they will be able to recognize a large number of words from an unlimited number of users. The capability of the computer talking back to remind personnel of needed care requirements is also being developed. It is theorized that robots designed like those used in industry can be in the patient's room to give the patient a drink, open the window, roll up the bed, and even empty a bedpan. These applications of computer technology will allow an overextended staff to spend more time in counseling, planning, and educating the patient.[18]

Artificial Cardiac Pacemakers

Many patients with acute myocardial infarctions develop high-degree heart block or significant bradycardia that may require intervention. Temporary and permanent pacemaker therapy may be necessary. (See Chapter 11 for additional information.)

Implantable Cardioverter-Defibrillator

During the past 3 years the automatic implantable defibrillator (AID) has been established as an effective treatment for those patients suffering from malignant ventricular arrhythmias. It has become apparent that the great majority of survivors of sudden cardiac death suffered from hemodynamically unstable ventricular tachycardias rather than from ventricular fibrillation.[20]

The growing clinical experience with the AID has shown clearly that it can reliably identify and correct both ventricular fibrillation and hemodynamically unstable ventricular tachycardias of patients in or out of the hospital. This new modality also appears to decrease significantly cardiac mortality in properly selected high-risk patients. There are no undue side effects or risks. Although a longer experience is necessary to reach definite conclusions, it is evident that the AID is adding a new dimension to the management of potentially lethal arrhythmias and to the prevention of sudden cardiac death.[20]

Electrical Hazards

The electrical equipment employed in a CCU increases the potential of electrical shock hazard for both the patient and the equipment operator. Therefore it is important that CCU personnel have a basic understanding of the principles of current flow, current source, and grounding.

When ground connections of equipment are not at the

Time 1220	Bed 7		Bed 8
Systolic	141	mmHG	124
Diastolic	77	mmHG	69
Mean	102	mmHG	91
Heart rate	96	/min	110
Right atrial	4	mmHG	5
Left atrial	4	mmHG	16
Blood	180	ml	0
Chest drainage	185	ml	12
Chest drainage	80	ml/hr	0
Urine output	526	ml	22
Urine output	172	ml/hr	0
Nipride	.0	ml	.0
Rectal temperature	35.1	deg. C.	25.0
Skin temperature	.0	deg. C.	.0
Respiration	10	/min	8
*** Messages ***		*** Messages ***	
		Rectal Temperature Low	

FIG. 12-6. Computer display of physiologic parameters. At 2-minute intervals current measurements are displayed on the video for two patients simultaneously.

same potential (zero volts or a few millivolts above zero), leakage current may flow between the source and its ground. Current will flow through the patient if he serves as a link in this circuit. Skin offers resistance to current flow and therefore protects the heart from electrical shock. If the voltage is high enough or skin resistance has been lowered or eliminated, ventricular fibrillation may result. On some equipment, built-in isolation circuits isolate patients from the ground and the power line, thus preventing any conductive pathways. However, an intracardiac catheter or fluid column bypasses the skin and the protection from current flow that it affords, making the patient highly vulnerable to electrical shock. Alternating current (AC) power-line current levels of only millionths of amperes, undetectable when applied to the skin, can induce ventricular fibrillation if contact with the myocardium is made.

Any AC power-line–operated device from which some of the current flows through the metal frame, case, or other exposed parts may serve as a current source. It may be an electric bed with a broken or missing ground connection or any device with two-wire power cords (two-pronged plugs) such as TV sets, bed lamps, or electric fans. The patient may lie in the path of the current source and ground directly by touching the electrical device, or the patient may ground indirectly by making physical contact with another person who touches the defectively grounded instrument. Either situation causes the patient to become a conductive pathway and allows current to flow through him to ground.

Equipment operators should be cautious when using electronic equipment near water, steam pipes, radiators, or plumbing fixtures. Such pipes and fittings are excellent electrical grounds. Consequently any electrical device near them, including the power cords, plugs, and wall receptacles, that exposes the user to live current can be extremely hazardous if the operator simultaneously contacts both the device and a grounded pipe or faucet. The operator then becomes the link between the current source and the ground that the current seeks. The resultant shock may not be fatal, but serious injury can result from the violent muscular reaction in "letting go" (Table 12-1).

Personnel may detect tingling sensations when touching or brushing against a piece of electronic equipment. The voltage necessary to produce this sensation is only one thousandth of an ampere. Under ordinary circumstances this is harmless; however, this voltage is nearly 50 times the amount necessary to produce ventricular fibrillation if current flows directly to the patient's heart.

Clearly, many considerations are necessary to ensure electrical safety. Awareness of potential hazards, prompt correction of faulty equipment, and regular safety inspection checks are all needed. Personnel should be thoroughly briefed in the following rules for electrical safety in the CCU:

A. All equipment should be grounded. This means that a pathway of least resistance is available for the currents within the machine to flow to ground.
   1. All equipment must have three-pronged plugs which connect the hospital ground to the equipment chassis.
   2. Adaptors fitting a three-prong plug into a two-slot electrical outlet should not be used.
   3. Extension cords should not be used to connect electronic equipment. If extensions are necessary, use only three-pronged grounding-type cords.
B. Wet surfaces conduct current. Therefore hazards such as wet sheets and wet floors should be eliminated.
C. Safety inspection checks should be routine. A qualified electrical technician should check all equipment for faulty or missing ground connections and hazardous voltages. (Remember that equipment can still operate with defective ground connections.)
D. When two instruments are in use near a patient, connect them to the same power receptacle.
E. Never plug or unplug equipment or turn on a light while any part of your body or the patient's is in contact

---

TABLE 12-1. Effects of electric current

60-Cycle Current (1-Second Duration) Delivered through Skin		60-Cycle Current (1-Second Duration) Leading to Heart	
Milliamperes	Effects	Microamperes	Effects
1	Threshold of perception; tingling	20 to 50	Ventricular fibrillation
16	"Let go" current; muscle contraction		
50	Pain; possible fainting; mechanical injury		
100-3000	Ventricular fibrillation		
6000 or greater	Sustained myocardial depolarization followed by normal rhythm; temporary respiratory paralysis; burns		

with water, steam pipes, radiators, or plumbing fixtures.

F. Prevent equipment cords from kinking, draping on pipes and plumbing, or lying on wet surfaces.

G. Report tingling sensations emitted from objects such as a bed frame or an instrument case. Unplug the equipment that is not necessary to support the life of the patient; correct this condition immediately in equipment necessary for life support.

H. When using a intracavitary lead, connect the electrode catheter to the V lead of the ECG machine, since this circuit has a high electrical resistance in relation to ground. Anyone or anything electrically grounded must not touch the V-lead electrode terminals.

I. Additional precautions should be taken for patients with temporary cardiac pacemakers.

1. The electrodes at the end of the pacemaker should be well insulated. On older models a rubber glove is used to cover the exposed terminals at the junction with the external power source. Most newer models are adequately insulated.

2. When possible, use external battery pacemakers that are isolated from the power-line sources.

3. Personnel should wear rubber gloves when connecting or disconnecting the battery pacemaker and when adjusting electrodes at the end of the catheter.

4. Personnel should not wear leather-soled shoes on conductive or carpeted floors.

5. Patients should not wear leather-soled shoes on conductive floors.

6. Patients should use battery-operated razors rather than razors that require electricity.

POTENTIAL PROBLEMS

Arrhythmias, myocardial dysfunction, and psychologic alterations are prominent among problems which may occur during hospitalization, particularly in the early hours or days following acute myocardial infarction.

Arrhythmias

Recurring arrhythmias compromise cardiac function by reducing cardiac output and coronary blood flow, increasing the myocardial need for oxygen, predisposing the patient to the development of more serious arrhythmias, and complicating therapy. Therefore prompt prevention and control of arrhythmias and the states predisposing to them (acidosis, electrolyte imbalance, early cardiac failure, pain, and anxiety) decrease the incidence of more serious arrhythmias and should improve the chances for survival after myocardial infarction. Awareness of these facts underscores the importance of detecting arrhythmias through the cardiac monitor.

Staff in the CCU should be skilled in arrhythmia interpretation and treatment. Most CCUs have established protocols for administering antiarrhythmic agents. Controversy continues regarding the prophylactic use of lidocaine and other antiarrhythmic agents in patients admitted with sinus rhythm. Although there is no consensus, it has been suggested that prophylactic use of antiarrhythmic agents *may* be helpful in preventing ventricular arrhythmias.[21] See Chapter 10 for further discussion of drugs useful in arrhythmia management.

Atrial or ventricular pacing is frequently used in the care of patients with tachyarrhythmias and bradyarrhythmias. (See Chapter 11 for description of therapeutic pacing modalities.)

It is necessary that the staff be certified in skills of basic cardiac life support (BCLS) as defined by the American Heart Association or the American Red Cross. Personnel must also be trained to perform other procedures, including preparation of medication, recording times of events and medication given, and assisting as necessary with activities during the resuscitation effort. Nurses who are well prepared in resuscitation techniques often successfully treat a patient who has had a cardiac arrest before the arrival of a physician.

Certification in the skills of advanced cardiac life support (ACLS) is also important for coronary care personnel. ACLS includes all the skills of basic cardiac life support in addition to the techniques of endotracheal intubation, venipuncture, arrhythmia interpretation, and drug administration.

In the development of a tachyarrhythmia the first and frequently the most important therapeutic maneuver is to slow the ventricular rate.[22] The speed with which this should be accomplished is determined by the patient's clinical status and the nature of the arrhythmia. Pharmacologic therapy for tachyarrhythmias consists of lengthy and potentially dangerous biologic titration of such drugs as digitalis, quinidine, and verapamil. The levels at which these drugs become toxic cannot be predicted with absolute certainty, and side effects may occur.

Electrical Cardioversion. Many of the problems caused by drug treatment may be avoided through electrical cardioversion. Under optimum conditions of supervision and monitoring, a precisely regulated "dose" of electricity can restore sinus rhythm immediately.

Transthoracic cardioversion delivers electrical energy to the heart by means of metal paddles placed on the intact chest or placed directly on the heart when the chest is opened, as during cardiac surgery. This procedure depolarizes the excitable myocardium, thereby interrupting reentrant circuits and discharging automatic pacemaker foci to establish electrical homogeneity. Cardioversion successfully restores sinus rhythm if the sinus node becomes the first automatic focus to fire after the electrical shock and thus controls the pacing function of the heart. Transvenous cardioversion using a catheter electrode placed in the right ventricle delivers very low energy levels and permits cardioversion in an awake, unsedated patient.[23]

By synchronizing the capacitor to discharge during the downslope of the R wave or with the S wave, the vulnerable period of the ventricle (an interval of 20 to 40 msecs near the apex of the T wave) may be avoided. This minimizes but does not completely eliminate the danger of precipitating ventricular fibrillation with the DC shock. However, if synchronization cannot be established rapidly and immediate cardioversion is indicated, the shock is delivered asynchronously. Immediate cardioversion using 200-300 joules without synchronization (defibrillation) is the mandatory treatment for ventricular fibrillation or ventricular flutter and for ventricular tachycardia if it produces cardiovascular collapse. If defibrillation is unsuccessful, IV drug therapy should begin with lidocaine, followed by procainamide or bretylium tosylate.[24]

However, if the tachyarrhythmia does not terminate promptly, cardioversion or defibrillation should be performed using 360 joules. Short, limited bursts of ventricular tachycardia are treated medically. As a general rule any supraventricular tachyarrhythmia that produces signs or symptoms, such as hypotension, angina, or congestive heart failure, and does not respond promptly to medical therapy should be terminated electrically. Cardiopulmonary resuscitation (CPR) is performed during this period as indicated by patient condition. See ACLS algorithms for ventricular tachycardia and fibrillation (Fig. 12-7).[24]

An elective cardioversion may be carried out wherever resuscitative aids, such as suction, intubation equipment, medications, and experienced personnel trained in airway management, are available. The cardioversion procedure is listed below.

1. Explain the procedure to the patient and obtain written *informed* consent.
2. Withhold diuretics and short-acting digitalis preparations for 24 to 36 hours. However, it has been suggested that discontinuing digitalis in nontoxic, normokalemic patients may not be necessary. If indicated, obtain a serum potassium or serum digitalis level. Hypokalemia enhances electrical instability and may increase arrhythmias after cardioversion.[25]
3. Keep the patient fasting for 6 to 8 hours before cardioversion.
4. Perform a thorough physical examination, including vital signs, mentation, and palpation of pulse (see Chapter 4).
5. Obtain a 12-lead ECG before and after cardioversion, as well as a rhythm strip or oscilloscopic monitoring (or both) during procedure.
6. Maintain a reliable IV site.

7. If patient has dentures, remove them.
8. Allow the patient to breathe oxygen for 5 to 15 minutes before and then immediately after DC shock if not contraindicated; this promotes myocardial oxygenation. During cardioversion the presence of oxygen with electrical arcing may encourage combustion.
9. Employ synchronous discharge mode on the difibrillator/cardioverter for elective procedures. The QRS complex recorded on the oscilloscope must be tall to ensure that it alone triggers the capacitor discharge. Determine the accuracy of synchronization by discharging several test shocks before applying the paddles to the patient.
10. Administer diazepam or other medication prescribed to produce transient amnesia or light sleep.
11. Apply electrode paste liberally but not excessively to the polished surface of the paddles, and then place them in firm contact with the chest wall at points distant from the monitoring electrodes. The paddles may be positioned (1) anteroposteriorly in the left infrascapular region and over the upper sternum at the third interspace, or (2) anteriorly to the right of the sternum at the second intercostal space and in the left midclavicular line at the fifth intercostal space.
12. Employing the minimum effective electrical energy level reduces complications; therefore the starting level for most arrhythmias is around 50 joules or less (Fig. 12-8). The energy necessary to terminate some arrhythmias, such as atrial flutter or ventricular tachycardia, may be considerably less. If unsuccessful, this initial level may be increased to 100 joules and then by 100-joule increments until a level of 360 joules is reached. Make sure that all personnel have moved away from the patient and the bed before discharging the defibrillator.
13. Record the postshock rhythm to determine whether the procedure was successful. V_1 or MCL_1 lead recording is preferable. An oscilloscope interpretation is frequently unreliable.
14. Continue rhythm monitoring and close observations of cardiovascular and pulmonary status for 2 to 3 hours until the patient's condition is stable after cardioversion.
15. Precautions
    a. When digitalis excess is suspected, electrical cardioversion should be deferred and the arrhythmia treated with medication initially to prevent production of serious ventricular tachyarrhythmias and failure to terminate the digitalis-related arrhythmia.
    b. Emergency drugs and equipment needed for pacing, intubation, or suction must be available.
    c. If using electrode paste, avoid coating the paddles

Unmonitored Ventricular Fibrillation

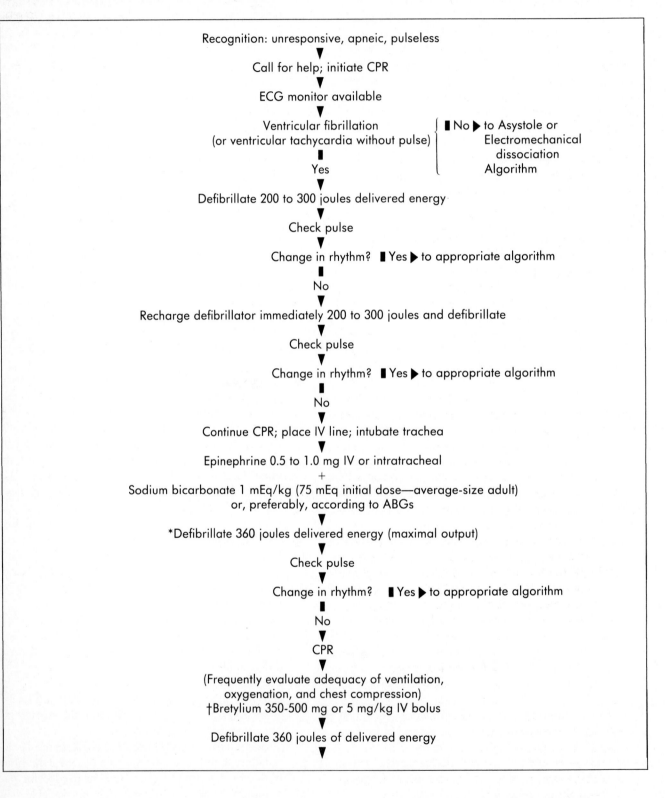

Recognition: unresponsive, apneic, pulseless

▼

Call for help; initiate CPR

▼

ECG monitor available

▼

Ventricular fibrillation   { ■ No ▶ to Asystole or
(or ventricular tachycardia without pulse) {   Electromechanical
■   dissociation
Yes   {   Algorithm

▼

Defibrillate 200 to 300 joules delivered energy

▼

Check pulse

▼

Change in rhythm?   ■ Yes ▶ to appropriate algorithm

■

No

▼

Recharge defibrillator immediately 200 to 300 joules and defibrillate

▼

Check pulse

▼

Change in rhythm?   ■ Yes ▶ to appropriate algorithm

■

No

▼

Continue CPR; place IV line; intubate trachea

▼

Epinephrine 0.5 to 1.0 mg IV or intratracheal

+

Sodium bicarbonate 1 mEq/kg (75 mEq initial dose—average-size adult)
or, preferably, according to ABGs

▼

*Defibrillate 360 joules delivered energy (maximal output)

▼

Check pulse

▼

Change in rhythm?   ■ Yes ▶ to appropriate algorithm

■

No

▼

CPR

▼

(Frequently evaluate adequacy of ventilation,
oxygenation, and chest compression)
†Bretylium 350-500 mg or 5 mg/kg IV bolus

▼

Defibrillate 360 joules of delivered energy

▼

Unmonitored Ventricular Fibrillation—cont'd

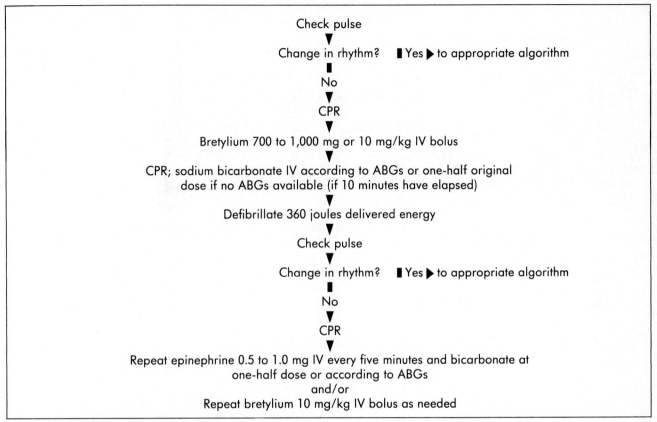

Check pulse
▼
Change in rhythm?   ▌Yes ▶ to appropriate algorithm
▪
No
▼
CPR
▼
Bretylium 700 to 1,000 mg or 10 mg/kg IV bolus
▼
CPR; sodium bicarbonate IV according to ABGs or one-half original dose if no ABGs available (if 10 minutes have elapsed)
▼
Defibrillate 360 joules delivered energy
▼
Check pulse
▼
Change in rhythm?   ▌Yes ▶ to appropriate algorithm
▪
No
▼
CPR
▼
Repeat epinephrine 0.5 to 1.0 mg IV every five minutes and bicarbonate at one-half dose or according to ABGs
and/or
Repeat bretylium 10 mg/kg IV bolus as needed

*Reference point for **Monitored Ventricular Fibrillation Algorithm.**
†Some may prefer at this point to use lidocaine 100 mg (or 1 mg/kg) IV bolus followed by additional bolus(es) 50 mg (or 0.5 mg/kg) at 5- to 10-minute intervals (total dose of boluses not to exceed 225 mg) and an infusion of 2-4 mg/min, or procainamide 20 mg/min (100 mg/5 min) up to 1 g followed by an infusion of 1-4 mg/min before proceeding to bretylium.

FIG. 12-7.   ACLS algorithms for ventricular tachycardia and fibrillation. (Reprinted with permission of American Heart Association, Dallas, Texas.)

Continued on p. 368.

excessively or placing them too near monitoring electrodes which may allow a spark to jump and burn the skin. Local skin inflammation caused by the paddles is best treated with a topical steroid preparation.

d. Certain arrhythmias may occur after cardioversion; therefore monitoring the rhythm must continue for 2 to 3 hours. Other complications may include embolic episodes which occur in 1% to 3% of patients after the arrhythmia is converted to sinus rhythm.

Electrophysiologic Monitoring. When the modified pulmonary artery catheter is in the right atrium at the junction of the superior vena cava, stable ECGs of high quality can be obtained. These high-fidelity ECGs allow rapid and accurate diagnosis of various complex arrhythmias. Because of the limited noise in the ECG signal, con-

tinuous quantitative interval measurements by a computerized system are possible. Moreover, the stable intracavitary electrode position provides a reliable atrial pacing site for converting supraventricular tachycardias, for maintaining an adequate rate during sinus bradycardia, and for suppressing ventricular premature beats by rapid atrial pacing rates.[28] This multipurpose catheter provides safe and convenient monitoring for long periods of time in patients with unstable cardiopulmonary problems.

Circulatory Arrest

Resuscitation begun during the first 3 to 4 minutes following circulatory arrest usually prevents irreversible cerebral damage. Ventricular fibrillation, rather than ventricular asystole, commonly precipitates the arrest. However, a recent study reported sudden death in ambulatory

Ventricular Tachycardia

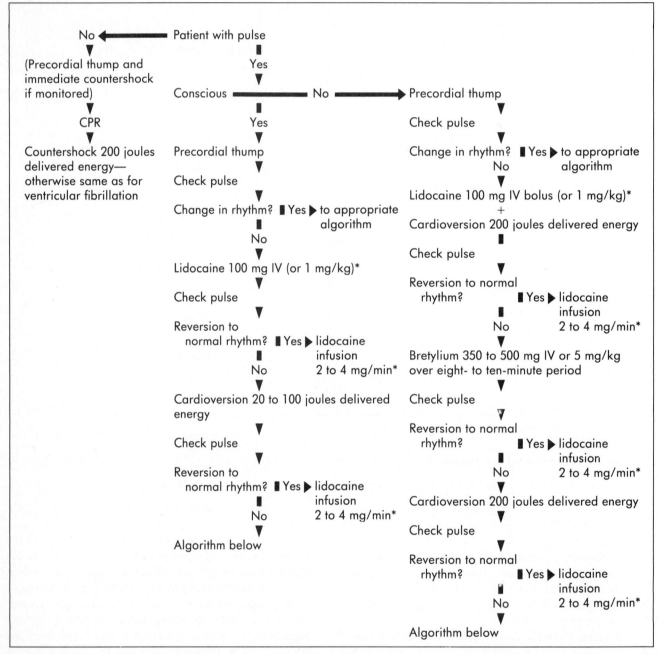

*A second loading dose of 0.5 mg/kg should be given in 5 to 10 minutes.

FIG. 12-7, cont'd. ACLS algorithms for ventricular tachycardia and fibrillation.

monitored patients secondary to bradyarrhythmias.[26] Defibrillation procedures should be initiated in a CCU within 30 seconds of onset of the arrest. Prompt reversion to sinus rhythm often prevents the biochemical derangements that accompany ventricular fibrillation, eliminates the need for endotracheal intubation, and significantly increases the success rate of resuscitation attempts. After a successful resuscitation, it is important that measures be taken to prevent recurrence of the cardiac arrest. Prophylactic lidocaine and cardiac pacing can be used to prevent extrasystole and/or bradycardia, since these arrhythmias may presage the occurrence of ventricular tachycardia/fibrillation.

Recurrent Ventricular Tachycardia (after Maximum Lidocaine Infusion)

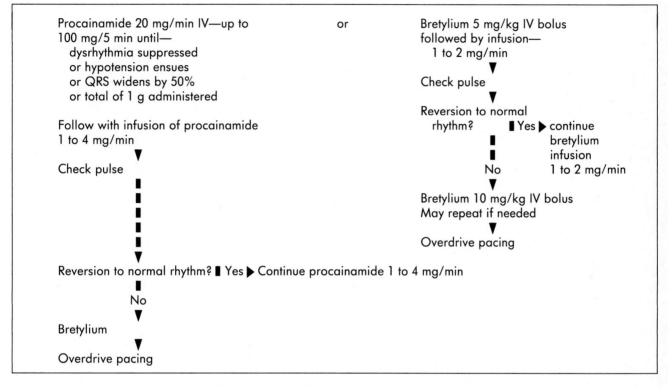

Procainamide 20 mg/min IV—up to
100 mg/5 min until—
   dysrhythmia suppressed
   or hypotension ensues
   or QRS widens by 50%
   or total of 1 g administered

Follow with infusion of procainamide
1 to 4 mg/min
   ▼
Check pulse

Reversion to normal rhythm? ▪ Yes ▶ Continue procainamide 1 to 4 mg/min

No

Bretylium

Overdrive pacing

or

Bretylium 5 mg/kg IV bolus
followed by infusion—
   1 to 2 mg/min
   ▼
Check pulse
   ▼
Reversion to normal
   rhythm?   ▪ Yes ▶ continue
              bretylium
              infusion
         No   1 to 2 mg/min
   ▼
Bretylium 10 mg/kg IV bolus
May repeat if needed
   ▼
Overdrive pacing

FIG. 12-7, cont'd.   ACLS algorithms for ventricular tachycardia and fibrillation.

When the monitor alarm is activated or the arrhythmia is observed on the oscilloscope, personnel must correlate the observed rhythm with the patient's clinical status by rapidly evaluating the patient's orientation, respirations, pupils, and carotid or femoral pulses. Loose leads can produce a rhythmic pattern simulating ventricular fibrillation. Moreover, a lidocaine reaction can mimic the disoriented state seen in tachyarrhythmias associated with inadequate cardiac output. The importance of careful diagnosis cannot be overemphasized.

Resuscitation*

1. Establish unresponsiveness by shaking the patient and calling his name. If there is no response, call for help.
2. Place patient in a supine position with a board or firm mattress under the chest.
3. Open the patient's airway using the head-tilt and chin-lift method or head-tilt and neck-lift method. The chin-lift method is preferred.

4. Look, listen, and feel for breathing. If the patient is breathing, keep the airway open, but do not begin other CPR techniques.
5. If the patient is not breathing, administer two breaths of about 1.5 seconds each into victim's mouth after pinching the nostrils and sealing the mouth.[27]
6. Check the patient's carotid pulse. If present, continue to administer only breathing at a rate of one breath every 5 seconds.
7. If the patient has no palpable pulse, begin cycles of 5 external cardiac compressions (at rate of 80 to 100/minute) and 1 breath if two people are resuscitating, or cycles of 15 compressions (at a rate of 80 to 100/minute) and 2 breaths if only one person is resuscitating the patient. Check for correct hand positioning.
8. After 4 cycles of ventilation and compression, check for return of patient's pulse and spontaneous breathing. If there is no pulse or spontaneous breathing, repeat the process.
9. Do not stop CPR for more than 7 seconds once it has begun. Pause every 4 cycles (after the initial pause noted in No. 8) to check for carotid pulse, spontaneous breathing, and pupillary reaction to light.

*For further information refer to the American Heart Association or the American Red Cross guidelines for cardiopulmonary resuscitation.

Monitored Ventricular Fibrillation

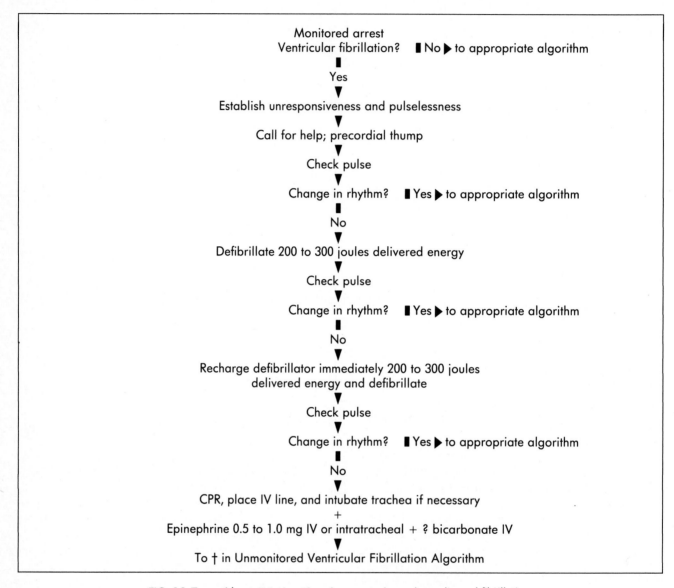

FIG. 12-7, cont'd.   ACLS algorithms for ventricular tachycardia and fibrillation.

10. At the same time one or more people provide cardio-respiratory support, someone else sets up the defibrillator if the patient's rhythm is unknown or is known to be ventricular tachycardia or fibrillation. If only one person is present, he or she must decide between instituting CPR and attempting to defibrillate the patient. If the defibrillator is close at hand and the patient can be treated with it in 15 to 30 seconds, it is probably best for the single resuscitator to choose defibrillation rather than beginning CPR alone. (*It is extremely critical that DC shock not be delayed when CPR has begun, an intubation attempted, an ECG recorded, or a physical examination [other than, for example, a brief palpation of pulses] performed. Rapid application of DC shock is usually the most important therapeutic maneuver in this situation.*)

11. IV fluid is started if it is not already running.

12. It is helpful to have a drug list such as the one shown in Table 12-2 taped to the emergency cart. Those medications most likely to be needed are prepared at the first opportunity.

13. If there is time and a sufficient number of people and

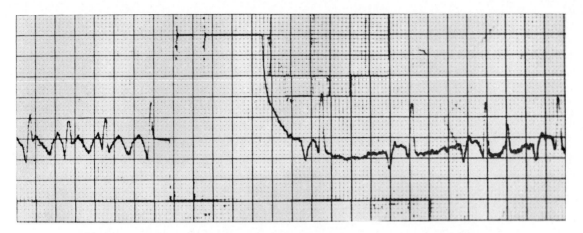

FIG. 12-8. Termination of atrial flutter. Direct current countershock was administered at 50 watt-seconds. The synchronized discharge occurred on R wave and terminated the flutter rhythm.

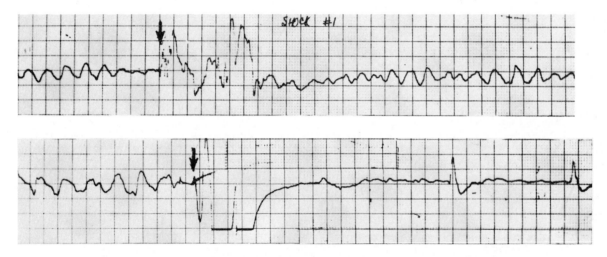

FIG. 12-9. Ventricular fibrillation was treated with application of unsynchronized countershock at 360 joules in top strip, noted by arrow. Since countershock was unsuccessful, as noted in continuous strip, countershock was again applied at 360 joules (arrow in second strip). Rhythm then converted to idioventricular mechanism.

if the mechanism of arrhythmia producing cardiac arrest is unknown, an ECG may be done following resuscitative measures. Most defibrillators have monitoring capability; their paddles act as electrodes that record the rhythm disturbance immediately before defibrillation.

14. As soon as the defibrillator is made ready (this should take no more than 30 seconds), the patient is shocked with the paddles in the same location as for cardioversion, at a peak energy level: 360 joules (Fig. 12-9). If this is not successful, defibrillation is repeated; the shock may be repeated again after lidocaine, procainamide, or bretylium tosylate administration.

15. Patients with ventricular fibrillation and ventricular tachycardia producing cardiovascular collapse are defibrillated or cardioverted immediately. Refer to appropriate algorithms for witnessed or unwitnessed ventricular tachycardia or fibrillation. Failure to restore an effective rhythm after delivery of a properly administered countershock at high intensity suggests that complicating problems such as hypoxia, acidosis, or drug toxicity may be present. If possible, these conditions should be corrected before the next countershock is delivered. If the cardiac arrest continues after several countershocks, sodium bicarbonate should be administered. Serial pH determinations

TABLE 12-2. Drugs commonly used in cardiac arrest: how supplied, usual dose (average adult)*

Drug	Concentration and Volume of Prefilled Syringe	Dose	Infusion Rate	Remarks
Atropine sulfate	0.1 mg mL in 10-ml syringe	0.5-1.0 mg = 5-10 mL		Repeat at 5-minute intervals to achieve desired rate. Generally, do *not* exceed 2 mg.
Bretylium tosylate	50 mg/mL in 10-mL ampule	5 mg/kg 350-500 mg as initial dose	500 mg in 5% dextrose in water (in 250 mL = 2 mg/mL; in 500 mL = 1 mg/mL) Infusion: 1-2 mg/min	Infusion started after loading dose to control recurrent ventricular tachycardia or ventricular fibrillation.
Calcium chloride 10%	100 mg/mL in 10-ml syringe	500 mg = 5 mL		May repeat dose every 10 minutes as needed.
Dopamine	200 mg in 5-mL ampule		200 mg in 250 mL dextrose in water = 800μg/mL Infusion: 2-10 μg/kg/min	
Epinephrine 1:10,000	0.1 mg/mL in 10-mL syringe	0.5 mg-1.0 mg = 5-10 mL IV or intratracheal	1 mg in 5% dextrose in water (in 250 mL = 4 μg/mL; in 500 mL = 2μg/mL) Infusion: 1 μg/min for maintenance of BP	Avoid intracardiac injection. Repeat dose every 5 minutes as needed in cardiac arrest.
Isoproterenol	0.2 mg/mL in 5-mL ampule		1 mg in 5% dextrose in water (in 250 mL = 4 μg/mL; in 500 mL = 2 μg/mL) Infusion: 2-20 μg/min. Titrate	Beware of PVCs.
Lidocaine	For IV bolus: 1% (10 mg/mL) in 10 mL = 100 mg 2% (20 mg/mL) in 5 mL = 100 mg For infusion after bolus: 4% (40 mg/mL) in 25 mL = 1 g	1%: 75 mg = 7.50 mL 2%: 75 mg = 3.75 mL	2 g in 500 mL 5% dextrose in water (or 1 g in 250 mL) = 4 mg/mL Infusion: 1-4 mg/min	For breakthrough ventricular ectopy: additional 50 mg bolus every 5 minutes to suppress, or total of 225 mg. Increase drip to 4 mg/min.
Procainamide	For IV bolus: 100 mg/mL in 10-mL ampule For infusion after bolus: 500 mg/mL in 2-mL ampules	20 mg/min until: a) Dysrhythmia suppressed b) Hypotension c) QRS widens by 50% d) Total 1 g administered	1 g in 250 mL 5% dextrose = 4 mg/mL Infusion: 1-4 mg/min	Monitor ECG and blood pressure. Administer cautiously in patients with acute myocardial infarction.
Sodium bicarbonate	1 mEq/mL in 50 mL = 50 mEq	1 mEq/kg or 75 mL initial dose (average-size adult) or preferably according to pH		Repeat according to pH. If not available, use ½ initial dose every 10 minutes.

From Textbook of advanced cardiac life support, American Heart Association, 1983. Reprinted with permission of the American Heart Association, Dallas, Texas.

*For additional information refer to "Standards and Guidelines for Cardiopulmonary Resuscitation and Emergency Cardiac Care," JAMA **255**(21):2938-2942, June 6, 1986.

should be performed to prevent overcorrection of acidosis (to alkalosis) and to determine whether enough sodium bicarbonate has been given. If pH determination is unavailable, give .5 mEq/kg sodium bicarbonate every 10 minutes.[24]

NOTE: Sodium bicarbonate should not be given without adequate oxygenation.[22] CPR must be continued between defibrillations or other procedures, since even a short interruption results in inadequate perfusion and increased anoxia. These complications in themselves may prevent successful resuscitation.

16. Repetitive shocks may not be effective in the presence of fine fibrillatory waves on the ECG. Giving the patient 5 ml of epinephrine 1:10,000 solution intravenously may convert these waves to large waves. In some cases lidocaine alone or in combination with epinephrine may assist in defibrillation. Procainamide IV and/or bretylium tosylate IV may also be tried.[24]

17. After successful conversion to sinus rhythm, continuous infusion with the antiarrhythmic drug, such as lidocaine, procainamide, or bretylium, should be instituted for maintenance therapy.[24]

18. If the rhythm is known to be ventricular asystole or slow idioventricular rhythm, atropine .5 mg may be given IV for a total of 2 mg. If the heart beat is not restored, CPR should be continued (see Nos. 1 to 9 and go to 19).

19. Epinephrine, 5 ml of a 1:10,000 solution, is administered intravenously. If this is unsuccessful, isoproterenol or calcium chloride may be administered.

20. Sodium bicarbonate should be given during the cardiac arrest, as described in No. 16.

21. Transvenous pacing equipment should be made ready for use. A direct percutaneous puncture of the heart may also be attempted.

22. At the first opportunity an episode sheet (Fig. 12-10) is completed, and clinical events and a drug tally are recorded.

Control of Environment. Regulation of the environment facilitates the rapidity and efficiency of the resuscitation procedure. The corridor to the patient's room must be free from obstacles. The patient's room should have adequate lighting with electrical outlets visible from the door. Furniture should not block traffic from the room door to the patient's bed. Flowers, if allowed in the CCU, should be set on a shelf away from the bed so that they will not be knocked off the table during an emergency.

Note: A fully stocked, adequately maintained emergency cart is imperative in every unit. It should include all drugs and equipment needed in an arrest and should not be cluttered with unnecessary items.

Postresuscitative Care. In the aftermath of a successful resuscitation it seems natural for CCU personnel to relax; however, meticulous attention to the patient's hemodynamic status, blood gas levels, and electrolyte balance continues to be important in maintaining clinical stability and in preventing recurrence. This is a time too during which the patient's family should be encouraged to visit when appropriate. The family should be prepared for changes in the patient or new equipment in use, such as a ventilator.

Inadequate Cardiac Output

The output of the heart may be inadequate to supply tissue needs as a result of myocardial dysfunction or arrhythmias.

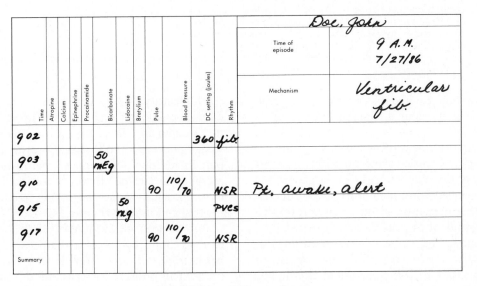

Time	Atropine	Calcium	Epinephrine	Procainamide	Bicarbonate	Lidocaine	Bretylium	Pulse	Blood Pressure	DC setting (joules)	Rhythm		
												Doe, John	
											Time of episode	9 A.M. 7/27/86	
											Mechanism	Ventricular fib.	
9 02										360	fib		
9 03		50 mEq											
9 10								90	110/70		NSR	Pt. awake, alert	
9 15					50 mg						PVCs		
9 17								90	110/70		NSR		
Summary													

FIG. 12-10. CCU episode sheet.

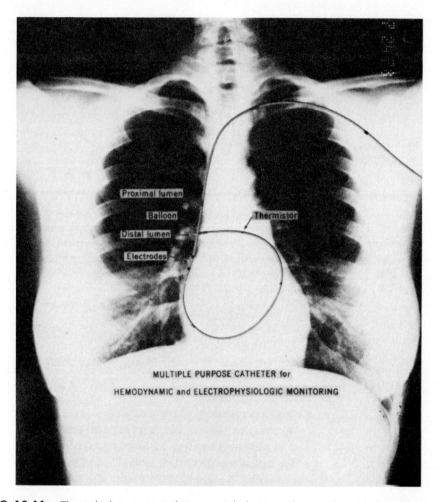

FIG. 12-11.   The multiple-purpose pulmonary triple-lumen catheter with atrial electrodes is shown superimposed on a chest x-ray film. The distal lumen records the pulmonary arterial or wedge pressure and is a useful site for withdrawing blood samples. The balloon can be inflated to facilitate passage through the right side of the heart. The thermistor permits measurements of the cardiac output by the thermal dilution technique. The electrodes record the atrial electrogram and can be used for atrial pacing. The proximal lumen records the CVP and is a useful site for infusing fluids and medications. The catheter tip should be kept in the proximal pulmonary artery except when a wedge pressure is being recorded. (From Mantle, J.A., and others: Chest 72:285, 1977.)

Invasive devices may be required for monitoring and treating the patient who develops a significant alteration in cardiac output.

Procedures for measuring cardiac output vary with the type of equipment used. Since the measurements are made with the pulmonary artery catheter, care of the patient and equipment is unchanged. Most pulmonary artery catheters are equipped with a thermistor in the distal portion that permits measurements of the cardiac output by the thermodilution technique (Fig. 12-11). Data regarding the cardiac output when combined with the left ventricular end-diastolic pressure (LVEDP) are useful in determining the adequacy of left ventricular function.[28]

Pulmonary Artery Catheters. A multipurpose flow-directed pulmonary arterial catheter permits monitoring of the pulmonary arterial pressure, pulmonary capillary wedge pressure, central venous pressure, and cardiac output. In addition, the standard thermistor catheter can be modified to include electrodes for atrial, ventricular, and atrioventricular sequential pacing and for recording intraatrial and intraventricular ECGs.

PULMONARY ARTERY (PA) PRESSURE. The pulmonary artery waveform evidences a sharp rise during ejection of blood from the right ventricle after the pulmonary valve opens. This pressure rise is followed by a slow decrease in pressure during the ejection of blood from the right ven-

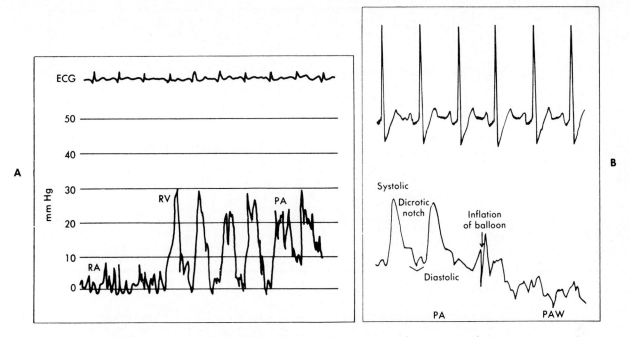

FIG. 12-12.   A, After inflation of balloon at tip of Swan-Ganz catheter, intracardiac pressure identifies right atrium *(RA)*, right ventricle *(RV)*, and pulmonary artery *(PA)* as catheter is advanced. Right ventricle is characterized by higher systolic but similar diastolic pressure value when compared to right atrial pressure. Pulmonary artery pressure shows same systolic value as that in right ventricle but diastolic pressure is higher than that in either right ventricle or atrium. Catheter whip or artifact is produced by exaggerated motion of catheter with inflated balloon and usually disappears with deflation of balloon. B, PA pressure waveform via balloon-tip catheter. Note balloon inflation and subsequent change to pulmonary artery wedge (PAW) waveform. (A modified from Rackley, C.W., and Russell, R.: Invasive techniques for hemodynamic monitoring, Dallas, 1973, by permission of the American Heart Association. B modified from Daily, E.K., and Schroeder, J.S.: Techniques in bedside hemodynamic monitoring, St. Louis, 1976, The C.V. Mosby Company.)

tricle until the pulmonic valve closes, indicated by the dicrotic notch. The pressure continues to decrease until systole occurs again.

Normal PA systolic pressure is 20 to 30 mm Hg, and normal PA diastolic pressure ranges from 5 to 16 mm Hg. The normal mean PA pressure ranges from 10 to 20 mm Hg. The PA systolic pressure normally equals the right ventricular systolic pressure (Fig. 12-12). The pulmonary artery end-diastolic pressure (PAEDP) should be almost equal to the mean pulmonary capillary wedge pressure (PCWP) in the absence of pulmonary vascular disease.

Elevation of PA pressure may occur during (1) increased pulmonary blood flow, as in a left-to-right shunt resulting from atrial or ventricular septal defect, (2) increased pulmonary arteriolar resistance resulting from primary pulmonary hypertension or mitral stenosis, and (3) left ventricular failure resulting from any cause.

PULMONARY CAPILLARY WEDGE PRESSURE (PCWP). Since there is normally a direct relationship among PAEDP, PCWP, and LVEDP, an elevated PAEDP or PCWP reflects the elevated LVEDP that occurs when the left ventricle can no longer adequately pump blood.

The PCWP is normally 4 to 12 mm Hg. PCWP exceeding 12 mm Hg may occur as a result of left ventricular failure, mitral stenosis, or mitral insufficiency, in addition to other possible causes.

PULMONARY ARTERY END-DIASTOLIC PRESSURE (PAEDP). Since the PAEDP is approximately equal to the PCWP and because the PAEDP is an accurate reflection of LVEDP (Fig. 12-13), the PAEDP can be used as an alternative measurement of LVEDP in most patients, even in the presence of pulmonary venous hypertension. At the time of catheter insertion, the PAEDP can be compared with the PCWP. If the difference is less than 5 mm Hg, the PAEDP can be used as an accurate estimation of the LVEDP,[28] eliminating the need for wedging the catheter.

Measurement of PA Pressure and PCWP. The method used to record PA pressure and/or PCWP from the standard strain gauge pressure transducer differs among institutions. Special points to consider in main-

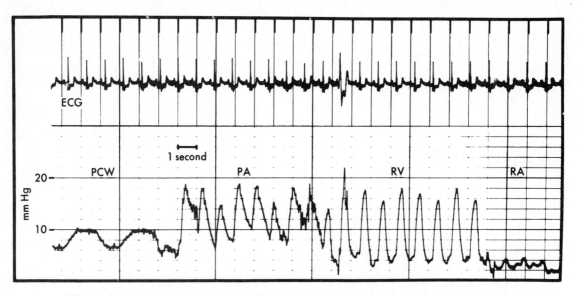

FIG. 12-13. Simultaneous recording of ECG and pulmonary capillary wedge *(PCW)*, pulmonary arterial *(PA)*, right ventricular *(RV)*, and right atrial *(RA)* pressures. The pulmonary arterial catheter was initially in a wedged position, with the balloon inflated. The balloon was then deflated, and the catheter was slowly withdrawn through the right heart chambers. Note the cyclic respiratory effects in the pressure signals. The PCW and PA end-diastolic pressures are equal. (From Mantle, J.A., and others: Advances in the treatment of heart failure. In Rackley, C.E., editor: Critical care cardiology: cardiovascular clinics, vol. 11, no. 3, Philadelphia, 1981, F.A. Davis Co.)

taining the catheter and measuring pressures include the following:

A. Obtaining measurements
  1. Record pressures at regular intervals as specified by the physician and as necessary. Evaluate changes and report to the physician as appropriate.
  2. Calibrate equipment before each measurement.
  3. Irrigate line before each measurement by pulling red rubber Intraflo plunger for 5 seconds (or manually if an Intraflo catheter is not used).
  4. Measurements should be taken using the phlebostatic axis, which is located at the midaxillary line at the sixth intercostal space.
B. Maintaining the catheter
  1. Maintain patency of the catheter.
    a. Irrigate automatically with 3 ml of D5W or normosol and heparin solution per hour, using an Intraflo catheter and maintaining pressure bag at 300 mm Hg.
    b. Irrigate manually every hour by pulling the red rubber Intraflo plunger for 5 seconds.
    c. Measure irrigating solution used at the end of each shift as part of IV intake.
    d. Change the dressing as described in section on arterial catheters.

  e. Observe for signs of infection and/or phlebitis at the insertion site.
  2. Observe the complexes for changes in fluctuations.
    a. Flattened complex: a possible wedging of the catheter in a pulmonary arteriole, which could result in pulmonary infarction. Turn the patient and ask the patient to cough and take some deep breaths; this may dislodge a catheter stuck in a wedge position. The physician should be notified so that the catheter can be repositioned.
    b. Irregular complex: an irregular fluctuation with no clear pressure wave form, indicating the need for irrigation with a 10-ml syringe. If this complex continues, the catheter is probably of no value and should be removed.
    c. Unobtainable wedge pattern: when the balloon is inflated and no wedge pattern is noted. Either the balloon is ruptured or the catheter is out of position. The physician should be notified to reposition or remove the catheter.
    d. No complex: check all stopcocks for proper position and follow with recalibration if needed.

CARE OF THE PATIENT AND PULMONARY ARTERY EQUIPMENT
1. Following insertion of the pulmonary artery catheter, apply a sterile dressing to the site and change it at least

every 48 hours. Note the condition of the site, including presence of active bleeding and signs of infection.

2. Immobilize the extremity to prevent accidental dislodgement of the catheter. Tape the catheter to the extremity to stabilize the catheter. A padded armboard or wooden device promotes comfort and immobilizes the extremity.

3. Check the extremity for circulatory insufficiency and bleeding at least every hour.

4. Observe the catheter frequently for leakage and proper stopcock position. Care should be taken to return the stopcock to the off position when drawing blood from the catheter.

5. The balloon should always remain deflated with a syringe attached, except when the PCWP is being read.

6. After the catheter is removed, observe the site closely for bleeding and infection until healing is complete. Apply a sterile dressing to the site.

Potential Problems in Use of Pulmonary Artery Catheters. There are several complications that may occur from the use of a pulmonary artery catheter. The major complication, pulmonary hemorrhage, may result if the balloon is inflated when the catheter tip is in a small arterial branch; however, careful adherence to proper procedures for balloon inflation will minimize this risk. The catheter tip may become wedged in a distal branch after repeated inflations, which may lead to a pulmonary infarction. When the catheter tip is withdrawn from the wedged position, it often recoils into the right ventricle or right atrium and must be repositioned.[28]

Measurement of Arterial Pressure. The uses and purposes of the arterial catheter are discussed in Chapter 7. When monitoring arterial pressure directly, personnel must carefully observe the following precautions to obtain meaningful values:

1. Standardize, balance, and calibrate the monitoring equipment at least once every 8 hours and after position changes or movements that might alter the calibration. Instructions for this procedure accompany the individual manufacturer's equipment.

2. An Intraflo device provides continuous flushing with a prescribed flow rate of a solution of D5W or normosol with heparin. The catheter should be flushed manually to clear the line after blood is drawn or if blood is in the line for any reason. The pulse waveform will become dampened or flattened somewhat if impairment of flow occurs.

3. Prevent catheter displacement by fastening the arterial catheter securely to the skin. The catheter may be sutured to the skin after insertion.

4. Prevent blood from entering the transducer. Blood in the transducer will dampen the pressure reading and may damage the transducer.

5. Observe the extremity in which the catheter is inserted every 1 to 2 hours for bleeding and check for circulatory insufficiency by capillary refill, skin temperature, and distal pulses. Check the arterial catheter frequently for leakage and proper stopcock position.

6. Apply a sterile dressing to the site, and change it at least once every 48 hours. Avoid the use of antimicrobial ointments at the insertion site. Povidone-iodine ointment at the insertion site is recommended to prevent infection. When a translucent dressing is applied, the dressing change can be done every 3 to 5 days unless conditions warrant more frequent changes.

7. Observe the site for infection when changing dressings. Should the catheter remain in the artery longer than 48 to 72 hours, observation of the site at least every 8 hours is imperative.

8. Immobilize the extremity to prevent accidental dislodgement of the catheter. If an armboard or wooden device is used, proper padding will prevent stasis changes of skin and increase comfort.

9. Exercise care when drawing blood from the catheter. The stopcock must be returned to the original position to ensure proper operation and prevent leakage.

10. After removing the catheter, apply direct pressure to the artery for 10 to 15 minutes or longer until bleeding ceases. The site should be covered with a sterile pressure dressing for 24 hours.

11. After the catheter is removed, observe the site for signs of bleeding, infection, and circulatory insufficiency until healing is complete. If any of these are noted, immediate attention should be given to correction of the condition.

Intraaortic Balloon Pump. The intraaortic balloon technique may be employed in patients with low output failure and is discussed in Chapter 7. Special points to be considered include the following:

1. Arrangement and preparation of equipment before insertion must be meticulous.

2. Pulses must be assessed before insertion to evaluate postinsertion complications.

3. The ECG or arterial pressure wave is the triggering stimulus for balloon activation.

4. Antibiotic therapy must be adequate.

5. Anticoagulation therapy may be desirable.

6. Angina and/or acute back pain may indicate complications of balloon insertion.

7. Timing of the balloon must be carefully monitored and adjusted as necessary.

8. A chest x-ray film may be used to verify the position of the balloon.

9. Strict aseptic technique must be maintained for dressing changes.

Thromboembolic Events

Anticoagulants. The need for anticoagulation therapy in patients who have a myocardial infarction continues to be controversial. Many physicians are not administering anticoagulants to patients in the acute phase following an infarction, but some patients are given antiplatelet drugs such as aspirin and dipyridamole. However, if the patient is receiving anticoagulant therapy, partial thromboplastin times and prothrombin times should be monitored. Any tendencies toward bleeding should be noted and treated immediately. Once the patient is out of the intensive care unit, oral anticoagulants may be prescribed to replace heparin if anticoagulation therapy is to be continued.

Thrombolytic Therapy and Percutaneous Transluminal Coronary Angioplasty (PTCA). A dramatic intervention for selected patients is the installation of a thrombolytic agent into the site of vascular occlusion. Streptokinase is an enzyme used in this capacity, and it triggers a chemical action, causing fibrin dissolution. This may be done in combination with PTCA and/or surgical intervention. There is still some controversy over whether the intracoronary administration of streptokinase is more beneficial than the intravenous administration.

The patient who receives streptokinase therapy must be observed closely for signs of bleeding. Vital signs and pulses in the extremities are checked frequently for adequacy of blood flow. Other nursing care required is based on protocol for patients with myocardial infarction undergoing cardiac catheterization. The patient continues on anticoagulation therapy for weeks to months.

PTCA has been introduced as an alternative to coronary artery bypass surgery for selected patients. The technique involves the use of a balloon-tipped catheter that is guided through the coronary artery lesion and inflated briefly. The pressure from the balloon compresses the atheromatous material against the vessel wall. Myocardial perfusion and performance are thus improved. (See Chapter 15 for further discussion.)

A recent advancement in fibrinolytic therapy is an experimental use of tissue plasinogen activator (t-PA) in the treatment of patients with acute myocardial infarctions. When coronary reperfusion is instituted within 6 hours of the occlusion, studies have shown reduced myocardial infarction size.[29] t-PA seems to have some advantages over streptokinase therapy in that its specific fibrin affinity reduces the possibility of hemorrhage as a side effect by eliminating the systemic lytic state noted with streptokinase, and it can be administered by peripheral intravenous access with good results.[30] Further investigation is needed before t-PA is available for general use.

Psychologic Alterations

Psychologic alterations in the patient may be noted at any point during the illness and should be evaluated on a continuing basis. For example, the intricate electronic equipment may contribute to the patient's psychologic stress. Patients should be encouraged to discuss their feelings about the monitor and other equipment. Continued simple explanations and reassurance should help relieve anxiety. Families should be included too because they often share patients' fears and increase their apprehension. Additional psychologic considerations are presented in Chapter 5.

CARE ISSUES
Sociocultural Considerations

Because the United States is a pluralistic society, health professionals must be prepared to work with patients from various cultures and to present health care in ways that are appropriate for individual patients. In addition, when professionals understand specific factors that influence individual health behaviors, they are in a better position to meet patients' needs. Knowledge of cultural backgrounds can help personnel anticipate differences in values, religion, dietary practices, lines of authority, family life patterns, and beliefs and practices related to health and illness. Total care can only become a reality when patients are seen in the framework of their individual cultural patterns.[31,32]

A minority culture frequently speaks English only as a second language. Persons who are bilingual may manifest a communication pattern that uses a combination of their native language and English, resulting in idiomatic speech. Because they have difficulty understanding and following medical jargon and staff directions, patients often feel devalued by staff members. Many patients express feelings of inferiority because of the inability to speak English or because they speak "wrong" English. Because of language difficulty, many patients are unable to read and comprehend consent forms or explanation of therapies.

Role expectations for the health professional vary. In general, they are based upon sex, age, educational preparation, and the ethnic identity of the staff. In nursing, the registered nurse has been regarded as having more status than the licensed practical nurse, and white nurses have more status than black or other minority nurses. Greater courtesy and deference have been accorded to female nurses than to their male counterparts, and disapproval has been expressed by patients when health professionals did not fulfill sex role expectations.[33]

Age is an important consideration in providing care. Many subcultures maintain a reverence for the elderly that has become minimized in our youth-dominated society. The elderly patient expects to be treated respectfully and in a formal manner, and the behavior of some younger staff has been viewed as callous and disrespectful.

In many subcultures health is not viewed as a high priority. The illness episode is viewed as a small part of a person's life. It is often difficult to gain cooperation for preventive health behaviors such as diet as part of blood pressure control and cessation of smoking to prevent heart and lung disease.

Daily Care

Once potential problems have been assessed, daily care of the patient can be based on the data obtained. Important components in daily care of the patient include relief of anxiety and pain, monitoring of blood gas levels and fluids, decreasing the myocardial work load, continuation of dietary recommendations, and prevention and/or early detection of complications.

If the patient experiences pain, it is important to note the frequency, duration, quality, quantity, location, associated factors such as diaphoresis and dyspnea, and alleviating factors. This information should be recorded on the patient's chart, accompanied by an ECG rhythm strip. Furthermore, a 12-lead ECG should be obtained and evaluated for changes from the initial ECG, and the patient's physician should be notified. If the physician has prescribed nitrates and analgesics, they should be given to the patient, and the nurse should monitor the patient's vital signs and respiratory characteristics. If the pain is not relieved, the physician should be notified so that the duration of pain and the increased oxygen demand on the heart can be decreased as soon as possible.

Once established, the need for supplemental oxygen should be evaluated often during the acute phase of the illness. Arterial blood gas samples should be drawn at intervals to evaluate acid-base balance.

Flow sheets that record many values are useful in maintaining a graphic representation of the patient's progress (Fig. 12-14). Some CCUs prefer a separate flow sheet for arterial blood gas levels, especially for people who require frequent arterial blood gas analysis.

Limiting myocardial work continues to be an important component of daily patient care. Activities should be gradually increased according to the plan of rehabilitation and the patient's stage of recovery. Patients are now being mobilized earlier than in previous years, since prolonged bed rest may not prevent but may actually promote development of complications following myocardial infarction. The patient must, however, be assisted in all activities, especially during the acute phase of the illness.

Initial dietary recommendations are usually maintained throughout the acute phase of illness and often throughout hospitalization and convalescence.

Fluid and electrolyte balance is vital during the acute phase of the myocardial infarction as previously discussed. Accurate measurement of intake and output levels, daily weight readings, evaluation of hydration, presence of pulmonary findings such as crackles, and edema are all important components in the evaluation of fluid and electrolyte balance.

Techniques such as recording daily weight and accurate intake and output measurements are aimed to prevent congestive heart failure or detect it early. Intake of routine IV fluids should be kept to a minimum of 20 ml/hour in the patient who has had a myocardial infarction, unless dehydration is present. All fluids, except in an emergency, should be administered via microdrip, and drugs such as lidocaine should be placed in a reliable automatic drip-control device and checked frequently to determine whether the proper amount of fluid is being delivered. A heparin lock may be substituted when it is necessary to continue IV medications.

Each of these components should be evaluated and care planned accordingly. Goals should be set with the patient for his care. Reevaluation and further planning are performed in relation to changes in the patient's status.

Elastic supports on the legs also may be used to prevent venous stasis. They must be applied with equal pressure from the foot to above the knee, checked frequently, and removed 2 or 3 times a day. Lotion or powder may be applied to the skin. The patient should be instructed not to cross his legs or ankles in order to prevent venous stasis. Sometimes the elastic stockings roll down over the knee and create a tourniquet effect on the leg; if this occurs, it should be corrected promptly. The legs should be observed for redness, swelling, heat, red streaks, and a positive Homans' sign. This sign occurs as a slight pain at the back of the knee or calf where the ankle is forcibly dorsiflexed and is indicative of incipient or established thrombosis in the veins of the leg. Should any evidence of embolization be observed, the patient's physician should be notified.

The exercise program is a necessary component of the total rehabilitation effort. An exercise program can help prevent the complications engendered by inactivity, such as respiratory complications, venous stasis, joint stiffness from immobility, and the weakness resulting from loss of muscle tone. Furthermore, exercise therapy promotes relaxation by decreasing tension and aids the patient psychologically.

An exercise program with appropriate program goals and priorities for implementation should be planned with the patient for use throughout hospitalization and after discharge (see Chapter 14). Structured in progressive stages, the exercise program should be individualized according to the patient's tolerance. Initially the patient may be assisted in performing passive exercises. A footboard is useful for the patient to exercise his leg muscles. Tolerance

	Date: Time:	7-3	3-11	11-7	7-3	3-11	11-7
Chest							
Chest pain		No					
R_x and response		–					
Gallops/murmurs		S3					
1 + edema		1+pedal					
Jugular venous distention		No					
Breath sounds		Bilateral					
Crackles		Inspiratory					
Rhonchi		No					
Wheezes		RUL					
Cough		Yes					
Dyspnea		No					
Cyanosis		No					
Other							
Abdomen							
Nausea/vomiting		No					
Appetite/diet		Not hungry					
Bowels/guaiac		No					
Abdominal distention		No					
Hepatomegaly		No					
Other							
Rhythm							
Basic rhythm		NSR					
Arrhythmias		Occ. PVCs					
Conduction defect		No					
Emotional status		Quiet Appears depressed					
Other							
Vital signs							
Bath/activity level		Bed bath/bed rest up to B.S.C.					
Temperature/weight		99.4°/206 lbs.					
Apical/radial pulse		82/82					
Respirations		20 at rest					
Blood pressure		138/84 R. arm					
Pedal pulses		3+bilateral					
Cardiac output		N.A.					
Right atrial pressure		N.A.					
Pulmonary artery pressure		N.A.					
Pulmonary capillary wedge pressure		N.A.					
Time		7 A.M.					
Laboratory data							
Enzymes		CK-MB-7%, LDH$_1$>LDH$_2$					
Blood gases		N.A.					
Other							
I and O							
Intake							
Oral		740 cc					
IV		280 cc					
Total		1020					
Total 24 hours							
Output							
Urine		530 cc					
Emesis/Gomco		N.A.					
Total							
Total 24 hours		530					
Signature							

FIG. 12-14. CCU summary flow sheet.

to exercise at each stage should be observed, evaluated, and recorded. When the patient is out of bed for the first time, medical personnel should record the patient's supine and standing blood pressures.

The complications most frequently encountered in patients who have a myocardial infarction are congestive heart failure and arrhythmias. The following sections outline methods of detecting and preventing these complications. For further discussion, see Chapter 7.

The patient should be assessed frequently to check for signs of possible congestive heart failure. The examination should include the following points:

1. Examine the heart, listening closely for the presence of a ventricular gallop (S_3) indicative of heart failure, and proceed with the other usual components of the cardiac examination. Special notice should also be given to the development of any tachyarrhythmias or bradyarrhythmias. These should be treated immediately.

2. Examine the lungs. Listen for crackles and if present previously compare their location, type, and amount. Note the presence of rhonchi that do not clear with coughing. Also, observe whether the patient is coughing (especially when lying flat), has Cheyne-Stokes respirations, or wheezes.

3. Search for peripheral edema or ascites. Although both are late signs of congestive heart failure, they can be correlated with earlier evidence such as unexplained gain in weight or oliguria during the day and increased urination during the night.

4. Evaluate dyspnea. Congestive heart failure should be suspected in the patient who has had a myocardial infarction and then develops dyspnea without another known cause.

5. Evaluation of jugular veins may reveal signs of elevated jugular venous pressure. The neck veins also may become distended when sustained pressure is applied on the liver (hepatojugular reflux). Systemic venous pressure is often abnormally elevated and may be recognized most easily by observing the extent of distension of the jugular veins.

The improved management of arrhythmias constitutes a significant advance in the treatment of myocardial infarction. The prevention of serious and life threatening arrhythmias depends on early recognition and aggressive management of their precursors. The most frequent arrhythmias noted in the acute phase of myocardial infarction are premature ventricular systoles, ventricular tachycardia, ventricular fibrillation, idioventricular rhythms, and AV blocks (see Chapter 8).

Transfer from CCU

Patients experiencing minimum or no complications are generally transferred to an intermediate care unit by the third day following myocardial infarction. Adequate preparations are important to minimize any emotional or physiologic reactions that may accompany transfer. Because the CCU is viewed by some patients as a safe atmosphere, they may be reluctant to leave. Others may anticipate moving to an environment they view as less restrictive. Whatever the reaction may be, it is important that the personnel in the CCU provide explanations of the regimens to be followed that can be reinforced by the staff in the intermediate care unit.

Since the actual transfer may be planned or sudden, the patient should be informed about the elements of transfer before the anticipated time of transfer. The patient should be aware that the staff in the intermediate care unit will be given a verbal report concerning his illness, progress, and potential problems for which they should be alert. The CCU nurse should accompany the patient to the intermediate care unit and introduce him to the primary nurse responsible for his care so that he is familiar enough with the person to call should he need assistance. Any information that the patient requests regarding the new unit can then be given by the intermediate care unit nurse.

The following suggestions will ease the patient's transition from the CCU to the intermediate care area:

1. Have the intermediate care area prepared with all the equipment needed by the patient and locate the patient close to bathroom facilities, nurses' station, and emergency equipment.

2. Monitor cardiac activity by telemetry to provide continuity of care and rapid detection of potential arrhythmic problems.

3. Provide a proposed guideline of educational activities for the patient to participate in during the remainder of hospitalization.

4. Provide the patient and family with information on routines appropriate to efficient operation of the unit, such as visiting policies, educational opportunities, activity routines, and the purpose of specialized equipment.

Several terms have evolved to describe an area designed to allow closely supervised convalescence for patients who have been transferred from the CCU. This area provides more intense observation and care than a routine medical unit but less than that provided in a CCU. Synonyms for this area include *step-down unit, liberalized cardiac unit,* and *intermediate care unit.* Regardless of the name selected, this unit has these multiple purposes:

1. Continued patient monitoring to allow for immediate recognition of cardiac arrhythmias and conduction disturbances

2. Immediate cardiopulmonary resuscitation

3. Safe, supervised, early mobilization

4. Reduction in costs

5. Environment conducive to psychologic and physical recovery
6. Education and reeducation concerning abilities and disabilities related to heart disease
7. Continuation of the planned rehabilitation program

Studies have shown that some patients who suffer acute myocardial infarction continue to be at risk even after surviving the first few hazardous days after onset.[34] In fact mortality during the later in-hospital phase of the illness, when the patient is usually no longer being cared for in the CCU, may be as high as that in the CCU for some groups of patients. This situation is the basis for the concept of intermediate coronary care, whereby patients can be located in an area that is usually close to the CCU. This unit has monitoring and resuscitative equipment and is staffed with personnel sufficiently prepared to provide routine as well as cardiopulmonary emergency care.

The following groups of patients have been shown to be at increased risk of catastrophic cardiac events during hospitalization and after discharge from the CCU:[34]

1. Patients with anterior infarctions involving large portions of the left ventricle and interventricular septum
2. Patients who while in the CCU exhibit circulatory failure in the form of cardiogenic shock, pulmonary edema, and congestive heart failure
3. Patients with preexisting cardiovascular disease, prior infarction, and fascicular block
4. Patients who exhibit arrhythmias that are primarily ventricular in origin, such as premature ventricular systoles, or are indicative of heart failure, such as atrial fibrillation or flutter and/or persistent sinus tachycardia
5. Patients with severe left ventricular dysfunction
6. Patients with functional abnormalities, such as exercise-induced ischemia noted as at least 2 mm of ST segment depression or angina at heart rates less that 135 and exercise intolerance noted as exercise capacity of less than 4 METs

Although current data indicate that people who fall within the categories listed above have a two to six times greater chance of late in-hospital sudden death, this cannot be predicted with complete accuracy. However, these patients have had a slightly longer stay in the CCU (1 to 2 days longer) and tend to be 3 to 4 years older than their counterparts who survive hospitalization. These facts alone support the need for accurate assessment and interpretation of data to prevent and treat the complications that contribute to this high late in-hospital mortality.[35]

Priorities during Intermediate Care

During the period of intermediate care, attention is focused on activity tolerance, educational strengths and deficits, and the patient's physical and psychologic status.

One goal of intermediate care is supervised early mobilization. Consistent with this expectation is a gradual increase in physical activity during the remainder of hospitalization, enabling the patient to reach the activity levels required for self-care when he returns home. The activities allowed include progressively increased self-care, increasing time spent sitting up in a chair, and body motion and strength-building exercises. The patient should increase his ambulation daily until he can walk about the hospital unit without tiring. (See Chapter 14 for specific rehabilitation recommendations.)

These physical activities are alternated with rest periods. Exercise should always be avoided after meals, when a large percentage of cardiac output is diverted to digest food. Criteria for decreasing the level of activity include the following:

1. Chest pain or dyspnea
2. Heart rate exceeding 120 beats/minute
3. Occurrence of a significant arrhythmia
4. Decrease in systolic blood pressure of 20 mm Hg
5. Increased ST segment displacement on the ECG or monitor[14]

Assessment of the patient's educational strengths and deficits should be determined soon after admission to the intermediate care unit so that planned teaching can be completed before discharge. In many instances personnel with special knowledge and skill in psychologic evaluation can be of tremendous assistance in determining how best to motivate patients and facilitate their learning. For some patients denial, depression, and despair are patterns of behavior that prevent optimum benefit from educational efforts. Individuals who have psychologic expertise can be of help in dealing with these exceptional patients and their families. This period immediately following the CCU experience has been recognized as the time when patients are most receptive to changes in life-style. Lifelong habits can be changed at this point more easily than later when the emotional impact of the acute event has subsided. Personnel must take full advantage of this receptive period.

Preparation for Discharge

Bauknecht reported in a study that investigated changes in patterns of referrals from hospitals to home health care that patients are being released from the hospital earlier in their convalescent period. Some patients are being discharged directly from intensive care units while still requiring respirators, suction machines, nasogastric tubes, urinary catheters, intravenous therapy, and continuous oxygen.[36,37]

The average length of stay for the uncomplicated myocardial infarction patient has decreased in the past 5 years.[38] Most patients in this treatment category are hospitalized between 9 and 10 days. The CCU phase of hospitalization is approximately 3 days.[14] The shortened hospital stay has impinged upon the time available for patient education and patient comprehension.

Written materials are especially useful to patients and families both in helping them to understand information that is given to them by personnel and in reminding them of the information once they are at home. Written materials should cover information needed by the patient to comply with prescriptions related to medications, diet, physical activity, and health behaviors. Although providing such information does not ensure compliance, it is necessary that the patient know how he can best contribute to his recovery.

Medications. Prescriptions and details of the drug regimen should be explained to both the patient and a responsible family member. Prescriptions should be labeled, and actions and side effects of each drug noted. The patient should be assisted to adjust the medication schedule to the usual life-style at home to ensure maximum adherence to the regimen.

Nutrition. The desired dietary modifications of calories, fats, and sodium should be explained. Demonstration of food preparation consistent with the dietary regimen and the patient's eating preferences and habits is desirable.

Physical Activity. An activity prescription should be individualized for each patient based on his prior level of activity and job requirements. It is the responsibility of the health team to prescribe and initially supervise the type of exercise, determine its duration and schedule, and warn against overexercising and describe its signs.

Smoking. Patients who smoke should be discouraged from continuing this practice. Many self-help programs are available to assist in smoking cessation. Moreover, health care personnel should set an example by not smoking.

Sexual Activity. It is important that the patient and partner receive information about resuming sexual relations. Often patients and their partners do not ask questions because of embarrassment or fear and make false assumptions about returning to previous sexual behavior. It is the responsibility of the health team to ensure that this information is provided and that the patient and partner be allowed to express concerns and ask any questions they may have. Patients and their partners should learn when it will be safe to engage in sexual intercourse and that sexual activity should commence when the patient is rested and not after a heavy meal or alcohol consumption.

Follow-up Care. Patients should receive information about a follow-up visit to the physician. In addition, the patient should know that chest pain, palpitations, shortness of breath, syncope or presyncope should be reported at once. It is important that family members learn about available community emergency services and how to obtain help if needed. Moreover, family members should be encouraged to acquire CPR skills.

Community Resources. The local heart association, vocational rehabilitation center, Veterans Administration, and other organizations may be of help to the patient. Other people, such as the social worker, public health nurse, dietitian, physical therapist, chaplain, occupational therapist, and psychologist may be asked for assistance and advice. Many communities have developed "coronary clubs," in which interested postmyocardial infarction patients, their families, and health care workers meet at regular times for guidance in care and education. This offers an opportunity to teach basic cardiac life support to the former patient and his family. Guest speakers may discuss topics such as nutrition, exercise, sexuality, basic cardiac life support, and antismoking techniques.

SUMMARY

Myocardial infarction is a major event in the life of a patient and his family. The care provided in the hospital and following hospitalization is important in assisting the patient to return to as normal a life as possible within the constraints of his heart disease. Each health team member has an opportunity to contribute to the cardiac patient's rehabilitation.

REFERENCES

1. McGregor, M.: Myocardial ischemia: towards better use of the coronary care unit, Am. J. Med. **76**:887, 1984.
2. Wheeler, D.J.: Unresolved questions concerning coronary care units, Clin. Invest. Med. **4**(1):13, 1981.
3. Hofvendahl, S.: Influence of treatment in a coronary care unit on prognosis in acute myocardial infarction, Acta Med. Scand. **519** (suppl.): 1, 1971.
4. Astvad, K., and others: Mortality from acute myocardial infarction before and after establishment of a coronary care unit, Br. Med. J. **1**:567, 1974.
5. Hill, J.D., Holdstock, G., and Hampton, J.R.: Comparison of mortality of patients with heart attacks admitted to a coronary care unit and an ordinary medical ward, Br. Med. J. **2**:81, 1977.
6. Armstrong, A., and others: Natural history of acute coronary heart attacks: a community study, Br. Heart J. **34**:67, 1972.
7. Goldman, L., and others: Evidence that hospital care for acute myocardial infarction has not contributed to the decline in coronary mortality between 1973-1974 and 1977-1978, Circulation **65**:936, 1982.
8. Gordis, L., Naggan, L., and Tonascia, J.: Pitfalls in evaluating the impact of coronary care units on mortality from myocardial infarctions, Johns Hopkins Med. J. **141**:287, 1977.
9. Pantridge, J.F., Webb, S.W., and Adgey, A.A.J.: Arrhythmias in the first hours of acute myocardial infarction, Prog. Cardiovasc. Dis. **23**:265, 1981.
10. Lazzara, R., and others: Ventricular arrhythmias and electrophysiological consequences of myocardial ischemia and infarction, Circ. Res. **42**:741, 1978.
11. Norris, R.M., and Sammel, N.L.: Predictors of late hospital death in acute myocardial infarction, Prog. Cardiovasc. Dis. **23**:129, 1980.
12. National Institutes of Health (NIH) Consensus Development Conference on Critical Care, vol. 4, no. 6, 1983.
13. Schuch, C.M., and Price, J.G.: Determination of time required for

blood gas homeostasis in the intubated, post open-heart surgery adult following a ventilator change, Heart Lung, 1987. (In press.)

14. Nelson, A.: Personal communication, Dec. 19, 1985.
15. Mathewson, M.: Rule: give only decaffeinated coffee to cardiac patients, Crit. Care Nurse 4:12, 1984.
16. Eberhart, R.C.: Changing perspectives in critical care computing, Crit. Care Med. 10:805, 1982.
17. Baer, A.R.: Design of large scale microcomputer software for the nursing environment. In Ackerman, M.J., editor: Computer applications in medical care, Washington, 1985, IEEE Computer Society Press.
18. Edmunds, L.: Hospital information systems for nursing problems and possibilities. In Ackerman, M.J., editor: Computer applications in medical care, Washington, 1985, IEEE Computer Society Press.
19. Sheppard, L.C.: Integration of computer-based clinical systems, AAMI Technol. Analyses Rev. 11:55, 1985.
20. Mirowski, M.: The implantable cardioverter-defibrillator: an update, J. Cardiovasc. Med. 9:191, 1984.
21. Harrison, D.C.: Should lidocaine be administered routinely to all patients with acute myocardial infarction, Circulation 58:581, 1978.
22. Gazes, P., and Gaddy, P.: Bedside management of acute myocardial infarction, Am. Heart J. 97:782, 1979.
23. Zipes, D.P.: Future directions: electrical therapy for cardiac tachyarrhythmias, PACE 7:606, 1984.
24. Textbook of advanced cardiac life support, Dallas, 1983, American Heart Association.
25. Spence, M: Cardioversion. In Miller, S., and others, editors: Methods in critical care, Philadelphia, 1980, W.B. Saunders Co.
26. Clark, M.B., Dwyer, E.M., and Greenberg, H.: Sudden death during ambulatory monitoring analysis of six cases, Am. J. Med. 75:801, 1983.
27. Standards & guidelines for cardiopulmonary resuscitation (CPR) and emergency cardiac care (ECC), JAMA 255:2905, 1986.
28. Mantle, J.: Cardiovascular evaluation and therapy in unstable patients. In Kinney, M., and others, editors: AACN's clinical reference for critical care nursing, New York, 1981, McGraw-Hill Book Co.
29. Kloner, R.A., and others: Studies of experimental coronary artery reperfusion, Circulation 68 (suppl. 1): 1, 1983.
30. Braunwald, E., TIMI Study Group: The thrombolysis in myocardial infarction (TIMI) trial, phase I findings, N. Engl. J. Med. 312::932, 1985.
31. Tripp-Reimer, T., Brink, P.J., and Saunders, J.M.: Cultural assessment: content and process, Nurs. Outlook 32:78, 1984.
32. Graison, B., O'Leary, L., and Wagner, J.: Cultural assessment . . . how well do we know our patients, J. Nephrol. Nurs. 1:132, 1984.
33. Archor, S.: Mexican Americans in a Dallas barrios, Tucson, 1978, University of Arizona Press.
34. Dennis, C.: Which MI patient has second-event risk? Hosp. Pract. 19(9):50, 1984.
35. Vedin, A., and others: Prediction of cardiovascular deaths and nonfatal reinfarctions after myocardial infarction, Scand. J. Rehabil. Med. 201:309, 1977.
36. Bauknecht, V.L.: Testimony cites impact of DRG system, Am. Nurse 17(10):3, 1985.
37. Andreoli, K.G., and Musser, L.A.: Trends that may affect nursing's future, Nurs. Health Care 6:47, 1985.
38. Hurst, J.W., and others: The heart, ed. 6, New York, 1986, McGraw-Hill Book Co.

CHAPTER 13

Psychologic Considerations in Coronary Artery Disease

James A. Blumenthal
Helene S. Mau

There has been a radical change in the epidemiologic characteristics of disease in the United States in the twentieth century. Infectious diseases, the chief cause of morbidity and mortality a 100 years ago, are no longer major factors. Chronic diseases are now the most prevalent causes of death, and cardiovascular disease in particular currently constitutes the single most frequent cause of death in adults in the United States.

A number of large-scale prospective studies have identified a set of characteristics that distinguish groups of people who are vulnerable to developing coronary heart disease (CHD) from people who remain healthy. These so-called risk factors include elevated blood pressure, hyperlipidemia, a positive family history, and cigarette smoking (see Chapters 2 and 3).[1,2,3] These risk factors, however, have been disappointing in their ability to predict individuals who develop CHD and offer only a partial explanation of why a given individual will develop CHD at a particular time. Moreover, these same risk factors have been even less useful in predicting subsequent mortality or morbidity once the disease has developed.[4] As a consequence, the role of psychologic, behavioral, and social factors in CHD has received growing recognition in the medical community and has been the subject of numerous scientific investigations. The purpose of this chapter is to provide a brief overview of the psychosocial aspects of coronary heart disease.

A HOLISTIC PERSPECTIVE

It is important to develop a conceptual framework for understanding human behavior as it relates to health and illness. Even Hippocrates observed that "the mode in which the inhabitants live, and what are their pursuits, whether they are fond of drinking and eating to excess, and given to indolence, or are fond of exercise and labor"—in effect, people's total lifestyle—must be considered when studying disease. Although an extended discussion about the various models of human behavior is beyond the scope of this chapter, mention should be made of the *biopsychosocial* model that is currently gaining widespread recognition in medicine and the behavioral sciences.[5] This model incorporates a holistic view of human functioning, emphasizing the need to understand the patient and his or her disease in a psychosocial context. On this view all disease is considered to have psychologic and social, as well as physical, aspects.

The biopsychosocial model extends the notion of disease beyond purely somatic parameters. The term "illness" is perhaps more inclusive and implies a necessary consideration of the social, cultural, and psychologic factors that contribute to the etiology, clinical manifestations, and subsequent outcome of the disease process. In any case the biopsychosocial model does not ignore biochemical, genetic, or other biologic influences. Rather, to understand the determinants of disease and to arrive at a rational and effective treatment regimen, it uses a holistic perspective. The patient, the social and cultural environment, and the complementary system devised by society to meet the patient's needs—that is, the health care system—all represent forces that influence the course of the disease.

ROLE OF LEARNING

The physician-patient relationship has typically been one in which the patient adopts a sick role and the physician adopts a professional one. These roles are learned behaviors that are transmitted by the culture. For the patient, sick behavior extends beyond the primary symptoms to include a set of behaviors that develop secondary to the disease. For example, the attention and sympathy a patient receives may serve to reinforce a pattern of illness behavior that may eventually be maintained independently of the disease itself.

Each role imposes certain responsibilities and obligations (see box on p. 386). The patient must be motivated to get well, must seek help, and must accept the physician as acting in his or her best interest. As a result of adopting these principles, the patient is often exempted from certain obligations and personal responsibilities. For example, the patient may not be required to return to work or to perform routine household duties. Moreover, the patient is frequently not held responsible for symptoms or for the behaviors that may result from the disease.

The physician, on the other hand, is obligated to act in the patient's best interests and to be ethically and morally responsible. As a result, physicians claim the privilege of having full access to patients' private lives and may assume

COMPLEMENTARY ROLES OF PATIENT AND PHYSICIAN	
Patient	Physician
SICK ROLE OBLIGATIONS	PROFESSIONAL ROLE OBLIGATIONS
Be motivated to get well	Act in the welfare of the patient in facilitating recovery
Seek technically competent help	Be guided by the roles of professional behavior
Cooperate with the physician and treatment regimen	Be affectively neutral and objective
PRIVILEGES	Engage in professional self-regulation
Exemption from normal social responsibilities	PRIVILEGES
Exemption from responsibility for one's own health	Access to physical and psychologic domains and to confidential information
	Professional authority and dominance

Modified from Parsons, T.: The social system, New York, 1951, The Free Press.

control of the relationship with the patient, as well as authority over other health care providers.

In the past two decades the role of social learning in the development of *illness behavior* has received growing attention. For example, Mechanic[7] has described illness behavior as the different ways in which patients perceive and respond to illness. He attempts to account for the reasons why some people ignore their symptoms and do not seek medical help, whereas others tend to overreact to symptoms and place excessive demands on physicians and medical care facilities.

Chronic illness behavior in patients represents a more long-standing pattern of response characterized by complaints of pain or dysfunction that seem disproportionate to objective medical evidence. Typical chronic illness behaviors include multiple somatic complaints, a constant search for diagnosis or more successful treatment, and behaviors designed to elicit attention from health care providers and family. Although there may be a physiologic basis for some symptoms, the perception of the symptoms and the resultant behaviors are considered to be subject to the laws of learning. Behavior that is followed by a desirable experience and/or behavior that is followed by the discontinuation of a negative or aversive experience tends to be reinforced; that is, the *consequences* of behavior affect the likelihood of its recurrence. Typical social reinforcers include sympathy, attention, and avoidance of embarrassment or pain. For example, a patient who develops chest pain while performing housework and then experiences pain relief on stopping makes an association of the behavior (resting) with the diminution of pain, which increases the likelihood of not performing such activities. When the patient also receives attention and sympathy for pain behaviors (i.e., verbal complaints, grimacing, or posturing), such social reinforcers may also serve to reinforce the pain behaviors. Furthermore, it is possible for a patient to avoid

routine responsibilities that may be assumed by others, such as family members. This situation is often referred to as *secondary gain*—that is, the social advantages of being ill. Money may also be a potent reinforcer. Thus disability payments for patients who are sick may serve to actually reinforce the sick role, and, in some cases, discourage resumption of previous activities such as return to work. The sick role thus can become an ingrained style of behaving that is highly resistant to change.

PSYCHOSOCIAL AND BEHAVIORIAL PRECURSORS

The psychologic and behavioral precursors of coronary disease have been observed for centuries. Dr. John Hunter, who suffered from angina pectoris, once observed, "My life is at the mercy of any rogue who chooses to provoke me." [8] Unfortunately, Dr. Hunter died after a heated board meeting at St. George's Hospital in London in 1793.[9] In 1897 Sir William Osler stated, "I believe the high pressure at which men live and the habit of working the machine to its maximum capacity are responsible [for arterial degeneration] rather than the excess of eating and drinking . . . ."[10]

In the past 50 years there has been a growing body of scientific data implicating a variety of social, psychologic, and behavioral factors in the pathogenesis and expression of clinical coronary artery disease (CAD).[11,12] For example, such factors as social mobility or social status incongruity (for example, the difference between aspiration and level of achievement), excessive life changes, absence of social support, depression, and chronic tension have all been suggested as playing an etiologic role in the development of CAD. Moreover, overt lifestyle behaviors such as overeating, cigarette smoking, and sedentary living have also been implicated (see Chapter 2).

A constellation of behaviors receiving much attention

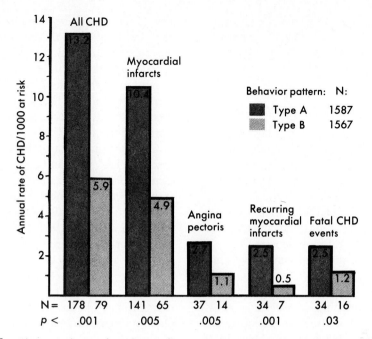

FIG. 13-1. The annual rate of incidence of coronary heart disease in 3154 subjects studied prospectively in the Western Collaborative Group Study (WCGS) project for 8½ years. The higher incidence of all forms of CHD in the Type A subject is shown. Note too that recurring myocardial infarcts occurred 5 times as often and fatal CHD attacks approximately twice as often in Type A than in Type B subjects. *N*, number of cases. (From Friedman, M., and Rosenmann, R.H.: Ann. Clin. Res. 3:300, 1971.)

is called the type A (coronary-prone) behavior pattern (TABP). TABP is characterized by excessive competitive drive, extreme desire for recognition and achievement, a chronic sense of time urgency, motoric hyperactivity, and underlying hostility. The converse, type B, behavior pattern is defined as a relative absence of these characteristics.[13]

The classification of individuals as type A or type B is usually determined by clinical judgments based on a series of specific questions. These questions are designed to elicit a particular *style* of response that is often displayed by type A individuals, as well as to acquire information regarding the individual's typical behavior based on self-reported attitudes and practices.[14] During an interview to determine type A behavior, the subject is asked approximately 20 to 25 questions dealing with feelings of ambition and competitiveness, past history of feelings of anger, sense of time urgency and impatience, and current feelings of irritation and frustration. The manner in which the interview is conducted attempts to create a situation whereby type A behaviors can be observed. For example, the interviewer purposefully interrupts the subject to elicit anger, asks questions rapidly to encourage a quick response, and slows a question, stumbling over words, to facilitate an interruption on the part of the respondent. Thus the assessment of the type A behavior pattern depends more on the basis

of *observed overt behaviors* than on the self-reported habitual behavior of the patient.

In a series of retrospective and prospective studies, individuals displaying the type A behavior pattern have been shown to have two to seven times the incidence of CAD as seen in their type B counterparts.[14-16] For example, the Western Collaborative Group Study identified 3154 healthy men who were studied annually over a mean period of 8½ years.[17] The results of this study are shown in Fig. 13-1. Of the 257 men that developed CHD during this period (1960 to 1970), 178 were classified as type A by the interview method, whereas only 79 were classified as type B. When traditional risk factors such as age, serum cholesterol, blood pressure, and smoking habits were statistically controlled, the relative risk of CHD for type A was about twice that of type Bs. Furthermore, despite a relatively small sample, a five-fold greater rate of recurrent myocardial infarctions in type A subjects compared with type B subjects was highly significant.

In 1981, the National Heart, Lung, and Blood Institute assembled a review panel of scientists to evaluate the TABP literature. They concluded:

The review panel accepts the available body of scientific evidence as demonstrating that Type A behavior . . . is associated with an increased risk of clinically apparent coronary heart disease in employed middle-aged U.S. citizens. The risk is greater than that imposed by age, elevated values of systolic blood pressure and serum cholesterol, and smoking, and appears to be of the same order of magnitude as the relative risk associated with the latter three of these other factors.[18]*

ROLE OF ANGER AND HOSTILITY

In an effort to identify components of TABP that may be especially pathogenic much attention has recently focused on the role of *hostility*. A measure of hostility known as the Cook-Medley Hostility (Ho) Scale has been shown to be directly related to TABP classification. Type A subjects score significantly higher on the Ho Scale than Type Bs. Moreover, high scorers on the Cook-Medley Scale also have greater levels of CHD than do low scorers.[19]

Fig. 13-2 shows that Ho scores and gender were independently and significantly related to severity of CAD in a sample of patients undergoing coronary angiography. Note for both men and women, high-hostile, type A individuals had the highest levels of CAD. Moreover, Dembroski and others[20] recently showed that high levels of "potential for hostility" were also related to increased levels of CAD, particularly if anger was kept in rather than expressed outwardly.

Interpretation of these relationships between hostility

*Recent studies have reported inconsistent associations between type A behavior and manifestations of CHD. (For review, see Matthews, K.A., and Haynes, S.G.: The type A behavior pattern and coronary risk: update and critical evaluation, Am. J. Epidemiol. **123:**923-960, 1986.

and CHD in patients referred for coronary angiography must be qualified by the fact they are based on *concurrent* observations in a clinical population with suspected CHD. Several *prospective* studies have now been completed in which scores from the Cook-Medley Ho Scale were obtained from initially healthy men whose health status has been followed for periods as long as 25 years after completion of the test.[21,22]

One such investigation by Shekelle and colleagues[21] was based on 1877 men in the Western Electric Study. These men, aged 40 to 55 years at time of intake, were employees at the Hawthorne Works of the Western Electric Company in Chicago and initially completed the Ho scale in 1957-1958 and again in 1961-1962 as part of a larger examination that included evaluation of blood pressure, cigarette smoking, and serum cholesterol. Men continuing in the study were reexamined annually until 1969, primarily to determine the occurrence of new CHD events. The most recent follow-up for mortality was carried out in 1978. One important finding was a correlation of 0.84 between Ho scores obtained at the initial examination and scores obtained 4 years later for 1653 men who took the Cook-Medley on both occasions. This suggests that Ho scores appear to be measuring a relatively stable personality characteristic. The 10-year incidence of major coronary events (myocardial infarction [MI] and CHD deaths) for high Ho scorers was associated with increased CHD morbidity relative to low scorers. After adjustment for blood pressure, serum cholesterol, smoking, alcohol use, and age, the risk of a major CHD event was 1.47 times greater in men with

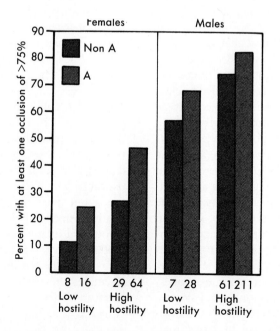

FIG. 13-2. Relation of gender, hostility score and Type A behavior to presence of significant coronary atherosclerosis.

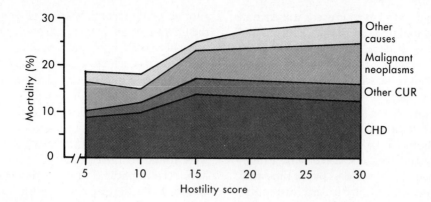

FIG. 13-3. Causes of mortality as a function of hostility scores in the Western Electric sample. (Based on data from Shekelle et al., 1983.)

Ho scores greater than 10 than in men with Ho scores less than 10. Fig. 13-3 shows that the Ho scale was also significantly and positively associated with a crude 20-year risk of death from CHD, malignant neoplasms, all causes except cardiovascular-renal (CVR) diseases and malignant neoplasms, and from all causes combined. After adjustment for age, cigarette smoking, intake of alcohol, systolic blood pressure, and serum cholesterol level by Cox-type regression analysis, the Ho scale maintained a statistically significant, positive association with 20-year total mortality and for mortality due to causes other than CVR diseases and malignant neoplasms. An increase of 23 points on the Ho scale, i.e., the difference between the mean Ho scores

for the first and fifth quintiles, was associated with a 42% increase in mortality risk during the 20 years of follow-up after adjustment for cholesterol, systolic blood pressure, smoking, age, and intake of alcohol.

The relationship between Ho scores and subsequent morbidity and mortality was also evaluated in a study by Barefoot, Dohlstrom, and Williams[22] of 255 male physicians who had completed the Cook-Medley Scale while in medical school at the University of North Carolina 25 years earlier, when their mean age was 25 years. Fig. 13-4 shows the impact of high hostility scores on subsequent total mortality. Over the entire 25-year follow-up period, 98% of the low-hostile group were still alive. In contrast, only

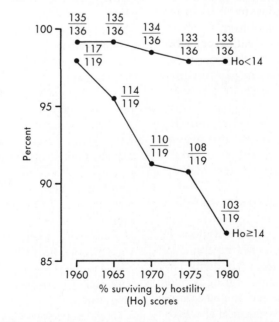

FIG. 13-4. Hostility and coronary heart disease incidence (myocardial infarction or cardiac death) over a 25-year follow-up period in 255 physicians who took the Minnesota Multiphasic Personality Inventory (MMPI) during medical school. (From Psychosomatic Medicine, 45:1 March, 1983.)

87% of those in the high-hostile group were still alive in 1980. Whereas among middle-aged cardiac patients and Western Electric employees the relative risk of significant CAD or CHD associated with a high hostility score was roughly 50% greater than those with low hostility scores, in this sample of healthy young physicians the relative risk of dying was six times greater for the high hostility group relative to the low hostility group. Inspection of the survival curve for the high-hostile group suggests one explanation for the lower relative risk associated with a high-hostile score among middle-aged persons: by the time middle-age is reached, those who are particularly susceptible to the consequences of hostility will have already died.

BIOBEHAVIORAL MECHANISMS

Currently the major biologic characteristics that are thought to be responsible for the association between TABP/hostility and CHD are the excessive cardiovascular and neuroendocrine responses shown by individuals displaying TABP.

It is generally believed that the initiating event in the atherosclerotic process is some type of damage to the inside lining (endothelium) of the artery wall.[23] This initial insult might be the result of hemodynamic factors in which turbulence and shear forces set the stage for the formation of atherosclerotic buildup, or perhaps the process depends on the presence of excessive amounts of certain hormones or other chemicals that make certain sites on the coronary arteries vulnerable to lesion (see Chapter 2).

Many of the cardiovascular and neuroendocrine factors that may be pathogenic have been shown to be associated with TABP. The earliest evidence comes from Friedman and others[24] who showed that persons with type A behavior excrete excessive amounts of catecholamines and other metabolites. Resting levels were found to be the same between type A and B persons; however, during work, levels of norepinephrine were greater in the type A men. This same phenomenon was noted under more controlled conditions whereby type A subjects increased their plasma norepinephrine levels by 30% in response to a specific challenge, while the response of the type Bs remained the same.[25]

In an experimental paradigm,[26] harassment was added to a competition task for both type A and B subjects. Type As responded to harassment with greater elevations in plasma epinephrine than did all the other experimental groups. Catecholamines are released from the adrenal medulla and from sympathetic nerve endings during periods of arousal. The hormones epinephrine and norepinephrine may have direct hemodynamic and biochemical effects relating to CHD. They serve to increase heart rate, blood pressure and platelet aggregation, while releasing lipids and free fatty acids into the bloodstream. Free fatty acids are another component of the circulating blood taken up by the atheromatous plaque, while platelet aggregation may contribute both to plaque formation and to certain clinical CHD events such as myocardial infarction.

Cholesterol metabolism has also been found to be affected in type A individuals with notable increases occurring during periods of stress. Clotting time and cholesterol levels were monitored in a group of accountants before and during the April 15th deadline for tax returns. Both were found to increase during periods of job stress and have been implicated in the pathogenesis of CHD.[27] Biochemical abnormalities have been found in both type A women[28] and men.[29] Fasting and postprandial serum triglyceride levels were also elevated in type A subjects,[30] along with postprandial sludging of erythrocytes[31] known to be associated with angina. Other neuroendocrine and biochemical characteristics associated with TABP and thought to be associated with the atherogenic process include: (1) elevated levels of ACTH (adrenocorticotropic hormone) and a depressed response to secreting 17-hydroxycorticosteroids following an injection of ACTH, (2) decreased level of growth hormone even following arginine challenge, (3) hyperinsulinemic response to glucose challenge in the absence of a positive glucose tolerance test, (4) excess cortisol secretion, and (5) excess testosterone during a typical day.[32-34] This latter finding is especially important in light of the recent observations of increased plasma estradiol levels among male heart attack victims compared to men free of coronary disease.[35,36] Since most of the plasma estradiol in men is derived from testosterone via aromatization—a conversion that is stimulated by norepinephrine—and since type A men appear to secrete more testosterone and norepinephrine in response to daily challenges, increased testosterone secretion among hostile type A men may play a pathogenic role in the development of CHD. Moreover, excessive cortisol secretion could also promote atherogenesis. Both epinephrine and cortisol are secreted during the experience of anger, which may occur with greater frequency and intensity among type A individuals. Cortisol is known to potentiate both the cardiovascular and metabolic effects of catecholamines, which could accelerate processes involved in the endothelial "injury" thought to be responsible for atherogenesis. In addition, the administration of corticosteroids has been associated with acceleration of atherosclerosis in patients with rheumatoid arthritis,[37] and patients with more severe angiographically documented CAD have been found to have higher morning cortisol levels than patients with minimal disease.[38]

Type A persons also exhibit enhanced cardiovascular reactivity. Individuals displaying TABP show a heightened response to sympathetically mediated processes like heart rate (HR) and blood pressure (BP), especially in the face of a challenging situation. For example, in a group of cardiac patients matched with patient controls, Dembroski and colleagues[39] monitored ECG and blood pressure while administering a structured interview (for assessing TABP) and a challenging history quiz. As predicted, not only were there more type As among the patient group but this group as a whole had significantly elevated systolic and diastolic blood pressures throughout the course of the interview when compared to the controls and this difference became even more pronounced during the challenge of the history quiz. Since the patients were all on propranolol (a drug that reduces HR response) at the time of the study, the data may be even more significant. Thus the greater cardiovascular and neuroendocrine responsivity observed among type A individuals could be the mechanism by which type A behavior and hostility contribute to increased risk of CHD.

PSYCHOLOGIC ADJUSTMENT TO CORONARY HEART DISEASE

The emotional, behavioral, and social impact of a heart attack is often profound and, for many patients, may be even more debilitating than the limitations imposed solely by the physical effects of the disease. Psychologic adaptation begins when symptoms are first noticed and continues throughout hospitalization and the subsequent return home. For the purposes of the present chapter, three phases of the illness will be discussed: prehospital, hospital, and posthospital.

Prehospital Phase

Probably the most common reaction of the patient to the first signs of illness is simply to do nothing and hope that the symptoms go away. The average time between symptom onset and admission to a medical facility is about 3 hours, although patients may delay seeking help for more than 24 hours.[40]

Approximately 55% to 65% of the time between symptom onset and hospital arrival involves what has been termed *decision time*. During this period patients become aware of their symptoms and may engage in various behaviors designed to provide themselves with relief: they may rest, take medication, or discuss the problem with spouse or friends. An additional 25% of the time between symptom onset and entry into the medical facility involves the period of *medical preparation*. It is during this time sequence that the physician is contacted and arrangements are made for subsequent hospital care. The remaining 10% is time required for transportation to the hospital and is typically referred to as *transportation time*.

Since more than half of all deaths following myocardial infarction occur within the first 4 hours, it is important that the interval between symptom onset and medical care

be reduced. Longer time to respond to symptoms appears to be unrelated to demographic factors such as age, sex, or socioeconomic status. Psychologic factors appear to play a predominant role, especially in the decision time. Denial, that is, the tendency to ignore or minimize the true significance of the symptoms, seems to be the most common reaction and often leads to incorrectly attributing the symptoms to such noncardiac factors as indigestion or dysfunction in other organ systems.[41]

Probably the most important remedy to the lengthy delay in response to cardiac symptoms is education of the patient, family, and physician. It is interesting to note that the available data suggest that the subgroup of patients who delay appropriate response the most are individuals with a past history of cardiac problems. Cardiac patients should be instructed to consult their physicians when symptoms first develop rather than waiting to see if their medication is effective. If their symptoms have progressed, patients should not be falsely reassured but should be encouraged to act quickly and decisively. Physicians are encouraged to get to know their patients so that they can better judge the significance of the patient's symptoms. Unfortunately, it is not uncommon for physicians to use the same maneuvers as their patients, blaming other organ systems or minimizing the symptoms—perhaps in the belief that the patient is exaggerating or overreacting to minor symptoms.

Hospital Phase

Admission to the hospital is an unmistakable sign to the patient that something is wrong and that medical intervention is required. The single most important emotional feature of patients in the initial acute phase of their illness is extreme fear and anxiety. The content of anxious thought usually focuses on the realization of the possibility of sudden death, concerns about being abandoned and out of control, and the conscious preoccupation with symptoms such as shortness of breath, chest pain, fatigue, or irregular heart rhythm. Depression, hostility, and agitation also are observed in many patients. Cassem and Hackett[42] have developed a model for the temporal sequence of emotional reactions in patients with CHD, based on reasons for psychiatric referral in the Coronary Care Unit (CCU). The sequence is graphically displayed in Fig. 13-5. The patient feels heightened anxiety during the first 2 days of hospitalization and subsequently becomes depressed for a few days. Anxiety and depression both decline after 5 or 6 days as a result of the mobilization of two main defense mechanisms: denial and repression. Isolation of affect is a third common defense mechanism that helps the patient cope with the illness. This process involves the acknowledgement of the reality of the situation, but the affective or emotional component of this awareness is unconscious.

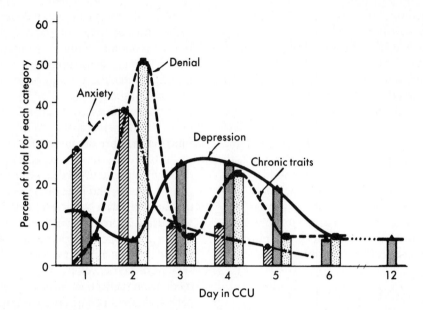

FIG. 13-5. Hypothesized course of emotional behavioral reactions in the CCU. (From Cassem, N.H., and Hackett, T.: Ann. Intern. Med. **75:**9, 1971.)

Although the majority of patients do not require formal psychiatric intervention, a substantial number do experience significant emotional distress. Many patients have confronted death for the first time, they are frightened and depressed over the perceived loss of physical health, they are prone to worry about future employment, family relations are disrupted, and their financial security may be threatened.

While patients with CHD often tend to avoid admitting fears and worries during brief interviews, more intensive contact in which the patient is given an opportunity and permission to discuss feelings and problems in a supportive, nonthreatening environment can be extremely therapeutic. Most patients will welcome a chance to "get things off their chest," and the process often promotes feelings of reassurance and relief.

Patient teaching is another important aspect of the hospital phase. Frequently patients have trouble assimilating and retaining all the information presented to them. However most want to know about their condition (in varying degrees of detail); so it is often useful to sit down with the patient and spouse to review the important aspects of cardiac care. It is imperative to *listen* as well as to talk with the patient. Patients will communicate what they know and what they want to know if given an opportunity. Disguised fears and anxieties and misconceptions about their illness also can become apparent. For example, the statement "I guess this means I'll never go back to work" may reflect apprehension about remaining autonomous, anxiety about being dependent on others, and uncertainty about the realistic limitations of the illness. Such statements should be explored and discussed with the patient.

Although each patient is different and needs to be treated as an individual, specific issues should be reviewed with every patient before discharge. The following outline presents objectives based on the American Nursing Standards of Cardiovascular Nursing Practice[43]:

A. Demonstrate a knowledge level that will enable the patients to make appropriate therapeutic judgments and seek medical help when indicated
   1. Accurately describe what to do if chest pain occurs
   2. Describe the signs and symptoms that necessitate medical advice
      a. Chest pain unrelieved by nitroglycerin and rest
      b. Increased shortness of breath
      c. Fainting
      d. Very slow or rapid heart rate
   3. Be able to accurately take own pulse
   4. State time, date, place, and person(s) to be seen for follow-up care
B. Maintain a pharmacologic regimen compatible with therapeutic and personal goals
   1. State when to take each medication
   2. Describe desired effects of each medication
   3. Describe possible adverse reactions to each medication
   4. Describe what to do if adverse reactions to medication occur
C. Maintain a dietary intake compatible with therapeutic and personal goals

1. Describe dietary restrictions
2. Describe rationale for restrictions
3. State examples of foods to avoid
4. State that excessive body weight increases the work of the heart
5. Describe the effects of alcohol on the heart
6. Describe the effects of caffeine on the heart

D. Demonstrate a knowledge level that enables the patients to appropriately modify their lifestyles
1. Describe the pathophysiology of myocardial infarction and angina pectoris
2. Identify risk factors and relate them to the development of coronary disease
3. Identify the patients' own risk factors
4. Indicate an understanding of the importance of providing the heart with adequate oxygen and rest by describing factors that decrease oxygen supply and/or increase workload
   a. Digestion of food
   b. Cigarette-smoking
   c. Emotional stress
   d. Very hot or cold weather
   e. Very hot or cold baths or showers
   f. Isometric exercises (give examples of these)
   g. Working with arms above shoulder level
   h. Sexual behavior

E. Participate in the planning to modify the patient's lifestyle
1. Describe own plan for the resumption of the following activities that is consistent with prescribed activity level
   a. Activities of daily living
   b. Household tasks
   c. Sexual activity
   d. Vocational activities
   e. Driving a car
   f. Recreation
2. Discuss plans to decrease or stop cigarette smoking
3. Discuss plans to minimize or eliminate sources of stress and tension
4. Discuss and implement plan to screen children for risk factors

F. Demonstrate coping mechanisms effective in adapting to patient's altered lifestyle
1. Ability to cope with anxiety as evidenced by the following
   a. Sleep at least 6 uninterrupted hours in a 24-hour period
   b. Relax body musculature during rest periods
   c. Talk about events other than those related to self or own illness
   d. Resume grooming behavior

G. Maintain activity pattern that is compatible with therapeutic and personal goals
1. Describe factors that should be taken into account when walking
   a. Distance
   b. Speed
   c. Weather
   d. Incline
2. Discuss plan for walking and outline stages of progression (see Chapter 14)

Patient instruction is an extremely important activity and has been shown to increase the patient's knowledge and to improve subsequent psychosocial and medical adjustment. An excellent review of the importance of the nursing staff and the stresses of the CCU experience can be found in an article by Cassem, Nelson, and Rich.[43] It should be noted, however, that patients differ in their receptivity to health information, and that the amount of responsibility and information given to a patient must be carefully determined by taking into account the patient's ability to comprehend and use the information.

A number of research investigations have attempted to relate stressful experiences on the CCU to subsequent recovery. In general, data suggest that the CCU equipment, activities, and procedures do not result in any long-term maladjustment in coronary patients.[44] However at least one study[45] has shown that witnessing a coronary crisis in the CCU can result in physiologic arousal (that is, heightened systolic blood pressure) and increased subjective anxiety.

The CCU is stressful for the staff as well as for the patients. Patients demand intense personal contact from the staff whom they do not know and may never see again after discharge from the hospital. The CCU nurse must be able to establish rapport quickly with patients, provide expert nursing care and emotional support, and then be able to maintain an emotional detachment and objectivity in making nursing decisions and in aiding the patients' release from the CCU.

Although emotional stresses require adjustment, the physical demands of work on the CCU can be equally challenging. For example, heavy lifting, unpredictable scheduling, and a hectic work pace are common conditions to which nurses are subjected. Regular group meetings can be extremely effective in helping staff cope more effectively with the intense job demands and deal more constructively with interpersonal conflicts.

Posthospital Phase

After about a week on the CCU the patient is transferred to a ward with less supervision but remains under intensive medical care for the next 1 to 2 weeks. The posthospital phase begins with the patient's discharge from the hospital and for all practical purposes continues indefinitely thereafter. During this phase the responsibility for the patient's care shifts from the hospital team of physicians, nurses, physical therapists, and others to the patient and family.

It has been widely documented that psychologic and behavioral factors affect the course of recovery and that psychologic problems are seldom resolved during the acute period of hospitalization. For example, research has documented that at 6 months to 1 year after discharge from the hospital, as many as 88% of the patients sampled were anxious or depressed, 50% reported disturbed sleep, 20% did not return to work, and 83% complained of excessive weakness.[46] Heart disease also affects the family, and marital conflicts, often centering around medical instructions (concerning such areas as diet, medication, and sexual activity), are not uncommon.[47]

Unlike the structured hospital setting, the return home often means that the patient is unsupervised and that no concrete, specific guidelines are made available. The patient may be uncertain about the extent to which physical activity is permissible, and the advice "take it easy" is too often misunderstood or is so general as to be of no real value. Concern about sexual functioning, apprehensiveness about returning to work, and awareness of diminished energy and strength are not uncommon.

In general, emotional distress reaches its peak during the patient's convalescence. There appear to be at least five main problem areas that affect a substantial number of coronary patients: (1) excessive concerns about health and the fear of dying, (2) organic problems, (3) emotional problems, (4) continuation of personality problems from the time before the illness, and (5) developmental issues and existential concerns.

Excessive Concerns about Health

Once a person has experienced a myocardial infarction (MI), good health can no longer be taken for granted. Many patients become sensitized to their bodily functioning. In extreme cases patients may become preoccupied with their health and overreact to even minor discomfort.

Fear and anxiety about death are common reactions to a heart attack. Most people do not think about their own deaths very much. However the occurrence of a heart attack serves as a reminder of our mortality and raises a cultural expectation of death. This expectation is founded in clinical fact, since patients with CHD have higher mortality rates than their healthy age-matched counterparts. Thus a diagnosis of coronary disease may be viewed as a "hex word," suggesting that death is imminent.[48]

Losses are considered to be less disruptive when they are "scheduled" or when the events are perceived as being subject to schedule.[49] Anxiety about death as a major loss is also related to attitudes about aging. Expectations for decline, loss, or death are far more inconsistent for the later

years of life than for the early years. Thus, for the young, society expects continued growth and the pattern of change is predictable. As people grow older, however, the pattern of development becomes ambiguous and expectations become unclear. The lack of clear positive expectations for development during the adult years also contributes to the attribution of normative loss. However, a myocardial infarction for a young person may be more traumatic than for the older individual whose myocardial infarction, which heralds aging, is more often expected. Disability and death are seen as more appropriate to the elderly than to the young and public policy decisions predictably follow this attitude.[50]

For many patients, a heart attack represents significant *loss:* loss of income, loss of family and friends, loss of job, loss of status, and loss of independence, as well as loss of health. As a result of these actual and/or threatened losses, grief reactions are not unusual. The patient's reactions may parallel the stages observed among patients with cancer: denial, anger, depression and, ultimately, acceptance.[51] These "stages of dying" have not been fully confirmed, however, and some of the conceptual and methodologic deficiencies have been described elsewhere.[52]

In the past, it was felt that health professionals should not talk with cardiac patients about anything that might disturb or excite them. As a consequence, the post-MI patient's fears and anxieties were often denied or ignored. More recently, however, the importance of effective communication with the coronary patient has been recognized. Specifically, affective empathy is considered extremely important along with acceptance of the patient's feelings. For a more extended discussion of death and dying, the interested reader may want to review other sources.[50,51,53]

Cardiac neurosis is a term often used to describe a situation in which the patient has become completely debilitated by the illness. Fear of leaving home or anxiety over physical exertion may be present, and even minor symptoms are thought to be emergencies or precursors of a fatal cardiac event. Although some hypochondriac patients are also depressed and the affective component is often minimized, the behavioral and biologic components are pronounced. The possibility that the patients' overconcern about the integrity of their body may reflect a *masked depression* (physical complaints hiding or obscuring the depression) or a *depressive equivalent* (physical complaints reflecting the clinical manifestations of depression) should not be overlooked. On rare occasions hypochondriasis may also reflect a prepsychotic condition in which the patient's ability to test reality is significantly impaired. Most hypochondriacs, however, while afraid of having a disease, do not have the bizarre ideation characteristic of the psychotic patient.

Hypochondriac patients share several basic characteristics. They are insecure and their self-concept is vulnerable; they feel incomplete and their identity often is overly dependent on others; they feel internal conflict about their need to depend on others. Encouragement and support, firm and concrete guidelines for progressive physical exercise, and regularly scheduled medical checkups appear to be very therapeutic for them.

Organic Problems

Impaired cognitive functioning is present in a small but not necessarily insignificant proportion of patients with coronary disease.[54-56] For patients who undergo bypass surgery, cognitive changes appear to be even more common. *Pump time,* that is, time on the cardiopulmonary bypass pump, has been suggested as one mechanism by which patients sustain impairment of cognitive functioning. Patients with preexisting organic impairment may be especially vulnerable; surgical survivors may have exhibited less dysfunction prior to surgery than those who died after surgery. Typical symptoms that patients report are memory loss, decline in intellectual functioning, or occasional aphasic signs (such as difficulty remembering a name, decreased fine-motor control, or problems performing routine arithmetic tasks). Occasionally patients may display a labile mood, apathy, or psychomotor retardation. These latter symptoms may not reflect organic impairment but rather an underlying depression that may require careful evaluation.

In addition to the effects that the disease process may have on cognitive functions, advancing age contributes to a general decline in mental abilities. Aging is associated with a decline in cognitive functioning, and cardiac disease is most common in the latter half of the life cycle. Research has suggested that "crystallized" abilities, such as a person's vocabulary or fund of information, may remain intact, whereas "fluid" abilities, such as problem-solving or verbal reasoning skills may deteriorate more quickly as a result of the combined effects of aging and organic damage.

Administration of neuropsychologic tests such as the Halstead-Reitan Neuropsychological Battery can be used to evaluate precisely the presence and extent of organic impairment. These procedures include a variety of behavioral tasks involving assessment of memory, reasoning and conceptual abilities, and psychomotor performance. Impaired functioning can often be inferred on the basis of patterns of scores or by the departure of scores from normative data. A comprehensive review of psychologic strategies for evaluating coronary patients is presented elsewhere.[57]

Postoperative psychosis is a related disorder that can be dramatic in its clinical manifestations. Estimates of the prevalence of delirium in postcardiotomy and coronary bypass patients range from 0.1% to as high as 30% to 40%, with the typical rate for any given hospital setting probably somewhere in between. The characteristic symptoms of psychosis include perceptual distortions, visual and auditory hallucinations, delusions, and disorientation. Somatic concomitants of anxiety are also common, including hyperventilation, elevated heart rate and blood pressure, and sweating. Although the etiology of the psychosis is not known, current research suggests that organic factors, of which cerebral ischemia is the most likely, may be important. Patients whose psychologic defenses, especially those of repression and denial, have deteriorated may be more likely to experience delirium than patients whose defenses remain effective.

Delirium is typically treated with the use of major tranquilizers such as chlorpromazine hydrochloride (Thorazine), chlordiazepoxide hydrochloride (Librium), or haloperidol (Haldol). Moreover, it has been suggested that a supportive environment in which patients are encouraged to talk about their fears and anxieties may reduce the frequency of postoperative psychosis and facilitate more rapid recovery.

Emotional Problems

As previously described, psychologic and behavioral factors affect the course of cardiac rehabilitation. Although available data are somewhat variable from one study to another, most studies report that the majority of patients experience anxiety and depression; yet there is also agreement that the extent of emotional distress declines substantially over the course of 1 to 2 years after the infarction. For an excellent review of the subject area, the reader is referred to an article by Doehrman.[44]

Depression is a common complaint that is often characterized by sadness, crying spells, sleep disturbance (such as early morning awakening), excessive fatigue and weakness, and low energy. Anxiety is also fairly common, although the defense mechanisms of repression, denial, and isolation of affect often protect the patient from consciously experiencing the subjective discomfort associated with anxiety. Most patients do not suffer from significant and debilitating anxiety a year after myocardial infarction. For patients whose symptoms persist, however, anxiolytic or antidepressant medication (such as doxepin hydrochloride [Sinequan] or Xanax) is often helpful in reducing symptoms.

CAD may evoke feelings of vulnerability and worthlessness. The patient may become dependent or unconsciously allow himself or herself to become passive as a result of the socially acceptable role as patient. Encouraging the patient to talk about feelings and to become more physically active are important aids to treatment. The importance of exercise therapy is now widely recognized and is discussed in Chapter 14.

Problems Continuing from Earlier Years

Most patients who develop CAD are not psychiatric patients. However patients with significant emotional problems also develop heart disease. Problems that have developed over the course of a lifetime rarely improve after a heart attack. People who are prone to depression can be extremely affected by a sudden decline in their health. Similarly, people who tend to act impulsively or who show an inability to tolerate life's frustrations may exhibit a continuation of past behaviors: they may continue to overeat, overdrink, or overindulge themselves in ways that have a negative effect on their health and on those around them.

In brief, those individuals who have problems before their illness are likely to have problems after their illness. Marriages are seldom improved when one member becomes sick, and often CAD may cause additional problems for couples and families.

Developmental Issues and Existential Concerns

Erik Erikson[58] has identified eight stages of human development. Each stage has its own salient issues that require resolution. The last stage, *ego integrity,* implies an acceptance of life as it has turned out and death as the inevitable outcome of human life. He notes, "Wisdom then is detached concern with life itself in the face of death itself. It maintains and conveys the integrity of experience in spite of the decline in bodily and mental functions."[59]

Familial, cultural, and spiritual values become more important as one grows older, and illness often brings about a reevaluation of what is meaningful, not just in terms of what happens after death but what happens before death. A myocardial infarction may make a patient seek to avoid feelings of helplessness and hopelessness and may stimulate a renewed interest in people. It is not uncommon for patients to review their lives and to reflect on opportunities chosen and neglected. Some patients adopt a new philosophy about life and shift from material to more spiritual interests.

Patients with CHD are often in their middle years and must face developmental issues common to middle age. The most important issues facing middle-aged and older adults is how to cope with loss; for the myocardial infarction patient, the most obvious loss is that of physical prowess and functional abilities. This may threaten the individual's self-concept and may lead to forced dependence on others.

As one gets older, the experience of illness becomes more frequent, and it is more difficult to compensate for lost friends. Patients may feel lonely, isolated, deserted, and experience the loss of shared memories. Retirement also can be traumatic. It means an end of a phase of life, and with loss of work is often a loss of a sense of autonomy and power. Loss of relationships with co-workers, of social status, and of income are also experienced.

Talking about life requires someone who is willing to listen. Although professional help is often useful, a patient should also be encouraged to talk with spouse, relatives, and friends.

Treatment Considerations

Most published research on the psychologic treatment of myocardial infarction patients has been about treatment in the form of group psychotherapy. To date, results have been mixed. Several studies have demonstrated improved psychologic well-being in the treatment group compared to a no-treatment control group, and at least one study[60] has reported a significantly lower mortality in the treated group. However, it has been noted that group treatment of cardiac patients does not follow a process similar to group treatment of psychiatric patients (see recent reviews by Blanchard and Miller[61] and Gil and Blumenthal[62]). Educational and supportive groups appear to be preferable to self-exploratory or psychoanalytically oriented groups.

Several recent studies have employed behavioral techniques, including progressive muscle relaxation training and stress management techniques. The main behavioral treatments for patients with coronary disease appear to be those that attempt to remove the source of stress or modify the patients' perceptions and reactions to stress. *Progressive muscle relaxation,* in which the patient is taught to tense and relax muscles, is an example of a technique counteracting the effects of a stressful environment. Other behavioral techniques for treating stress reactions include *cognitive restructuring,* in which the patient is taught to reinterpret events to make them less stressful, and *systematic desensitization,* in which the patient learns to relax to counteract the emotional or physical symptoms during exposure to situations that evoke symptoms. *Biofeedback,* a treatment designed to teach patients control of autonomic nervous system functions, has been used successfully to treat a variety of cardiovascular disorders including cardiac arrhythmias, hypertension, and peripheral vascular disease. However the effectiveness of behavioral techniques in actually prolonging the life of patients with coronary disease has not been established. *Type A modification* has also gained widespread recognition, and recent data have suggested that reductions in type A behavior may be associated with decreased risk of recurrent CAD events.[63]

Recovery from heart attack is a complex process. Social, psychologic, and medical factors are all important and interrelated. Successful treatment is most likely to be achieved by the collaborative efforts of nurses, physicians, psychologists, physical therapists, and vocational counselors. The key ingredient is an interest in and commitment to victims of a disease with important psychosocial as well as physical consequences.

REFERENCES

1. Epstein, F.: The epidemiology of coronary heart disease: a review, J. Chronic Dis. 18:735, 1965.
2. Keys, A.: The individual risk of coronary heart disease, Ann. NY Acad. Sci. 134:1064, 1966.
3. Simborg, D.W.: The status of risk factors and coronary heart disease, J. Chronic Dis. 22:515, 1970.
4. Blumenthal, J.A., and others: Cardiac rehabilitation: a new frontier for behavioral medicine, J. Cardiac Rehab. 3:637, 1983.
5. Engel, G.L.: The need for a new medical model: a challenge for biomedicine, Science 196:129, 1977.
6. Parsons, T.: The social system, New York, 1951, The Free Press.
7. Mechanic, D.: Social psychologic factors affecting the presentation of bodily complaints, N. Engl. J. Med. 286:1132, 1972.
8. Kobler, J.: The reluctant surgeon: a biography of John Hunter, New York, 1960, Doubleday & Co., Inc.
9. Kligfield, P., and Hunter, J.: Angina pectoris and medical education, Am. J. Cardiol. 45:367, 1980.
10. Osler, W.: Lectures on angina pectoris and allied states, New York, 1897, D. Appleton.
11. Jenkins, C.D.: Psychologic and social precursors of coronary disease, N. Engl. J. Med. 284:244, 307, 1971.
12. Jenkins, C.D.: Recent evidence supporting psychologic and social risk factors for coronary disease, N. Engl. J. Med. 294:987, 1033, 1976.
13. Friedman, M., and Rosenman, R.H.: Association of specific overt behavior pattern with blood and cardiovascular findings, JAMA 169:1286, 1959.
14. Rosenman, R.H.: The interview method of assessment of the coronary-prone behavior pattern. In Dembroski, T.M., and others, editors: Coronary-prone behavior, New York, 1978, Springer-Verlag New York, Inc.
15. Rosenman, R.H., and others: A predictive study of coronary heart disease: the Western Collaborative Group Study, JAMA 189:15, 1964.
16. Jenkins, C.D., Rosenman, R.H., and Zyzanski, S.J.: Prediction of clinical coronary heart disease by a test for the coronary-prone behavior pattern, N. Engl. J. Med. 290:1271, 1974.
17. Rosenman, R.H., and others: Coronary heart disease in the Western Collaborative Group Study: final follow-up experience of 8½ years, JAMA 233:872, 1975.
18. The Review Panel on Coronary Prone Behavior and Coronary Heart Disease: A critical review, Circulation 63:1199, 1981.
19. Williams, R.B., and others: Type A behavior, hostility, and atherosclerosis, Psychosom. Med. 42:539, 1982.
20. Dembroski, T.M., and others: Components of Type A, hostility, and anger: relationship to angiographic findings, Psychosom. Med. 47:219, 1985.
21. Shekelle, R.B., and others: Hostility, risk of coronary heart disease, and mortality, Psychosom. Med. 45:109, 1983.
22. Barefoot, J.C., Dahlstrom, G., and Williams, R.B.: Hostility, CHD incidence, and total mortality: a 25-year follow-up of 255 physicians, Psychosom. Med. 45:59, 1983.
23. Ross, R., and Glomset, J.A.: The pathogenesis of atherosclerosis, N. Engl. J. Med. 295:396, 1976.
24. Friedman, M., and others: Excretion of catecholamines, 17-ketosteroids, 17-hydroxycorticoids, and 5-hydroxindole in men exhibiting a particular behavior pattern (A) associated with high incidence of clinical coronary heart disease, J. Clin. Invest. 39:758, 1960.
25. Friedman, M., and others: Coronary-prone individuals (Type A behavior pattern) growth hormone responses, JAMA 217:929, 1971.
26. Glass, D.C., and others: Effects of harassment and competition upon cardiovascular and plasma catecholamine responses in Type A and B individuals, Psychophysiology 17:453, 1980.
27. Friedman, M., Rosenman, R.H., and Carroll, V.: Changes in the serum cholesterol and blood-clotting time in men subjected to cyclic variation of occupational stress, Circulation 17:825, 1958.
28. Rosenman, R.H., and Friedman, M.: Association of specific behavior pattern in women with blood and cardiovascular findings, Circulation 24:1173, 1961.
29. Friedman, M., and Rosenman, R.H.: Association of specific overt behavior pattern with blood and cardiovascular findings, JAMA 169:1286, 1959.
30. Friedman, M., and Rosenman, R.H.: Serum lipids and conjunctival circulation after fat ingestion in men exhibiting type A behavior pattern, Circulation 29:874, 1964.
31. Friedman, M., Byers, S.O., and Rosenman, R.H.: Effects of saturated fats upon lipidemia and conjunctival circulation, JAMA 193:882, 1965.
32. Friedman, M., Byers, S.O., and Rosenman, R.H.: Plasma ACTH and cortical concentration of coronary-prone subjects, Proc. Sci. Exp. Biol. Med. 140:681, 1972.
33. Friedman, M., and others: Coronary-prone individuals (Type A behavior pattern): some biochemical characteristics, JAMA 212:1030, 1970.
34. Zumoff, B., and others: Elevated daytime urinary excretion of testosterone glucuronide in men with the type A behavior pattern, Psychosom. Med. 46:223, 1984.
35. Klaiber, E.L., and others: Serum-estrogen levels in men with acute myocardial infarction, Am. J. Med. 73:872, 1982.
36. Luria, M.H., and others: Relationship between sex hormones, myocardial infarction, and occlusive coronary disease, Arch. Int. Med. 142:42, 1982.
37. Kalbak, K.: Incidence of atherosclerosis in patients with rheumatoid arthritis receiving long-term corticosteroid therapy, Ann. Rheuma. Dis. 31:196, 1972.
38. Troxler, R.G., and others: The association of elevated plasma cortisol and early atherosclerosis as demonstrated by coronary angiography, Atherosclerosis 26:151, 1977.
39. Dembroski, T.M., MacDougall, J.M., and Lushene, R.: Interpersonal interaction and cardiovascular responses in type A subjects and coronary patients, J. Human Stress 5:28, 1979.
40. Gentry, W.D., and Haney, T.: Emotional and behavioral reaction to acute myocardial infarction, Heart Lung 4:738, 1975.
41. Hackett, T.P., and Cassem, N.H.: Factors contributing to delay in responding to the signs and symptoms of acute myocardial infarction, Am. J. Cardiol. 24:651, 1969.
42. Cassem, N.H., and Hackett, T.P.: Psychiatric consultation in a coronary care unit, Ann. Intern. Med. 75:9, 1971.
43. Cassem, N.H., Nelson, K., and Rich, R.R.: The nurse in the coronary care unit. In Gentry, W.D., and Williams, R.B., editors: Psychological aspects of myocardial infarction and coronary care, ed. 2, St. Louis, 1979, The C.V. Mosby Co.
44. Doehrman, S.R.: Psychosocial aspects of recovery from coronary heart disease: a review, Soc. Sci. Med. 11:199, 1970.
45. Bruhn, J.G., and others: Patients' reaction to death in a coronary care unit, J. Psychosom. Res. 14:65, 1970.
46. Wishnie, H.A., Hackett, T.P., and Cassem, N.H.: Psychological hazards of convalescence following myocardial infarction, JAMA 215:1292, 1971.
47. Cassem, N.H., and Hackett, T.P.: Psychological rehabilitation of myocardial infarction patients in the acute phase, Heart Lung 2:382, 1973.
48. Weisman, A.D., and Hackett, T.P.: Predilection to death: death and dying as a psychiatric pattern, Psychosom. Med. 23:232, 1961.
49. Glasser, B.G., and Strauss, A.L.: Time for dying, Chicago, 1967, Aldine Publishing Co.
50. Kastenbaum, R.: Dying and death: a life span approach. In Birren,

J.E., and Shaie, K.W., editors: The handbook of the psychology of aging, New York, 1986, Van Nostrand Reinhold Co., Inc.

51. Kübler-Ross, E.: On death and dying, New York, 1969, Macmillan Publishing Co., Inc.

52. Kastenbaum, R., and Costa, P.T.: Psychological perspectives on death. In Rosenwage, M.R., and Porter, L.W., editors: Annual review of psychology, Palo Alto, CA, 1977, Stanford University Press.

53. Schwartz, A.M., and Karasu, T.B.: Psychotherapy with dying patients, Am. J. Psychother. **31**:19, 1977.

54. Gilberstadt, H., and Sako, Y.: Intellectual and personality changes following open-heart surgery, Arch. Gen. Psychiatry **16**:210, 1967.

55. Kornfeld, D.S., Zimberg, S., and Malm, J.R.: Psychiatric complication of open-heart surgery, N. Engl. J. Med. **273**:287, 1965.

56. Heller, S.S., and others: Psychiatric complications of open-heart surgery: a reexamination, N. Engl. J. Med. **283**:1015, 1970.

57. Blumenthal, J.A.: Assessment of patients with coronary heart disease. In Keefe, F.J., and Blumenthal, J.A., editors: Assessment strategies in behavioral medicine, New York, 1982, Grune & Stratton, Inc.

58. Erikson, E.H.: Identity and the life cycle: psychological issues, Monograph 1, New York, 1959, International Universities Press, Inc.

59. Erikson, E.H.: Insight and responsibility: letters on the ethical implications of psychoanalytic insight, New York, 1964, W.W. Norton & Co., Inc.

60. Ibrahim, M.A., and others: Management after myocardial infarction: a controlled trial of the effects of group psychotherapy, Int. J. Psychiatry Med. **5**:253, 1974.

61. Blanchard, E.B., and Miller, S.T.: Psychological treatment of cardiovascular disease, Arch. Gen. Psychiatry **34**:1402, 1977.

62. Gil, K., and Blumenthal, J.A.: Behavior modification in the primary and secondary prevention of coronary heart disease, Cardiol. Pract. **1**:274, 1985.

63. Friedman, M., and others: Alteration of type A behavior and reduction in cardiac recurrences in postmyocardial infarction patients, Am. Heart J. **108**:237, 1984.

CHAPTER 14

Rehabilitation after Myocardial Infarction

Elizabeth Wagner
R. Sanders Williams

BASIC PRINCIPLES AND GOALS OF REHABILITATION PROCESS

There are two basic goals in approaching the patient who has experienced a myocardial infarction: (1) to eliminate any physical or psychologic barriers that impede the patient's resumption of a satisfying and productive life; and (2) to minimize the patient's risk for subsequent adverse cardiovascular events such as sudden cardiac death, progressive angina pectoris, and recurrent myocardial infarction. Although these goals have served as a standard for medical management of the postinfarction patient for half a century, physicians and nurses have recently made some radical changes in the management of patients experiencing a heart attack.

One dramatic change has been the increasingly widespread application of therapies designed to restore coronary blood flow during the early hours of myocardial infarction, thereby limiting the ultimate amount of myocardium that becomes infarcted. This approach has added a new dimension to coronary care, which previously was limited to therapies designed to treat the complications of an infarct but not the underlying process.

The rationale for such acute intervention comes from solid evidence that acute coronary thrombosis occurring at the site of a preexisting atherosclerotic plaque is usually the immediate event that precipitates myocardial infarction,[1] and that, if blood flow can be restored within a certain critical period of time (1 to 6 hours), myocardium that otherwise would become infarcted can be saved from infarction[2] (often termed *salvaged*). Since the mass of infarcted myocardium relative to the remaining normal myocardium has a major influence on subsequent survival rates, both in terms of early (hospital) survival and in terms of survival in the months and years following an infarct,[3] this strategy has a sound physiologic basis.

Three general types of interventions have been used for this purpose: administration of thrombolytic drugs such as streptokinase and tissue plasminogen activator (TPA), mechanical dilatation of occluded or stenotic coronary vessels by percutaneous transluminal coronary angioplasty (PTCA), and acute surgical coronary artery bypass grafting (CABG).

It is beyond the scope of this chapter to discuss these new forms of therapy in detail (see Chapters 5 and 15). In addition, although each strategy has been demonstrated to restore blood flow to previously occluded coronary arteries, additional research is needed to determine the optimal manner in which these techniques should be employed. However the application of these management strategies has already had a major impact on both in-hospital and postdischarge management of myocardial infarction patients in many centers.

A second development that has changed the practice of cardiac rehabilitation has been the recognition that the majority of patients who are likely to suffer sudden death or reinfarction in the first year after discharge following an initial event can be identified on the basis of clinical variables and exercise testing performed before discharge.[4] Even asymptomatic patients with physical findings of ventricular dysfunction (S3 gallop), electrocardiographic evidence for extensive infarction (Q waves in multiple anatomic regions of the heart), abnormal exercise tests (low exercise capacity, exertional hypotension, ST segment changes at low workloads or heart rates), abnormal left ventricular function detected by echocardiography or by radionuclide studies, or large areas of residual myocardium supplied by severely stenosed arteries (major perfusion defects on thallium studies or multivessel disease shown by coronary arteriography) have a high risk for death or reinfarction after discharge and should be managed differently than patients without such findings. Formerly, patients that can now be identified as low risk would have been managed in an identical manner to other patients that can now be identified as high risk. Today these categories of patients are generally managed in different ways, as will be discussed in more detail in a subsequent section.

A third development in cardiac rehabilitation, and one that antedates the two factors described above, has been a trend over two decades toward increasingly faster schedules of hospital discharge, resumption of physical activity, and return to work for most patients recovering from myocardial infarction.

For at least 30 years, from the 1930s until the late 1960s, physicians placed tremendous restrictions on the activities of their postinfarction patients. Standard medical practice recommended a month or more of hospitalization after an infarction, much of which was spent on complete bed rest. After discharge even moderate physical exercise, sexual activity, and return to full employment were often prohibited for periods up to a year or, in some cases, indefinitely. These recommendations were based on concerns that even routine activities constituted undue stress on a damaged heart and exposed the patient to excessive risk of further life-threatening cardiac events. More often than not, these restrictions were placed arbitrarily, without reference to the results of functional testing or other pertinent clinical variables in individual patients.

In the 1980s sudden arrhythmic death and recurrent infarction still remain serious risks to individuals who have experienced an initial infarction. However the restrictions formerly placed on all patients recovering from a myocardial infarction are currently viewed as generally excessive; for most individuals, a far more aggressive approach is not only safe but more likely to facilitate the patient's return to an active and productive mode of living.

Many major medical centers, as well as an increasing number of community hospitals, have instituted formal programs of cardiac rehabilitation for their patients surviving myocardial infarction.[5] To address the two major clinical goals stated previously, most cardiac rehabilitation programs have emphasized three basic principles: (1) early and repeated functional testing of the patient (generally, graded treadmill exercise tests) to provide a rational basis for recommending or proscribing specific activities in the recovery period and to help identify patients who are in need of drug treatment or surgical treatment of complicating features such as arrhythmias or angina pectoris; (2) individually prescribed, graduated programs of exercise training to augment functional work capacity; and (3) a rehabilitation team approach involving health professionals skilled at psychologic, dietary, and vocational evaluation and counseling. The remainder of this chapter focuses on the specifics of cardiac rehabilitation programs organized around these three principles.

SEQUENTIAL STEPS IN CARDIAC REHABILITATION

It is important that the rehabilitation of the patient who has suffered a myocardial infarction be viewed as a continuous and logical process that begins in the Coronary Care Unit (CCU) and extends to a lifetime program of prudent activity and risk-factor control. The potential efficacy of the rehabilitation process is compromised when rehabilitation efforts are delayed until weeks or months after the patient has left the hospital.

To provide a convenient framework for discussion, the management of the postinfarction patient can be divided into four phases (Fig. 14-1): (1) inpatient management in the CCU and hospital ward, (2) the transition period in the 3 to 6 weeks following hospital discharge, (3) the later

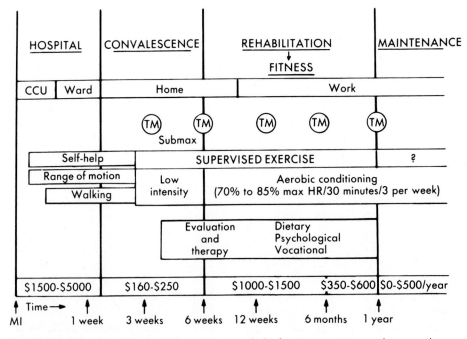

FIG. 14-1. Rehabilitation following myocardial infarction: an integrated approach.

rehabilitation period commencing approximately 6 weeks from the date of the infarction, and (4) the maintenance phase, wherein the subject seeks to maintain the highest possible level of the functional capacity and risk-factor control that has been achievable during the active rehabilitation phase. It should be emphasized, however, that this identification of "phases" or "steps" is somewhat arbitrary; future research may dictate changes in the length of time subjects spend in each phase or in the activities that are deemed safe and effective in each time period. Likewise, the major emphasis should be placed on the continuity of care as the patient passes through the initial weeks and months of recovery rather than on specific features of each rehabilitation phase.

Phase I—Inpatient Management

Once the pain associated with acute infarction has been relieved and the patient has been stabilized and is free from life-threatening complications, the rehabilitation process should begin. For patients with no complications, the use of bedside toilet facilities or short walks to a private bathroom, as well as other self-care activities such as shaving, dressing, and bathing, are appropriate even within the first 24 to 48 hours. Excessive dependence on the CCU staff for routine self-care activities should be strongly discouraged. Range of motion exercise or chair-sitting minimizes the deleterious effects of bed rest[6] and forestalls the excessive and unwarranted fear of even minimal physical activity that persists in many patients for extended periods following their infarction. Early activity also minimizes the risk of venous thrombosis and pulmonary embolus.[7]

Gradually increasing periods of walking about the room or in the ward corridor can be started by the third hospital day for most patients. It is obvious that activity schedules must be modified in patients experiencing ventricular or atrial arrhythmias, postinfarction angina, or congestive heart failure. The walking performed by postinfarction patients in the inpatient phase should in no way be designed to constitute aerobic training. Its purpose is to minimize physical deconditioning, prevent venous thrombosis, prepare the patient for predischarge functional testing, and foster a positive psychologic outlook. Walking sessions should be short (5 to 20 minutes) and of low intensity (heart rates elevated no more than 20 bpm above resting level in most subjects). Multiple short walks during the day are probably preferable to a single longer walk.

Whenever possible the patient should be introduced during the hospital stay to the physicians and/or nurses who will be managing the postdischarge rehabilitation. This establishes continuity for postinfarction management and guards against the patient receiving conflicting instructions about postdischarge activities. Educational efforts should routinely include specific instructions about med-

ications and their potential side effects, amount of physical activity after discharge, sexual counseling, smoking cessation, and dietary modification. It is important to involve the spouse or other family members in these educational sessions.

In addition to progressive physical activity and patient education, a major goal of the inpatient rehabilitation process should be risk stratification,[4] based routinely on the results of the physical examination, ECG, predischarge exercise test, and in some cases other studies such as 24-hour electrocardiographic monitoring, radionuclide ventriculography, isotope perfusion studies, echocardiography, or cardiac catheterization with coronary arteriography.

Emphasis on characterizing risk status for postinfarction patients *before* hospital discharge is based on evidence that the highest rate of fatal arrhythmias or reinfarctions occurs in the first few weeks and months after the initial event.[4] Failure to identify high-risk patients before discharge may deny such patients potentially life-saving therapies or may result in inappropriate decisions concerning posthospital rehabilitation. Failure to properly identify low-risk patients may result in unnecessary restrictions on activity or delayed return to work.

Certain complications in patients occurring in the first 24 hours after myocardial infarction, such as ventricular fibrillation or other transient arrhythmias, do not necessitate special management in subsequent rehabilitation that is different from that for uncomplicated patients. However other complications, particularly congestive heart failure or postinfarction angina, require that physical activity be advanced more slowly and that advice concerning postdischarge activities be modified accordingly.

Phase II—Immediate Postdischarge Period

The first few weeks after hospital discharge are a critical period for the rehabilitation process. Not only is this the period of highest mortality rates, but patients are extremely vulnerable to anxiety over the safety of routine activities, morbidity in outlook toward the future, and depression. The rehabilitation process should address the special requirements of this stage by:

1. Monitoring patients carefully for symptoms or physical signs of progressive angina, arrhythmias, or ventricular dysfunction
2. Allaying irrational fears and fostering a positive psychologic outlook
3. Facilitating return to work and leisure activities in a manner appropriate to the individual clinical situation of each patient
4. Extending the educational efforts that were begun in the hospital

It is essential that rehabilitation efforts be initiated immediately following hospital discharge and that patients not be denied frequent contact with the health personnel managing their rehabilitation during this vulnerable period. The previous policy of enrolling patients in formal rehabilitation programs only after 6 weeks of home convalescence has now been replaced by a much more aggressive approach during this early stage of rehabilitation.

Accordingly, enrolling patients in supervised exercise classes immediately after hospital discharge seems preferable for a number of reasons. Close contact with the patient is maintained by the rehabilitation team, which allows prompt identification of complicating medical events, facilitates proper interpretation of new symptoms, and provides reassurance to patients and their families. Specific attention should be given to the adjustment of spouses in this difficult period. Getting the patient out of the home and into a group setting reinforces a positive outlook toward the eventual resumption of full activities and allows for close monitoring of daily exercise prescriptions. In terms of educational efforts, most patients are given extensive instructions about home activities before hospital discharge; however their receptivity for understanding detailed activity schedules during their hospitalization is often low unless instructions can be reinforced frequently after the patient returns home. Office visits to the physician often are not sufficient to reinforce the educational efforts provided in the hospital.

In addition to the surveillance and educational goals described above, enrolling patients in supervised exercise classes during the first 3 to 4 weeks after hospital discharge has essentially the same rationale as that for exercise prescribed during the inpatient phase: limiting the deleterious effects of physical deconditioning and maintaining a psychologic climate favorable for a return to normal activities. In contrast to physical training regimens described in the section entitled "Exercise prescriptions," medically supervised exercise in the immediate postdischarge period usually is prescribed at lower intensities, with no attempt to have patients exercise in an aerobic training range. Additionally, extremely close medical supervision of patients during exercise is mandatory.

Phase III—Later Cardiac Rehabilitation: Aerobic Training and Return to Work

The specific features of cardiac rehabilitation programs serving patients from 3 weeks to 1 year after infarction are detailed in the following sections. The goals of phase III cardiac rehabilitation build on and extend the more limited goals of phases I and II. Patients need a realistic reassessment of the limitations, if any, that are imposed on them by cardiac disease and a specific plan of action to reduce these limitations as much as possible. The specific goals of treatment continue to be optimizing drug therapy, identifying patients whose clinical outlook is likely to be improved by angioplasty or by surgical intervention, limiting depression or excessive anxiety in patients in whom such psychologic features impede functioning in vocational or leisure activities, and minimizing risk factors for recurrent catastrophic cardiac events.

The central focus of most cardiac rehabilitation programs is medically supervised aerobic exercise in a group setting. The psychologic benefits of this type of program have already been discussed. Additional physiologic benefits offered by aerobic conditioning in postinfarction patients are considerable and are well established by quantitative data from several centers.[8,9] Functional work capacity is enhanced, and favorable changes may occur in several major coronary risk factors including hypertension, hyperlipidemia, obesity, diabetes mellitus and, perhaps, coronary-prone behavior patterns (type A). These results can be expected even in subjects with severely damaged ventricles or with postinfarction angina.[10]

Based on histologic studies of the time course of scar formation in infarcted myocardium, a convention of beginning vigorous aerobic training 6 weeks after a myocardial infarction has become the established norm. However there are no firm data that earlier institution of vigorous exercise has deleterious effects, and, in fact, it is probably reasonable to begin such training earlier in patients with normal ventricular function and without evidence of exertional ischemia in residual noninfarcted myocardium. For the patient who has undergone a submaximal exercise test at the 9th to 21st day, a symptom-limited exercise test is recommended 6 weeks after infarction to allow for further individualized exercise prescription and to base the decision about return either to work or to specific leisure activities on pertinent physiologic data. Psychologic, dietary, and vocational evaluations should also be completed at this time. If either specific interventions for psychologic problems or major changes in dietary habits are to be recommended, they are often easier to implement before the patient returns to full-time employment.

Symptom-limited exercise tests are recommended to monitor the responses to exercise training and to identify patients with worsening myocardial ischemia; such tests should be administered after 6 weeks of aerobic training, and then after 6 months and after 1 year. In addition to functional testing, monitoring of the patient's overall clinical condition by a medical history and a physical examination and the assessment of risk-factor control are recommended at these intervals.

Phase IV—Maintenance Programs

A number of criteria have been presented to define patients who have been fully rehabilitated from their myocardial infarctions. These include (1) return to gainful employment if this is medically feasible, (2) achievement of an acceptable level of functional capacity that allows the patient to perform desired work or leisure activity (9 METs* is a conventional threshold), (3) optimal control of all risk factors for recurrent cardiac events, (4) successful patient education regarding necessary restrictions on activity, proper medication usage, and continued risk-factor control. Some patients may meet these criteria within a few months after infarction, whereas other patients either have medical limitations that render rehabilitation to completely normal activity impossible, or they are unable to adhere to prescribed treatment regimens that would facilitate complete rehabilitation. Patients successfully achieving criteria for complete rehabilitation should be encouraged to continue a program of regular exercise and risk-factor control. Many patients are able to accomplish this on their own without further specialized assistance from the rehabilitation team. (A more detailed discussion of medically unsupervised exercise training for coronary patients is presented later.) On the other hand, many other patients either enjoy participation in a group cardiac fitness program or lack the self-motivation to maintain an unsupervised exercise training program. Many rehabilitation programs offer low-cost, minimally supervised, "maintenance" programs for these types of individuals.

PROGRESSIVE ACTIVITY PROGRAM

Physiologic rationale for exercise training in patients with coronary artery disease (CAD): Medically supervised physical training sessions constitute the central focus of most comprehensive management programs for myocardial infarction survivors. The rationale for this emphasis on exercise training is twofold: (1) such programs clearly lead to substantial augmentation of functional work capacity in coronary patients either in the presence or absence of angina pectoris or ventricular dysfunction, and (2) such programs induce favorable changes in psychologic function and in risk factors for recurrent cardiac events.[9,11]

A consideration of some basic concepts of exercise physiology illustrates the effects of physical conditioning on exercise performance. Fig. 14-2 depicts the heart rate response to treadmill exercise in a subject who had experienced a myocardial infarction that produced substantial ventricular damage. The resting left ventricular ejection fraction of 20% determined from radionuclide angiography is substantially reduced from the normal range of 50% or greater. Two months after this patient's infarction and

before beginning an aerobic conditioning program, his heart rate rose rapidly with only minimal exertion, and he was forced to discontinue exercise because of shortness of breath. After 2 months of exercise training he was again forced to discontinue exercise because of shortness of breath and had the same heart rate as on the pretraining study; but he was able to exercise to a peak workload comparable to that of most healthy males in his age group. Note also that his heart rate was considerably lower on the posttraining treadmill test than on his baseline test at any given level of work. Since heart rate is the major factor determining the oxygen requirements of the heart itself, the occurrence of this "training bradycardia" means that trained subjects can perform any task with lower myocardial oxygen costs and at reduced coronary blood flows. This effect of physical training can produce substantial, sometimes dramatic, changes in the level of activity coronary patients can perform before the onset of angina pectoris or fatigue.

In most normal subjects exercise training produces increased exercise capacity and training bradycardia both by increasing the maximal pumping capacity of the heart (peak cardiac output during exercise) and by increasing the ability of the exercising skeletal muscle to extract and use oxygen from the blood. Although similar effects occur in some cardiac patients, other patients achieve increases in exercise capacity without changes in maximal cardiac output.[8] The observation that the training effect in myocardial infarction patients may be predominantly caused by effects of exercise training on skeletal muscle rather than on the heart itself has encouraged investigators to use exercise training as a form of therapy for patients with severely damaged ventricles.[10] Clearly, even these subjects can increase their exercise capacity and develop training-induced sinus bradycardia.

The manner in which exercise training may improve the quality of life in infarction patients is illustrated in Fig. 14-3, A, which depicts the maximal work capacity in METs of 11 patients before and after 6 months of exercise training. The arrow to the right illustrates the approximate work capacity required for common activities such as light gardening or doubles tennis. Since most persons cannot sustain activities requiring greater than 85% of maximal work capacity for more than a few minutes, the majority of these subjects would have been unable to perform even these simple activities before the training program. However, following training most of these subjects could perform these types of activities without difficulty.

Fig. 14-3, B, shows the effects of physical training on exercise heart rate at a standard workload in the same subjects depicted in Fig. 14-3, A. Even those subjects who failed to augment their maximal work capacities developed training-induced sinus bradycardia.

---

*An understandable and useful method of measuring the energy cost of certain activities is through the use of the unit called the MET, or metabolic equivalent of the task. A MET is defined as the rate of energy expenditure requiring an oxygen consumption of 3.5 ml/minute/kg body weight. One MET is equal to the energy cost of a person sitting quietly on a chair. Five METs therefore means that an activity of this level requires five times the oxygen costs of sitting quietly in a chair.

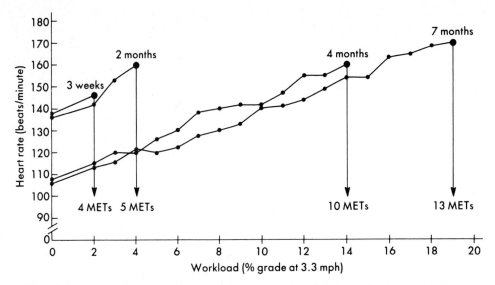

FIG. 14-2. Heart rate as a function of work load during serial treadmill exercise tests in a 43-year-old patient who suffered an extensive anterior myocardial infarction. Tests were performed at the stated intervals following his infarct. The exercise test performed 3 weeks after infarct was a submaximal test. Following 5 more weeks of low-level exercise *(2 months)*, a symptom-limited (dyspnea) test revealed no conditioning effect and a persistently low exercise capacity. The patient then participated in a carefully graduated aerobic training program. Subsequent treadmills at 4 months and 7 months after infarct demonstrate major cardiovascular conditioning effects: increased work capacity and bradycardia at submaximal workloads. He returned to full-time employment 6 months following his infarct. The vertical arrows point to the MET equivalent of his treadmill performance at each testing interval. The left ventricular ejection fraction is 20%.

In addition to these effects on work capacity, the "physical training effect" includes favorable changes in a number of medical problems that are prevalent in myocardial infarction patients. Physical training aids in the management of hypertension[12] and obesity[13] and improves glucose tolerance in subjects with diabetes mellitus.[14] According to most reports, it lowers plasma triglycerides and low-density lipoprotein cholesterol levels and increases levels of high-density lipoprotein cholesterol,[15] concentration of which has a strong inverse correlation with risk of cardiac events in large-scale population studies. Exercise training may also enhance the fibrinolytic activity of blood plasma,[16] perhaps reducing the risk of intravascular thrombus formation.

Despite evidence linking physical activity to reduced cardiac mortality in population studies,[17] it has not been demonstrated conclusively that exercise training and risk-factor control indeed reduce the incidence of further major cardiac events in patients who have experienced a previous myocardial infarction.[18] However, even in the absence of conclusive data regarding the effects of exercise training on longevity in infarction survivors, a persuasive case can be made for physical conditioning programs purely on the basis of well-documented improvements in exercise capacity and for the less quantifiable but widely substantiated

psychologic benefits of this type of intervention. It is perhaps pertinent to note that conclusive evidence for beneficial effects on patient survival is also lacking for two other widely-prescribed cardiac treatment modalities: antiarrhythmic drug therapy for ventricular arrhythmias and coronary artery bypass grafting for coronary occlusive disease not involving the left main vessel.

Exercise Prescriptions

To achieve cardiovascular fitness or conditioning in the cardiac patient, an exercise prescription geared to the needs and capabilities of the individual must be formulated.[19] In large measure, exercise prescription should be based on careful analysis of the graded exercise test. The duration of the test and the maximum heart rate attained by the patient, as well as blood pressure response and signs of ischemia, arrhythmias, and other problems must be evaluated before the prescription is formulated. The level of activity in the first few weeks of aerobic training should be kept low to prevent undue muscle soreness, to decrease orthopedic problems, and to allow a safe adaptation period with minimum risk. Another important feature is regular review (often weekly) of the exercise prescription, with changes recommended on the basis of observation of the

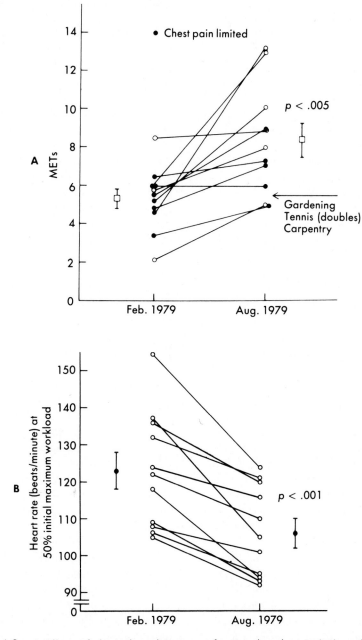

FIG. 14-3. A, Effects of physical conditioning on functional work capacity in patients following myocardial infarction. Each circle represents the results of symptom-limited treadmill testing before *(left)* and following *(right)* 6 months of physical conditioning in an individual patient. The squares depict mean values (±S.E.M.). The horizontal arrow demonstrates the approximate oxygen demands required for the indicated activities. Most subjects cannot perform sustained work requiring more than 85% of their maximal work capacity. B, Heart rates at a standard treadmill submaximal work load (50% of the initial maximum) before and following physical conditioning in the same subjects shown in A. It is important to note that all these subjects demonstrated training bradycardia (and therefore would be expected to perform routine activities with lower myocardial oxygen requirements), although several did not elevate their maximum work capacities.

subject during training sessions and analysis of the results of repeat exercise testing performed at the previously stated intervals in the activity program.

Exercise prescription for the cardiac patient has four main characteristics which need to be analyzed individually: type, intensity, duration, and frequency of physical activity.

Type of Activity. The exercises selected for physical conditioning in the cardiac patient should generally be repetitive, rhythmic, low-resistance contractions of the large muscle groups of the body. Activities that may be included in this group are brisk walking, jogging, stationary and regular cycling, stair climbing, swimming, and other selected exercises. Whichever activity is selected, it should be pleasurable to the patient and not produce prolonged fatigue or discomfort. Highly competitive activities are to be avoided by cardiac patients, except carefully selected, low-risk individuals.

Intensity of Activity. The work intensity of the cardiac patient during the exercise session must be determined by the most recent stress test. Studies in both normal subjects and coronary patients suggest that the previously described exercise training effects occur most readily if the intensity of the training stimulus is sufficient to increase oxygen consumption to 70% to 85% of maximum.[9] Since heart rate increases linearly with increases in oxygen consumption, simple measurements of heart rate during exercise constitute a readily available measure of the adequacy of the training stimulus. One can approximate 70% to 85% of maximum oxygen consumption by adding 70% to 85% of the increment between resting heart rate and maximum heart rate to the resting heart rate. For example, if the resting heart rate is 80 beats/minute and the peak exercise heart rate is 180 beats/minute, 70% of maximal oxygen consumption will occur at a heart rate of 150 beats/minute (70% of (180 − 80) + 80) and 85% of maximal oxygen consumption will occur at 165 beats/minute (85% of (180 − 80) + 80). A proper training range for a patient limited by angina at a heart rate of 130 beats/minute who is taking a β-adrenergic antagonist drug and who has a resting heart rate of 60 would, therefore, be 108 to 120. In practice patients should count their pulses for 10-second intervals and multiply by 6; the training ranges are therefore rounded off to the nearest multiple of 6.

To ensure against the occurrence of potentially dangerous myocardial ischemia during training sessions, exercise should be limited to heart rates of 10 to 15 beats/minute below the heart rates at which angina or other signs of myocardial hypoperfusion are evident during stress testing.

Previously sedentary patients should probably begin at a low level of work intensity, gradually increasing the intensity level over several weeks to the calculated training range. Signs of excessive fatigue, breathlessness, and other adverse symptoms must be watched for and carefully avoided. The use of the concept of the maximum safe heart rate limit and target heart rate zones during the conditioning activity is probably the safest way of calculating the work of the heart and thus the intensity of the exercise prescription.

Duration of Activity. Any activity chosen by cardiac patients should be begun slowly at a low intensity for several minutes. Following this warm-up phase of 5 to 10 minutes, a stimulus period of 20 to 40 minutes with the heart rate in the target zone has been shown to be effective in producing aerobic training effects in cardiac patients. Several minutes should also be allowed for cooling down at the end of the stimulus activity when a gradual return of the metabolic and circulatory systems to baseline activity occurs. The warm-up and cool-down periods have been shown to be most likely times for exercise-related ventricular fibrillation to occur and should therefore take place in close physical proximity to the medical staff and emergency equipment.

Frequency of Activity. An endurance activity must be continued on a regular basis to achieve the proper conditioning response. Usually three times per week is sufficient and may limit the risk of orthopedic injury. At lower levels of activity, or if a more rapid achievement of training effects is desired, a schedule of 5 days per week is preferable. Rapid achievement of training effects may be a motivational stimulus to continue regular activity in the cardiac rehabilitation program.

In creating an exercise prescription for use by the cardiac patient, individual preferences, goals, and personal safety must be taken into consideration. Getting patients involved in the planning phases may increase their adherence to and satisfaction with the experience.

Supervised Versus Unsupervised Exercise

It is unfortunate that in the United States formal cardiac rehabilitation programs are available only to a minority of patients. Furthermore, the availability of such programs is often dictated more by economic and geographic than by medical considerations. This is not the case in several other western nations such as Canada or West Germany.

The preferred setting for the conditioning or training of the cardiac patient is the supervised setting of the cardiac rehabilitation program. This setting allows for close observation and facilitates patient education and the initiation of the conditioning response in the individual. These effects in turn should produce a more favorable compliance rate. Although the risk of controlled exercise in myocardial infarction survivors[20] appears to be very small (less than one death per 100,000 patient-hours in supervised programs), serious problems such as ventricular fibrillation and myocardial infarction do occur. Over 75% of cardiac arrest victims in medically supervised exercise programs are successfully resuscitated, whereas such events are almost uniformly lethal when they occur outside of medical supervision.

A supervised program is not economically and logistically feasible for all cardiac patients. Williams and associates[21] have formulated the following guidelines to identify patients who may be at particularly high risk during unsupervised exercise:

1. Patients with low maximal functional capacity (<6 METs)
2. Those with severely depressed left ventricular function
3. Those with complex ventricular arrhythmias
4. Those with QT prolongation on the ECG
5. Those with exercise-induced hypotension
6. Those unable to perform effective self-monitoring of their exercise heart rate

These authors recommend that patients with coronary artery disease who lack these high-risk features may perform conditioning exercises in an unsupervised setting if they have demonstrated a clear understanding of the principles of safe physical conditioning. Patients should demonstrate knowledge of their maximum safe heart rate limit and the target heart rate zone prescribed for them at the most recent treadmill test; they should also be reliable observers of their own heart rates during exercise. In our experience over 50% of cardiac patients are good candidates for exercise programs in which the daily exercise sessions are not medically supervised. However, regardless of the issue of safety, many patients require the structure of a supervised exercise program to achieve and maintain physiologic training effects and are unlikely to adhere to an unsupervised program.

Somewhat paradoxically, the actual practice of cardiac rehabilitation in this country has emphasized the care of the patient without complications. In a major U.S. study of the effects of supervised exercise programs on subsequent mortality and reinfarction, high-risk patients were excluded.[22] A more rational use of resources would provide a short term (3 to 12 week) period of formal rehabilitation efforts directed at the relatively uncomplicated low-risk patient but would also support long-term rehabilitation efforts for high-risk or severely impaired but ambulatory patients.

Energy Requirements of Common Activities

Some cardiac rehabilitation programs allow participants to perform certain activities depending on the MET expenditure of the exercise (see footnote on p. 403) in relation to the patient's functional capacity. This is a rational method, but allowances should be made for the individual's

skill in sports, proper medication usage (especially proper use of sublingual nitroglycerin), and knowledge of the danger signs that merit immediate attention.

OTHER MEMBERS OF REHABILITATION TEAM

Physicians and nurses who manage patients recovering from myocardial infarction should be aware of the special contributions that other allied health professionals may make to the rehabilitation effort. Cardiac rehabilitation centers incorporate exercise physiologists, clinical nutritionists, clinical psychologists, and vocational specialists along with physicians and nurses on a rehabilitation team. By this approach, specialists from each of these areas assist in the evaluation of the patient and provide reports to the managing physician. Moreover, they often have specific roles in the educational aspects of the rehabilitation program. The high prevalence of coronary-prone lifestyles, of maladaptive behavioral responses to environmental stresses, and of acute or chronic emotional distress in coronary patients provides the main reason for including these types of allied health specialists in the rehabilitation process on a nearly routine basis.

Adherence to a prudent lifestyle sometimes requires changes in ingrained habits. Individual instruction and formal classes geared to understanding the principles of physical conditioning and the personal limits of each patient's performance are important educational elements in the cardiac rehabilitation program. Environmental influences affecting exercise, especially outdoor exercise, are components the patient needs to understand thoroughly. How to recognize limiting symptoms during physical activity must be thoroughly explained by staff members and understood by patients.

DIETARY EDUCATION

Several of the risk factors for CAD are amenable to dietary modification. Most noteworthy of these are lipid abnormalities, hypertension, obesity, and diabetes. Dietary education, therefore, should center around reducing the intake of saturated fats, cholesterol, and simple sugars; restriction of sodium ingestion; and limiting total caloric consumption to that required to maintain ideal body weight. Another goal of dietary therapy should be to reduce total plasma cholesterol to levels below 200 mg/dl or to reduce total cholesterol to a level not more than 4.1 times that of high-density lipoprotein cholesterol.

A skilled dietitian can contribute by analyzing each patient's dietary habits and making specific suggestions that allow the diet to remain palatable to the individual, affordable, nutritionally adequate, and yet capable of achieving the desired effects.

A dietary change of major importance for many cardiac

patients is restricting total calories to control obesity. In addition to the deleterious effects obesity may have on diabetes, hypertension, and lipoprotein levels, excessive body weight may greatly impair functional work capacity in subjects limited by angina pectoris or congestive heart failure.

The group setting of a supervised exercise program along with specialized dietary counseling can help an individual adjust to reduced caloric intake until the ideal body weight is achieved and maintained. Ideal body weight can be calculated from standard nomograms or from body density determinations—the goal is 16% to 19% body fat composition in adult men and 22% to 25% in adult women.[23] This information can be best ascertained by underwater weight determinations (if the facilities are available) or by use of skin calipers to estimate body fat composition. The reduction diet chosen for the patient must be reasonable and allow for increasing activities, such as regular exercise and return to work. A weight loss of 1 to 3 pounds per week without symptoms of ketosis can be expected for most subjects consuming 700 to 1000 calories daily. Family involvement is important, and emphasis on the prevention of cardiovascular disease for the entire family and the generalized use of a prudent diet—limited in sodium, saturated fats, and cholesterol and high in complex carbohydrates—should be stressed.

CIGARETTE SMOKING

Continued cigarette smoking is a major risk factor for secondary cardiac events[11] and thus cannot be overlooked in any multifactorial approach to this problem. The program for smoking cessation starts with instruction from the physician or nurse about the deleterious effects of smoking. Individual and group counseling, including the use of behavior modification techniques, may prove useful in many instances. By these methods up to 50% of subjects can permanently discontinue smoking[24] (see Chapter 3).

PSYCHOLOGIC ASPECTS OF CARDIAC REHABILITATION

Patients respond to a cardiac event with a large diversity of coping mechanisms. Some patients appear to deny the gravity of the situation, whereas others exaggerate the problem and may never return to routine activities despite minimal limitations on physiologic cardiac function. Situational depression is almost uniformly present to some degree. For an understanding of these varied responses and adaptations, a thorough psychologic evaluation when the patient initially enters a supervised cardiac rehabilitation program is useful (see Chapter 13). The medical evaluation conducted by physicians or nurses should specifically address psychologic issues, and psychologic test procedures and individual interview sessions with a psychologist can often contribute a great deal to patient management. Attention should usually be paid to the patient's reaction to environmental stresses, basic personality traits, present level of anxiety and depression, and other behavioral characteristics. Appropriate recommendations concerning stress management and behavioral modification may be made, and referral for psychiatric intervention or psychotropic medication may be advised.

SEXUAL ACTIVITY

A point of great concern to patients after a cardiac event is the resumption of sexual activity.[25] Although sudden death during sexual intercourse has been reported[26] and is greatly feared, the risk of sexual activity for cardiac patients with familiar sexual partners has probably been overemphasized. Most patients free from angina at heart rates up to 130 beats/minute during exercise testing can safely resume sexual activity soon after hospital discharge, but individual counseling with the physician is desirable after the patient's functional capacity has been evaluated. The patient should be encouraged to report any symptoms experienced during intercourse. It may be encouraging to the patient entering a cardiac rehabilitation program to know that exercise training or conditioning may enhance sexual performance,[27] especially if an increased angina threshold and reduced anxiety over other activities can be achieved. Adjustments in medications such as prophylactic nitroglycerin may also decrease symptoms during sexual activity. Impotence is common in male patients after myocardial infarction and may be exacerbated by drugs or depression. Since patients may be reluctant to initiate discussion about such problems, it is important that a member of the rehabilitation team make specific inquiries about this problem so that medication adjustments, more aggressive psychologic intervention, or specific sexual counseling can be employed appropriately.

RETURN TO WORK

Another area of great concern to infarction patients is when and if they should return to work. This decision, of course, should be made by the personal physician and the patient, with the assistance of a vocational counselor after the patient's functional capacity has been properly evaluated by treadmill or other tests.[1,4] Selected uncomplicated low-risk patients may return to work as early as 3 weeks following their infarction, although 6 weeks remains a more typical duration of convalescence. For reasons that may be unrelated to the severity of their cardiac disease (for example, secondary gain, financial renumeration) persons who remain out of work for more than 34 months are more likely to remain on permanent disability. The vocational counselor is usually able to offer valuable suggestions after collecting data about the patient's present job. In addition to the functional capacity of the patient and the demands of the job, other variables to consider are age, skill, emotional tension, and environmental factors. Vocational recommendations should also consider the specific nature of work activities requiring physical labor. The capacity of a subject to perform an occupation requiring work with the arms may not be directly assessable by treadmill exercise testing only. Also, since most cardiac rehabilitation programs achieve cardiovascular conditioning with motion involving the large muscles of the legs and hips, fitness of the arms and shoulders may not be improved. Individualized programs designed to increase the endurance of the upper body may need to be developed for these patients.

LONG-TERM PATIENT ADHERENCE TO REHABILITATION PROGRAMS

Despite the favorable physiologic adaptations that occur with exercise conditioning and despite the best efforts of the rehabilitation team, a sizable proportion of postinfarction patients fail to continue dietary and exercise habits that have been prescribed for them. Based on data from Duke University's Cardiac Rehabilitation Program, Blumenthal and associates[28] demonstrated that noncompliers could be distinguished from compliers by a certain set of physical and psychologic parameters obtained at the time of entry into the program. Compliers were those who attended 75% of the sessions over a 1-year period, whereas noncompliers were those who ceased attending the rehabilitation program during this period of time. Dropouts had greater cardiac disability with lower left ventricular ejection fraction as evaluated by radionuclide angiography. However, no other risk factors such as obesity, hypertension, or elevated serum lipids distinguished these noncompliers. The psychologic factors common to the individuals who dropped out of the program indicated that this group experienced more psychologic stress. These individuals were most concerned about their health, had higher scores on anxiety and depression, and were socially introverted. Their ego strength was lower, and testing indicated inadequate coping mechanisms. Efforts to identify strategies to increase compliance in patients with these characteristics are under way.

SUMMARY

The rehabilitation of the patient recovering from a myocardial infarction involves two major goals: (1) to eliminate any potentially reversible physical or psychologic barriers that impede resumption of a satisfying and productive life, and (2) to minimize risk for subsequent catastrophic cardiac events. Modern concepts of cardiac rehabilitation emphasize early functional testing to facilitate rational, individualized patient management; progressive exercise conditioning programs; intensive and repeated patient ed-ucation and counseling regarding psychologic, social, sexual, and vocational aspects of the recovery from myocardial infarction; and addressing modification of risk factors for subsequent adverse events.

For a fuller discussion regarding specific issues in cardiac rehabilitation than that provided in this chapter, the reader is referred to several recent textbooks and reviews.[5,9,29,30] Other publications designed for patient education are also available.[31-34]

REFERENCES

1. Roberts, W.C., and Muja, M.: The frequency and significance of coronary arterial thrombi and other observations in fatal myocardial infarction, Am. J. Med. **52**:425, 1972.
2. Markis, J.E., and others: Myocardial salvage after intracoronary thrombolysis with streptokinase in acute myocardial infarction, N. Engl. J. Med. **305**:777, 1981.
3. Sobel, B.E.: Infarct size, prognosis, and causal contiguity, Circulation **53**:1-146, 1976.
4. DeBusk, R.F., and others: Identification and treatment of low-risk patients after acute myocardial infarction and coronary-artery bypass graft surgery, N. Engl. J. Med. **314**:161, 1986.
5. Pollock, M.L., and others: Exercise in health and disease, Philadelphia, 1984, W.B. Saunders Co.
6. DeBusk, R.F., and others: Cardiovascular responses to dynamic and static effort soon after myocardial infarction, Circulation **58**:368, 1978.
7. Miller, R.R., and others: Prevention of lower extremity venous thrombosis by early mobilization, Ann. Intern. Med. **84**:700, 1976.
8. Williams, R.S., and others: Effects of physical conditioning upon left ventricular ejection fraction in subjects with coronary artery disease, Circulation **70**:69, 1984.
9. Wenger, N.K.: Exercise and the heart, Philadelphia, 1985, F.A. Davis Co.
10. Conn, E., and others: Physical conditioning in patients with severely depressed left ventricular function, Am. J. Cardiol. **49**:296, 1982.
11. Kaplan, N.M., and Stamler, J.: Prevention of coronary heart disease, Philadelphia, 1984, W.B. Saunders Co.
12. Black, H.R.: Nonpharmacologic therapy for hypertension, Am. J. Med. **66**:837, 1979.
13. Bjorntorp, P.: Exercise in the treatment of obesity, Clin. Endocrinol. Metab. **5**:431, 1976.
14. Pederson, O., and others: Increased insulin receptors after exercise in patients with insulin-dependent diabetes mellitus, N. Engl. J. Med. **302**:886, 1980.
15. Hartung, G.H., and others: Relation of diet to high-density lipoprotein cholesterol in middle-aged marathon runners, joggers, and inactive men, N. Engl. J. Med. **302**:357, 1980.
16. Williams, R.S., and others: Physical conditioning augments endothelial release of plasminogen activators in healthy adults, N. Engl. J. Med. **302**:987, 1980.
17. Paffenbarger, R.S., Jr., and others: Physical activity as an index of heart attack risk in college alumni, Am. J. Epidemiol. **108**:161, 1978.
18. May, G.S., and others: Secondary prevention after myocardial infarction, Prog. Cardiovasc. Dis. **24**:331, 1982.
19. American College of Sports Medicine: Guidelines for exercise testing and exercise prescription, Philadelphia, 1980, Lea & Febiger.
20. Haskell, W.K.: Cardiovascular complications during exercise training on cardiac patients, Circulation **57**:920, 1978.
21. Williams, R.S., and others: Guidelines for unsupervised exercise in patients with ischemic heart disease, J. Cardiol. Rehab. **1**:213, 1981.

22. The National Exercise and Heart Disease Project: Effects of a prescribed supervised exercise program on mortality and cardiovascular morbidity in patients after a myocardial infarction, Am. J. Cardiol. **48:**39, 1981.

23. Pollack, M., and others: Health and fitness through physical activity, New York, 1978, John Wiley & Sons, Inc.

24. Scott, R.R., and Lamparski, D.: Variables related to long-term smoking status following cardiac events, Addictive Behav. **10:**257, 1985.

25. McLane, M., and others: Psychosexual adjustment and counseling after myocardial infarction, Ann. Intern. Med. **92:**514, 1980.

26. Ueno, M.: The so-called coition death, Japanese J. Leg. Med. **17:**333, 1963.

27. Stein, R.A.: The effect of exercise training on heart rate during coitus in the post-myocardial infarction patient, Circulation **56:**738, 1977.

28. Blumenthal, J.A., and others: Determinants of exercise compliance in coronary rehabilitation: a prospective study, Psychosom. Med. **43:**93, 1981.

29. Oberman, A.: Key references: cardiac rehabilitation, Circulation **62:**909, 1980.

30. Kulbertus, H.E., and Wellens, H.J.J.: The first year after a myocardial infarction, Mount Kisco, NY, 1983, Futura Publishing Co., Inc.

31. Warren, J.V., and others: Surviving your heart attack, Garden City, NY, 1984, Doubleday and Co., Inc.

32. Heyden, S.: The heart book, New York, 1981, Delair Publishing Co., Inc.

33. Shipley, R.: Quit smart: a guide to freedom from cigarettes, Durham, NC, 1985, J.B. Press.

34. The American Heart Association Cookbook, New York, 1984, David McKay Co., Inc.

CHAPTER 15

Surgical Management and Angioplasty for Coronary Heart Disease

Elaine G. Martin
Susan J. Hasselman

When medical management can no longer control the pain and related sequelae of coronary artery disease, additional intervention may be necessary. This chapter will describe four such procedures: coronary angioplasty, bypass, transplantation, and the use of artificial hearts.

PERCUTANEOUS TRANSLUMINAL CORONARY ANGIOPLASTY

Percutaneous transluminal coronary angioplasty (PTCA) is a nonoperative procedure that uses a balloon catheter to increase the luminal diameter of stenotic coronary arteries and thereby increase blood flow distal to the stenosis. Improvement in coronary blood flow following PTCA is associated with decreased symptoms and increased exercise tolerance in patients with angina pectoris.[1] PTCA may also prevent reocclusion following thrombolytic therapy for acute myocardial infarction (MI). Consequently, PTCA has gained wide acceptance as an effective therapy for selected patients with symptomatic coronary artery disease.

Dotter and Judkins first used a percutaneously introduced catheter in 1964 to dilate peripheral atherosclerotic lesions.[2] In 1977 Gruentzig applied percutaneous transluminal angioplasty to a highly selected subgroup of patients with stable angina and a discrete proximal, noncalcific stenosis of a single coronary artery.[3] Technical advancements in percutaneous catheters, guidewires, and balloons have expanded the range of indications for PTCA; many lesions once thought contraindicated are now safely and successfully dilated. In 1984, 70,000 PTCAs were performed,[4] including some in patients with unstable angina, multivessel disease, multiple stenoses in single vessels, and stenoses in coronary artery bypass grafts. Recent investigations suggest that PTCA in association with thrombolytic therapy will be useful in reestablishing coronary blood flow after acute myocardial infarction.

PTCA has grown popular for many reasons. When compared with coronary artery bypass grafting (CABG), PTCA is psychologically and physically much less traumatic. The recovery period for PTCA is short: less than 24 hours of bed rest is required after the procedure. The patient is usually discharged from the hospital within 3 days after angioplasty. Although the number of patients who return to work after successful angioplasty is not significantly different from patients who have undergone CABG, the length of time until return to work is shorter in PTCA patients.[5]

Equipment

Basic equipment used during angioplasty includes a balloon, pacing and guiding catheters, and a transducer system for monitoring ventricular and coronary artery pressures. The balloon catheter has two lumens; the central lumen is used for injection of contrast media and for pressure monitoring, and the outer lumen is used for balloon inflation and deflation. Maximal balloon inflation diameters range from 2 mm to 4.2 mm, and the balloon can withstand pressures from 2 to 10 atmospheres. Gold markers, visible under fluoroscopy, are positioned at both ends of the balloon to define its alignment within the lesion.

As a precautionary measure, a pacing catheter is placed prior to angioplasty. If the right coronary artery is to be dilated, third-degree AV block may result while the artery is occluded. If the left anterior descending artery is occluded during angioplasty, an idioventricular rhythm may occur.

The guiding catheter is a large, single-lumen one used to position the balloon catheter. A modern angioplasty catheter system is shown in Fig. 15-1.

Mechanism

Initially, the main mechanism of PTCA was thought to be the compression and relocation of atherosclerotic plaque. Several human cadaver and animal studies now suggest that balloon inflation during angioplasty causes the plaque to split at its thinnest and weakest point.[6-9] This split may extend into internal elastic membrane, and further balloon dilatation may stretch the media and adventitia of the vessel,[10] causing an arterial wall tear to occur in the direction of blood flow. The subsequent healing process is not well understood; presently it is thought that some of the plaque may dissolve in the bloodstream. Arterial wall fibers may cause retraction of the split, and endothelial cells may promote healing of the exposed inner surface of the vessel.[11]

Selection of Patients for PTCA

The results of the history, treadmill test, and coronary angiogram are used to determine a patient's suitability for PTCA. Ideally, the stenosis should be less than 10 mm in

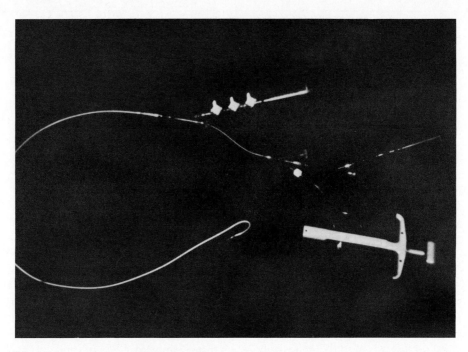

FIG. 15-1.   Modern steerable guidewire equipment used for coronary angioplasty. (Courtesy of Dr. Richard Stack, Duke University Medical Center.)

length, not involve a major vessel bifurcation, and be free of angiographic filling defects.[2] The ideal candidate for PTCA has a single, proximal, concentric, noncalcific coronary artery lesion in the setting of persistent angina despite medical therapy. Patients whose symptoms are controlled by medical therapy may do just as well on medical therapy as they would with PTCA.

With the development of steerable guidewires, better guiding catheters, and low-profile balloons, patient selection has broadened to include multivessel disease. For best results, it is not clear whether all stenoses or only the most stenotic lesion should be dilated.[12]

Stenoses in coronary artery bypass grafts have been successfully dilated. Grafts have no side branches for the tip of the dilating catheter to advance into, so the success rate is high. The complication rate is correspondingly low; only 2.5% of patients require emergency CABG. The risk of emergent CABG for PTCA of native arteries is higher. Coronary artery bypass grafts that are older than 5 years generally have degenerated atherosclerotic plaques that make angioplasty impossible.[12]

Totally occluded coronary arteries may be approached with PTCA if functioning myocardium exists distal to the occlusion. For example, the situation may occur where two coronary arteries supply one area of myocardium. If one of these arteries is totally occluded and the other is severely stenosed, the total lesion may be dilated to protect func-

tioning myocardium that would otherwise be in jeopardy if the stenotic lesion occluded.

PTCA may be performed in patients over 65 years of age, although the success rate is lower in this age group than in younger patients. The complication rate of PTCA in the elderly is higher than in younger patients, with death occurring in 2.2% of all patients over the age of 65 according to the National Heart, Lung, and Blood Institute Registry as compared with 0.7% of patients under 65. Excluding death, the complication rate for both age groups is the same.[13]

Not all lesions are considered for angioplasty. An increased frequency of coronary occlusion and an inability to localize and effectively use the dilating balloon make lesions that are excessive in number and length and distal in location high risk. If tortuosity of the vessel precludes easy placement of the steerable guidewire, the patient should not be considered a candidate for angioplasty. In most centers patients with left main disease are not candidates. Individual patients' coronary arteriograms must be evaluated to make these decisions. The box on p. 413 lists indications and precautions for PTCA.

Procedure

Before the procedure, indications, risks, and benefits are explained to the patient and informed consent is obtained. Patients should understand that when signing consent for

INDICATIONS AND PRECAUTIONS FOR PTCA

Indications	Precautions

1. Stenosis that is:
   a. less than 10 minutes in length
   b. proximal
   c. single
   d. concentric
   e. noncalcific
	1. Stenosis that:
	   a. involves a major vessel bifurcation
	   b. has angiographic filling defects
	   c. is tortuous
	2. Multivessel disease
	3. Coronary artery bypass grafts
	4. Excessive number of stenoses
	5. Chronic total coronary artery lesions
	6. Left main disease (contraindicated in most medical centers)

PTCA, they are also consenting to emergency CABG should it be required. If patients are unable to give consent, their legal next-of-kin must act for them. If no family member is available, the physician may declare the need for PTCA an emergency and proceed without consent.

In most cases a diagnostic cardiac catheterization precedes PTCA by one or more days. Although the angioplasty procedure is very similar to cardiac catheterization, the patient may express new fears concerning balloon dilatation and possible emergent coronary artery bypass grafting. Therefore it is important to thoroughly explain the procedure to the patient. The family or support system of the patient should be included in the teaching so they have an understanding of the procedure and can provide the support the patient needs.

The patient is allowed nothing by mouth from midnight until after angioplasty to minimize the risk of emesis and aspiration during the procedure. Both groins are cleansed and shaved. Routine laboratory tests obtained prior to angioplasty include hemoglobin, hematocrit, coagulation studies, electrolytes, BUN and creatinine. Blood is typed and screened in case emergency surgery is required.

The operating suite should be notified in advance of all angioplasty cases. A room should be prepared and a cardiothoracic team must be mobilized in the event of any complications of angioplasty that require immediate surgery.

Because platelet adhesion is thought to be the cause of early restenosis after angioplasty, low molecular weight dextran or a combination of aspirin and dipyridamole may be given before the procedure. However, the effectiveness of these drugs has not been proved. Diphenhydramine is commonly administered before angiography to reduce the risk of allergic reaction to contrast media. Long-acting nitrates and calcium channel blockers may be given the day before angioplasty.

Once in the angiography laboratory, the patient is prepped and draped in a sterile fashion. After the femoral vein is located with a large-bore needle, an introducer sheath is inserted and the pacing catheter is advanced to the level of the inferior vena cava. A second needle is used to locate the femoral artery. An introducer sheath is placed in the artery, and the guiding catheter is advanced to the level of the coronary ostium. To prevent spasm, 200 mcg to 300 mcg of intracoronary nitroglycerin and/or sublingual nifedipine may be given. A steering device on the distal end of the guidewire system directs the guidewire into the coronary circulation and across the atherosclerotic lesion. Once in place and verified by fluoroscopy, the balloon is advanced along the guidewire and across the lesion. Gold markers at each end of the balloon assist in determining proper placement within the vessel, and pressure gradients across the lesion may then be measured. The guiding catheter measures proximal pressure while the dilating catheter measures distal pressures; the difference in pressures is termed the *pressure gradient*. A large lesion that significantly obstructs blood flow causes a greater decrease in pressure distal to the lesion and, consequently, a greater pressure gradient.

The balloon is then inflated at pressures from 2 to 10 atmospheres for 10 to 60 seconds (Fig. 15-2). One or more inflations at varying pressures may be performed. With the guidewire across the lesion in case of sudden reocclusion, the results are assessed by arteriography. The pressure gradient measured after successful angioplasty should be significantly lower. Pressure gradients may be distorted by the presence of the balloon catheter or guidewire across the lesion, contrast media, or collateral blood flow.[10] With these limitations in mind, some investigators do not rely on pressure gradients to determine success after PTCA. Fig. 15-3 shows coronary arteriograms before and after PTCA.

If angioplasty is successful, the catheters are removed. Because heparin is given during angioplasty, clotting times will be elevated after the procedure. The sheaths are left in place to prevent bleeding, and the patient is returned to his or her room. To decrease the risk of sudden arterial reocclusion after PTCA, intravenous heparin may also be given after the procedure. The heparin may be discontinued several hours to 24 hours after PTCA. When coagulation times return to normal, the sheaths may be removed, after which the patient should lie flat for approximately 6 hours to promote healing of the femoral artery puncture site. The patient should be watched closely for signs of bleeding in the groin area. Pedal pulses should be checked

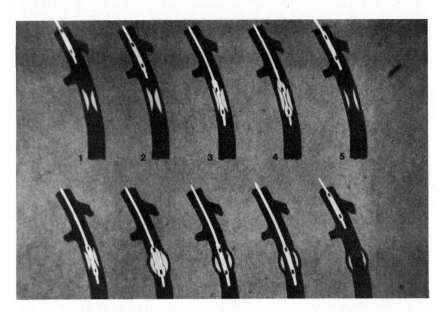

FIG. 15-2.   Balloon compression of atherosclerotic lesion. (Courtesy of Dr. Richard Stack, Duke University Medical Center.)

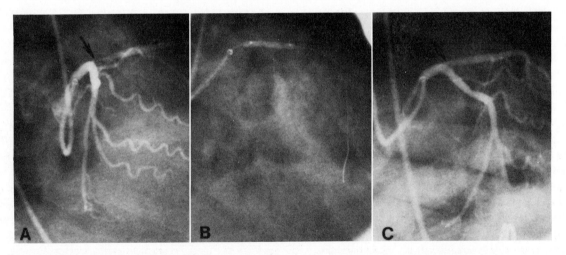

FIG. 15-3.   Coronary arteriograms during PTCA. Arrows denote the lesion before (A) and after (C) dilation. B, The balloon inflated within the lesion. (Courtesy of Dr. Richard Stack, Duke University Medical Center.)

frequently in case thrombosis of the femoral artery occurs. Blood pressure is taken frequently to monitor for hypotension.

Most important, the patient should be monitored for chest pain, which is common after PTCA and may be caused by abrupt occlusion or restenosis of the dilated coronary artery, coronary artery spasm, or pulmonary embolism. When chest pain occurs, an ECG should be obtained and nitrates and calcium-channel blockers should

be administered. If the ECG reveals ST segment elevations and chest pain is not relieved by medication, occlusion should be suspected and emergent repeat PTCA or CABG should be performed. After medication, if ST elevations return to baseline and pain subsides, spasm should be considered and medication continued. Since ST depressions on ECG indicate possible restenosis, urgent repeat PTCA should be performed. Pulmonary embolism should be considered if no cardiac source of chest pain is found. The usual source of pulmonary emboli after PTCA is the femoral vein puncture site. When pulmonary embolism is documented, systemic anticoagulation should be initiated. If no organic source of chest pain is found, anxiety is probably the cause and the patient should be reassured.

Complications

Complications associated with PTCA are similar to those of cardiac catheterization. Dye reaction, hypotension, bradycardia, blood loss, and hematoma may occur. Each of these can usually be treated effectively and results in minor morbidity.

Although increased physician experience may reduce the incidence of minor complications, the incidence of major complications does not change with physician experience.[14,15] The National Heart, Lung, and Blood Institute registry[14,16] reports a 13.6% incidence of an acute coronary vascular event with PTCA, including dissection, occlusion, spasm, embolism, perforation, or rupture. An ischemic event, including myocardial infarction or prolonged angina, may also occur during PTCA. Prolonged angina occurred in 6.8% of patients and myocardial infarction occurred in 5.5%. Major complications such as myocardial infarction, emergency surgery, and in-hospital death occurred in 9.4% of patients. Minor complications consisting of prolonged angina, bradycardia, transient ventricular dysrhythmias, or excessive blood loss occurred in 11.8% of patients.

A catheter has recently been developed for use in the abrupt occlusion that can occur during PTCA. This reperfusion catheter (or bail-out catheter) is advanced along the guidewire until its end is distal to the stenosis. Small holes in the catheter wall allow blood to pass from a site proximal to the occlusion, through and distal to the occlusion. The catheter must be flushed with streptokinase before and during placement to prevent clots from forming in it. The patient must then be taken directly to surgery.

Restenosis is a significant long-term complication associated with PTCA. It is defined as greater than 30% in the narrowing of the stenotic site at follow-up angiography, or a 50% reduction in luminal diameter when compared with the initial improvement obtained at angioplasty.[17] Restenosis occurs in approximately 25% to 30% of patients, but a wide range (13% to 47%) has been reported.[17-19] Restenosis can only be documented by coronary arteriography, but recurrence of symptoms after PTCA may suggest restenosis.[17] Most coronary restenosis after successful PTCA occurs in the first 8 months after the procedure.[12]

Several antiplatelet agents are used routinely to help prevent restenosis, although their effectiveness has not yet been documented. A combination of aspirin and dipyridamole is frequently used to reduce platelet adhesion to the endothelium of the dilated coronary vessel.

Thrombus caused by the rupture of atherosclerotic plaque is felt to be the usual cause of myocardial infarction.[20-22] Once thrombosis occurs, myocardial necrosis begins in the subendocardium and proceeds outward to the epicardium causing a transmural infarct. Within 6 hours myocardial necrosis is nearly complete. Since the development of PTCA, researchers have investigated the possibility of reperfusing an occluded coronary artery within the first few hours of myocardial infarction. Several studies suggest that if blood flow to the ischemic area can be reestablished within the first 6 hours of coronary thrombosis, myocardium in jeopardy of necrosis may be salvaged and infarct size decreased.[23,24]

Other investigators have described the use of intravenous and intracoronary thrombolytic agents to reestablish coronary blood flow.[25-27] Streptokinase is presently the thrombolytic agent of choice. Other agents, such as a tissue-type plasminogen activator (t-PA), which is a natural human enzyme used to lyse clots, are under investigation but have not yet been approved by the FDA.

Thrombolytic agents may be given intravenously or via the intracoronary route. Intravenous thrombolytic therapy has enabled community hospitals without angiographic facilities to initiate reperfusion therapy. If reperfusion occurs with thrombolytic therapy alone, the patient may be watched and treated medically at that institution or transferred to a medical facility where cardiac catheterization is available. The limitation of using thrombolytic therapy alone is the high incidence of residual high-grade stenosis after reperfusion; the potential for reocclusion in these patients is great. Consequently, most researchers believe PTCA should follow intravenous streptokinase, although when to perform PTCA after reperfusion with thrombolytic agents has not been defined. However, most patients are transferred to a hospital with angiographic and PTCA facilities within the first 48 hours after acute infarction.

If reperfusion is not accomplished with thrombolytic therapy, emergency PTCA may be performed. Almost half of the patients who have myocardial infarction have single-vessel disease, making them good candidates for PTCA.[2] The procedure for emergency PTCA is very similar to routine angioplasty, and most investigators believe that a degree of spasm occurs in the coronary artery during acute myocardial infarction.[28] Therefore most operators will administer intracoronary nitroglycerin before administering intracoronary streptokinase. If no intravenous streptokinase was given, intracoronary streptokinase may be infused in an attempt to lyse the thrombus. If the lesion remains occluded, the guidewire and catheter are used to directly cross the vessel. Usually a stenosis greater than 50% remains and angioplasty is performed immediately.

The efficacy of PTCA during acute myocardial infarction is being investigated; most researchers now use ejection fraction measured by ventriculography to assess left ventricular function before and after PTCA.[12]

Thrombolytic therapy cannot be given to all patients. Contraindications include active internal bleeding, cerebral vascular accident within the past 2 months, postpartum period, puncture of a noncompressible blood vessel, and recent major surgery or organ biopsy.[29]

Complications of streptokinase include bleeding at the site of arterial catheterization, hematoma, gastrointestinal bleeding, gingival bleeding, and oozing from recent skin puncture sites. Patients may also have an allergic response to streptokinase. Premedication to reduce the risk of an allergic response includes cimetidine and diphenhydramine.

Reperfusion often causes increased ventricular arrhythmias in the form of an accelerated idioventricular rhythm. Ventricular tachycardia and ventricular fibrillation occur only rarely. Since a reperfused right coronary artery rarely causes third-degree AV block, a pacing catheter is placed before angioplasty for this reason. Relief of chest pain, gradual return of the ST segment to baseline on the ECG, and the development of abnormal Q waves on the ECG indicating some myocardial necrosis demonstrate that the acutely occluded coronary artery has been reperfused.[30,31] Serum CPK and CPK-MB levels peak 6 to 10 hours earlier than in the absence of reperfusion.

PTCA is an established therapy for coronary artery disease. Criteria for patient selection have broadened, allowing more patients the option of PTCA. Although restenosis is a major obstacle of PTCA, attempts are being made to overcome it. New therapies involving laser energy and the development of microsurgical instruments to remove plaque may produce effective alternative therapies for the treatment of coronary artery disease.

CORONARY ARTERY BYPASS SURGERY
Indications for Surgery

The decision to perform coronary artery bypass surgery is based on what is possible and desirable to achieve by it as opposed to what can and should be achieved by medical therapy alone. If an improvement in the patient's quality of life is foreseeable with surgical intervention, then coronary artery surgery is an effective alternative. The general intent of coronary artery bypass surgery is to increase myocardial oxygen supply by increasing coronary blood flow. There are no standardized indications for revascularization, although certain conditions seem to warrant surgical intervention more than others.[32-34]

In general, potential candidates for coronary artery bypass surgery are those patients with significant coronary artery stenosis—obstruction greater than 70% of the artery

---

NEW YORK HEART ASSOCIATION
PATIENT CLASSIFICATION

Class I
Asymptomatic with ordinary physical exertion

Class II
Symptomatic with ordinary physical exertion

Class III
Symptomatic with less than ordinary physical exertion

Class IV
Symptomatic at rest

---

diameter—and with good distal run-off. This is demonstrated when the artery distal to the obstruction is seen during arteriography to be patent and capable of carrying blood should it be revascularized.[35] Coronary artery grafting is usually not performed for single-vessel disease unless that vessel is a major coronary artery supplying a large segment of the myocardium, for example, the left main coronary artery.

The principal indication for coronary artery bypass is chronic angina despite vigorous medical management (NYHA Class III, IV; see box above). Although still debated in the medical literature, the operation seems to provide effective relief of angina in the majority of patients.[36]

Unstable angina (preinfarction angina) is also an indication for coronary artery surgery. In this syndrome angina may be so prolonged and severe at rest that it is unresponsive to any treatment except narcotics and/or IV nitroglycerin.

Coronary artery surgery may be recommended for ongoing ischemia following an acute myocardial infarction. In this situation, surgery may prove valuable in salvaging threatened myocardium, but when an infarction results in persistent ventricular arrhythmias, revascularization may also be warranted.

History and Physical Examination

Successful cardiac surgery is predicated on a comprehensive, organized preoperative medical history and examination (see chapter 14). This information helps in the formation of tentative diagnoses as well as in the definition of therapeutic goals. Components of the medical history include identifying data, source of referral, present illness, past medical history, family history, psychosocial history, and reviewing all body systems.

During the history-taking, particular attention should be paid to medication usage because the patient with coronary artery disease frequently has been taking many types of medication to control symptoms, prevent complications, and improve cardiac function. Whether diuretics, cardiotonics, antiarrhythmics, antibiotics, antihypertensives, steroids, or anticoagulants are being used or not is information that is critical to include in the patient record. Drug sensitivities or allergic reactions should be noted and fully described.

A thorough, systematic physical examination will establish the patient's baseline as well as identify any factors capable of affecting the outcome of the surgery. For each body system assessed, detailed documentation describing any anatomic or physiologic abnormality must follow. Not only is it of paramount importance to evaluate the patient's cardiac function; it is also essential to evaluate the patient's respiratory, neurologic, gastrointestinal, and renal status. The skin and musculoskeletal systems offer important clues about the general health and nutrition of such a patient.

Nothing in the physical examination should be overlooked as unimportant. Most practitioners of cardiac surgery can recall situations when what was considered "insignificant" before surgery became of "critical" importance in the prostoperative management of the patient. Assessment of oral hygiene, for example, may lead to the discovery of recent major dental repairs and the potential for oral infections. Incomplete wound healing or skin abrasions may be deemed risky enough to warrant postponing elective surgery until healing is complete. The use of illicit drugs, if undetected, can present major problems in postoperative pain control.

Laboratory Studies

The box at right lists commonly performed laboratory studies for an adult patient admitted for cardiac surgery. The schedule of tests should be modified according to specific needs. Not every test should be performed on each patient and additional tests may be required for some. In general, preoperative blood studies assess formed elements, oxygen-carrying capacity, and coagulation tendencies.

Specific tests for hepatic, renal, pulmonary, metabolic, and cardiac function provide information about organ physiology for postoperative comparison.[35] A general pattern of improvement in hepatic and renal function, for example, is anticipated following cardiac surgery because congestive heart failure is reduced and cardiac output is improved. Cardiac enzymes, which indicate injured myocardial cells, assist in determining the significance of any postoperative angina and the need for further diagnostic tests. Pulmonary pathology requires careful follow-up, since normal pulmonary functioning is interrupted during surgery and residual effects of cardiopulmonary bypass may

COMMON LABORATORY STUDIES

General
Blood typing and crossmatch

Pulmonary
Arterial blood gases
Pulmonary function tests

Cardiac
Serum enzymes (SGOT, LDH, CPK isoenzymes)

Renal-Metabolic
Urinalysis
BUN
Creatinine
Urine electrolytes
Serum electrolytes
Serum lipids
Serum cholesterol
FBS

Liver
Serum bilirubin
Serum proteins
Alkaline phosphatase
SGOT
LDH
SGPT

Hematologic
CBC (RBC, WBC, Hgb, Hct)
Platelet count
PT
PTT
Fibrinogin

persist to some degree in the immediate postoperative period.

Chest X-ray (CXR)

A baseline CXR is ordered immediately before surgery whether or not previous films exist. Visualization of the heart yields valuable information about overall cardiac size and function. Analysis of the lung fields and pulmonary vessels can detect changes in pulmonary vasculature indicative of venous or arterial hypertension and increased or decreased blood flow.[35] Identification of a pneumothorax, pleural effusion, or atelectasis is very significant in preoperative management and, if necessary, should be treated before proceeding with surgery. Many patients having coronary bypass surgery have had a history of cigarette-smoking, and the CXR is vital in assessing pulmonary changes that would lead to inadequate ventilation and CO_2 retention postoperatively.

Electrocardiogram

An ECG is performed on all patients before cardiac surgery because any disturbances in rate, rhythm, and conduction are noteworthy, as are changes indicative of ischemia. An ECG may also reveal any evidence of digitalis or other cardiotonic drug toxicity (that is, atrial or ventricular dysrhythmias, varying degrees of heart block), which should be remedied before surgical intervention. A baseline ECG is of particular value during postoperative management as a comparison for evaluating the electrophysiologic state of the heart.

Arteriography

Coronary arteriography provides a means of accurately determining the presence and extent of coronary artery disease. Arteriography provides visualization of the coronary arteries including the site and severity of stenotic lesions; characteristics of the distal coronary vessels in terms of size, disease state, and the amount of viable myocardium; an estimate of coronary blood flow; and information about collateral vessels and their functional importance.[37] Measurement of left ventricular pressure at rest or after introduction of pharmacologic agents is made possible with left ventricular catheterization, which also provides a visual analysis of wall motion, ventricular volume, and ejection fraction.

Wall motion can be further evaluated by the addition of stress (such as with atrial pacing). Left ventricular contraction can be augmented by nitrates or catecholamines to enhance identification of wall segments having potential for improved function following revascularization. Correlation of the coronary arteriogram and left ventriculogram permits delineation of bypassable coronary arteries.[37] The information is necessary in determining operability, operative risk, and probability of operative success.

Medications

All patient medications should be evaluated before surgery. There are varying opinions regarding when and if preoperative medication should be discontinued. The practice of administering most medicines up to the time of surgery is gaining popularity; therefore the following suggestions should be considered while the needs of each patient are determined individually.

Antibiotics. Although the value of prophylactic antibiotics is debatable and their effectiveness is difficult to establish, physicians at many centers believe that their use is warranted in cardiac surgery.[38] Administration of a broad-spectrum agent such as cephalosporin is begun the night before surgery, when the patient is on call to the O.R., and then continued postoperatively until invasive lines and tubes are discontinued. This ensures that the antibiotic reaches the required blood level during the period when the patient is most vulnerable to infection.

Digoxin. Digoxin is commonly administered up to the time of surgery. There is little consensus in the medical literature about prophylactic digitalization of preoperative patients, but the drug is advantageous to patients who suffer heart failure or experience atrial fibrillation. A short-acting preparation such as digoxin permits more readily controllable drug levels than other preparations and is not washed out or removed from the tissues during cardiopulmonary bypass.

Diuretics. Fluid restriction is preferable to diuretic therapy in the preoperative treatment of milder forms of fluid retention because of the tendency for diuretics to produce electrolyte abnormalities. If fluid restriction alone is inadequate, then a diuretic is administered, furosemide (Lasix) being the drug of choice.

Propranolol. Beta-blocking agents such as propranalol (Inderal) are usually continued up to the time of surgery.

Calcium Channel Blockers. Because the therapeutic potential for verapamil and nifedipine extends to the management of cardiac dysrhythmias, angina, hypertension, cardiomyopathy, and myocardial infarction, its continuation until surgery may be indicated, but the decision is made on an individual basis.

Warfarin. Anticoagulants are discontinued several days before surgery to allow time for clotting mechanisms to return to normal.

Aspirin. Aspirin can interfere with coagulation by preventing normal platelet aggregation, which is responsible for the formation of a platelet plug. The effect of aspirin persists for the life of the platelet, so it is desirable to withhold aspirin administration for at least 1 week before surgery.

Preoperative Teaching

Preoperative teaching is done by the members of the surgical and nursing staff involved in the patient's care. Each covers information from his or her area of expertise: the surgeon reviews the patient's condition, operative plans, potential risks, and expected outcomes; the anesthesiologist discusses the type of anesthetic and the events that will take place during induction and immediately after surgery; the nurse describes postoperative nursing care, procedures, and monitoring devices.

Patient and family teaching begins on admission and continues throughout hospitalization and discharge. Effective teaching must be geared to the patient's level of understanding; teaching must be designed to alleviate anxiety rather than induce it. Teaching cardiac surgery patients is highly individualized and should be timed according to when the patient is ready to listen and learn. Family members or others who play an important part in the patient's life need to be included in the teaching sessions, since they will provide psychologic and emotional support during the recovery phase. Teaching sessions can be complemented by the use of audiovisual aids such as models of the heart, slide presentations, and visits to the intensive care unit.

Preparation for Surgery

Skin preparation for surgery starts with a shower using a germicidal agent (such as pHisoHex) to decrease skin bacteria. On the evening before surgery, the patient is shaved from chin to toes to decrease contamination from hair. Care is taken to avoid nicks or skin abrasions because these serve as potential sites of infection.

The night before surgery the patient is kept NPO. A laxative or enema is used to empty the lower bowel and prevent a bowel movement during the immediate postoperative phase. A mild sedative is made available to the patient the night before surgery to reduce anxiety and promote sleep.

Intraoperative Management
ANESTHESIA AND MONITORING

Anesthetic requirements are determined by the health status and particular needs of each surgical patient. Many agents are available for cardiac surgical procedures and each is used according to its ability to facilitate the surgery and reduce morbidity.[39-41] The reader is advised to refer to cardiovascular anesthesia references for a detailed list of the advantages and disadvantages of specific narcotics (i.e., morphine sulfate, fentanyl, Sufentanil), inhalational agents (i.e., nitrous oxide, halothane, Enflurane, Isoflurane), muscle relaxants (i.e., curare, Pavulon, Atacurium, metocurine) and benzodiazepines (Valium).

Continuous monitoring of the ECG and arterial, central venous, and pulmonary artery pressures is part of intraoperative management. Peripheral IV lines are started for additional volume and medication administration. A nasogastric tube is inserted to prevent gastric distention and a Foley catheter to measure urinary output. After the patient is intubated, arterial blood gases and serum electrolytes are measured at regular intervals. All parameters indicative of hemodynamic performance are frequently evaluated to allow for early recognition of trends or potential complications throughout the surgery.

EXTRACORPOREAL CIRCULATION

Intracardiac surgery employs the technique of cardiopulmonary bypass (CPB).[34,42,43,44] During CPB the heart and lungs are bypassed to allow for surgical repair while their function is performed by the cardiopulmonary bypass machine (also called the pump-oxygenator or heart-lung machine). Venous blood is removed from the patient via cannulae in the venae cavae, circulated through an oxygenator where gas exchange occurs, and returned to the arterial circulation via a catheter in the ascending aorta or, on occasion, in the femoral artery (Figs. 15-4 and 15-5).

There are pronounced risks during cardiac surgery because of the mechanisms of CPB. Most patients do not evidence long-term dysfunction following bypass, but the transient effects that are most clinically apparent postoperatively include the following:

1. Damage to formed blood elements—Direct contact of the blood with tubing surfaces, compression from roller pumps, and the blood-gas interface causes cellular damage to plasma proteins, RBCs, WBCs, and clotting factors. Platelets are particularly vulnerable to destruction, so their viability and effectiveness decrease following CPB.

2. Microemboli—Incorporation of microfilters in the bypass system reduces but does not completely eliminate the possibility of embolic complications. The presence of particulate matter, microbubbles, and lipids can affect blood flow through the microcirculation.

3. Electrolyte and ion shifts—Ionic shifts (namely, Na^+, K^+, Ca^+, Mg^{++}) caused by extracorporeal circulation can produce a state of metabolic acidosis postoperatively. Potassium levels are significantly altered by diuresis, which occurs as a result of hemodilution and diuretics present in the pump-priming solutions.

4. Altered immune response—The concentration of WBCs and plasma antibodies is reduced because of hemodilution, sequestering, and direct cellular trauma. There is also evidence that the phagocytic activity of circulating leukocytes is decreased in the immediate postoperative period.

5. Hemodilution—Prior to initiating bypass, pump oxygenators are primed with an isotonic solution, which is responsible for hemodilution of the patient's blood. Hemodilution reduces blood viscosity, thus improving microcirculation, reducing hemolysis, reducing the usage of blood products, and promoting diuresis. Conversely, hemodilution leads to increases in extracellular water and interstitial fluid, both of which must be carefully monitored and managed postoperatively.

6. Hypothermia—A state of hypothermia (20° C to 30° C) is routinely produced during CPB to reduce systemic and myocardial oxygen demands: there is a reduction in metabolic rate by 7% per degree lowering of temperature. It is important to realize that rewarming does not occur uniformly immediately

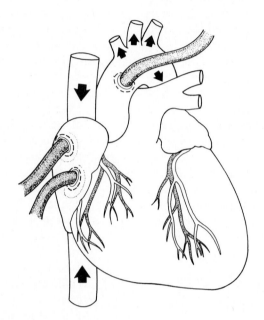

FIG. 15-4. Venous connections remove blood from the right heart; arterial connections return oxygenated blood via the ascending aorta while on cardiopulmonary bypass.

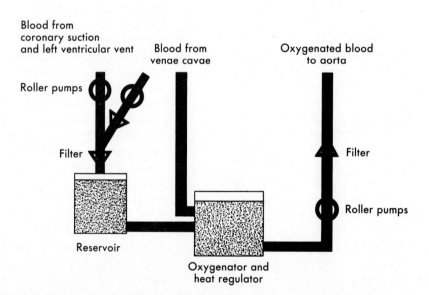

FIG. 15-5. The basic components required for extracorporeal circulation include 1, connecting tubing and roller pumps for venous blood flow from the patient; 2, an aspirating system for retrieving blood from the surgical field; 3, filters within the system to remove particulate material, lipids, and gaseous emboli; 4, reservoir; 5, oxygenator for gas exchange; 6, heat exchanger for controlling blood temperature; and 7, connecting tubing and roller pumps to return oxygenated blood to the patient. This system delivers a nonpulsatile blood flow with an ideal mean pressure between 50 and 85 mm Hg.

after surgery, i.e., organs with high blood-flow will rewarm faster than muscle and skin. This is evidenced by temperature variations and changes in hemodynamic stability as the periphery begins to warm.

7. Coagulation—Heparinization is required at the onset of CPB to achieve a clotting time of 6 to 8 minutes (300 units/kg) and is maintained throughout the surgery with additional doses of heparin. The actions of heparin are reversed with protamine sulfate after CPB is terminated; the amount of CPB administered depends on clotting times and the dosage of heparin given. The combined effect of the heparin and protamine administration, altered clotting factors, and a state of hypothermia renders a patient's clotting ability relatively unstable immediately after surgery.

8. Reduced lung compliance—While gas exchange is being performed by the oxygenator, the lungs remain inactive. Surfactant production is decreased

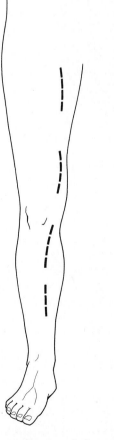

FIG. 15-6. The greater saphenous vein is commonly used in coronary artery bypass surgery. Healing is facilitated by making several small incisions along the course of the vessel. Other sources of conduits include the cephalic and basilic veins and mammary artery.

during this time, intensifying the chances of local lung edema and reduced lung compliance following bypass.

Revascularization

As the sternum is being longitudinally opened, the greater saphenous vein is removed, inspected, and tested for leakage (Fig. 15-6). After heparinization is completed, cannulation of the venae cavae and aorta is performed and CPB is started. With good visualization of the coronary arteries, a segment of the saphenous vein is anastomosed to the distal vessel followed by graft anastomosis to the aorta. The internal mammary artery may also be used as an arterial conduit and creates an artery-to-artery graft with good patency results (Fig. 15-7). Once the surgeon has completed grafting and is satisfied with the operative procedure—including the lengths of the grafts—CPB is weaned and discontinued. Great care is taken to evacuate air from the aorta and grafts before discontinuing CPB. Prior to leaving the O.R., mediastinal tubes are placed to facilitate postoperative drainage, epicardiac pacing wires are attached, and the sternum is rewired with stainless steel sutures (Figs. 15-8 and 15-9).

Postoperative Management
TRANSFER TO THE INTENSIVE CARE UNIT

The surgeon and anesthesiologist transport patients from the O.R. directly to the recovery room or cardiothoracic intensive care unit, where they stay until they are extubated, made hemodynamically stable, and arterial and venous lines are removed. Just as the operative period requires highly trained and skilled professionals, the immediate postoperative interval is one of major change, demanding optimum attention and management.

Once in the ICU, the patient is reconnected to the ventilator and hemodynamic monitoring is established. A continuous ECG via lead I, II, or III is displayed. All pressure lines (CVP, PA, LA) are assessed and quickly connected to the unit's transducing system and monitors. Depending on the type of pulmonary artery catheter used, cardiac output and continuous oxygen saturation are established. A rectal temperature is taken and correlated with the core temperature that is obtained from the distal portion of the pulmonary artery catheter.

Chest tubes are connected to 15 to 20 cm of continuous suction, stripped to maintain system patency, and marked for initial drainage. Chest tube stripping should be done with extreme care because very high negative pressures can be created by this procedure. Urinary output is measured via a Foley catheter, and the nasogastric tube is checked for patency and connected to low suction. All volume lines are assessed, and fluids and medications are regulated accordingly. Pacing wires inserted at the time of surgery are

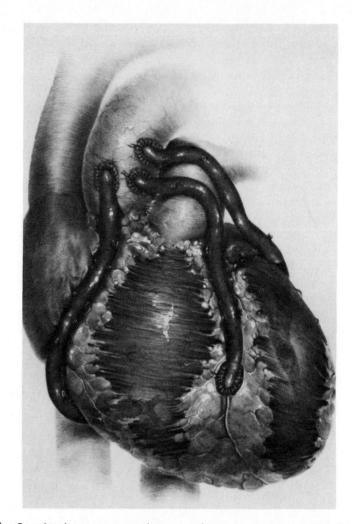

FIG. 15-7.   Completed coronary artery bypass grafting using saphenous veins. (From Harlan, B., Starr, A., and Harwin, F.: Manual of cardiac surgery, New York, 1980, Springer-Verlag New York, Inc.)

connected to an AV sequential pacemaker and used as needed. A chest x-ray examination and ECG are done, and the first set of lab work is drawn (ABG, CBC, chemistry, PT, and PTT). A quick head-to-toe assessment is performed by the admitting nurse and physician to establish the patient's baseline condition upon arrival in the ICU. Pages 428 to 430 elaborate on the nursing care plan for the adult postoperative patient.

MANAGEMENT OF CARDIOVASCULAR PERFORMANCE

Postoperative efforts are directed toward maintaining optimum cardiovascular performance.[38,42,45,46] This is viewed in terms of how well the heart is able to constantly deliver adequate amounts of oxygenated blood to the peripheral system. For adults, a minimum cardiac index of 2.0 L/min/M² is required to meet these demands. Cardiac rate, rhythm, preload, afterload, and contractility govern cardiovascular performance; manipulation of these determinants is a major part of postoperative management.

RATE AND RHYTHM. Normal sinus rhythm is most desirable to optimize cardiac output following coronary artery bypass surgery. Disturbances in rate and rhythm are commonly encountered after cardiac surgery and are prone to occur in the first 48 hours. Factors that predispose to dysrhythmias include advanced heart disease, renal disturbances, incisional or ischemic trauma, hypokalemia, drug toxicity, acid-base imbalance, hypoxemia, anesthetic agents, hypothermia, hypovolemia, and pain.

After coronary artery bypass surgery, premature ventricular contractions (PVCs) are the most frequent dysrhythmia. They are particularly important because of their potential to advance to ventricular tachycardia or fibrillation. PVCs of more than 6 per minute, multifocal PVCs, or those close to the T wave are treated with a lidocaine

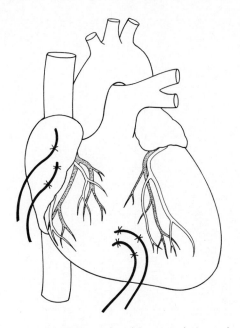

FIG. 15-8. Epicardial pacing wires (2 atrial and 2 ventricular) are shown in place. They are brought out to the surface of the skin as the chest is closed.

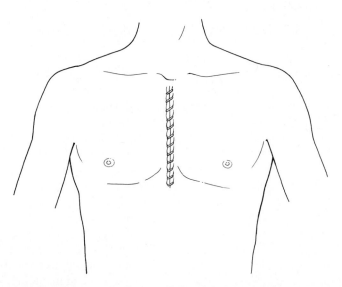

FIG. 15-9. Most cardiac procedures are performed using a median sternotomy, since it provides the best visualization and access to heart chambers and the least respiratory impairment and patient discomfort following surgery. The incision is made from below the sternal notch to just below the xiphoid process.

bolus and drip; other antiarrhythmic agents may also be employed.

Atrial pacing, commonly and safely performed via epicardial wires, is used to suppress unifocal PVCs resulting from bradycardia. In this instance atrial pacing is preferred over ventricular pacing to synchronize atrial and ventricular contraction, which increases the cardiac output by ap-

proximately 15%. If atrial wires are not present, overriding the patient's heart rate via ventricular pacing wires is an effective means of controlling ectopy from bradycardia. If there are no pacing wires available, chronotropic agents like atropine and isoproterenol can be used.

Atrial dysrhythmias commonly occur after coronary artery bypass surgery. Premature atrial contractions (PACs)

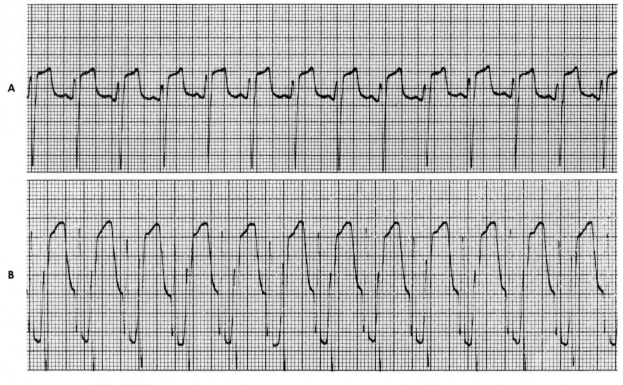

FIG. 15-10.   A, Normal bedside monitoring using lead III. B, Atrial ECG. Note pronounced P waves with atrial ECG.

often herald atrial fibrillation. If atrial fibrillation or atrial flutter does occur, treatment includes digitalization, rapid atrial pacing, or cardioversion, depending on the patient's situation. If digoxin was taken preoperatively, toxicity must be considered and a serum digoxin level must be drawn. When atrial activity is difficult to analyze, such as in many supraventricular tachycardias, an atrial ECG is employed (Fig. 15-10).

Junctional rhythm and AV heart block can occur post-operatively but are uncommon. When such disturbances do occur, they are often a result of injury to the conduction system from edema or local hemorrhage. Although usually transient, treatment may be warranted and includes cardiac pacing and an Isuprel drip titrated according to heart rate.

PRELOAD. Preload is routinely assessed by right and left atrial pressures following cardiac surgery.[38,45,46,47] If a left atrial line was not placed during surgery, then left-sided filling pressures are evaluated by pulmonary artery diastolic and wedge pressures. The principal method of enhancing preload postoperatively is by expanding vascular volume, which may be in the form of crystalloid or colloid infusion. The amount and type of infusion are dependent on ventricular function, renal and pulmonary status, coagulation, and hematocrit.

When filling pressures are low, infusion of volume assists in improving the cardiac output up to a certain point.

However, there is little or no response in cardiac output if cardiac filling pressures are already elevated, which is an expression of the Frank Starling principle. (See Chapter 1.) The rate of volume infusion depends upon the myocardial response to volume; too rapid an infusion can lead to ventricular failure even in the face of hypovolemia. Nitroprusside is often used to provide necessary vasodilatation while building an adequate circulatory blood volume. By continually evaluating the central venous, pulmonary artery, and left atrial pressures, progression of volume through the vascular system can be evaluated and volume infusion adjusted accordingly.

There is a distinct possibility that patients may develop hypovolemia and low cardiac output after coronary artery surgery. Factors contributing to this tendency include fluid shifts from the vascular spaces, changes in arterial and venous vessel capacity, excessive bleeding, and inadequate volume replacement. The possibility of cardiac tamponade must always be a major consideration while managing a patient with a low cardiac output. The collection of fluid in the posterior pericardial sac or in the mediastinal space interferes with cardiac filling by obstructing the return of blood from the great vessels and the ejection of blood from the ventricles. In addition to decreased cardiac output, classic indicators of tamponade include rising filling pressures, decreasing arterial pressure, marked decrease in chest tube output, mediastinal widening by chest x-ray, distant heart sounds, narrowing pulse pressure, and a decrease in ECG voltage. This is an emergency situation and requires rapid surgical evacuation and exploration.

AFTERLOAD. Afterload, or impedance to left ventricular ejection, is managed postoperatively primarily by controlling arterial blood pressure.[38,45,46,47] Hypertension is undesirable following cardiac surgery, whereas lowering the systemic blood pressure (1) improves myocardial performance, that is, increases cardiac output and reduces left ventricular end diastolic pressure; (2) reduces myocardial oxygen requirements; and (3) reduces the potential for bleeding from suture lines and chest tubes. There are two modalities commonly used for reducing afterload: vasodilating agents and intraaortic balloon pumping.

Intravenous vasodilating drugs can have arterial and venous activity. Nitroprusside is commonly used for afterload reduction because of its balanced activity; it also has a rapid effect with brief duration and can be precisely titrated. Other reduction agents include hydralazine (Apresoline), phentolamine (Regitine), chlorpromazine (Thorazine), and nitroglycerin. Assessing systemic vascular resistance (SVR) helps to determine if afterload is high or low while titrating reduction agents. A value over 1500 dynes/sec/cm^5 may indicate enough impedance to decrease cardiac output; a value below 800 dynes/sec/cm^5 may cause extreme vasodilatation and low cardiac index.

The intraaortic balloon pump is a temporary circulatory-assist device that is useful in managing the cardiac patient postoperatively by improving hemodynamic status, reducing congestive heart failure, and controlling serious dysrhythmias. The balloon is threaded in a retrograde fashion through the femoral artery to the descending thoracic aorta. According to proper timing, it will inflate during diastole and deflate during systole. As the balloon inflates, blood is propelled onward increasing the diastolic pressure and coronary artery perfusion. Upon balloon deflation, the potential space filled by the balloon is filled with blood from the aortic root. As this happens, the pressure facing the aortic valve is decreased, allowing it to open more easily at lower pressures, thus helping to reduce cardiac workload (Fig. 15-11).

CONTRACTILITY. The only direct means of augmenting the inotropic state of the heart is the use of pharmacologic agents.[38,45,46,47] Their proper use is invaluable for effective myocardial support following cardiac surgery. The following drugs have been widely used for strengthening myocardial contractility: isoproterenol (Isuprel), dopamine (Intropin), epinephrine (Adrenalin), dobutamine (Dobutrex), digoxin, calcium chloride, norepinephrine (Levophed), calcium glucagon, and phenylephrine (Neo-Synephrine). Specific drug actions and patient perfusion needs determine which drug is recommended; each drug has unique effects on heart rate, contractility, renal blood flow, and oxygen expenditure. In general, inotropic drugs are not used to augment myocardial contractility until manipulation of other variables, such as heart rate, preload, and afterload, has been attempted.

MANAGEMENT OF RESPIRATORY PERFORMANCE

Most patients experience some degree of transient respiratory dysfunction in the immediate postoperative period. This generally takes the form of decreased oxygenation and ventilatory depression, which appears as hypoxemia, alveolar hypoventilation, and reduced ventilatory reserve.

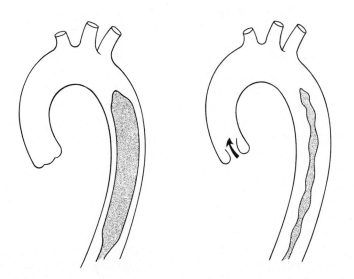

FIG. 15-11.   The intra-aortic balloon is properly positioned in the descending thoracic aorta distal to the left subclavian artery. Inflation during diastole increases systemic and coronary perfusion; deflation during systole reduces afterload.

The basic components of postoperative respiratory care are (1) optimizing ventilation and pulmonary mechanics; (2) improving blood gas exchange; (3) reducing metabolic needs and oxygen consumption; (4) assessing cardiovascular performance as it affects perfusion and the oxygen transport system; and (5) avoiding prolonged intubation and mechanical ventilation.[48]

Patients are mechanically ventilated during the first 12 to 48 hours following coronary artery surgery. The level of surveillance and support is related to preexisting pulmonary disease, the nature and patient's response to the cardiac repair, duration of the cardiopulmonary bypass, and any coexisting system disorders such as of the liver or kidneys.

Ventilator management during the postoperative period includes regulation of oxygen concentration, providing a tidal volume of 15 to 20 ml/kg, controlling respiratory rate to maintain acceptable $PaCO_2$, and adding positive-end-expiratory-pressure (PEEP) when needed. Arterial blood gases and chest x-ray films are frequently examined while the patient remains intubated; in addition, tissue perfusion and sensorium are carefully monitored. Since it is desirable to ventilate patients who are not struggling, shivering, coughing, gagging, or fighting the ventilator, appropriate interventions are taken when these occur.

Criteria for extubation differ from patient to patient, but extubation is favored when the patient is alert and responsive, when arterial blood gases are stable with good pulmonary mechanics, and when the patient's cardiac, pulmonary, and renal systems are performing satisfactorily. Following extubation, patients are supplemented with humidified oxygen via a face mask or nasal cannula for 24 to 48 hours. A program of vigorous pulmonary toilette, which includes frequent deep breathing and coughing, chest physiotherapy, turning in bed, and ambulating as soon as possible, is employed.

Although most patients experience acceptable spontaneous respirations by 24 to 48 hours postoperatively, some require prolonged ventilation. Often these patients have experienced respiratory complications that necessitate further support to sustain life. Excessive secretions, pneumonia, segmental or lobar atelectasis, pleural effusions, pulmonary edema, and acute respiratory failure require highly specialized, comprehensive management.

MANAGEMENT OF RENAL PERFORMANCE

Postoperative treatment centers around maintaining adequate intravascular volume and cardiac output to ensure adequate renal perfusion and urinary output while balancing electrolyte levels.[49] Adequacy of renal performance is assessed by monitoring urinary output, specific gravity, BUN, and creatinine. Other indications are daily weights,

skin turgor, edema, sensorium, serum chemistries, and intravascular pressure measurements.

Electrolyte disturbances are common after cardiac surgery, but with proper management their detrimental effects can be avoided. Retention of sodium and excretion of potassium can be expected. Sodium supplements are usually not necessary, but potassium is lost in sufficient quantities to require replacement therapy. Metabolic acidosis and alkalosis may also be encountered along with occasional disturbances in calcium and magnesium concentrations.

A measurable alteration of renal function accompanies cardiac surgery. Preoperative apprehension, fluid restrictions, and surgical trauma promote increased secretion of antidiuretic hormone (ADH) and aldosterone. During the immediate postoperative period, the renal tubules must also handle products of tissue breakdown from surgery and free hemoglobin from bypass perfusion. The combined effect of these variables is responsible for the oliguria that commonly occurs after surgery. Treatment of oliguria usually consists of volume administration and if the patient is well hydrated, a diuretic such as furosemide (Lasix).

Acute renal failure is a serious complication following surgery. A low urinary osmolarity, high urinary sodium level, and the failure to respond to diuretics are early signs of acute renal failure. The most frequent contributing factor to acute renal failure is low cardiac output and accompanying reduction in renal blood flow. It is therefore important to ensure hydration that promotes a urinary output of at least 30 cc/hour in adults. Other factors that seem to render patients vulnerable to acute renal failure are severe cardiac dysfunction, renal disease, and advanced age.

If acute renal failure does occur, the administration of fluids must be restricted, potassium administration must be curtailed, clearance of medications must be carefully considered, blood and urine studies must be frequently monitored, and hypertension must be controlled. Peritoneal dialysis may also be necessary during the oliguric phase of acute renal failure to reduce fluid overload, hyperkalemia, and uremic symptoms. Diuresis may occur after the oliguric phase. Patients who are supported well and survive the oliguric and polyuric phases will ultimately regain function, although it may be months before recovery is complete.

MANAGEMENT OF NEUROLOGIC FUNCTION

Major neurologic complications have significantly declined because of the modern advances in cardiac surgery and cardiopulmonary bypass.[50] Nevertheless, level of consciousness is continually assessed until the patient recovers from the anesthetic and is awake. Neurologic checks, which include pupillary size and reaction, gross motor movement and sensation, and orientation to person, place, and time are performed. Any noted disorders such as failure to respond, seizures, or unilateral weakness warrant a neurologic consultation and full work-up. Management of any complication is directed toward relief of symptoms, prevention of further injury, and restoration to maximum function.

It is estimated that a large majority of adults who have open heart surgery experience some form of transient sensory disturbance postoperatively. These disturbances can be as minor as anxiety or as severe as hallucinations and delusions. If the sensory distortions are severe, the patient may cause self-harm by disrupting monitoring cables, pulling out tubes, and disturbing life-support lines. Sensory alterations in postcardiotomy patients are difficult to deal with because there are so many factors that seem to render patients vulnerable. Some of these are anesthetic agents, cardiopulmonary bypass, the ICU environment, sleep deprivation, surgical stress, advanced age, and degree of morbidity. Because of this tendency toward sensory disturbances, postoperative care must include attention to safety factors (that is, close attendance, side rails, wrist restraints prn), reorientation techniques (verbal information to patient, clocks, calendars), and normalizing the ICU environment as much as possible (family visits, day/night cycles).

MANAGEMENT OF GASTROINTESTINAL FUNCTION

Gastric distention, which can place undue pressure on the lungs and heart, is avoided postoperatively by the use of a nasogastric tube connected to low intermittent suction or left to gravity. All patients, particularly those with a history of gastric bleeding, should have their gastric pH checked routinely and antacids should be administered accordingly. The abdomen is assessed for distention, pain, ascites, and bowel sounds. When normal peristalsis returns and the patient is able to take liquids by mouth, a diet is resumed and advanced as tolerated (usually a regular diet with no added salt or a 2 g low-sodium diet). Most patients eat without difficulty by 24 hours after surgery.

BLEEDING

Some bleeding is normal in every patient following cardiac surgery, but persistent bleeding requires special attention. The amount of bleeding that warrants concern is contingent upon hemodynamic response, patient size, clotting studies, and the nature and extent of surgery.[51,52] Usually more than 100 ml of blood every hour from the mediastinal tubes over several hours is considered excessive. In such a case the primary strategy in patient management is to determine the cause: is the bleeding caused by a coagulation disorder or by a surgical bleeder?

All clotting parameters are evaluated. If clotting factors, such as platelets, are deficient, they are replaced. An activated clotting time (ACT) helps to determine if additional protamine is needed. If the ACT is normal, fresh frozen plasma may be administered to provide additional clotting factors. Aminocaproic acid (Amicar), which causes diffuse clotting, may also be considered a pharmacologic modality. As therapy is initiated to control the bleeding, clotting studies are repeated to determine the success of treatment. Any oozing from incision sites is carefully watched, marked, and possibly treated with Surgicel.

If bleeding continues despite normal coagulation studies, a surgical bleed is probable. Some bleeders seal themselves off without major intervention. Excessive bleeding, however, must be treated promptly. Rapid infusion of blood, plasma, and plasma expanders may be required to prevent severe depletion of circulatory volume until the patient is returned to surgery for exploration and repair.

INFECTION

Infections following coronary artery surgery can be systemic, operative, or involve any body system.[53] A variety of organisms—bacterial, fungal, viral, and protozoal—have been found to be responsible for these infections. It is crucial that meticulous attention be paid to aseptic technique while performing all care routines, especially wound care, suctioning, and maintenance of invasive lines.

A low-grade fever is common following surgery, but a temperature elevation beyond 24 to 48 hours after surgery is unusual and requires specific attention. Antipyretics, steroids, tepid baths, and cooling blankets may be used in addition to culturing blood, urine, and sputum for potential infectious agents.

A serious complication requiring aggressive treatment is a sternal wound infection and mediastinitis. This is a potentially life-threatening complication because of the possibility of extension to the heart, aorta, and suture lines. Initial signs and symptoms of infection may be mild but progress to purulent drainage and dehiscence. When this condition occurs, drainage, debridement, and irrigation of the mediastinum are required. Following debridement, wound care is usually extensive and appropriate antibiotic therapy is critical.

Rehabilitation

Rehabilitation and discharge planning commence actively once the patient is transferred out of the intensive care unit.[54,55] At this point most patients are performing self-care, are capable of getting up and rising freely, and are ready to regain their independence. As preparation for discharge begins, limitations or restrictions on daily activities should be considered and discussed.

Medication schedules, rest, gradual exercise, sexual activity, diet therapy, coping mechanisms, and psychologic adjustments are vital elements in long-term recovery and must be addressed. Most patients are greatly concerned about returning to work and need guidance in setting realistic goals and time-frames. Because the underlying pathology of atherosclerosis has not been eliminated by surgery, modification of risk factors is preeminent in trying to achieve the healthiest life-style possible following discharge.

NURSING CARE PLAN FOR ADULT POSTOPERATIVE CARDIOTHORACIC SURGERY PATIENT*

Problem

Potential for dysrhythmias related to surgery, hypoxia, acid-base imbalance, electrolyte imbalance.

Goal

1. Patient will remain free from dysrhythmias.
2. If dysrhythmias occur, patient will remain hemodynamically stable.

Interventions

1. Anticipate potential dysrhythmias based on past medical history, surgery, and/or medications. Observe closely for PVCs following CABG.
2. Monitor ECG continuously with alarms on at all times.
3. Monitor lab values for factors that predispose patient to arrhythmias. Maintain serum K+ and Po_2 within normal limits.
4. Keep AV sequential pacemaker connected to patient with pacing wires for use prn. Monitor pacemaker when in use.
5. Document dysrhythmias and patient response to the dysrhythmia.
6. Notify physician of dysrhythmias and patient response to them.
7. Administer antiarrhythmic drugs and assist with cardioversion and defibrillation as needed.
8. Auscultate for pericardial friction rub.

Problem

Potential for compromised respiratory status related to anesthesia, surgery, immobility, pain, and mechanical ventilation.

*Modified from the Cardiothoracic Unit, Duke University.

Goal

Patient will achieve and maintain adequate respiratory status.

Interventions

1. Anticipate potential respiratory problems related to past medical history (smoking, COPD, asthma).
2. Maintain patent airway at all times and administer oxygen as prescribed. Verify ventilator settings frequently.
3. Auscultate lung fields for change in breath sounds or presence of pleural rub and adventitious sounds.
4. Monitor ABGs and CXR as indicated and prescribed. Notify physician of abnormal ABG results.
5. Perform endotracheal suction every 2 hours, and prn to control secretions while patient is intubated; document character of secretions.
6. Turn patient every 2 hours and percuss when extubated. Encourage coughing and deep breathing.
7. Use pain medications as necessary to promote increased pulmonary toilette.
8. Care for pleural chest tubes in accordance with unit policy. Assess and document drainage, air leaks, etc.

Problem

Potential for hemodynamic instability related to surgical insults, postoperative bleeding, dysrhythmias, hypothermia, low cardiac output.

Goal

Patient will achieve and maintain hemodynamic stability.

Interventions

1. Anticipate CV problems related to past medical history (PVD, stroke, clotting disorders).
2. Monitor hemodynamic parameters every 30 minutes to 1 hour prn (CO, CVP, O_2 Sat, PAD, PCWP, LAP). Monitor blood pressure and MAP every 15 minutes. Correlate cuff pressures with monitor every 4 hours.
3. Monitor ECG continuously and notify physician of dysrhythmias; treat dysrhythmias as indicated and ordered. Consider possibility of ischemia or infarction.
4. Assess peripheral perfusion (pulses, capillary refill temperature) every hour and prn.
5. Assess sensorium for changes.
6. Monitor UO every hour; notify physician if less than 30 cc per hour.
7. Monitor CT drainage every hour and notify physician for CT output greater than 100 cc per hour.

Maintain patency of CT and monitor for signs and symptoms of cardiac tamponade.

8. Administer vasoactive medications and colloid volume as needed.

9. Monitor body temperature every hour and maintain normothermia using overbed warmer, blankets, Tylenol, tepid bathing, or cooling blanket as ordered.

10. If pain is present, differentiate between incisional pain or angina, and treat accordingly.

Problem

Potential for fluid and electrolyte imbalance related to cardiopulmonary bypass, diuretic therapy, blood transfusions, or postoperative bleeding.

Goal

Patient will achieve and maintain adequate fluid and electrolyte status:

a. electrolytes within normal ranges
b. adequate output and fluid balance

Interventions

1. Anticipate potential fluid and electrolyte problems related to O.R. course (serum K^+ depletion, increased urine output).

2. Monitor I and O every hour, and specific gravity every 2 to 4 hours.

3. Monitor hemodynamic parameters continuously.

4. Inspect for signs of hypervolemia and hypovolemia (skin turgor, edema, neck vein distention).

5. Monitor lab values for signs of hypervolemia or hypovolemia (PO_2, BUN, creatinine, Hct) and for abnormal electrolyte values.

6. Administer/restrict fluids as indicated.

7. Administer diurectics and supplemental electrolytes as indicated.

8. Weigh daily.

Problem

Potential for altered neurologic status/neurologic deficit related to anesthesia, hypoxia, medication, cerebral microemboli, low cardiac output, ICU environment.

Goal

Patient will achieve and maintain normal neurologic function.

Interventions

1. Assess neurologic function and compare to preoperative neurologic function (pupils, grips, movement, orientation).

2. Reorient to time and place frequently. Use clocks, radios, and TVs as appropriate.

3. Document and notify physician of neurologic deterioration and abnormality.

4. Monitor laboratory values that affect neurologic status as indicated, including ABG, electrolytes, liver enzymes, and ammonia level.

5. Administer volume and pharmacologic agents to increase cardiac output and cerebral perfusion as indicated.

6. Use soft restraints to protect from injury; keep side rails up at all times.

7. Organize nursing care to provide periods of rest and sleep.

8. Allow family visits as frequently as possible.

9. Reduce noxious stimuli (loud conversations, lights, etc.).

Problem

Potential GI distress related to surgical stress, NPO, and medications.

Goal

Patient will exhibit normal GI functioning.

Interventions

1. Anticipate GI problems from patient history (coping mechanisms, response to stress, ulcers, bleeding tendencies).

2. Check patency of NG tube and connect to low suction or gravity. Note characteristics of drainage. Check gastric pH every 2 hours, administer antacids as per protocol.

3. Keep NPO until NG tube is discontinued/withdrawn and bowel sounds are present.

4. Assess for signs of abdominal tenderness or distention.

5. Note return of flatus, character or absence of BM.

Problem

Potential for altered coagulation caused by surgical insult, heparin/protomine, hypothermia, hemolysis.

Goal

Normal hemostasis will be maintained.

Interventions

1. Monitor VS and hemodynamic pressures continually.

2. Strip chest tubes upon arrival to ICU and notify physician of excessive drainage.

3. Obtain hemoglobin and hematocrit studies every 2 to 4 hours and prn.

4. Evaluate clotting studies (PT, PTT, platelets, ACT) and administer coagulation agents as prescribed.

5. Have fresh blood and blood products available and administer as needed and as prescribed.

Problem

Potential for infection related to surgical incisions, invasive lines, and intubation.

Goals

Patient will remain free from infection.

Interventions

1. Monitor temperature per unit policy. Notify physician of temperature greater then 38.5° C and administer antipyretics as prescribed.
2. Assess all surgical sites and invasive lines every shift and prn for signs or symptoms of infection. Change fluid and IV lines per protocol.
3. Monitor for signs of UTI (urinary tract infection) and perform Foley catheter care every shift.
4. Monitor for signs of pulmonary infection and perform pulmonary toilette frequently.
5. Maintain strict aseptic technique when performing all patient care.
6. Notify physician if signs or symptoms of infection develop. Assist with drawing cultures.
7. Administer antibiotics adhering closely to time schedule.

Problem

Potential for pain and discomfort related to incisions, chest tubes, and invasive lines.

Goals

Patient will receive adequate pain control.

Interventions

1. Assess patient for pain (signs, symptoms, and verbalization by patient) and need for pain medication.
2. Attempt to identify cause of pain.
3. Use comfort measures to relieve pain (positioning, back rubs).
4. Medicate for pain or discomfort as prescribed. Evaluate effectiveness.
5. Medicate for pain 1 to 1½ hours before pain-producing procedures.

Problem

Potential for anxiety in patient's family because of critical condition of patient, ICU environment, and restricted visiting hours.

Goal

Family will be supported emotionally during patient's ICU stay.

Interventions

1. Prior to family's first postoperative visit, orient them to environment (monitors, ventilator, IVs, drainage tubes, alarms).
2. Explain ICU visitation policy and rationale to family.
3. Encourage verbalization of anxiety and questions.
4. Obtain family emergency phone number and offer unit phone number to family.
5. Provide comfort measures for family as appropriate.

Cardiac Transplantation
RECIPIENT SELECTION

Cardiac transplantation is indicated for end-stage cardiac disease that is refractory to conventional medical and surgical therapy. Advanced functional disability (NYHA Class IV) is present and the probability of surviving more than 6 months to 1 year without transplantation is exceedingly low. Patients selected for transplantation who have not been transplanted at the end of one year have a mortality rate of 100%, indicative of the severity of cardiac disease.[56] Most patients being considered for transplantation are being treated for congestive heart failure, low cardiac output, and major dysrhythmias (see box below).

Cardiac transplantation is most likely to benefit a selected group of people who meet the above description.[57-59] Criteria have evolved to identify patients with significant potential for physical recovery and emotional rehabilitation.

Selection guidelines vary slightly from institution to institution, but cardiac transplantation is generally contraindicated by the following:

1. Advanced age—Patients should be no older than 55. Older patients are less likely to survive the surgery and do not tolerate prolonged immunosuppression well; specifically, resistance to infection may be lower and side effects from steroid therapy may develop.
2. Any other system disease—Any system disease or dysfunction will compromise recovery and predispose the transplant patient to postoperative morbidity. Some renal, pulmonary, or hepatic insufficiency

---

PRIMARY DIAGNOSIS LEADING TO END-STAGE MYOCARDIAL DISEASE

Coronary artery disease
Idiopathic cardiomyopathy
Valvular disease with ventricular dysfunction
Post-traumatic aneurysm
Congenital heart disease

may be present in association with end-stage cardiac disease, but it must be considered reversible with restoration of a healthy, normally functioning heart.

3. Insulin-dependent diabetes—This condition would be exacerbated in the presence of postoperative steroid therapy. There is also the tendency for prolonged wound healing and thus an increased risk of infection as in the case of anyone suffering from diabetes.

4. Severe pulmonary hypertension—Chronically elevated pulmonary vascular resistance would interfere with the performance of the donor heart. The healthy right ventricle could not acutely adjust to the workload needed to overcome the excessive resistance. Ultimately, this would lead to right ventricular failure and early postoperative death.

5. Recent pulmonary embolism or infarction—These disorders increase the patient's susceptibility to disastrous pulmonary infections when immunosuppressive therapy is initiated. In addition, surgery is contraindicated because of the risks of anticoagulation necessary for cardiopulmonary bypass.

6. Infection—Selection for cardiac transplantation cannot be considered in the presence of infection. The recipient's immune system would not be able to oppose the progression of an existing infection while at the level of immunosuppression required immediately following surgery.

7. Emotional instability and poor compliance to medication schedules—Severe psychosocial problems and noncomplaint behaviors are major negative factors affecting the outcome of cardiac transplantation.

Patients are identified by analyzing the results from the history and physical exams, hematologic studies, x-rays, and cardiac catheterization. If the cardiologist and surgeon conclude that further therapy cannot benefit the patient and that no contraindicating factors are present, cardiac transplantation may be offered to the patient as a treatment alternative.

PREPARATION OF PATIENT AND FAMILY

Candidates for transplantation are placed on a waiting list until a suitable donor is found. A computer communication system makes long distance donor heart information available. Donor organs may be removed and transplanted locally or removed in the city where the death occurred and transported via aircraft to the waiting site. During the days or sometimes weeks of waiting, the transplant candidates may be hospitalized or may remain out-patients, whichever is warranted by their condition.

Members of the transplant team work together to allay apprehension and to support the patient and family during this preoperative waiting phase. The goal in working with the patient and family is preparing them with realistic and factual information about the procedure, intensive care, recovery, and long-term follow-up. They must understand that the surgery is not a final solution and that rigid routines will follow. Adherence to diet and exercise should be stressed and the impact of maintenance immunosuppressive therapy should be clearly described. The associated risks of rejection and infection must be carefully explained to enable the patient and family to fully comprehend and knowingly pursue the option of transplantation.

DONOR SELECTION AND ORGAN PROCUREMENT

Criteria for donor selection are clearly delineated.[57,58] The individual being considered must have irreversible and total cessation of brain function. Most donors are victims of traumatic accidents resulting in neurologic catastrophes such as closed head injuries or intracranial hemorrhage. The potential donor should be no older than 35 years and have no prior history of cardiac disease. There should be no significant injury to the myocardium such as might result from severe chest trauma or prolonged cardiopulmonary resuscitation. In addition, there must be no evidence of infection; potential donors must be screened for hepatitis and HTLV-III.

Once the family has consented to organ donation, cardiac status should be thoroughly evaluated. A detailed history is obtained and a physical examination is performed with special attention to cardiovascular functioning. The heart should be of normal size and shape by x-ray and in normal sinus rhythm. Murmurs, ventricular hypertrophy, or evidence of ischemia would prevent organ donation. Cardiac catheterization *may* be performed to validate suspected abnormalities or rule out coronary artery disease. If the donor heart is deemed suitable for transplantation, and if there is size, weight, and ABO compatibility with a recipient, plans for organ procurement can begin.

Aggressive management of donors awaiting organ retrieval is essential. Most are cared for in the intensive care unit, where they can be mechanically ventilated and monitored. In addition to supportive measures, particular attention is paid to the maintenance of serum electrolytes and the prevention of hypotension. Volume replacement with colloids or crystalloids and vasopressors is often necessary to maintain a blood pressure adequate for organ perfusion. Diabetes insipidus, resulting from the loss of pituitary function, is treated with vasopressin to control diuresis. Loss of thermoregulatory mechanisms may require the use of warming techniques to maintain an acceptable body temperature. Prophylactic antibiotics are started along with an immunosuppressive agent to prepare the organ for transplantation.

OPERATIVE PROCEDURE

If the donor heart is to be removed and transplanted on site, two adjacent operating rooms are used. In one the donor heart is excised, with great care taken to preserve the sinoatrial node, passed through a series of cooled saline baths, and transferred into the recipient's room, where it is sutured in place.

In many instances the donor heart needs to be transported to another center for transplantation, in which case the organ is removed and placed in a saline solution at 4° C, which provides topical hypothermia during transport. An ischemic time for the donor heart of less than 4 hours generally results in satisfactory organ functioning.

Regardless of the donor's geographic vicinity, the operative procedure is not started on the recipient until the donor heart has been directly evaluated by a member of the donor transplant team. Once the donor heart is deemed suitable, anesthetic induction of the recipient begins.

In orthotopic cardiac transplantation, the heart of the recipient is exposed via median sternotomy, and standard cardiopulmonary bypass is initiated. The venae cavae are tied off and the aorta is clamped. The heart of the recipient is excised leaving a right and left atrial cuff and the atrial septum and great vessels are transected distal to the semilunar valves.[58,59,60]

Implantation of the new heart begins with anastomosis of the left and right atria. Approximation and suturing of the aorta and pulmonary artery follows (Fig. 15-12). At the conclusion of the grafting, it is critical to evacuate air from the heart chambers. When the transplanted heart warms and normothermia returns, the heart often resumes a spontaneous rhythm; if it does not, electrical defibrillation is required. Although the conduction system of the donor heart is normal and has been preserved, epicardial pacing wires are attached and mediastinal chest tubes are inserted prior to closing the chest. An isoproterenol infusion is commonly used and titrated to ensure an acceptable cardiac rate and output.

A second technique for performing transplantation is a heterotopic or piggy-back approach.[57] In this instance the donor heart is placed in the right chest without removing the recipient heart. Anastomosis should allow blood to flow through both hearts.

POSTOPERATIVE CARE

Whether orthotopic or heterotopic, the immediate postoperative care of the transplant patient is very similar to that of any patient who has undergone open heart surgery except for immunosuppression and isolation. The patient is transferred from the operating room to a protective isolation environment in the cardiothoracic intensive care unit. A complete assessment is performed on admission. Mechanical ventilation is provided via an endotracheal tube for approximately 24 hours. Continuous monitoring of ECG, arterial and pulmonary artery pressures, and chest drainage is part of routine postoperative care. One or two peripheral IV lines are usually in place to provide venous access for volume replacement and drug administration. The transplant patient will also have a urinary catheter to straight drainage and a nasogastric tube to low intermit-

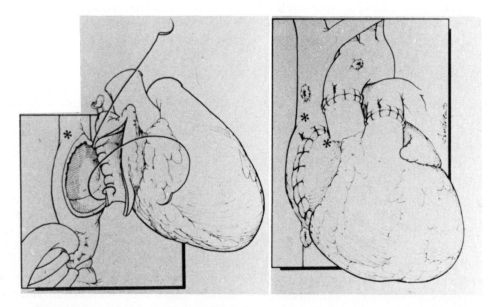

FIG. 15-12. Anastomosis of donor heart. (From Cooley, D.: Techniques in cardiac surgery, Philadelphia, 1984, W.B. Saunders Co.)

tent suction or gravity. A major postoperative goal is to direct meticulous attention to maintaining the sterility of all invasive lines, tubes, or catheters, and to discontinue them as soon as possible to avoid the hazards of infection.

Problems that may diminish the cardiac output may occur in the acute postoperative phase, including bleeding, tamponade, and rhythm disturbances. Bleeding disorders following heart transplantation may be intensified by a preexisting coagulopathy caused by liver dysfunction or as a result of extensive suture lines. Excessive chest tube bleeding necessitates the infusion of blood products to provide coagulation factors and protamine sulfate or aminocaproic acid to reverse anticoagulation agents. Additional surgery may be required for patients who do not respond to medication and colloid infusions.

There is a risk of tamponade following heart transplantation. Because of the gradual enlargement of the pericardium that occurs in the preoperative period to accommodate the hypertrophied heart, blood may accumulate following transplantation and may be concealed within the enlarged pericardium. Drainage of this blood is promoted by turning the patient from side to side every 2 hours with frequent milking and gentle stripping of the chest tubes to maintain patency. If the accumulation of blood is rapid, it will severely compromise cardiac output and is an emergency requiring surgical evacuation.

Rhythm disturbances are uncommon in the initial postoperative period if the donor heart has not been subjected to prolonged ischemia. An interesting change that may be noted on the ECG following transplantation is the appearance of activity from the SA node of the recipient's right atrium in addition to the new heart's cardiac complex.[61] The impulse, a *p* wave from the atrial remnant, has no clinical significance because it is not conducted along the electrical pathway, but it should be noted, however, in order to avoid confusion in rhythm interpretation.

Following cardiac transplantation there is no direct neural control of the conduction system; instead, the adrenal hormones exert primary stimulation by exciting the adrenergic receptors of the donor myocardium with circulating catecholamines. Epicardial pacing wires, placed on the right atrium and ventricle, may be used to override atrial or junctional bradycardia in the early postoperative period if necessary. An isoproterenol infusion may also be used for 3 to 5 days to augment the cardiac output with its chronotropic and inotropic properties. It is important to remember that the denervated heart may be less sensitive to certain drugs, such as atropine and digoxin, than the innervated heart and that all drugs given to affect cardiac performance should be given in balanced doses and closely monitored.

DRUG THERAPY

Vasoactive drugs—Inotropic support and vasodilator therapy may be indicated in the early postoperative period as in the case of any patient who has undergone open heart surgery.

Antibiotics. A broad-spectrum antibiotic is given before surgery and continued postoperatively until the patient is extubated and invasive lines are removed. Because of the immunosuppressed state, prolonged prophylactic antibody therapy is avoided to reduce the risks of fungal overgrowth and the emergence of resistant bacteria. Should signs and symptoms of infection occur, antibiotics specific for the causative organism may be resumed.

Digoxin. The patient may have been on digoxin prior to surgery, but the drug is usually not required after transplantation.

Anticoagulants. Anticoagulation is unnecessary following orthotopic transplantation unless it is prescribed for a specific postoperative development.

Diuretics. Patients who suffered from severe cardiac failure preoperatively may require a diuretic for several days after surgery. Lasix, administered intravenously, is the initial drug of choice.

Antacids. As a means of preventing steroid-induced gastric irritation and ulceration, an antacid regimen may be employed. Cimetidine (administered intravenously and then orally) provides additional protection and is begun immediately following surgery.

Narcotics. As long as the patient remains intubated, small doses of morphine or other narcotics are needed to facilitate ventilation and to control pain. Once extubated, the patient should have access to some type of oral pain medication and he or she receives vigorous pulmonary toilette and increases physical activity.

IMMUNOSUPPRESSION

When a foreign material gains access to the tissues of a living host, an immune response is mounted to destroy the offending material and maintain hemostasis. This can occur either by humoral immune response or by cell-mediated response, both of which are derived from different kinds of lymphocytes.

Lymphocytes are continually exported from the bone marrow and differentiate into T-lymphocytes and B-lymphocytes; exposure to an antigen stimulates their production. B-lymphocytes, responsible for humoral immunity, enlarge, divide, and develop into plasma cells. The mature cells produce and secrete antibodies or antigen-specific immunoglobulins. The result of the antibody-antigen reaction may be a precipitate, or an agglutination that renders the cell easily phagocytosed, or neutralization of the

TABLE 15-1. Commonly used immunosuppressive drugs in cardiac transplantation

Drug	Azathioprine (Imuran)	Corticosteroids	Antithymocyte Globulin (ATG)	Cyclosporin-A (Sandimmune)
Use in trans- plantation	1962	1963	1966	1978
Mechanism of action	An antimetabolite that competes for and blocks specific receptors, affecting DNA and RNA synthesis and interfering with protein synthesis	Anti-inflammatory properties reduce capillary permeability, vasodilatation, and edema. May also inhibit movement of T-lymphocytes from blood to graft	ATG prepared by immunizing rabbits or horses with human lymphocytes. ATG binds to T-lymphocytes and reduces their number in circulation	Acts selectively on T-lymphocytes, preventing production of effector T-cells. Does not depress bone marrow as antimetabolites. Immune activity is specific and reversible
Metabolism	Liver	Liver	—	Liver
Side effects	Bone marrow depression resulting in leukopenia, thrombocytopenia, and anemia. Recovery of bone marrow usually rapid following withdrawal or reduction of drug Pancreatitis Muscle-wasting in conjunction with steroids	Infection Diabetes GI bleeding Cushingoid appearance Steroid psychosis	Chills, fever Hypotension Anaphylaxis	Nausea, vomiting, diarrhea Hepatotoxicity (elevated liver enzymes, alkaline phosphatase) Nephrotoxicity (elevated BUN, creatinine, decreased creatinine clearance) Hypertension
Dosage	Loading: 3-5 mg/kg/day p.o. Maintenance: Tapered to 1-2 mg/kg/day p.o.	Loading: Methylprednisone 0.5 g IV intraoperative, with 125 mg IV × 3 doses Maintenance: Prednisone 100 mg p.o. every day. Taper to 0.2-0.5 mg/kg/day by 2 months	Loading: Rabbit ATG 2 mg/kg/day IM every day × 3 days, then every other day × 3 days Equine ATG 10-15 mg/kg/day p.o. Maintenance: Adjusted according to circulating T-cells	Loading: 14-18 mg/kg/day p.o. IV dose ⅓ of oral dose Maintenance: 5-10 mg/kg. Adjusted to maintain therapeutic levels
Other	Maximum tolerated level judged by absence of complications. WBC should be maintained at 500/mm³	High doses of steroids are started when rejection is diagnosed in attempt to save graft	Goal of therapy is to suppress circulating lymphocytes to less than 10% of normal (100/mm³). These are assessed daily and dose adjusted. Rises above therapeutic range herald impending graft rejection. T-cells will elevate without rejection (approx. 6 wk) and this immunologic monitoring is no longer sensitive	Blood should be drawn just before drug is given to determine trough level and 2-4 hours later to determine peak levels. Levels: Blood 250-800 mg/cc. Plasma 50-300 mg/cc. Drugs that affect CVA blood levels: (1) Cimetidine increases concentration; (2) Phenytoin, Rifampin, Phenobarbital decrease concentration
Acute rejection	Dose may be increased but in accordance with WBC, platelet count, and any clinical complications	Methylprednisone 1 g every day × 3 days	Repeat course of ATG	Dose may be increased but in accordance with serum levels and any clinical complications
Specific nursing care	Monitoring WBC and platelets Good oral hygiene	Anticipate multiple adverse effects of steroid therapy and plan care accordingly	Skin test prior to injection "Z" tract technique for IM injections Pain and inflammation from injection lessened by heat to site before and after injection, massage, exercise Tylenol and Benedryl prior to injection to minimize anaphylactic response	Careful attention to functioning of renal and hepatic systems Punctual lab drawing for trough and peak levels Awareness of effects from other drugs

toxin.[32] The humoral response produces vascular damage to the transplanted heart.

Sensitized T-lymphocytes, important in cellular immunity, are capable of attacking and destroying the invading antigen. Some T-lymphocytes are described as effector cells, which contain cytotoxic substances capable of accelerating antigen destruction. Damage to the heart from this response is made evident by platelet aggregation and thrombosis.

The goal of immunosuppression after cardiac transplantation is to prevent graft rejection without forfeiting the host's ability to ward off infectious diseases. Careful monitoring of the recipient's immune response and adjusting pharmacologic agents to maintain therapeutic drug levels become a central focus in postoperative management. Table 15-1 compares the four most common immunosuppressive drugs used today: azathioprine, corticosteroids, antithymocyte globulin, and cyclosporine A.[60,62,63,64]

Variations of immunosuppressive agents and protocols are currently in use. Conventional therapy includes corticosteroids, azathioprine (Imuran), and antithymocyte globulin (ATG) as adjuncts when there is evidence of rejection. Cyclosporine is a more selective immunosuppressive drug; current therapy involves concomitant use of only cyclosporine and corticosteroids. The dosage of steroids is tapered as soon as the patient can tolerate it, in an attempt to achieve the lowest possible maintenance dosage while reducing its multiple side-effects.

Isolation. Isolation is necessary to reduce the risk of transmitting infectious organisms via personnel, equipment, visitors, and others while the patient is severely immunosuppressed. Following surgery, the patient is transferred to a specially equipped isolation room and remains there until endomyocardial biopsy reports and drug levels indicate an adequate immune response. At that time isolation techniques are reduced and the patient's environment is made more natural.

In preparation for the heart transplant patient, the room is vigorously cleaned with a bactericidal agent and re-stocked with clean supplies. Many items necessary for patient care cannot be sterilized and therefore should be new or as clean as possible. All equipment (ECG machine, ventilator, x-ray machine) must be cleaned with a bactericidal agent before being taken into the isolation room. Traffic in the room is kept to a minimum, and everyone entering the isolation room (physicians, nurses, technicians, and family members) must undergo proper scrubbing and gowning procedures.

Infection. Infection constitutes the major cause of morbidity and mortality among cardiac transplant recipients.[56] Early after transplantation when immunosuppressive therapy is intense, patients are at risk for infection from opportunistic organisms. According to Stanford University Medical Center statistics, bacterial infections are most common (89%), followed by viral infections (63%). Fungal (17%), protozoan (3%), and nocardia (3%) infections also occur. There seems to be a broad range of involvement, but the majority of infectious episodes (50%) affect the pulmonary system. Herpes simplex, cytomegalic virus, septicemia, and urinary tract infections also appear frequently.

With the high incidence of infection and its potentially devastating results, meticulous surveillance is necessary to detect early signs and symptoms of an infectious process. Surgical incisions, chest tube and pacemaker wire sites, and invasive lines are carefully evaluated for redness, oozing, or inflammation. Aseptic technique is closely adhered to for any invasive procedure. Following extubation, vigorous pulmonary toilette is initiated as are daily chest films. Routine sputum and urine cultures are obtained, and the patient's temperature is carefully watched.

Successful management of an infection requires aggressive diagnosis and specific follow-up. Immunosuppressive agents required to control the infection should be administered at the lowest possible dosage necessary for graft survival. Once the causative organism has been identified, appropriate antibiotics are administered and the infectious process is evaluated until it is resolved.

REJECTION

Rejection is an expected phenomenon within the first months following cardiac transplantation; approximately one half of patients will have had a rejection episode by 1 month and 80% by 3 months.[58] However, with early diagnosis and treatment, rejection is usually reversible.

Careful monitoring for signs and symptoms of rejection is extremely important after transplantation. Physical examination to detect the development of graft dysfunction is ongoing.[62,63] Clinical findings indicative of rejection in-

STANFORD CARDIAC TRANSPLANTATION INFECTIOUS EPISODES (DECEMBER 15, 1980—MARCH 31, 1984)	
Pulmonary	50
Septicemia	20
Urinary tract	20
Mediastinum	8
Herpes simplex	30
Herpes zoster	10
CMV	23
Retinitis	2
Empyema	1
CNS	1

From Stanford Cardiac Transplantation Statistics, Stanford University Medical Center, Stanford, Calif., 1984, Unpublished data.

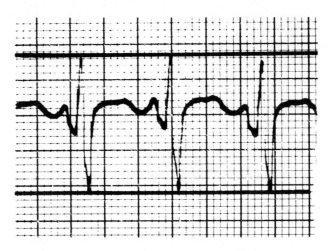

FIG. 15-13. ECG voltage is determined by the height of the QRS and is measured by: (1) identifying the maximum positive deflection and maximum negative deflection; (2) counting the millimeters or small blocks in the height of the complex; and (3) assessing and totaling voltage similarly in leads I, II, III, and V_5. A 20% or greater decrease in QRS voltage is suggestive of rejection.

clude: (1) development of S^3 or S^4; (2) weakness, fatigue, malaise; (3) hypotension; (4) reduced cardiac output; (5) decreased urinary output; (6) weight gain; (7) changes in peripheral perfusion; (8) elevated CVP; and (9) dysrhythmias such as premature atrial contractions, atrial fibrillation, or atrial flutter. A 20% decrease in the QRS voltage on the ECG is a nonspecific though highly sensitive indicator of graft rejection (Fig. 15-13). ECGs are performed every 4 to 6 hours during the initial postoperative period and daily thereafter or as the patient's condition dictates.

Immunologic monitoring is a central component in detecting the onset of rejection. The laboratory technique of determining circulating T-lymphocytes is among the most useful. Elevation of these levels has been found to correlate with rejection episodes, and daily evaluation is recommended.

The most reliable indicator of cardiac rejection is histologic examination of the endomyocardium via serial biopsies. These are begun approximately 5 to 6 days after surgery and then weekly thereafter according to the patient's status (Fig. 15-14). Histologic appearance of the myocardium undergoing rejection is characterized by intracellular and interstitial edema, lymphocyte infiltration, and vascular congestion (Fig. 15-15). Severe rejection can cause irreversible damage to the myocardium as a result of cellular degeneration, necrosis, and interstitial hemorrhage.

Acute rejection is managed by altering and augmenting immunosuppressive therapy. Treatment with ATG and methylprednisone is instituted, and Imuran or cyclosporine doses are increased accordingly. Strict protective isolation may be initiated because the intensity of immunosuppression poses greater risks of major infection.

Retransplantation may be an alternative for recurrent and intractable acute rejection because of irreversible and devastating injury to the myocardium. It may also be indicated for coronary atherosclerosis of the transplanted heart following episodes of chronic rejection.

PSYCHOLOGIC SUPPORT

It is difficult to generalize about the impact cardiac transplantation has on individual patients and their families. Psychologic conflict may arise from (1) fear of death; (2) fear of morbidity; (3) the idea of receiving another person's heart following his or her death; (4) unfamiliar people, environment, and procedures; (5) isolation; (6) lack of privacy; (7) mood-altering steroids; (8) lifelong dependency on drugs; (9) alterations in life-style; and (10) financial concerns. A major objective in the postoperative period is to minimize any psychologic injury and assist the patient and family to work through such conflicts. This entails using other family members, friends, and hospital support systems and services. Providing consistent caregivers helps to establish a relationship amenable to open communication and resolution of anxieties or fears. Maintaining as "normal" an isolation environment as possible may prevent the feeling of total isolation; the availability of magazines, books, get-well cards, family pictures, a telephone, and a television reinforces the patient's self-image and prevents boredom during hospitalization. Long-term psychologic support and consultation may be necessary, depending on the individual's adjustment to the transplantation.

SURVIVAL AND REHABILITATION

According to Stanford's statistics, survival rates following cardiac transplantation have steadily improved during the

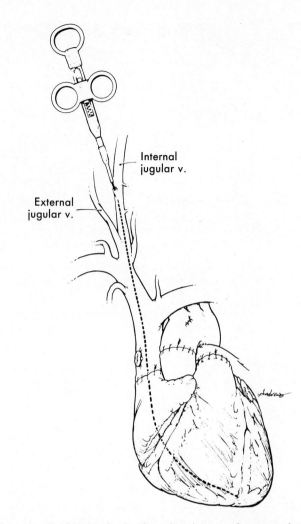

Internal
jugular v.

External
jugular v.

FIG. 15-14.   A myocardial biopsy obtains direct histologic confirmation of rejection. A bioptome is passed to the apex of the right ventricle and specimens of tissue are removed. PVCs may occur as the instrument comes in contact with the endocardium. The procedure is performed under local anesthesia in the operating room or cardiac cath lab with relatively few risks. (From Cooley, D.: Techniques in cardiac surgery, Philadelphia, 1984, W.B. Saunders Company.)

last 12 to 15 years.[56,65,66] After the first year of the program, the 1-year survival rate was 22%, increasing to 62% after 7 years, and 88% after 15 years. The 5-year survival rates have also improved. Successful rehabilitation of survivors continues. Of Stanford's transplant population, 84% of 1-year survivors are rehabilitated at 1 year. Most have returned to some form of work, but others have chosen to retire.

The Artificial Heart
HISTORICAL PERSPECTIVE

The concept of implanting a mechanical device to replace the heart dates back to the 1800s. In 1812 Julien-Jean-Cesar La Gallois noted that "if one could substitute for the heart a kind of injection (of arterial blood), one would

succeed easily in maintaining alive indefinitely any part of the body." In 1928 Dale and Schuster, working in England, developed the first diaphragm heart pump.

In the early 1900s, inspired by his sister-in-law's severe valvular heart disease, Charles Lindbergh began to study methods of cardiac support. In 1935, 8 years after his solo transatlantic flight, Lindbergh and associate Alex Carrell developed a pump oxygenator and demonstrated the feasibility of total body perfusion with a pump.[67-69]

In 1934 Michael DeBakey developed the first roller pump for assisted circulation, and in 1953 Gibbon introduced his heart-lung machine for clinical use.[70] This machine was first used successfully to close an atrial septal defect under direct visualization. In 1957 Drs. Akutsu and Kolff, working at the Cleveland Clinic, presented the first

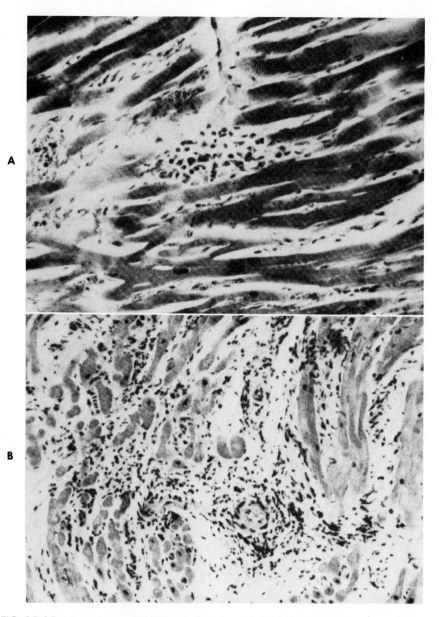

FIG. 15-15. Endomyocardial biopsies show A, mild, B, moderate, and C, severe rejection. Histologic findings consist of myocardial edema and cellular infiltrate. (From Cooper, D., and Lanza, R.: Heart transplantation, Boston, 1984, MTP Press Limited.)

total artificial heart model.[71] It was made of polyvinyl chloride and had two ventricles and four valves. The heart, powered by an extracorporeal compressed air source, was orthotopically inserted into the chest of a dog and maintained the dog's circulation for 90 minutes. From the late 1960s to the early 1970s, Kwan-Gett and associates developed several pneumatically driven hearts, one of which kept a dog alive for 50 hours.[72] In 1967 A. Kantrowitz first used the intraaortic balloon pump clinically as a method of partial support for the failing heart.[73]

EARLY HUMAN IMPLANTS

In 1969 at the Texas Heart Institute, a 47-year-old man with diffuse coronary artery disease and left ventricular dyskinesia had surgery for his disease. Unable to wean the patient from cardiopulmonary bypass, Cooley implanted a total artificial heart designed by Liotta.[74,75] This total artificial heart (TAH) was powered by a bedside pneumatic pump. After 64 hours of use, the cardiac prosthesis was replaced with a cardiac transplant. The patient died 32 hours later from pneumonia.

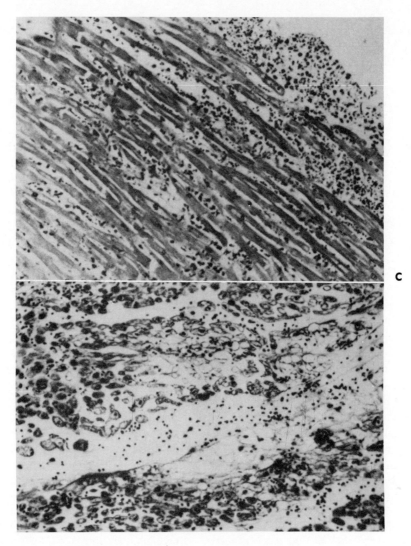

c

FIG. 15-15, cont'd. For legend see opposite page.

In 1981 a second TAH implantation was performed by Cooley.[76] A 36-year-old man suffered cardiac arrest after a three-vessel coronary artery bypass graft (CABG) operation. The patient was returned to the operating room, and a pneumatically driven Akutsu TAH was inserted. After 54 hours of circulatory support by the TAH, cardiac transplantation was performed; the patient died 10 days later from multiple organ failure.

The Jarvik total artificial hearts have been the most widely used and publicized. The Jarvik-3 was introduced by its developer, Dr. Robert Jarvik, at the University of Utah in 1972. This model showed advanced design, improved blood component compatibility, and an increased cardiac output.[77] This model was further modified, and in 1981 Olsen, Jarvik, and Kolff implanted a Jarvik-5 TAH into a calf. The calf lived for 268 days. The Jarvik-5 was built larger to meet the cardiac output needs of the calf. A scaled-down model, the Jarvik-7, with a stroke volume of 104 milliliters, was built to fit into the human mediastinum.[78]

COMPLICATIONS

Problems associated with total artificial hearts have included design, fabrication, implantation, coagulation, hemolysis, thrombus formation, disseminated intravascular coagulation, and respiratory distress syndrome.[77] The cause of death in animals implanted with total artificial hearts is often infection. Other complications observed in animals with artificial heart implantations include thrombus, pannus, embolization, and mechanical failure.[79] Bacteria may lodge in the crevices of the inflow or outflow tracts, cre-

TABLE 15-2. Survival rates and causes of death in calves with artificial hearts (76 calves with utah tah, 1976-1980)

Time	No. Surviving
0-30 d	32
30-150 d (avg. 64 d)	35
Early deaths:	
Technical problems	
Bleeding	
Thromboembolic	
Infection	
>150 d (avg. 181 d)	9
Late deaths:	
Pannus	5
Hemorrhage	2
Endocarditis	1
Severe LV failure	1

ating an endocarditis-like picture.[77] Septic emboli may be spread to other organs and may compromise blood flow in the TAH. Antimicrobial agents are usually ineffective in the treatment of bacteria harbored in a foreign body. Potentially successful treatment for infection requires surgical replacement of the infected part of the TAH and long-term use of synergistic antibiotics.

Pannus is a dense, fibrous connective tissue similar to the intimal hyperplasia found in vascular grafts. This tissue has shown preference for growth on the inflow parts of the artificial heart in animal recipients.[80] This growth may cause an inflow obstruction similar to mitral stenosis. Calcification of the flexing diaphragm has been a serious problem in calves with the TAH, but postmortem examination of a human recipient showed no signs of calcification.[81] Mechanical failure is an infrequent cause of death in animals.[77] Table 15-2 lists survival rates and causes of deaths in calves.

MECHANICS OF THE MODERN ARTIFICIAL HEART

Alterations in structure and design of the TAH have slowly resolved some of these problems. The Jarvik-7 is a 20-year culmination of these alterations at the University of Utah; it is designed to provide maximum internal volume, accommodate space limitations within the adult human mediastinum, and eliminate turbulence, stagnation, and destruction of red blood cells.[77] The current heart consists of the ventricles, four prosthetic valves and Dacron connections that attach to the native atria, pulmonary artery, and aorta.

The ventricles are spherical and made of segmented polyurethane (Biomer), which provides a smooth thromboresistant surface. The outer housing of the ventricles is reinforced with Dacron mesh, and the base of each ventricle is composed of aluminum. Each ventricle is powered by pulsing air, separated from the circulating blood by a pliable diaphragm made of four layers of Biomer, with dry graphite between each layer to provide lubrication. This construction offers minimum resistance during systole and diastole.[77]

For insertion, Dacron-felt cuffs are sutured to the native atria and Dacron vascular prosthetic grafts are sewn to the native great vessels. Quick-connects, made of coated rigid polycarbonate segments, are found at the open ends of the Dacron connections and the total artificial heart. These quick-connects mold together and form an airtight seal between the artificial heart and the Dacron connections. Should ventricular or valvular malfunction occur, the quick-connects allow easy removal and replacement of the malfunctioning artificial ventricle. Four valves, consisting of clinical-grade pyrolitic carbon discs, ensure unidirectional blood flow through the artificial heart.

An external console, or heart driver, is connected to a source of air, electricity, and vacuum. Pulsed compressed air, at adjustable rates, provides the driving power for the TAH. The vacuum line is optional and appears to have minimum impact on chamber emptying during clinical trials.[67] The console has rechargeable batteries to supply energy in case of power failure. Presently, the console is large and weighs about 323 pounds. A smaller portable unit that may be carried on the shoulder is now under trial.[67] Reinforced polyurethane tubing, connecting the artificial heart to the console channels pulsed air in and out of the ventricles. This tubing, or drive line, exits the body through two stab wounds in the left periumbilical area. Teflon-felt skin buttons enhance tissue growth around the drive lines despite movement of the lines during patient activity. An abdominal belt assists in securing the drive lines.[75] One goal of artificial heart research is to develop a heart that is totally implantable, including a power source. Eliminating the drive lines, and thus the stab wounds they exit, would decrease the chance of infection. Also, eliminating the driving console would increase patient mobility and satisfaction with the prosthesis.

Pulsation of air in and out of the ventricles causes the diaphragm to expand and collapse. Air pulsed into the airspace under the diaphragm causes the diaphragm to expand and create systole. Movement of the diaphragm in systole is influenced by pneumatic driving pressures, end-diastolic blood volumes, and systemic vascular resistance. Console driving pressures must be strong enough to overcome pulmonary and peripheral vascular resistance as well as the higher than normal resistance of the artificial valves. Diastole is the collapse of the diaphragm that allows blood to pass through the remnant atria and prosthetic valves into the ventricle. The diaphragm collapses in direct proportion to the volume of blood that enters the ventricle.[77]

A characteristic of the artificial heart is its sensitivity to preload and afterload. As inflow pressure changes, stroke volume of the prosthesis changes following the Frank-Starling law of the heart. Atrial inflow pressures of 5 to 7 mm Hg increase cardiac output to 12 to 13 L/minute, and inflow pressures of 10 to 15 mm Hg increase cardiac output to 12 to 13 L/minute without adjustment of heart rate.[78] Maximum stroke volume of each Jarvik-7 ventricle is 104 ml. Once this capacity is reached, changes in heart rate are required within the console to improve cardiac output.

PATIENT SELECTION

The University of Utah and the Humana Audubon Hospital in Louisville, Kentucky, have been awarded permission from the Food and Drug Administration to implant the Jarvik-7 TAH. The experimental nature of this project demands strict patient-selection criteria. Two subgroups of patients are presently being considered for TAH implantation. The first group consists of patients who, after corrective cardiac surgery, cannot be weaned from cardiopulmonary bypass. If medications and intraaortic balloon pumping fail to promote weaning from the bypass machine and the patient had given previous consent, the TAH may be implanted.[82]

The second group includes patients with chronic, nonoperative, end-stage congestive heart failure or cardiomyopathy. The New York Heart Association Class IV criteria for myocardial dysfunction must be met for 8 weeks, in which time no evidence of recovery should be seen. These criteria include a cardiac ejection fraction of less than 18% with a cardiac index less than 1.5 L/minute/m² and congestive symptoms at rest not relieved by medications or amenable to surgical correction (such as valvular lesions, ventricular aneurysm, or patent ductus arteriosus). Percutaneous myocardial biopsy must confirm that no inflammatory disease from which a patient may recover is present. The patient must also display slow deterioration with no response to medical therapy.[82] Patients eligible for transplant who begin to deteriorate while waiting for a donor heart may be considered candidates for artificial heart implantation.[67]

Patients must be at least 18 years old and have a stable home situation with a reliable person to provide the necessary home care. They must live less than 45 minutes from the hospital where the implantation is to be performed to ensure proper follow-up care. Patients must have an understanding of their disease process and the ability to understand the mechanism of the artificial heart drive system. They must demonstrate a stable psychologic profile, stable coping mechanisms, and be free of drug and alcohol ad-

diction. Finally, they must be free of any additional major medical problems and show no evidence of infection.[82]

An 11-page consent form with the procedure, risks, and benefits is explained to the patient. The consent must be signed by the patient once and then signed again 24 hours later to reaffirm the patient's intent. Routine open-heart preparations are performed before the artificial heart implantation takes place.

IMPLANTING THE ARTIFICIAL HEART

A median sternotomy incision allows the chest to be opened and the heart visualized. The patient is given anticoagulants, and cannulation is done for cardiopulmonary bypass. Total body hypothermia is used to decrease the metabolic rate of the patient during full cardiac arrest.[77] Once adequate cardiopulmonary bypass flow is established, the aorta is cross-clamped and the venae cavae are occluded with tourniquets. Because the ventricles are being replaced, no cardioplegia is needed.[83] After the heart is arrested, the right and left ventricles are excised at the atrioventricular groove.[77] The pulmonary artery and aorta are divided above the valves, and the leaflets of the pulmonic and aortic valves are excised. The four Dacron connections are sewn into the remnant atria, pulmonary artery, and aorta. Graft material that is too long may cause kinks and disturb the hemodynamic function of the prosthetic ventricle.[77] Therefore the grafts are individually measured to ensure proper fit. Plastic quick-connect rings at the bottom of the atrial cuffs and the vessel grafts should meet with the quick-connect rings on the artificial ventricles and vessels.

Before the ventricles are placed, the sutures of the anastomoses are tested by injecting blood under physiologic pressure through covers that snap into the quick-connect rings. The anastomoses are observed for signs of leaks. After the covers are removed, the artificial ventricles are snapped into the quick-connect rings of the atria and ventricles and pressure drive lines are brought through two separate stab wounds in the skin. Air that was in the ventricles before implantation is aspirated by a venting port in the ventricle. The ventricles are primed with blood, the clamps and tourniquets on the aorta and venae cavae are released, and pumping is initiated. Heart rate and driving pressures are gradually increased and the patient is weaned from cardiopulmonary bypass. Left atrial and pulmonary artery pressure lines are brought out through the chest wall. Two mediastinal chest tubes are placed and exited through the chest incision as usual, and the medial sternotomy is closed.

POSTOPERATIVE COURSE

A normal postoperative open-heart course is expected but often not realized. Hemodynamic pressures are obtained

TAH CHARACTERISTICS

No HIS bundle
No beta receptors
No coronary arteries
No myocardial blood flow

from the pulmonary artery and the left atrial pressure lines. The TAH is without a conduction system and myocardial blood flow (see box above). Therefore monitoring, which takes place outside the TAH, includes the monitoring and treatment of arrhythmias, standard cardiopulmonary resuscitation, use of a pulmonary artery catheter, and administration of support catecholamine drugs.[77] The ECG is flat. Nurses caring for the patient must monitor drive line pressures and use the cardiac output monitoring device.

Driving pressures from the pneumatic console are individualized to each ventricle and adjusted to the lowest value that completely empties the ventricle. The wave form representative of TAH functioning has characteristic landmarks for the onset of mechanical systole, ventricular ejection and aortic blood flow, the end of ventricular ejection, peak driving pressure and end of mechanical systole, and complete emptying and filling of the ventricles.

Underdriving is the incomplete emptying of the end-diastolic blood volume. Clinically, systemic venous overload and/or pulmonary vascular overload are seen in an underdriving situation. Increased end-diastolic volume, afterload increase, development of outflow obstruction and stiffening of the diaphragm because of rupture or calcification may cause underdriving. *Overdriving* is an excessive pressure for the volume of blood that needs displacing. A change in vascular pressure, systemic resistance, systemic hypovolemia, or inadequate delivery of blood to the affected ventricle may cause overdriving.[77]

Cardiac output is used to assess the function of the TAH. The COMDU unit, used with the Jarvik-7, was developed to provide continuous monitoring of stroke volume and cardiac output.[84] A pneumotachometer and a computer sense the rate and amount of ventricular air exhausted during diastole. The airflow signal integrated over time gives the amount of air displaced during diastole, which equals the blood volume entering the ventricle at that time. A calibration constant is used to convert the amount of ventricular air displaced into volume in milliliters, or stroke volume. The computer then calculates cardiac output. An average of eight diastolic periods is taken over 30 seconds and displayed on the COMDU. High filling pressures of the ventricles may cause high exhaust air flow rates. Low flow rates may be the result of hypovolemia or valvular inflow obstruction.[77]

Several patients have received the Jarvik-7 TAH. Barney Clark, D.D.S., at age 62, was the first person to receive an artificial replacement heart. He survived 112 days with the TAH in place. Death was attributed to peripheral vascular collapse caused by *Clostridium difficile* pseudomembranous enterocolitis.[67] Clark's postoperative course was complicated by several noncardiac problems, including acute tubular necrosis, persistent nosebleeds, and respiratory insufficiency.[67,85] Only one postoperative complication was related to the artificial heart. A fracture of the major strut of the prosthetic mitral valve requiring replacement of the left ventricle occurred on the thirteenth postoperative day.[83]

Improvements necessary for future artificial hearts include efficiency, cosmetic and psychologic concerns, and reduction of cost.[81] Experiments with the pneumatically driven hearts placed heterotopically without removing the failing heart are under way. Heterotopic placement of an artificial heart may allow the diseased heart to partially recover.[67] Several other artificial hearts, developed at medical facilities around the world, are not potentially implantable.

REFERENCES

1. Kent, K., and others: Improved myocardial function during exercise after successful percutaneous transluminal coronary angioplasty, N. Engl. J. Med. **306:**441, 1982.
2. Dotter, C.T., and Judkins, M.P.: Transmittal treatment of arteriosclerotic obstruction: description of a new technique and a preliminary report of its application, Circulation **30:**654, 1964.
3. Gruentzig, A.R., Senning, A., and Siegenthaler, W.E.: Nonoperative dilatation of coronary artery stenosis: percutaneous transluminal coronary angioplasty, N. Engl. J. Med. **301:**61, 1979.
4. Kent, K.M.: Indications for transluminal coronary angioplasty, Circulation **72**(6):166, 1985.
5. Holmes, D.R., and others: Return to work after coronary angioplasty: a report from the National Heart, Lung, and Blood Institute Percutaneous Transluminal Coronary Angioplasty Registry, Am. J. Cardiol. **53:**48C, 1984.
6. Pasternak, R.C., and others: Scanning electron microscopy after coronary transluminal angioplasty of normal canine coronary arteries, Am. J. Cardiol. **45:**591, 1980.
7. Simpson, J.B., and others: Coronary transluminal angioplasty in human cadaver hearts (abstract), Circulation **58**(suppl. II): 11, 1978.
8. Block, P.C., and others: Morphology after transluminal angioplasty in human beings, N. Engl. J. Med. **305:**382, 1981.
9. Block, P.C., and others: Transluminal angioplasty: correlation of morphologic and angiographic findings in an experimental model, Circulation **61:**778, 1980.
10. Stack, R.S., and others: Interventional cardiac catheterization, Invest. Radiol. **20:**333, 1985.
11. Zarins, C.K., and others: Arterial disruption and remodeling following balloon dilatation, Surgery **92:**1086, 1982.
12. Block, P.: Percutaneous transluminal coronary angioplasty: role in the treatment of coronary artery disease, Circulation **72**(6):161, 1985.

13. Mock, M.B., and others: Percutaneous transluminal coronary angioplasty (PTCA) in the elderly patient: experience in the National Heart, Lung, and Blood Institute PTCA Registry, Am. J. Cardiol. 53:890, 1984.

14. Cowley, M.G., and others: Acute coronary events associated with percutaneous transluminal coronary angioplasty, Am. J. Cardiol. 53:12C, 1984.

15. Kelsey, S.F., and others: Effect of investigator experience on PTCA, Am. J. Cardiol. 53:56C, 1984.

16. Corros, G., and others: Percutaneous transluminal coronary angioplasty: report of complications from the National Heart, Lung, and Blood Institute PTCA Registry, Circulation 67:723, 1983.

17. Holmes, D.R., and others: Restenosis after percutaneous transluminal coronary angioplasty (PTCA): a report from the PTCA Registry of the National Heart, Lung, and Blood Institute, Am. J. Cardiol. 53:77C, 1984.

18. Scholl, J.M., and others: Recurrence of stenosis following percutaneous transluminal coronary angioplasty, Circulation 64 (suppl. IV):193, 1981.

19. Jutzy, K.R., and others: Coronary restenosis rates in a consecutive patient series one year post successful angioplasty, Circulation 66: (suppl. II) 331, 1982.

20. DeWood, M.A., and others: Prevalence of total coronary occlusion during the early hours of transmural myocardial infarction, N. Engl. J. Med. 303:897, 1980.

21. Buja, L.M., and Willerson, J.T.: Clinicopathologic correlates of acute ischemic heart disease syndromes, Am. J. Cardiol. 57:343, 1981.

22. Ridolf, R.L., and Hutchins, G.M.: The relationship between coronary artery lesions in myocardial infarction: ulceration of atherosclerotic plaques precipitating coronary artery thrombosis, Am. Heart J. 93:468, 1977.

23. Reimer, K.A., and Jennings, R.B.: The wavefront phenomenon of myocardial ischemic cell death. II. Transmural progression of microsis within the framework of ischemic bed size (myocardium at risk) and collateral flow, Lab. Invest. 40:633, 1979.

24. Reimer, K.A., and others: The wavvefront phenomenon of myocardial ischemic cell death. I. Myocardial infarct size versus duration of coronary occlusion in dogs, Circulation 56:786, 1977.

25. Chazov, E.I., and others: Intracoronary administration of fibrinolysin in acute myocardial infarction, Ter Arkh 48:8, 1976.

26. Rentrop, K.P., and others: Initial experience with transluminal recanalization of the recently occluded infarct-related coronary artery in acute myocardial infarction: comparison with conventionally treated patients, Clin. Cardiol. 2:92, 1979.

27. Schroder, R., and others: Intravenous short-term infusion of streptokinase in acute myocardial infarction, Circulation 67:536, 1983.

28. Oliva, P.B., and Breckenridge, J.C.: Arteriographic evidence of coronary spasm in acute myocardial infarction, Circulation 56:366, 1977.

29. Sharma, G.V.R.K., and others: Thrombolytic therapy, N. Engl. J. Med. 302:1268, 1982.

30. Ganz, W.: Intracoronary thrombolysis in acute myocardial infarction, Am. J. Cardiol. 52:92, 1983.

31. Ganz, W., and others: Intracoronary thrombolysis in evolving myocardial infarction, Am. Heart J. 101:4, 1981.

32. Price, S., and Wilson, L.: Pathophysiology: clinical concepts of disease processes, New York, 1982, McGraw-Hill Book Co.

33. Harlan, B., Starr, A., and Harwin, F.: Manual of cardiac surgery, New York, 1980, Springer-Verlag.

34. Sadler, D.: Secondary interventions: care of the person undergoing heart surgery. In Sadler, D., editor: Nursing for cardiovascular health East Norwalk, Ct., 1984, Appleton-Century-Crofts.

35. Jurado, R.: Preoperative evaluation and care. In Litwak, R., and Jurado, R., editors: Care of the cardiac surgical patient, East Norwalk, Ct., 1982, Appleton-Century-Crofts.

36. Tyra, D., and others: Left main equivalents: results of surgical therapy, Circulation 64 (suppl. II):7, 1981.

37. Franch, R.: Cardiac catheterization. In Hurst, W., and others, editors: The Heart, New York, 1978, McGraw-Hill Book Co.

38. Behrendt, D., and Austen, W.: Patient care in cardiac surgery, Boston, 1980, Little, Brown & Co.

39. Hug, C.: Anesthetic agents and the patient with cardiovascular disease. In Ream, A., and Fogdall, R., editors: Acute cardiovascular management, Philadelphia, 1982, J.B. Lippincott Co.

40. Hug, C.: Anesthesia and the patient with cardiovascular disease. In Hurst, J., editor: The Heart, New York, 1985, McGraw-Hill Book Co.

41. Bland, J., and Lappas, D.: Anesthesia for cardiac surgery. In Litwak, R. and Jurado, R., editors: Care of the cardiac surgical patient, East Norwalk, Ct., 1982, Appleton-Century-Crofts.

42. Fogdall, R.: The post-bypass period. In Ream, A., and Fogdall, R., editors: Acute cardiovascular management, Philadelphia, 1982, J.B. Lippincott Co.

43. Ream, A.: Cardiopulmonary bypass. In Ream, A., and Fogdall, R., editors: Acute cardiovascular management, Philadelphia, 1982, J.B. Lippincott Co.

44. Litwak, R., and Giannelli, S.: Open intracardiac operations employing extracorporeal circulation. In Litwak, R., and Jurado, R., editors: Care of the cardiac surgical patient, East Norwalk, Ct., 1982, Appleton-Century-Crofts.

45. Sladen, R.: Management of the adult cardiac patient in the intensive care unit. In Ream, A., and Fogdall, R., editors: Acute cardiovascular management, Philadelphia, 1982, J.B. Lippincott Co.

46. Litwak, R.: Analysis, maintenance, and support of cardiac function after cardiac surgery. In Litwak, R., and Jurado, R., editors: Care of the cardiac surgical patient, East Norwalk, Ct., 1982, Appleton-Century-Crofts.

47. Kehler, C., and Fogdall, R.: Inotropic agonists and antagonists. In Ream, A., and Fogdall, R., editors: Acute cardiovascular management, Philadelphia, 1982, J.B. Lippincott Co.

48. Laver, M.: Lung function following open heart surgery. In Litwak, R., and Jurado, R., editors: Care of the cardiac surgical patient, East Norwalk, Ct., 1982, Appleton-Century-Crofts.

49. Glabman, S., von Albertini, B., and Litwak, R.: Renal failure in cardiac surgery. In Litwak, R., and Jurado, R., editors: Care of the cardiac surgical patient, East Norwalk, Ct. 1982, Appleton-Century-Crofts.

50. Budabin, M.: Neurologic complications of cardiac surgery. In Litwak, R., and Jurado, R., editors: Care of the cardiac surgical patient, East Norwalk, Ct., 1982, Appleton-Century-Crofts.

51. Hill, J., Rodvien, R., and Mielke, C.: Bleeding and hemorrhage complications. In Litwak, R., and Jurado, R., editors: Care of the cardiac surgery patient, East Norwalk, Ct., 1982, Appleton-Century-Crofts.

52. Ellison, N.: Coagulation evaluation and management. In Ream, A., and Fogdall, R., editors: Acute cardiovascular management, Philadelphia, 1982, J.B. Lippincott Co.

53. Meyers, B., and Jurado, R.: Infections associated with open heart surgery. In Litwak, R., and Jurado, R., editors: Care of the cardiac surgical patient, East Norwalk, Ct., 1982, Appleton-Century-Crofts.

54. Smith, D.: Nursing care of the surgical cardiac patient: intermediate phase to discharge. In McCauley, K., and Brest, A., editors: McGoon's cardiac surgery: an interprofessional approach to patient care, Philadelphia, 1984, F.A. Davis Co.

55. Tantum, J.: Nursing care: long-term adaptation after cardiac surgery. In McCauley, K., and Brest, A., editors: McGoon's cardiac surgery:

an interprofessional approach to patient care, Philadelphia, 1984, F.A. Davis Co.

56. Stanford Cardiac Transplantation Statistics, Stanford University Medical Center, Stanford, Calif., 1984, Unpublished data.

57. Cooper, D., and Lanza, R.: Heart transplantation, Boston, 1984, MTP Press Limited.

58. Baldwin, J., and others: Technique of cardiac transplantation. In Hurst, J., editor: The Heart, New York, 1985, McGraw-Hill Book Co.

59. Shumway, N.: Recent advances in cardiac transplantation, Transplant. Proc. 75:1223, 1983.

60. Lower, R., and others: Cardiac transplantation: should its use be expanded? In McCauley, K., and Brest, A., editors: McGoon's cardiac surgery: an interprofessional approach to patient care, Philadelphia, 1985, F.A. Davis Co.

61. Thornby, D.: Cardiac transplantation: nursing during the acute period, Dimens. Crit. Care Nurs. 2:212, 1983.

62. Shinn, J.: Heart transplantation. In Woods, S., editor: Critical care nursing, New York, 1983, Churchill Livingstone.

63. Harwood, D., and Cook, D.: Cyclosporine in transplantation, Heart Lung 14:520, 1985.

64. Painvin, G., and others: Cardiac transplantation: indications, procurement, operation, and management, Heart Lung 14:484, 1985.

65. Jamieson, S., and others: The heart transplant: eleven year progress report, Vasc. Surg. 15:225, 1981.

66. Heimbecker, R., and others: Heart and heart-lung transplantation, Heart Lung, 13:1, 1984.

67. Devries, W., and Joyce, L.: The artificial heart, Clin. Symp. 35, 1983.

68. Dale, H.H., and Schuster, E.H.J.: A double perfusion pump, J. Physiol. 64:356, 1928.

69. Lindbergh, C.: History of medicine, New York, 1976, Simon & Schuster, Inc.

70. Gibbons, H.J., Jr.: Application of a mechanical heart and lung apparatus to cardiac surgery, Minn. Med. 37:171, 1954.

71. Akutsu, T., and Kolff, W.J.: Permanent substitutes for valves and hearts, Trans. Am. Soc. Artif. Intern. Organs 4:230, 1958.

72. Kwan-Gett, C.S., Wy, Y., and Collan, R.: Total replacement artificial heart and driving system with inherent regulation of cardiac output, Trans. Am. Soc. Artif. Intern. Organs 15:245, 1969.

73. Kantrowitz, A., and others: Initial clinical experience with intra-aortic balloon pumping in cardiogenic shock, JAMA 203:113, 1968.

74. Cooley, D.A., and others: Orthotopic cardiac prosthesis for 2 staged cardiac replacement, Am. J. Cardiol. 24:723, 1969.

75. Cooley, D.A.: Heart substitution: transplantation and total artificial heart, the Texas Heart Institute experience, Artif. Organs 9:12, 1985.

76. Cooley, D.A., and others: Total artificial heart in two-staged cardiac transplantation, Cardiovasc. Dis. Bull., Texas Heart Institute 8:305, 1981.

77. Quall, S.J.: The artificial heart, Heart Lung 14:317, 1985.

78. Cowart, V.: Improvements predicted in artificial heart by 1990, JAMA 253:2621, 1985.

79. Murshita, J.: Current major problems in long survival animals with pneumatic total artificial hearts, Trans. Am. Soc. Artif. Intern. Organs 29:530, 1983.

80. Kessler, T.R.: Elimination of predilection sites for thrombus formation in the total artificial heart—before and after, Trans. Am. Soc. Artif. Intern. Organs 24:532, 1978.

81. DeVries, W.C., and others: Clinical use of the total artificial heart, NEJM 310:273, 1984.

82. Joyce, L.D., and others: Response of the human body to the first permanent implant of the Jarvik-7 total artificial heart, Trans. Am. Soc. Artif. Organs 29:81, 1983.

83. Patterson, P.: Replacing a human heart, AORN J. 37(2):183, 1983.

84. Wilshaw, P., and others: A cardiac output monitor and diagnostic unit for pneumatically driven artificial hearts, Artif. Organs 8:215, 1984.

CHAPTER 16

Coronary Artery Disease in the Elderly

Kathleen Gainor Andreoli
Leigh Anne Musser
John C. McMahon

In the past two decades, the number of persons over the age of 65 in the U.S. population has grown twice as fast as the rest of the population. This dramatic growth rate will continue to accelerate throughout the first three decades of the next century. As a result, the elderly, who represent over 11.7% of the population today, will comprise nearly 21% by the year 2030. At the same time, the elderly population itself is growing older: those age 75 and over, the "old-old," are expected to represent the majority of the elderly by 2040 and those age 85 and older, the "very-old," will increase seven-fold.[1] The *graying of America,* as it has been termed, will present significant challenges to the health care system by increasing the demand for health services in a fiscally austere health care market and shifting the primary focus of health care away from acute, curative care to long-term chronic care and rehabilitation. The potential impact of the growing number of elderly on the health care system can be extrapolated from the current situation in which those over age 65 account for 40% of acute hospital bed days, 30% of the total health care budget, and 50% of federal health expenditures.[2] Thus with an elderly population twice as large as it is today, by the twenty-first century the U.S. health care system will be increasingly oriented to the needs of the older consumer.

Although the majority of elderly consider themselves in excellent or good health,[3] nearly 80% have one or more chronic health problems, including heart conditions, hypertension, arthritis, and sensory impairments.[4] As a result of chronic disease, nearly one half of noninstitutionalized elderly people are limited in some way in their usual activities.[5]

This chapter focuses on one of the major chronic diseases in the elderly, coronary artery disease, with specific reference to differences in incidence, risk, symptomatology, treatment, and management of problems between older and younger population subgroups.

EPIDEMIOLOGY OF CORONARY ARTERY DISEASE IN THE ELDERLY

Data on the epidemiology of heart disease from the Framingham longitudinal study indicate that approximately 40% of individuals between the ages of 65 and 74 and 50% of those 75 and over have one or more cardiovascular disease.[6] The most prevalent form of heart disease among the elderly, coronary artery disease, affects approximately one half of men age 70 and older.[7] For women, the incidence of coronary artery disease is lower at all ages.[8] However, the difference in incidence between men and women decreases with age.

Like most chronic diseases, coronary artery disease is more debilitating for the elderly than for the young because of the existence of concurrent functional limitations of other organ systems, which often lead to activity restrictions or disability. According to the Bureau of the Census,[9] approximately 25% of men and 22% of women over age 65 have some activity limitation as a result of heart conditions, with an additional 6% of men and 11% of women having some activity limitation attributable to the increased cardiac workload imposed by hypertension.

Heart disease is the leading cause of death among those 65 and older, followed by cancer, stroke, influenza and pneumonia, and arteriosclerosis.[10] Age-associated physiologic decline in all organ systems and the interaction of coronary artery disease with other disease processes are, in part, reasons that the mortality rate from coronary artery disease is much higher for the elderly than for the young. The relationship between heart disease mortality and age is clear: death from heart attacks and stroke doubles each decade after age 30[11] and approximately 70% of sudden cardiac deaths occur among those 65 and older.[12]

In short, whether characterized as morbidity, disability, or death, coronary artery disease is more prevalent and has a greater impact on the health status and quality of life of the elderly than it does on the young.

RISK FACTORS AND PREVENTIVE STRATEGIES

A number of the major risk factors for coronary heart disease in younger populations (see Chapter 3) are also significant risk factors for older individuals. These factors include hypertension, high dietary levels of salt, long-term/heavy smoking, and lack of exercise. Obesity, one of the major preventable risk factors in younger age groups, does not appear to be significant in the elderly. Indeed, a number of studies have revealed higher coronary mortality in older adults at low relative weights.[13-15] There are data, however, suggesting that a history of previous obesity may be a more important risk factor for the elderly than existing obesity.[16] Total cholesterol levels and diabetes seem to decrease in importance with age (although when broken into components, low-density lipoproteins (LDL) remain a significant risk factor and high-density lipoproteins (HDL) a significant protective factor for coronary heart disease).[6,8,13] For older women, menopause may also be a risk factor, although its association with heart disease is not well understood.

A number of physical conditions that are often present in elderly individuals also increase their risk of heart disease. These include infection, anemia, pneumonia, recent surgery, fever, diarrhea, malnutrition, circulatory overload, hypoglycemia, and drug-induced and noncardiac illnesses such as renal disease and prostatic obstruction.[17]

Hypertension

Hypertension is the major controllable risk factor for coronary artery disease in the elderly.[6,18] Among older individuals, elevated blood pressure has been associated with accelerated arteriosclerosis and increased myocardial work, both of which may contribute to cardiac failure. As in all age groups, systolic pressure is more uniformly associated with cardiovascular disease in the elderly than is diastolic pressure.[6,19,20] Evidence from the Framingham Study indicates that among individuals aged 55 to 74, the risks of cardiovascular death for those with systolic pressures at or above 160 mm Hg with diastolic pressures below 95 mm Hg are almost twice as high for men and five times as high for women than for normotensive men and women.[21]

There is no uniform definition for hypertension, and accepted standards continue to change. Although elevated blood pressure and systolic hypertension are more prevalent in the elderly population,[22] the Framingham investigators concluded that "normal" blood pressure does not increase with age and that the standards for hypertension should remain the same regardless of age.[6] If hypertension is defined as a systolic blood pressure of 160 mm Hg or greater and diastolic blood pressure at 95 mm Hg or greater (as defined by the World Health Organization), then between 40% and 50% of individuals over age 65 are hypertensive.[18,23-25] Another 7% have isolated systolic hypertension, defined as systolic pressure greater than 160 mm Hg, accompanied by diastolic pressure less than 90 mm Hg. The prevalence of isolated systolic hypertension increases with age after age 55, with a greater rate of increase among older women than men.[21]

Attempts to reduce high blood pressure in the "young-old", those aged 60 to 70, are fairly common and have demonstrated success.[20,23,26] Treatment of hypertension in individuals over age 75 remains controversial.[18,20] There is little evidence to suggest that reduction of blood pressure in adults over age 75 provides any substantial benefit.[27]

Indeed, some studies suggest that treatment of high blood pressure in the elderly should be tapered off as patients approach age 75 and that no new treatment should begin after that age.[28,29] One problem with attempts at reducing blood pressure in older individuals arises in those who have cerebrovascular disease, dementia, or evidence of myocardial ischemia. Because vessels that have been permanently narrowed by the deposition of plaque often require a minimum driving pressure to maintain adequate perfusion to the brain or heart, an aggressive reduction in blood pressure may negatively affect these patients.[30]

One criterion for initiating hypertensive therapy in the older patient is the presence of congestive heart failure,[18] which may be seen as evidence that the metabolic demands of the heart are not being met. When management of blood pressure is deemed appropriate and necessary, intervention should focus on those hypertensive risk factors that have a behavioral component, such as overweight, dietary sodium, smoking, and diabetes mellitus. In addition, meditation, relaxation therapy, and other efforts to help the hypertensive older person control stress may be beneficial.[31]

For older individuals, drug therapy should be prescribed only if behavioral modification programs fail.[18] It is important that renal function assessment, diabetic testing, and urinalysis precede administration of any drugs. Drug therapy may consist of daily doses of diuretics or beta-blocking agents, either alone or in combination with diuretics.[30] Because elderly patients are more sensitive to volume depletion and sympathetic inhibition, and thus are more prone to hypotension than younger patients, antihypertensive treatment should be initiated with smaller-than-usual doses.[32] Patients with chronic obstructive airway disease should not be treated with beta-blockers because bronchial dilatation depends on a beta-receptor mediated reaction, and elderly patients with chronic obstructive airway disease may experience respiratory distress when given a beta-adrenergic blocking drug.[30] The Joint National Commission on Detection, Evaluation, and Treatment of High Blood Pressure recommends that isolated systolic hypertension in most elderly patients should be treated with dietary sodium restriction and weight reduction, if necessary. Treatment with drugs, if deemed appropriate, should lower systolic blood pressure, with caution, to a goal of 140 to 160 mm Hg and, if this level is well-tolerated and there are no side effects, to below 140 mm Hg.[32]

Diet

Although obesity is not significantly correlated with coronary artery disease in the elderly, a number of nutritional factors contribute to both hypertension and heart disease in this population. For one, older individuals, who have a history of high dietary fat and cholesterol intake may have a higher risk of heart disease mortality.[33] As discussed previously, LDL remains a significant risk factor for heart disease in the elderly and HDL is a significant protective factor, as for all age groups. Although high sodium intake is not singularly associated with hypertension in the elderly, reduction of dietary sodium has been shown to reduce high blood pressure in these individuals.[33] Sodium restriction is often recommended for elderly patients with hypertension or symptomatic heart disease. Restricted cholesterol intake may be advisable in elderly diabetics, and weight reduction in the obese elderly may also lower blood pressure.

Cigarette Smoking

For the population as a whole, an estimated one third of all cardiac deaths are associated with cigarette smoking.[34] For the elderly, the relationship between smoking and heart disease has not been clearly established, principally because of the lack of substantive research. One study revealed a positive correlation between cigarette smoking (both current and total lifelong consumption) and the presence of ischemic heart disease (presence of angina and/or documented history of cardiac infarction and/or abnormal ECG reading) in individuals over age 65[13] and concluded that "cigarette smoking is the only one of the commonly demonstrable risk factors for ischemic heart disease which can be positively identified in the elderly." Another study found that elderly smokers had a 52% higher risk of coronary mortality than nonsmokers.[35] In the Framingham study, although no significant relationship was found between cigarette smoking and the *incidence* of cardiovascular disease in individuals over age 55, there was a significant relationship between smoking and cardiovascular *mortality*.[6] Although the relationship between cigarette smoking and cardiovascular disease is not well defined in the elderly, the documented physiologic effects of smoking are all detrimental in terms of cardiopulmonary function. Smoking decreases pulmonary exchange of oxygen and carbon dioxide, decreases oxygen-carrying capacity of blood because of carbon monoxide, and increases vascular resistance due to nicotine, which compromises the ability of the heart to pump. This is especially significant for the older heart, which typically has greater physiologic limitations than the younger heart.

Smoking-cessation has been associated with a rapid and sustained reduction in the risk of coronary disease in the elderly.[35] Thus the risk of heart disease for elderly people who used to smoke, even those who have not smoked for the last 1 to 5 years, is equivalent to that of nonsmokers. These data suggest that even among older persons who have smoked for decades, the effects of smoking on coronary artery disease risk are at least partly reversible within 1 to 5 years after quitting.[35]

Most smoking-cessation research has been conducted on younger age groups, thus safe and effective smoking reduction methods for the elderly have not been clearly established. Careful consideration of the older individual's physical and mental health status must be made before a smoking-cessation program is begun.

Physical Inactivity

The Framingham Study demonstrated that moderate exercise had a beneficial impact on the incidence of cardiovascular disease for all age groups.[6] A number of studies have demonstrated that more strenuous activity, usually referred to as physical training, enhances cardiopulmonary function in the elderly.[36-42] Cardiac improvement occurs at a lower threshold in the old than in the young, and exercise that elevates the heart rate by as little as 40% of the available range (maximal heart rate to resting heart rate) results in some cardiac conditioning.[43] Thus, for individuals in their 60s and older, there is a significant benefit from walking for 30 minutes at a speed sufficient to raise the heart rate to 100.

Major benefits from both moderate and more strenuous activity include reduced percentage body fat, improved physical work capacity, reduced systolic and diastolic blood pressures at rest, improved oxygen transport capacity, reduced blood lactase levels, increased total blood volume, and increased total hemoglobin content.[38,41] Although most exercise research has been conducted on men, Adams and deVries[36] found similar improvements in a group of older women, including improved physical work capacity and lower resting heart rate. No significant changes, however, were noted in blood pressure or oxygen consumption.

It is generally accepted that some level of physical activity is necessary in the elderly in order to maintain adequate circulation, mobility, and body fitness and that moderate physical activity is generally safe for healthy older individuals. Yet an estimated 57% of individuals 65 and older do not exercise on a regular basis.[44] All elderly individuals, regardless of their health status, should have a complete physical examination before beginning an exercise program. In establishing an effective activity regimen for the elderly patient, the individual's mobility, desires, and tolerance should be the most important considerations. The patient should be taught to "listen to his/her body signals." Specifically, physical activity should not produce shortness of breath, angina, or tachycardia. It has been suggested that a target heart rate be 75% of the predicted maximum heart rate (220 − age) for unsupervised activity in healthy older adults.[43,45]

Menopause

As discussed earlier, women at all ages have a lower incidence of coronary artery disease; however, the difference in incidence between men and women decreases with age. Endogenous female hormones are believed to provide some protective benefit from heart disease in premenopausal women, although the relationship is not clear. In older women, however, there is a decrease in estrogen production and a concommitant reduction in progesterone. Menopause has been associated with an increased risk for atherosclerosis.[46] In fact, data from the Framingham Study revealed that the incidence of heart disease among postmenopausal women aged 45 to 55 was more than 2.4 times that observed in premenopausal women the same age.[47] However, studies of the relationship between treatment with exogenous estrogen and heart disease incidence have not established a clear positive relationship between female hormones and heart disease. In the Framingham Study, the use of estrogen therapy after menopause was actually associated with a doubling in heart disease incidence.[47,48] In another study, however, estrogen therapy was found to protect postmenopausal women from nonfatal infarction and fatal coronary heart disease.[49] Clearly, there is a need for more research to define the role of estrogen therapy in coronary artery disease morbidity and mortality in postmenopausal women.

Preventive Strategies

Prevention of coronary artery disease and promotion of healthy heart habits among the elderly are controversial subjects. On the one hand, because coronary artery disease risk factors are established over time, preventive strategies in the elderly seldom yield the long-term health benefits or economic benefits (lives saved, increased productivity, or reduced medical expenditures) that can be attained in younger age groups. On the other hand, it has been shown that of all age groups, the elderly are more likely to be motivated to alter their behavior to improve their health, because they are concerned about health care costs and maintenance of functional independence.[4] Furthermore, any improvements in the quality of life are reason enough to pursue prevention and promotion programs in elderly populations.

A government report, *Healthy People,* set out the national goals for health promotion and disease prevention for the elderly as "not only to achieve further increases in longevity, but also to allow each individual to seek an independent and rewarding life in old age, unlimited by many health problems that are within his or her capacity to control."[50] The major difference in the focus of health promotion and disease prevention programs for older and younger individuals is the need to address preexisting chronic conditions when dealing with the elderly. In some cases, the most realistic goal is only to achieve partial functional independence. This should not deter the health team, however, from seeking ideal interventions for the older individual.

The paucity of norms and baseline data on health promotion and disease prevention programs in the elderly makes it difficult to design behavioral interventions appropriate and safe for large groups of elders. For example, little is known about the nutritional requirements of the elderly. The Recommended Dietary Allowances of the National Research Council classify all persons between ages 51 and 74 in a single category and those 75 and older in another, with recommendations based on studies conducted on younger subjects. The 1980 Recommended Dietary Allowances proposed that "energy allowances for this group (51 to 75) be reduced to about 90% of the amount required as a young adult and for persons beyond 75 years about 75 to 80% of that amount."[51] Furthermore the majority of data available on the impact of promotion/prevention activities are based on research on men, despite the fact that in older age groups, women outnumber men and there appear to be significant, functional sex-specific differences.

Common health promotion activities for the elderly include education about diet, exercise, smoking, safe use of drugs, proper foot care, maximizing dental function, safety promotion and injury prevention, and identifying sensory deficits.[19] Community services for the elderly—such as nutrition programs, homemaker and volunteer services, and adult daycare programs, which often incorporate exercise, nutrition, and social activities—are also health promotion activities in that they allow the elderly to remain optimally independent.

In general, large-scale prevention activities for the elderly focus on screening programs and influenza immunizations. Specific to coronary artery disease, there is one preventive strategy that has proven to be simple and cost-effective in identifying individuals at risk of cardiovascular disease: the Cardiovascular Risk Function Score, which uses baseline data from the Framingham Study.[8] This score is based on age, sex, family history, cigarette-smoking history, and laboratory values for lipid and glucose levels, blood pressure, and resting ECG. A multiple logistic formulation is generated from these values to estimate the conditional probability of a major cardiovascular event for any given set of risk factors. The Risk Function Score has been effective in detecting coronary risk factors in the elderly and in providing a reference for managing patients with hypertension, diabetes, hyperlipidemia, and excessive cigarette smoking.[52]

ASSESSMENT OF THE ELDERLY PATIENT

Although the health care provider's approach to the geriatric patient is similar to the approach for the younger patient, a number of factors make accurate comprehensive assessment more difficult in the older patient and require additional considerations and modifications to the process described in Chapter 4. First, the occurrence of multiple symptoms makes it difficult to identify a single underlying disease process. Second, 10% of the elderly have some form of intellectual impairment or dementia,[53] which may interfere with the effective communication of medical complaints or mask or modify many symptoms of disease. Third, impaired hearing and vision, affecting 22% and 15% of the elderly respectively, can interfere with effective communication during the evaluation process.[53] Fourth, many older individuals often expect increasing levels of illness to occur as a normal part of aging, a fact which is often tacitly accepted by the medical community and which may lead to the underreporting of potentially important symptoms.[46] Finally, the impact of polypharmacy, the interaction of numerous prescription and nonprescription drugs, may also alter the geriatric patient's ability to sense, interpret, and communicate during the health assessment process and may make evaluation difficult. In a recent study, approximately one third of individuals over age 65 took from four to six different drugs at a time, with 12% of hospital admissions among the sample resulting from drug-induced causes.[54] The elderly are more susceptible to both side effects and exaggerated therapeutic effects of drugs because of such factors as reduced muscle mass, decreased renal flow and creatinine clearance, lower levels of liver enzymes, and fewer brain neurons.[55]

In the interview and assessment process, patience, sensitivity to concerns of the individual, and an awareness of the environmental problems and unique medical conditions of the geriatric patient are paramount. It is essential to remain alert for these specific limitations and make adjustments in the environment and diagnostic procedures to assure effective evaluation. For example, lighting becomes a much more important factor when assessing older patients, who are more prone to visual impairment than the young. Possible problems may be alleviated by the use of well-lighted, glare-free examining rooms. The elderly patient with a hearing impairment will benefit from elimination of extraneous noises and from the interviewer using slower, more pronounced speech, and face-to-face conversation. In the older patient, limited mobility, flexibility, and thermoregulation necessitate attention to the discomforts of a hard examining table, cool room temperature, and a prolonged assessment session. Shorter, more frequent interview sessions may also assist the older patient with recall.[18,56] Reliance upon alternate sources of information such as relatives, friends, and other caregivers can enhance the evaluation process. When family members or friends accompany the older patient, however, it is important to address questions to the patient and rely on the second party only for substantiation or assistance. Too often, impatience leads one to question a younger family member or friend and ignore the older patient. A conscious effort must be made to eliminate the many "ageist" tendencies, such as talking down to the patient, calling the

patient by the first name, and dismissing symptoms and/or complaints as being attributable to "old age."

Functional Assessment

Assessment of functional ability should be the central focus of health evaluation for the geriatric patient. Determining whether individuals are able to perform their usual activities provides vital diagnostic information, facilitates design of appropriate treatment protocols, and enhances compliance. Effective functional assessment requires an understanding of the elderly patient's "typical day" activity patterns, recent changes in those patterns, and potential underlying causes of change.[57] Functional ability information—such as the fact that the patient cannot walk to the mailbox, make his or her bed, or go shopping without becoming fatigued—can prove especially useful in identifying limitations of cardiac origin. One measure of functional status is the Index of Activities of Daily Living (ADL), developed by Katz and colleagues.[58] This widely-used instrument identifies an individual's ability to perform a number of specific "usual" activities, such as feeding, dressing, ambulation, bathing, toileting, and grooming.

The second dimension of functional assessment in the elderly patient is assessment of cognitive function. This is especially important in older individuals because they are more vulnerable to functional impairment stemming from psychologic factors, interaction between physiologic and psychologic disorders, and potential mental problems caused by polypharmacy. A brief examination of mental status may be performed using such instruments as the Mini-Mental state examination or the Blessed Dementia Scale.[18]

The third dimension of the functional assessment should address sociologic, economic, and environmental factors. The geriatric patient's social and physical environment, including living arrangement (that is, alone, with spouse, with children), type of residence, proximity to essential services, safety of neighborhood, and proximity to and relationship with friends, family, and neighbors, is vital information for determining the mode of care, making decisions about institutionalization, and facilitating compliance.[59]

Health History

The elderly patient is more likely than the younger patient to have had past surgeries, medical treatments, and prescription drugs. Medication history is especially important because symptomatology in the elderly is often altered by the interactions of the variety of drugs taken. Obtaining this information can be facilitated by asking the patient to bring in a list of medications, which some pharmacies provide from their computerized records. Since many patients use more than one physician or pharmacy, however, a more thorough approach is to ask the patient to bring in all drugs currently being taken, both prescription and non-prescription, at the time of the appointment.

The presence of multiple pathologies in the elderly requires careful attention to each disease state, because many may mimic coronary artery problems. For example, ankle-swelling, frequently seen in older individuals, may be a symptom of heart failure or may also be caused by varicose veins, gravitational edema, or hypoproteinemia.[60]

Common complaints which are often related to cardiovascular disease in the elderly include: (1) confusion, dizziness, and blackouts; (2) ectopic beats described as palpations, butterflies, or skipped heart beats; (3) coughing and wheezing; (4) shortness of breath, especially after exertion or waking from sleep; (5) fatigue; (6) edema of the legs; and (7) chest pain.[52,61] Other less common complaints of elderly patients that may involve heart disease include: (1) acute abdominal pain (from liver enlargement and congestion); (2) anorexia; (3) insomnia (often caused by Cheyne-Stokes respiration or orthopnea); (4) vomiting; and (5) nocturia and urinary frequency.[52] Because the elderly often delay seeking medical attention, health practitioners often see advanced cases of heart disease in this age group.[62]

Physical Assessment

The physical evaluation procedures for the elderly patient should be the same as for the younger patient (see Chapter 4). There are, however, differences in interpretations of the findings since the norms and base values for the elderly vary from those in younger populations.

Temperature. Decreased body temperature is a manifestation of lower metabolic rate in the elderly. Thus, fever in the older patient may exist at a lower body temperature than in the young and hypothermia is an ever-present danger. Mean values ranging from 96.8 to 98.2 degrees Fahrenheit have been found in studies of body temperature in the well elderly.[63-65] In one study, 10% of the sample of older individuals had a deep body temperature less than 95.9 degrees Fahrenheit.[64] It is also important to recognize that body temperature continues to decrease with age among the elderly, with the oldest old having the lowest temperature.[65]

Pulse. When palpating the arterial pulse in the older adult, the evaluator will notice, especially with the distal pulses, that the arterial wall is hard to the touch. This finding is frequently associated with the age-associated rigidity of the arterial system, which decreases the shock-absorbing capacity of the arterial tree, causing the more abrupt pulse characteristic of the older adult.

Average resting heart rate decreases with age, ranging from 44 to 108 beats per minute.[61] The pulse may be either regular or irregular caused by the occurrence of sinus ar-

rhythmia which is common in the older adult. Maximal achievable heart rate decreases with age after age 25,[66] apparently because of reduced sympathetic activity,[67] or decreased numbers of receptors and/or receptor sensitivity.[68]

Cardiac reserve also declines with age.[69] Tachycardia, produced only under exertional situations (for example, exercise or emotional strain) in younger individuals, may exist at rest in older adults. The increased metabolic demands and shortened filling times associated with tachycardia that may be brought on by emotional strain, fever, exercise, or other benign conditions may precipitate heart failure in older people.[70] Cardiac recovery time increases with age,[69] with more time required for the heart rate, once elevated, to return to normal level. Thus many older people do not tolerate sudden physical or mental stresses.

Blood Pressure. As discussed in the Risk Factors section of this chapter, 40% to 50% of the elderly have blood pressures greater than 160 mm Hg systolic and/or 95 mm Hg diastolic. Differences of 10 to 15 mm Hg in systolic or of 5 mm Hg diastolic pressure between successive previous examinations are not unusual in the elderly and usually require no treatment or lifestyle changes.[52] Because arterial pressure typically rises on exertion in older individuals,[71,72] the physical and emotional strain associated with visiting the physician may in itself provoke significant increases in blood pressure.

Because of the cumulative detrimental effects of high blood pressure on the entire cardiovascular system, the Joint National Committee on Detection, Evaluation, and Treatment of High Blood Pressure recommends follow-up blood pressure measurements every six to nine months for adults over age 50 whose blood pressure is between 140/90 and 160/95.[32] The patient may consider buying a stethoscope and sphygmomanometer or a newer, automated device for home measurement of blood pressure. Variations in blood pressure should be communicated to the physician by the patient who measures his or her own pressure.

Auscultation. Auscultatory findings in the elderly may be unique. An irregular pulse is relatively common and systolic murmurs resulting from rigidity of major vessels and heart valves occur frequently.[18] In fact, over 60% of those between ages 55 and 64 exhibit some cardiac valve calcification.[73] In addition, structural changes in connective tissue in the aged heart make it more susceptible to stretching, thereby contributing to mitral valve cusp prolapse or dilatation of the aortic root, leading to regurgitant murmurs.

Heart sounds in the older person may be as loud as in younger individuals, or they may be faint because of co-existence of skeletal deformities and chronic pulmonary disease such as emphysema, more commonly found in the elderly.[60,74] In patients with these conditions, the position of the apex beat is an unreliable guide to heart size.

As a result of sclerotic changes in the aortic valve, a soft systolic ejection murmur can be heard at the apex in 60% of older adults.[75] Age-related changes in the aortic valve which cause narrowing of the passageway and increased blood flow velocity, may produce a loud aortic murmur which usually reaches maximal intensity during the first half of systole.[52] Systolic murmurs in the elderly are usually no cause for concern because about one third to one half of aortic systolic murmurs are attributable to greater flow velocity from kinking, lengthening, and tortuosity of the aorta with age. Loud systolic aortic murmurs radiating into the neck, accompanied by a thrill, however, suggest obstructive organic aortic stenosis.[52]

Diastolic murmurs indicate an incompetent pulmonic or aortic valve and are always abnormal. Isolated diastolic aortic murmurs may be found in older persons with aortic insufficiency, syphilis, atherosclerotic heart disease, or functional dilatation of the aortic ring.[52] Regurgitant murmurs such as holosystolic murmurs originate from incompetent mitral or tricuspid valves and are heard throughout systole. In rare instances, as a consequence of myocardial infarction, the ventricular septum may rupture, causing a murmur.

There is some evidence of decreased cardiac output of approximately 1% per year between the ages of 20 and 80, resulting largely from stroke volume decreases of approximately 0.7% per year.[43] Other research, however, has suggested that the decline in cardiac output at rest and during exercise is not significant.[76-79] The discrepancy in data on cardiac output in the elderly may be attributed to the fact that, when confronted with increased vascular impedence, the aged myocardium may continue to provide adequate output by prolonging the duration of systole.[17]

COMPLICATIONS
Ischemic Heart Disease

Incidence. Approximately one fourth of all individuals over age 65 have some form of ischemic heart disease (IHD), making it the single most important form of coronary artery disease and the most common pathologic finding associated with symptoms of congestive heart failure in the elderly.[13,75] Arrhythmias, angina, and/or myocardial infarction are also a frequent consequence of a myocardial ischemic condition. Arrhythmias may not be recognized or may be ignored by the older adult until symptoms of clinical significance such as dizziness or falls become obvious. Although complaints of angina occur less frequently than would be expected given the overall incidence of IHD,[57] mortality rates from acute myocardial infarction increase significantly with age. For this reason, the term "silent MI" is frequently applied.[18] Data from the

Framingham Study indicate that by age 60, males have a 20% chance of having a first heart attack. The probability increases to about 41% by age 75, and is several times greater for men than for women,[8] in whom the incidence of first myocardial infarction lags behind men by 20 years.[12]

Symptoms. In those cases of IHD with no chest pain, typical symptoms in the elderly may include: (1) shortness of breath; (2) apparent gastrointestinal complaints; and (3) mental and neurologic symptoms caused by cerebrovascular insufficiency.[52] When chest pain is present, the symptoms that characterize angina pectoris are the same for the elderly as for the younger patient, including changes in blood pressure, retrosternal pain on exertion that is relieved by rest, and apprehension. These patients may also experience dizziness, lightheadedness, and a rapid pulse rate.[52,60] In older adults, it is also more common for such symptoms to be produced by esophagitis, ulcer, gallbladder disease, and hiatal hernia.[61,62]

The most common presenting symptom of myocardial infarction in the elderly as well as the young is substernal chest pain/pressure. There has been much controversy about the incidence of painless myocardial infarction in those age 65 and older. One study found atypical or absent chest pain in 38% of individuals over age 65 with acute myocardial infarction,[80] while another revealed that only 11.5% of elderly patients with diagnosed myocardial infarction presented without chest pain.[81] The Framingham study found that 25% of the total population experienced painless or atypical myocardial infarction.[6] Symptomatic elderly individuals are distinctive in that they tend to experience symptoms at rest—when asleep or inactive—more frequently than the young;[81] this could, however, be a result of their more sedentary lifestyle.

A diagnosis of myocardial infarction should always be considered in older patients with sudden unconsciousness, heart failure, or cardiac arrythmias.[52] Other diseases mimicking myocardial infarction in the elderly include acute pericarditis, acute cholecystitis, and herpes zoster.[60]

Assessment of ischemic heart disease in the elderly, as in the young, is based, in part, on interpretation of electrocardiographic changes. Interpreting ECG readings is more complicated in elderly patients than in younger patients. Although no ECG abnormalities are typical of the older heart, 19% of elderly men and 13% of elderly women have T wave changes and 7% of men and 10% of women have left axis deviation, consistent with left ventricular hypertrophy.[82] Although at younger ages, analysis of Q/QS and ST/T wave patterns can identify IHD, among the elderly, the implications of T wave changes are not so well documented. Furthermore, many of these patients are receiving digitalis, which distorts the ECG making ST evaluation meaningless.[83] For this reason, diagnosis of myocardial infarction is typically made based on history, and corroborated by clinical examination, ECG, and blood enzymes. Thus no unusual significance should be attached to any ECG finding, and each must be evaluated in the context of all other clinical data.

Management. In younger patients, the goal of IHD therapy focuses on prolonging life and allowing the patient to return to work. In the elderly, the goal is less ambitious, not seeking to increase life expectancy, but seeking to improve quality of life through control or reduction of symptoms, improved function, and continued independence.[84] Nitrites are the primary treatment modality for angina in older patients;[28] vasodilators have not demonstrated long-term benefit for patients over age 65.[62] After successful stress testing, older patients with stable angina may begin a sustained program of regular walking for at least 20 minutes per day.

Management of myocardial infarction usually consists of admission to the coronary care unit for monitoring, pain control, and supplemental oxygen administration.[85] Complications, including arrhythmias with possible pump failure, aneurysm of the myocardial wall which may progress to free wall rupture (causing cardiac tamponade), and sudden death all occur more frequently in the elderly than in younger patients.[61] The usage of analgesics and morphine is common for control of pain; morphine also dilates the great veins and, therefore, relieves some cardiac congestion precipitated by the ventricular failure. Caution should be used, however, when administering morphine drugs to older patients since they may obtain effective levels at lower doses than younger patients.

Nitrate preparations, beta-blocking drugs, and calcium-channel blockers may be used to decrease myocardial oxygen demand. Care should be taken when using nitrates in the older patient to prevent decreases in blood pressure that may result in postural hypotension. The decreased baroreceptor response in the older patient increases susceptibility to orthostatic hypotension. In addition, the patient also may be taking antihypertensives, diuretics or tricyclic antidepressants, which also cause hypotension and could lead to cerebrovascular insufficiency as well as myocardial ischemia. While some studies have demonstrated the effectiveness of beta-blockers in reducing mortality from myocardial infarction in the elderly (for example, The Norway Multi-Center Study Group which revealed a 35% decrease in mortality),[86] very little data are available on the therapeutic value or possible side effects from channel blockers in older patients.[84] The immediate goal in treatment of myocardial infarction is to decrease cardiac work, not enhance performance. For this reason, digoxin should not be prescribed unless atrial fibrillation is present.[60]

Coronary artery bypass surgery is another method of restoring blood flow and oxygen supply, but it holds a greater risk for older than for younger patients. In the postoperative period, the older patient has a greater probability of stroke, dysrhythmias, heart block, pulmonary embolism, perioperative psychosis, and/or the need for an intra-aortic balloon.[84] The success rate for coronary artery bypass surgery in the elderly has ranged from 0% to 21%.[87] Major complications related to angiography are also more common in the elderly, but mortality and incidence of nonfatal myocardial infarction as a result of arteriography in older patients are low.[87]

It is important to be aware that older patients who suffer from myocardial infarction frequently exhibit disordered behavior while in the coronary care unit. Drug reactions, hypoxia, brain disorders, pain, poor nutritional state, electrolyte imbalances, hypotension, anemia, hypothermia, infection, and multiple disease states may all serve to affect the elderly patient's orientation and behavior. In addition, the fear of permanent loss of independence and the fear of death are dominant in the elderly patient in the CCU. Unfortunately, access to a data base that adequately depicts the normal behavior or physiologic norms of an elderly patient is rarely available. The older person's decreased ability to regulate his/her body termperature, for example, is an especially important factor in the CCU or ICU where, in many cases, the temperatures are kept lower than in other parts of the hospital.[88] Also, the sleeping behavior of older adults differs from younger people, with less total sleep time, altered sleep distribution patterns, more frequent napping during the day, and more frequent interruptions of REM sleep.[88]

After discharge from the coronary care unit, patients with myocardial infarction should be encouraged to lead as active a life as possible.[57] The principal focus at this point is cardiac rehabilitation, reduction of fear, and counseling the patient and family.[19] The patient should be encouraged to rest when tired and to seek health care immediately upon onset of symptoms—including shortness of breath, confusion, fever, changes in urination pattern—or on a regular basis.

Arrhythmias

Incidence. Disorders of cardiac rhythm are extremely common in the elderly, but often they have no functional consequence. The development of Holter ambulatory electrocardiographic recording has demonstrated a number of ECG changes which typically accompany aging. These include sinus bradycardia and sinus pause, atrial fibrillation, ectopic beats, prolonged PR interval, QRS widening, and ST/T wave changes. Since at least one of these abnormalities may be present in 50% to 67% of ambulant, apparently healthy older individuals, they have little prognostic or diagnostic significance.[89]

Clinically significant arrhythmias may be associated with toxicity from drugs such as digitalis, and disturbances of the cardiovascular system, including congestive heart failure, arteriosclerosis, and fluid and electrolyte disorders.[61] For example, sinus node dysfunction is frequently encountered in the elderly and may result from ischemia.[90] Atrial arrhythmias occur because of nonspecific inflammation, degenerative and fibrotic processes, valvular lesions, ischemic heart disease, senile amyloid disease, or acute coronary thrombosis, which reduce sinus node blood supply.[52,61] Although atrial fibrillation occurs in 5% to 10% of asymptomatic ambulatory older adults,[18,90] it is a frequent preamble to, or early manifestation of, left atrial dilatation associated with congestive heart failure.[31] As the atrium enlarges, atrial fibrillation may become more sustained. Atrioventricular node dysfunction and impaired conduction in the bundle of His may lead to partial or complete block and symptomatically slow ventricular rates.

The impact of arrhythmias on the older individual depends on the degree of cardiac pump dysfunction.[31] In general, cardiac arrhythmias present clinically significant problems for the elderly who are not able to tolerate them as well or as long as younger individuals. Arrhythmias reduce an already compromised cardiac output, thus limiting blood flow to coronary vessels as well as to other vital organs that may be previously impaired by the aging process and disease. In addition, arrhythmias may cause anxiety, resulting in a greater outpouring of catecholamines, causing further increases in vascular resistance and cardiac work, as well as cardiac excitability.[52]

Symptoms. Older individuals, unlike younger patients, frequently present with symptoms related to disturbances of heart rhythm. The most common symptoms of arrhythmia in the elderly are palpitations and symptoms of disordered brain function, including giddiness and unsteady gait. The existence of cerebrovascular disease compounded by heart rhythm disturbances negatively affects cerebration.

The "sick sinus node syndrome" is particularly common among elderly patients[18] and should be considered in those with fatigue, lightheadedness, dizziness, recurrent transient arrhythmias, sudden falls, syncopal attacks, or congestive failure. About one fourth of these patients have detectable coronary artery disease.[52] There are, however, many other possible causes of these signs and symptoms in the elderly, such as organic brain disease or sudden fracture of bones weakened by osteoporosis, that first must be excluded from diagnosis.[91]

Management. Treatment of symptoms of atrial fibrillation is discussed in Chapter 8. Although digoxin is the principal drug treatment,[31] the maintenance dose is usually lower in the elderly because of decreased muscle mass, decreased creatinine clearance, and impaired renal function.[18,62] Lidocaine, which is effective for treatment of ventricular arrhythmias in the elderly, may have adverse effects in this population, including lightheadedness, drowsiness, disorientation, hypotension, convulsions, cardiovascular collapse or serious bradycardia which may even lead to cardiac arrest.[52] Artificial cardiac pacemakers (see Chapter 11) may benefit the elderly with certain arrhythmias, but pacemaker implantation is associated with certain complications, which may occur more frequently in the elderly than in younger patients. For example, the older patient has poor tissue turgor with impaired vessel contraction. Inasmuch as many patients have pacemakers implanted as a semi-emergency measure, drugs such as aspirin, routinely used in the elderly, also may contribute to impaired platelet function, hemorrhage, and postoperative hematomas in this situation. Ultimately, a large hematoma may contribute to battery pocket breakdown—a complication which is also more frequent in the geriatric population.[90]

Heart Failure

Incidence. Congestive heart failure is more prevalent among older individuals than among the young (see Chapter 7). Data from the Framingham Study revealed that the incidence of heart failure is low among young adults, but rises steadily with age. In men aged 50 to 54, the annual incidence rate of heart failure is approximately 3.0 per 1000; by ages 70 to 74, it rises to 8.7 per 1000.[92] Older women have heart failure incidence rates that are typically one third of men's.[16] Although congestive heart failure is prevalent in the elderly, it appears to be overdiagnosed.[18] This may be attributed to the fact that many elderly are obese, breathless, and have ankle edema caused by immobility or varicose veins—all apparent symptoms of heart failure.[83]

Coronary artery disease, which interferes with the metabolic nourishment of the myocardium is most often the physiologic basis of heart failure in the elderly. Hypertension, valvular disease, and chronic pulmonary lesions, all of which increase the resting work load of the heart, may also be responsible.[52] Whereas heart failure in the young typically results from a single cause, the elderly frequently have more than one cause and it may be precipitated or aggravated by, or mimic, failure of other organ systems.[93]

Symptoms. Some of the common complaints of older patients with heart failure include: fatigue, mental confusion, failure to thrive, loss of weight, dyspnea or nocturnal dyspnea, orthopnea, cough, hemoptysis (also indicative of pulmonary emboli), weakness, and edema.[31,52] Other, less common complaints include agitation, anorexia, insomnia, depression, and changes in mental state.[61] Anorexia may result because of congestive changes in the mucous membranes of the stomach and congestive changes in the liver and pancreas that cause a loss of nitrogen and vitamins.[94] Nutritional dificiencies also may occur in the elderly patient with congestive heart disease because of the difficulty in breathing while eating.[33] Pulmonary insufficiency caused by noncardiac factors is often misdiagnosed as heart failure in the elderly. Other diseases with similar symptoms include pulmonary thromboembolism, renal insufficiency or failure, peripheral venous insufficiency, and constrictive pericarditis.[93]

The patient history, physical examination, ECG, auscultation, chest x-ray, echocardiogram, and laboratory data are all used in the diagnosis of heart failure. The ECG demonstrates arrhythmias, as well as the mean QRS axis. Diagnosis may, however, be obscured by the left axis shift and decrease in QRS amplitude normally seen with aging.[95,96] Pulse abnormalities in rate, rhythm, or strength may be caused by dysrhythmias such as atrial fibrillation, premature ventricular or atrial contractions, sinus tachycardia, or pulsus alternans. Third and fourth heart sounds are also common.[31] Most murmurs associated with heart failure in older individuals arise from the left side of the heart.[93] Chest x-rays provide information on cardiac size and pulmonary congestion indicative of left-sided heart failure, pulmonary infection, and infiltrates.[19] The echocardiogram can be used to measure chamber size and wall thickness as well as abnormal wall motion which could be signs of dilatation, hypertrophy, and failure. Complete blood count, urinalysis, and tests for electrolytes and renal function may also be appropriate diagnostic approaches.[31]

The preponderance of cases of heart failure in the elderly originate with left-sided failure (see Chapter 7). As the condition worsens, however, the entire body, including lungs, neck veins, liver, abdomen and lower extremities, show manifestations of progression to right congestive heart failure. In the elderly patient, heart failure should be diagnosed when the following five symptoms are present: (1) dyspnea; (2) elevated venous pressure; (3) bilateral basal rales; (4) liver enlargement; and (5) bilateral symmetrical ankle edema.[82] The presence of dyspnea, orthopnea or paroxysmal nocturnal dyspnea accompanied by gallop rhythm or murmurs of aortic or mitral valves should be considered strong evidence of left-sided heart failure in the older person.[82]

Management. Effective management of the elderly patient with heart failure is similar to management in younger patients (see Chapter 7), including rest, reduction of heart work, prevention of salt and water retention, improvement of cardiac output, and education about underlying causes.[19,52] Moderately or severely ill older patients with chronic heart disease may require hospital care in a monitored environment.[31]

Medical treatment is aimed at improving cardiac performance and correcting underlying dysrhythmias (digoxin and parenteral inotropes) and decreasing cardiac work by decreasing vascular resistance (vasodilators) or by decreasing circulating blood volume(diuretics).[93] Diuretics, combined with salt restriction, are the chief medical modality for treatment of the older patient with heart failure. Specific potassium-sparing diuretics may be appropriate to prevent hypokalemia. The importance of using care when treating elderly patients with diuretics is underscored by the British Multicenter study finding in 1980 that diuretics caused the largest number of side effects in the elderly.[97]

Digitalis preparations, such as digoxin, must be used with caution in the elderly. Subtle signs of toxicity, such as dysrhythmias and impaired cardiac impulse conduction at the atrioventricular node may be overlooked as the drug accumulates in the presence of decreased renal function, a common occurrence among the elderly with heart failure. Digitalis is usually not indicated in elderly patients with slow ventricular response.[31]

COMPLIANCE TO TREATMENT

It has been suggested that of all age groups, individuals over age 65 are the least likely to comply with physician advice.[98] Many of the factors that make assessment and diagnosis of coronary artery disease difficult in the elderly may also negatively affect compliance. Impaired memory, poor eyesight, treatment with multiple drugs, and the involvement of several health practitioners without adequate communication and consultation with the patient and family all serve to make compliance more difficult for the elderly patient. Deeply entrenched behaviors and fear of loss of independence also often make the older patient less likely to comply.[99]

Pharmacologic compliance is a specific problem when the drug dose is critical; such is the case for many cardiovascular medications. With some cardiovascular drugs, such as warfarin, the risks associated with incorrect dosage are so great that their use may be unjustified despite strong clinical indication for them.[100]

To simplify the patient's routine, the drug regimen should be as simple as possible, with doses being given only once or twice daily rather than three, four, or more times. Diminished renal excretory capacity in the elderly may present a significant risk when administering drugs such as digoxin, which have a narrow margin of safety (that is, the difference between therapeutic and toxic levels). Supervision of medication administration by a relative, friend, or community nurse, where possible, should be encouraged.

Patient and family education are important nursing roles that assure compliance of the elderly patient in management and treatment of coronary artery disease. Poor compliance to cardiac rehabilitation programs among the elderly have been attributed to lack of motivation and incomplete or inadequate information.[101] Depending upon the management strategy selected, the patient and family should be provided information on minimizing unnecessary demands of cardiac function, proper food selection with emphasis on specific dietary limitations (especially salt restriction), the role of exercise in prevention and rehabilitation, relaxation techniques, and smoking-cessation. Because many elderly are often entrenched in their cultural and ethnic customs, the patient's preferences should be given appropriate consideration.[102]

RESEARCH NEEDS

A recurring theme throughout this chapter has been the relative scarcity of data on risk factors, prevention, incidence, and treatment of coronary artery disease in individuals over age 65. Unless such data are available, it is impossible to establish norms on which to base decisions for caring for the elderly patient with coronary artery disease.

More studies need to be conducted on the factors that increase risk of coronary artery disease in older persons. Evidence from the Framingham Study becomes increasingly important in this regard, with the original cohort now reaching older ages. Research on effective and safe methods of altering behavior—including eating, smoking, and exercise—and of improving compliance with behavioral and medical management among older population groups is also needed. In this vein, a new National Institute of Aging-funded study being conducted at Duke University Medical Center on the impact of intense exercise on the cardiovascular and psychologic functioning of healthy elderly will make an important contribution.[103]

Studies comparing the symptoms of coronary artery diseases in older and younger populations would do much to establish criteria for diagnosis and specialized treatment protocols. Research on the appropriate doses and unique side effects of medications used for the treatment of coronary disease in older patients remains an important need.

Specific issues aside, it is imperative that future studies of coronary artery disease address the elderly segmented by age, sex, and ethnicity. The elderly are not a homogeneous group and should not be treated as such. Rather than lumping all individuals in a single category, specific age groups beyond age 65 need to be studied. The Institute of Medicine recommends the collection and publication of statistical data on the elderly in 3- or 5-year age categories.[104] As discussed earlier, most studies of the relationship between the aging process and coronary artery disease have included only male subjects. Future research protocols should be designed to include both sexes in the sample population, with specific emphasis given to sex differences. An increasing amount of attention should be given particularly to the specific coronary problems of women as they relate to menopause, endogenous female hormones, and to estrogen therapy. Ethnic, economic, and social differences are as important for the elderly as they are for younger population subgroups and should receive specific research attention as well.

REFERENCES

1. U.S. Department of Commerce, Bureau of the Census: Projection of the population of the U.S.: 1982 to 2050 (advance report), P-25, No. 922, Washington, D.C., 1982, U.S. Government Printing Office.
2. Institute of Medicine: Health and behavior: a research agenda—Interim report #5: health, behavior, and aging, Washington, D.C., 1981, National Academy Press.
3. National Center for Health Statistics and Ries, P.W.: Americans assess their health, 1978, Vital and Health Statistics, 10(142), Washington, D.C., 1983, U.S. Government Printing Officie, DHHS Pub. No. (PHS) 83-1570.
4. Heckler, M.M.: Health promotion for older Americans, Public Health Rep. 100:225, 1985.
5. National Center for Health Statistics and Jack, S.S.: Current estimates from the National Health Interview Survey: United States, 1979, Vital and Health Statistics, 10(136), Washington, D.C., 1981, U.S. Government Printing Office, DHHS Pub. No. (PHS) 81-1564.
6. Kannel, W.B.: The Framingham study: a 30-year retrospective, Am. Coll. Cardiol. Audio Tape J., Program No. 50, 1984.
7. Gerstenblith, G., and others: Stress testing redefines the prevalence of coronary artery disease in epidemiological studies, Circulation 62(suppl III):III-308, 1980.
8. Kannel, W.B., McGee, D., and Gordon, T.: A general cardiovascular risk profile: The Framingham study, Am. J. Cardiol. 38:46, 1976.
9. U.S. Department of Commerce, Bureau of the Census: Activity limitation due to chronic conditions. Reproted in Stafstrom, A.: The elderly and their health care, Ambulatory Care 5(10):8, 1985.
10. National Center for Health Statistics: Health: United States, 1983, Washington, D.C., 1983, U.S. Government Printing Office, DHHS Pub. No. (PHS)84-1232.
11. Blackburn, H.: Risk factors and cardiovascular disease. In American Heart Association: Heartbook, New York, 1980, E.P. Dutton.
12. U.S. Department of Health and Human Services: Tenth report of the director: National Heart, Lung, and Blood Institute ten-year review and five-year plan, vol. 1, Progress and promise, Washington, D.C., 1982, U.S. Department of Health and Human Services, NIH Pub. No. 84-2356.
13. Kennedy, R.D., Andrews, G.R., and Caird, F.I.: Ischaemic heart disease in the elderly, Br. Heart J. 39:1121, 1977.
14. Andres, R.: Influence of obesity on longevity in the aged. In Danon, D., and others, editors: Ageing: a challenge to science and society, vol. 1, Biology, Oxford, U.K., 1981, Oxford University Press.
15. Pooling Project Research Group: Relationship of blood pressure, serum cholesterol, smoking habit, relative weight, and ECG abnormalities to incidence of major coronary events: final report of the Pooling Project, J. Chronic Dis. 31:201, 1978.
16. Evans, J.G.: Epidemiology. In Martin, A., and Camm, A.J., editors: Heart disease in the elderly, New York, 1984, John Wiley & Sons, Inc.
17. Harris, R.: Cardiac problems: treating the geriatric patient. In Busse, E.W., editor: Theory and therapeutics of aging, New York, 1973, Medcom, Inc.
18. Kane, R.L., Ouslander, J.G., and Abrass, I.B.: Essentials of clinical geriatrics, New York, 1984, McGraw-Hill Book Co.
19. Futrell, M., and others: Primary health care of the older adult, North Scituate, Mass., 1980, Duxbury Press.
20. Rowe, J.W.: Systolic hypertension in the elderly, N. Eng. J. Med. 309:1246, 1983.

21. Kannel, W.B., Dawber, T.R., and McGee, D.L.: Perspectives on systolic hypertension: the Framingham study, Circulation 61:1179, 1980.

22. Kannel, W.B., and others: Systolic blood pressure, arterial rigidity, and risk of stroke: the Framingham study, JAMA 245:1225, 1981.

23. Hypertension Detection and Follow-up Program Cooperative Group: Five-year findings of the Hypertension Detection and Follow-up Program II: mortality by race, sex, and age, JAMA 242:2572, 1979.

24. Harlan, W.R., and others: High blood pressure in older Americans: the first National Health and Nutritional Examination Survey, Hypertension 6:802, 1984.

25. Curb, J.D., Borhani, N.O., and Entwide, G.: Isolated systolic hypertension in 14 communities, Am. J. Epidemiol. 121:362, 1985.

26. VA Cooperative Study Group on Antihypertensive Agents: Effects of treatment on morbidity in hypertension. III. Influence of age, diastolic pressure, and prior cardiovascular disease: further analysis of side effects, Circulation 56:991, 1972.

27. Sprackling, M.E., and others: Blood pressure reduction in the elderly: a randomised controlled trial of methyldopa, Br. Med. J. 283:1151, 1981.

28. Isaacs, B: Should we treat hypertension in the elderly? Age and Ageing 8:115, 1979.

29. Martin, A.: Hypertension in the elderly, Omen 8, London, 1980, Update Publications.

30. Martin, A.: Hypertension. In Martin, A., and Camm,. A.J., editors: Heart disease in the elderly, New York, 1984, John Wiley & Sons, Inc.

31. Fowkes, W.C., and Fowkes, V.: Cardiovascular system. In O'Hara-Devereaux, M., Andrus, L.H., and Scott, C.D., editors: Eldercare: a guide to clinical geriatrics, New York, 1981, Grune & Stratton.

32. The Joint National Committee on Detection, Evaluation, and Treatment of High Blood Pressure: Special report—the 1984 report of the Joint National Committee on Detection, Evaluation, and Treatment of High Blood Pressure, Arch. Intern. Med. 144:1045, 1984.

33. Roe, D.A.: Geriatric nutrition, Englewood Cliffs, N.J., 1983, Prentice-Hall, Inc.

34. Coalition on Smoking or Health: Smoking or health: a briefing book, 1985, unpublished.

35. Jajich, C.L., and others: Smoking and coronary heart disease mortality in the elderly, JAMA 252:2831, 1984.

36. Adams, G.M., and deVries, H.A.: Physiologic effects of an exercise training regimen upon women aged 59 to 74, J. Gerontol. 28:50, 1973.

37. Benestad, A.M.: Trainability of old men, Acta Med. Scand. 178:321, 1965.

38. deVries, H.A.: Physiological effects of an exercise training program upon men aged 52 to 88, J. Gerontol. 25:325, 1970.

39. Hodgson, J.L., and Bushirk, E.R.: Physical fitness and age, with emphasis on cardiovascular function in the elderly. J. Am. Geriatr. Soc. 25:385, 1977.

40. Schurer, J., and Tipton, C.M.: Cardiovascular adaptation to physical training, Annu. Rev. Physiol. 39:221, 1977.

41. Sidney, K.H., and Shephard, R.J.: Frequency and intensity of exercise training for elderly subjects, Med. Sci. Sports 10:125, 1978.

42. Sidney, K.H.: Cardiovascular benefits of physical activity in the exercising aged. In Smith, E.L., and Surfass, R.C., editors: Exercise and aging: the scientific basis, Hillside, N.J., 1981, Euslow Publishers.

43. Kenney, R.A.: Physiology of aging: a synopsis, Chicago, 1982, Year Book Medical Publishers.

44. Maloney, S.K., and others: Aging and health promotion: market research for public education (executive summary), Washington, D.C., 1984, U.S. Public Health Service, Office of Disease Prevention and Health Promotion.

45. deVries, H.A.: Tips on prescribing exercise regimens for your older patient, Geriatrics 34:75, 1979.

46. Rowe, J.W.: Health care of the elderly, N. Engl. J. Med. 312:827, 1985.

47. Gordon, T., and others: Menopause and coronary heart disease: the Framingham study, Ann. Intern. Med. 89:157, 1978.

48. Wilson, P.W.F., Garrison, R.J., and Castelli, W.P.: Postmenopausal estrogen use, cigarette smoking, and cardiovascular morbidity in women over 50: the Framingham study, N. Engl. J. Med. 313:1038, 1985.

49. Stampfer, M.J., and others: A prospective study of postmenopausal estrogen therapy and coronary heart disease, N. Engl. J. Med. 313:1044, 1985.

50. U.S. Department of Health and Human Services: Healthy people, Washington, D.C., 1979, U.S. Government Printing Office.

51. National Academy of Sciences, Food and Nutrition Board: National Research Council Recommended Daily Dietary Allowances, Washington, D.C., 1980 (revision), The Academy.

52. Harris, R.: Special problems of geriatric patients with heart disease. In Reichel, W., editor: Clinical aspects of aging, Baltimore, Md., 1978, Williams & Wilkins.

53. Linn, B.S., and Linn, M.W.: Objective and self-assessed health in the old and very old, Soc. Sci. Med. 14A:311, 1980.

54. Shaw, M.W.: The challenge of ageing: a multidisciplinary approach to extended care, Melbourne, Australia, 1984, Churchill Livingstone.

55. Besdine, R.W.: Geriatric medicine: an overview. In Eisdorfer, C., editor: Annual review of gerontology and geriatrics, New York, 1980, Springer Publishing Co.

56. Yurick, A.G.: The nursing process and the aged person. In Yurick, A.G., editor: The aged person and the nursing process, ed. 2, Norwalk, Ct., 1984, Appleton-Century-Crofts.

57. Burggraf, V., and Donlon, B.: Assessing the elderly. I. System by system, Am. J. Nurs. 85:974, 1985.

58. Katz, S., and others: The index of ADL: A standardized measure of biological and psychosocial function, JAMA 185:914, 1963.

59. Caplis, J.: Assessment of social function. In Eliopoulos, C., editor: Health assessment of the older adult, Reading, Mass., 1984, Addison-Wesley Publishing Co.

60. Martin, A.: Ischaemic heart disease. In Martin, A., and Camm, A.J., editors: Heart disease in the elderly, New York, 1984, John Wiley & Sons, Inc.

61. Orem, S.E., Assessment of the cardiovascular system. In Eliopoulos, C., editor: Health assessment of the older adult, Reading, Mass., 1984, Addison-Wesley Publishing Co.

62. Hodkinson, H.M.: An outline of geriatrics, ed. 2, London, 1981, Academic Press.

63. Eriksson, H., and others: Body temperature in general population samples: the study of men born in 1983 and 1923, Acta Med. Scand. 217:347, 1985.

64. Fox, R.H., and others: Body temperature in the elderly: a national study of physiological, social, and environmental conditions, Br. Med. J. 1:200, 1973.

65. Higgins, P.: Can 98.6 be a fever in disguise? Ger. Nurs. 4:101, 1983.

66. Habasevich, R.A.: Implications of cardiovascular aging. In Lewis, C.B., editor: Aging: the health care challenge—an interdisciplinary approach to assessment and rehabilitative management of the elderly, Philadelphia, 1985, F.A. Davis Co.

67. Shephard, R.J.: Cardiovascular limitations in the aged. In Smith, E.L., and Surfass, R.L., editors: Exercise and aging: the scientific basis, Hillside, N.J., 1980, Euslow Publishers.

68. Rodstein, M.: Heart disease in the aged. In Rossman, I., editor: Clinical geriatrics, ed. 2, Philadelphia, 1979, J.B. Lippincott Co.

69. Harris, R.: The management of geriatric cardiovascular disease, Philadelphia, 1970, J.B. Lippincott Co.

70. Dock, W.: Aging of the myocardium, Bull. N.Y. Acad. Med. **32**:173, 1956.

71. Granath, A., Johnsson, B., and Strandell, T.: Circulation in healthy old men studied by right heart catheterization at rest and during exercise in supine and sitting position, Acta Med. Scand. **176**:425, 1964.

72. Granath, A., Johnsson, B., and Strandell, T.: Studies on the central circulation at rest and during exercise in the supine and sitting body position in old men—a preliminary report, Acta Med. Scand. **169**:125, 1961.

73. Lakatta, E.G.: Health, disease, and cardiovascular aging. In Institute of Medicine: Committee on an aging society: America's aging, Washington, D.C., 1985, IOM.

74. Harris, R., and Aravanis, C.: The normal phonocardiogram of the aged, Dis. Chest. **33**:214, 1958.

75. Forbes, E.J., and Fitzsimons, V.M.: The older adult: a process for wellness, St. Louis, Missouri, 1981, The C.V. Mosby Co.

76. Gerstenblith, G., Lakatta, E.G., and Weisfeldt, M.L.: Age changes in myocardial function and exercise response, Prog. Cardiovas. Dis. **19**:1, 1976.

77. Rodeheffer, R.J., and others: Exercise cardiac output is maintained with advancing age in healthy human subjects: cardiac dilatation and increased stroke volume compensate for a diminished heart rate, Circulation **69**:203, 1984.

78. Strandell, T.: Cardiac output in old age. In Caird, F.I., Dall, J.L.C., and Kennedy, R.D., editors: Cardiology in old age, New York, 1976, Plenum Press.

79. Williams, T.F.: Health promotion and the elderly: why and where does it lead? In Andreoli, K.G., Musser, L.A., and Reiser, S.J., editors: Health care for the elderly: regional responses to national policy issues, New York, 1986, Haworth Press.

80. Elderly heart attack symptoms more subtle—Geriatrics: what's new? Geriatrics **38**(3):13, 1983.

81. Semple, T., and Williams, B.O.: Coronary care for the elderly. In Caird, F.I., Dall, J.L.C., and Kennedy, R.D., editors: Cardiology in old age, New York, 1976, Plenum Press.

82. Caird, F.I., and Judge, T.G.: Assessment of the elderly patient, ed. 2, Philadelphia, 1979, J.B. Lippincott Co.

83. Mankin, H.T.: Value limitations of exercise testing. In Brandenburg, R.O., editor: Office cardiology, Philadelphia, 1980, F.A. Davis Co.

84. Glazer, M.D., Hill, R.D., and Wenger, N.K.: Dx and Tx of the elderly patient with atheroslcerotic coronary heart disease, Geriatrics **40**(10):45, 1985.

85. Ackman, D.: Treatment of acute myocardial infarction in the elderly, Geriatrics **38**(3):46, 1983.

86. Gunderson, T., and others: Timolol related reduction in mortality and reinfarction in patients ages 65-75 years surviving acute myocardial infarction, Circulation **66**:1179, 1982.

87. Gersh, B.J., and others: Coronary arteriography and coronary artery bypass surgery: morbidity and mortality in patients ages 65 years or older: a report from the Coronary Artery Surgery Study, Circulation **67**(3):483, 1983.

88. Baldwin, P.J., and Kaseman, D.F.: The needs of the older patient in critical care units. In Noble, M.A., editor: The ICU environment: directions for nursing, Reston, Va., 1982, Reston Publishing Co., Inc.

89. Camm, A.J., and Ward, D.E.: Clinical electrocardiography. In Martin, A., and Camm, A.J., editors: Heart disease in the elderly, New York, 1984, John Wiley & Sons, Inc.

90. Moss, A.J.: Pacemakers in the elderly. In Reichel, W., editor: Clinical aspects of aging, Baltimore, Md., 1978, Williams & Wilkins Co.

91. Martin, A.: Problems in geriatric medicine, Philadelphia, 1981, F.A. Davis Co.

92. McKee, P.A., and others: The natural history of congestive heart failure: the Framingham study, N. Engl. J. Med. **286**:1441, 1971.

93. Shocken, D.D.: Congestive heart failure: Dx and Rx in the elderly, Geriatrics **39**(11):77, 1984.

94. Wohl, M.G., Shuman, C.R., and Alper, C.: Nutritional and metabolic aspects of congestive heart failure, Arch. Intern. Med. **96**:116, 1955.

95. Mihalick, M.J., and Fisch, C.: Electrocardiographic findings in the aged, Am. Heart J. **84**:117, 1974.

96. Spodick, D.H., and Quarry-Pigott, V.M.: Fourth heart sounds as a normal finding in older persons, N. Engl. J. Med. **288**:140, 1973.

97. Lamy, P.P.: Side effects of diuretics a danger for aged, J. Geront. Nurs. **11**(6):44, 1985.

98. Haug, M.R., Ford, A.B., and Sheafor, M.: The physical and mental health of aged women, New York, 1985, Springer Publishing Co.

99. Butler, R.: Why survive? Being old in America, New York, 1975, Harper & Row.

100. Warrington, S.J., and Turner, P.: Clinical pharmacology. In Martin, A., and Camm, A.J., editors: Heart disease in the elderly, New York, 1984, John Wiley & Sons, Inc.

101. Gori, P., and others: Compliance with cardiac rehabilitation in the elderly, Eur. Heart J. **5**(suppl. E):109, 1984.

102. Ebersole, P.A., and Hess, P.: Toward healthy aging: human needs and nursing response, St. Louis, 1981, The C.V. Mosby Co.

103. News notes: Do not go gentle, Perspectives, Duke University Medical Center **6**(2):28, 1986.

104. Institute of Medicine: America's aging: health in an older society, Washington, D.C., 1985, National Academy Press.

INDEX

A

A wave, 6
Abdomen, postoperative assessment of, 427
Aberrant ventricular conduction, 216
Accelerated idioventricular rhythm, 196-197
  treatment of, 197
Accessory pathways, 160, 163
  tachycardia associated with, 164
Acebutolol (Seetral), clinical features of, 313
Acetylcholine in cardiac function, 6-7
Acidosis in cardiogenic shock, 127
Action potentials, 84
Activated clotting time (ACT), 427
Activities of Daily Living, Index of, 449
Acute myocardial infarction, 118-121
  complicated vs. uncomplicated, 119
  diagnosis of, 118
  medical management of, 119-121
  mortality rate of patients with, 119
  symptoms of, 118
  thrombolytic agents and, 316
Acute renal failure, postoperative, 426
Adams-Stokes syncope, 208
Adrenalin; see Epinephrine
Adrenergic nerve terminal, 309, 310
Adrenergic pharmacology, 309-314
Adrenergic receptors, 309
Advanced cardiac life support (ACLS), 364
Aerobic exercise; see also Exercise
  heart rate during, 406
Afterload, postoperative management of, 425
Agonist activity, intrinsic, 313
AH interval, 223
Air trapping, defined, 36
Alcohol and coronary artery disease, 18
Alpha-adrenergic blocking agents, 312
  action of, 312
  administration of, 312
  clinical uses of, 312
  side effects and toxicity of, 312
Alpha-adrenergic receptors
  subclassification of, 309
  drugs that stimulate, 309-312
Alprenolol and risk of sudden death, 288
Amicar; see Aminocaproic acid
Aminocaproic acid (Amicar), 427
Amiodarone (Cordarone), 188, 192
  administration of, 322
  clinical pharmacology of, 318
  electrophysiologic effects of, 317, 322

Amiodarone (Cordarone)—cont'd
  pharmacokinetics of, 322
  side effects and toxicity of, 322-323
  and sinus arrest, 148
Amplitude of QRS complex, 86-87
Amrinone, 123
  actions of, 303
Anacrotic notch, 31
Analog electrocardiography machine, 12-lead, for evaluating pacemaker, 342
Anaphylactic reaction in hemolytic transfusion reaction, 471
Anesthesia for bypass surgery, 419
Aneurysms, ventricular; see Ventricular aneurysms
Anger as factor in coronary artery disease, 388-390
Angina pectoris, 116-118
  atypical or variant (Prinzmetal), 116, 237, 272
  beta-adrenergic blocking agents and, 313
  characteristics of, 114
  diagnosis of, 116
  as indication for coronary artery bypass surgery, 416
  medical management of, 117-118
  during percutaneous transluminal coronary angioplasty, 415
  preinfarction, 416
  and risk of sudden death, 285
  unstable, 416
  variant; see Angina pectoris, atypical
Angiography, cardiac, 76-78
Angioplasty, percutaneous transluminal coronary; see Percutaneous transluminal coronary angioplasty
Annulus of heart, 2
Antiarrhythmic drugs, 317-326
  clinical electrophysiologic effects of, 317
  and sudden death, 289-290
Antibiotics
  and bypass surgery, 418
  after transplantation, 433
Anticoagulants, 314-315
  action of, 314
  controversy over, 378
  indications for, 314
Antithymocyte globulin (ATG) in transplantation, 434, 435
Anturane; see Sulfinpyrazone
Anxiety, 395
  of patient's family, nursing care plan for, 430
  relief of, 353
Aortic regurgitation
  echocardiographic evaluation of, 70, 72
  murmurs of, 49
Aortic stenosis
  echocardiographic evaluation of, 70

459